AF683736

Antituberculosis Chemotherapy

# Progress in Respiratory Research

## Vol. 40

Series Editor

Chris T. Bolliger Cape Town

# Antituberculosis Chemotherapy

Volume Editors

Peter R. Donald Tygerberg
Paul D. van Helden Tygerberg

53 figures, 2 in color, 50 tables, 2011

KARGER

Basel · Freiburg · Paris · London · New York · New Delhi · Bangkok · Beijing · Tokyo · Kuala Lumpur · Singapore · Sydney

**Prof. Dr. Peter R. Donald**
Desmond Tutu Tuberculosis Centre
Department of Paediatrics and Child Health
Faculty of Health Sciences
Stellenbosch University
PO Box 19063
Tygerberg 7505 (South Africa)

**Prof. Dr. Paul D. van Helden**
Director
DST/NRF Centre for Excellence for Biomedical Tuberculosis Research
MRC Centre for Molecular and Cellular Biology
Division of Molecular Biology and Human Genetics
Faculty of Health Sciences
Stellenbosch University
PO Box 19063
Tygerberg 7505 (South Africa)

Library of Congress Cataloging-in-Publication Data

A catalog record for this book is available from the Library of Congress

Bibliographic Indices. This publication is listed in bibliographic services, including Current Contents®.

Disclaimer. The statements, opinions and data contained in this publication are solely those of the individual authors and contributors and not of the publisher and the editor(s). The appearance of advertisements in the book is not a warranty, endorsement, or approval of the products or services advertised or of their effectiveness, quality or safety. The publisher and the editor(s) disclaim responsibility for any injury to persons or property resulting from any ideas, methods, instructions or products referred to in the content or advertisements.

Drug Dosage. The authors and the publisher have exerted every effort to ensure that drug selection and dosage set forth in this text are in accord with current recommendations and practice at the time of publication. However, in view of ongoing research, changes in government regulations, and the constant flow of information relating to drug therapy and drug reactions, the reader is urged to check the package insert for each drug for any change in indications and dosage and for added warnings and precautions. This is particularly important when the recommended agent is a new and/or infrequently employed drug.

All rights reserved. No part of this publication may be translated into other languages, reproduced or utilized in any form or by any means electronic or mechanical, including photocopying, recording, microcopying, or by any information storage and retrieval system, without permission in writing from the publisher.

© Copyright 2011 by S. Karger AG, P.O. Box, CH–4009 Basel (Switzerland)
www.karger.com
Printed in Switzerland on acid-free and non-aging paper (ISO 9706) by Reinhardt Druck, Basel
ISSN 1422–2140
ISBN 978–3–8055–9627–5
e-ISBN 978–3–8055–9628–2

# Contents

# Foreword

As series editor of *Progress in Respiratory Research*, it has always been my aim to cover the complete field of diseases of the chest which involve the lung. Up to now we have had many different topics but there has been one big gap concerning infectious diseases. Practising in Cape Town for more than a decade, I enjoy many fantastic aspects of the 'mother city' of South Africa, but sadly I am also acutely aware that Cape Town is also known as the 'tuberculosis capital of the world'. Tuberculosis together with HIV is one of the top medical priorities of South Africa, but this is also true for many developing countries, a fact which is often ignored in first-world set-ups. In the modern, extremely mobile world, it is however of great importance to follow global trends in communicable diseases closely, as air travel can spread highly infectious agents quickly or change the approach to treatment drastically, as recently shown with the emergence of multidrug resistance or even extremely resistant tuberculous strains.

Luckily we have many leading researchers in the field of tuberculosis in South Africa, and the team at the Faculty of Health Sciences, University of Stellenbosch, is arguably one of the leading tuberculosis research set-ups on a global level. This is true for clinical as well as for basic science. It was therefore a logical choice for me to ask two eminent senior researchers from my own faculty to compile a volume for the 'blue series' on drug therapy of tuberculosis. Professors Peter Donald and Paul van Helden assembled some of the best-known specialists in the field and were instrumental to cover all aspects of modern antituberculous chemotherapy, as they explain in their preface following this foreword.

Once again the main people responsible at the publishing house S. Karger AG, Basel, were Linda Haas and Stefan Sessler, who helped processing the various chapters, but also reminded some authors of delayed submissions to speed up delivery. Their input greatly facilitated the volume editors' and my task to come up with the finished product on time.

The final product is a must for all involved in the treatment of tuberculosis irrespective of whether one lives in highly industrialized or emerging countries: tuberculosis is of importance to all.

*C.T. Bolliger*, Cape Town

# Preface

Drugs for the treatment of tuberculosis have been available for nearly 60 years, and yet tuberculosis remains one of the major infectious diseases of mankind causing immeasurable suffering and mortality, and placing an enormous financial burden on countries and individuals. Since approximately 1980, short-course 6-month treatment regimens based on the use of isoniazid, rifampicin and pyrazinamide have been available and used extensively throughout the world to successfully treat millions of tuberculosis patients. Nonetheless, despite this long usage, it is clear that our understanding of these drugs and their optimal use is deficient in many respects. Part of the reason for this is the lack of interest in tuberculosis as a rewarding and stimulating research subject that followed the successful introduction of these drugs and the resulting lack of younger researchers entering the tuberculosis field. Under the influence of HIV and its devastating interaction with tuberculosis, this has changed over the last 2 decades with increasing interest in tuberculosis research and the development of a number of promising new candidate antituberculosis drugs. It used to be remarked that knowledge of syphilis would lead one into knowledge of every important aspect of medicine; perhaps this role is now being fulfilled by tuberculosis? Within the field of tuberculosis almost every aspect of the medical sciences is covered from sociology and human behaviour to the very foundations of the immune response. This volume reviews one aspect of tuberculosis and is devoted to the field of tuberculosis chemotherapy with the emphasis on new developments regarding our existing drugs and the prospects for the introduction of new drugs and their evaluation.

However, there is also still much to be learnt from experience with our existing drugs, and in compiling this volume we have not hesitated to look over our shoulders at experience with the evaluation and clinical use of existing drugs in the past. The most appropriate pathway to evaluate new antituberculosis drugs and regimens remains uncertain so that several of the methodologies currently in use are reviewed, and we hope that this will generate more discussion of these important subjects. Our current 'essential' drugs isoniazid, rifampicin and pyrazinamide are likely to remain in use for the foreseeable future, and aspects of their optimal use are discussed. Drug resistance remains an ever-present threat to patients and tuberculosis control programmes. As this volume demonstrates, the discovery, development and evaluation of antituberculosis drugs make a lengthy process, and we cannot allow our new drugs to follow the same path to resistance that has befallen our current drugs in many parts of the world. Several papers thus address the problems associated with drug resistance, its spread and diagnosis. Lastly childhood tuberculosis has recently been recognized as an important, but neglected, part of the tuberculosis problem; the pharmacokinetics and toxicity of antituberculosis agents in children can differ significantly from that in adults and may require adjustments in dosages to ensure an optimal safe and effective therapy in children with tuberculosis. Some of these issues and the evaluation of antituberculosis drugs in children are discussed by experts in the field of paediatric pharmacokinetics.

As editors we must offer our sincere thanks to our colleagues who have contributed so generously of their time

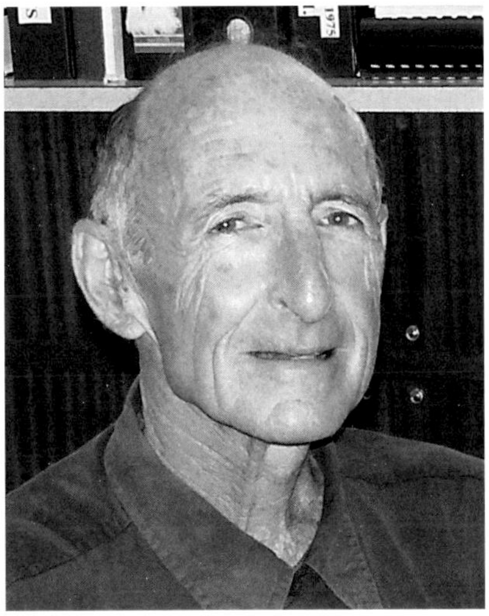

Peter R. Donald

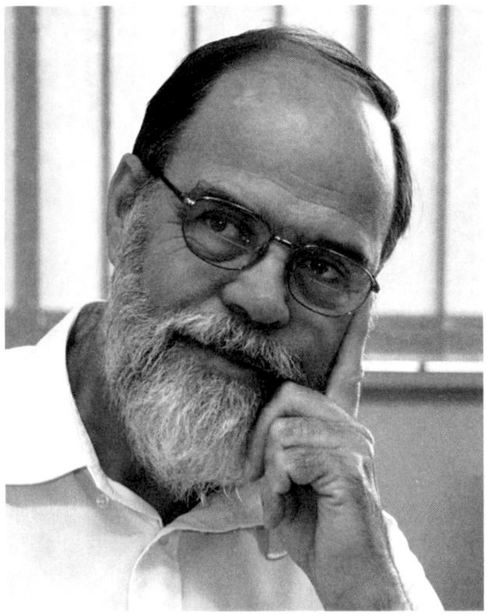

Paul D. van Helden

and expertise in helping compile this volume; as academics we are only too aware of the pressures of time and the time it takes to write a paper. Finally we appreciate the willingness of the publishers to accept our proposal of antituberculosis chemotherapy as a suitable subject to review in the belief that this can increase the dissemination of new knowledge about this important subject and so contribute to the better management of tuberculosis throughout the world.

*Peter R. Donald, Paul D. van Helden*, Tygerberg

# Retrospectoscope

Chapter 1

Donald PR, van Helden PD (eds): Antituberculosis Chemotherapy.
Prog Respir Res. Basel, Karger, 2011, vol 40, pp 2–9

# History of Drug Discovery: Early Evaluation Studies and Lessons Learnt from Them

Zahoor Ahmad[a,b] · Nusrat Habib Makaya[a] · Jacques Grosset[a]

[a]Center for Tuberculosis Research, Department of Medicine, Johns Hopkins University School of Medicine, Baltimore, Md., USA; [b]Indian Institute of Integrative Medicine, Srinagar, India

**Abstract**

The discovery of antituberculosis drugs was the outcome of concerted efforts made between 1930 and 1970 to identify antimicrobial drugs. Streptomycin (1943) and rifampicin (1967), the first and the last of the great antituberculosis drugs currently in use, were discovered by screening of the products of soil bacteria. While streptomycin is a natural product, rifampicin is a semisynthetic drug resulting from extensive structural manipulations designed to render rifamycin SV more bioavailable. On the other hand, isoniazid and pyrazinamide are both derivatives of nicotinamide whose antituberculosis activity was quite accidentally discovered in 1945. Para-aminosalicylic acid or PAS is also a synthetic drug but was synthesized, not to improve an existing compound but as a hypothetical antagonist of salicylates which were known to increase respiration, and thus the growth of *Mycobacterium tuberculosis*. Like isoniazid, pyrazinamide and PAS, ethambutol is a product of organic synthesis. Perhaps the most striking feature of the history of antituberculosis drug discovery is the rational way the drugs have been tested and the drug combinations assessed as soon as the drugs became available.

Copyright © 2011 S. Karger AG, Basel

On March 24, 1882, after relating before the Society of Physiology in Berlin the experiences that had led him to identify and cultivate the bacillus responsible for tuberculosis, Robert Koch [1] claimed that. . . 'Above all, one must consider all means available to humanely eliminate sources of the infectious material. One of these sources, certainly the most important, is the sputum of consumptive patients'. The first positive answer to Koch's claim was given 62 years later in January 1944, by Albert Schatz, Elizabeth Bugie and Selman Waksman, and was named streptomycin. The objective of the present paper is to describe the sequential steps that led from the discovery of streptomycin to the development of the 18-month standard treatment of tuberculosis and its implementation in the field, and then to the 6-month short-course chemotherapy. The discovery and testing of second-line drugs and of the new drugs currently in development will be covered in the other papers.

## Before the Streptomycin Era

Research conducted by Oswald Avery and René Dubos on the enzymatic digestion of the *Pneumococcus* capsule at the Rockefeller Institute in New York [2] and by Gerhard Domagk on the antibacterial activity of derivatives of dyes in Bayer Laboratories in Elberfeld, Germany, played an important role in the development of tuberculosis drugs. They led to the discovery in 1931 of the antimicrobial activity of Prontosil®, the first sulphonamide [3], and encouraged the systematic search for antibiotic substances secreted by soil bacteria. The synthesis of the first antituberculosis drug resulted from Domagk's wish in 1938 to change the core of sulphonamides to make them active for tuberculosis. Actually, the work began in Bayer Laboratories in 1941, and in late November 1941, the antituberculosis activity of benzaldehyde-thiosemicarbazone and then of the thiosemicarbazone constituent alone became evident. The bacteriostatic and inexpensive drug that would become the companion of streptomycin and isoniazid for the treatment of tuberculosis in developing countries was born. However, because of the numerous war-related issues, the new drug, thiacetazone, named Conteben® in Germany and Tibione® in the USA, was successfully tested only in 1946 [4].

## From the Discovery of Streptomycin to the 18-Month Standard Treatment of Tuberculosis

*Reducing Tuberculosis Short-Term Mortality*

In June 1943, Albert Schatz, a student in soil microbiology at Cook College in Rutgers University (New Brunswick, N.J., USA) agreed to conduct his doctoral studies under the supervision of Selman Waksman with the following 2 objectives: first, isolate antibacterial substances from soil micro-organisms with a broader spectrum of activity than streptothricin (tyrothricine) discovered by René Dubos in 1939 [5]; second, find an antibiotic with specific activity against *Mycobacterium tuberculosis.* After less than 6 months of intensive 'screening', Schatz isolated 2 strains of *Actinomyces griseus* (later renamed as *Streptomyces griseus*) which secreted a substance, streptomycin, with activity against Gram-negative and Gram-positive bacteria, including *M. tuberculosis* [6]. By the Spring of 1944, he was able to extract enough streptomycin to permit Feldman and Hinshaw [7] to test its effect on 4 guinea pigs infected with *M. tuberculosis* and convincingly demonstrate, by comparison with untreated controls, the promising antituberculosis activity of streptomycin. After subsequent guinea pig experiments [8], the treatment of 100 patients [9] confirmed the activity of streptomycin against *M. tuberculosis.*

Though very encouraging, the results of streptomycin treatment for pulmonary tuberculosis were inconclusive because some patients did not respond as well as others and the overall benefit of streptomycin treatment was not enduring for many. This led the British Medical Research Council (BMRC) to launch the first controlled clinical trial in the history of medicine [10], based on the procedure suggested by Hinshaw and Feldman [11] to use an untreated control group of patients in addition to the treated group. Between January and September 1947, 107 cases of bacteriologically confirmed, recent cases of bilateral pulmonary tuberculosis, aged 15–30 years, were randomly allocated to 1 of 2 arms, 55 to receive streptomycin (2 g/day given in 4 intramuscular injections at 6-hourly intervals) plus bed rest and 52 bed rest alone. All patients were treated by bed rest for 6 months but streptomycin was mainly given for the first 4 months only. At 6 months, 27% of the patients treated with bed rest only died whereas only 7% of patients receiving streptomycin died. Such a significant difference in the mortality rate demonstrated the antituberculosis activity of streptomycin. However, 3 negative findings were observed: first, major clinical and laboratory improvements were seen during the first 2–3 months of treatment only; second, clinical and laboratory deterioration was observed in 21 (38%) of streptomycin-treated patients, and, third, streptomycin resistance developed in 35 (85%) of the 41 streptomycin-treated patients for whom the streptomycin susceptibility testing was performed. Because of acquired resistance to streptomycin, it was therefore clear that there was no hope to cure patients with cavitary pulmonary tuberculosis with streptomycin alone.

*Preventing the Development of Bacterial Resistance to Streptomycin*

The first step towards the prevention of streptomycin resistance became possible when para-aminosalicylic acid (PAS) was developed by Jörgen Lehmann [12]. Unlike streptomycin, the discovery of PAS did not result from extensive screening of soil bacteria for antibiotic production but, rather, from rational design. Because sodium salicylate (*o*-hydroxybenzoate) and sodium benzoate increased the oxygen uptake of tubercle bacilli [13], Lehman, a master of competitive inhibition who discovered the antagonism between dicoumarol and vitamin K, postulated that antagonists of salicylate and benzoate should decrease the oxygen uptake and have an antituberculosis activity. Synthesized in 1943 by K.G. Rosdahl in Sweden, PAS demonstrated antituberculosis activity in guinea pigs and in the first 20 patients who received 10–15 g/day in Sweden after March 1944; however, PAS became readily available only in 1946. Its role in the treatment of tuberculosis was rationally assessed by the BMRC in a controlled clinical trial initiated at the end of 1948 [14]. After randomization, 59 patients were treated with PAS alone (20 g/day in 4 doses of 5 g), 54 with streptomycin alone (1 g/day in 1 dose because such a dosage had been demonstrated to be as active as and more convenient to administer than the previous schedule of 0.5 g every 6 h [15]) and 53 with streptomycin + PAS. At the 4-month time point, patients treated with any drug regimen improved clinically with a significant advantage for those treated with streptomycin alone or in combination with PAS. But the most outstanding findings were the higher rate of culture conversion, the lower rate of clinical deterioration and the lower rate of streptomycin resistance in the streptomycin-PAS-treated patients (table 1). These results provided the first evidence of the importance

**Table 1.** Results of the BMRC trial comparing streptomycin and PAS, alone and in combination (SP) against pulmonary tuberculosis [14]

| Drug regimen | Patients included | After 4 months of treatment | | |
|---|---|---|---|---|
| | | total | number culture negative | culture-positive patients with streptomycin-resistant bacteria |
| PAS 20 g/day | 59 | 57 | 6 (11%) | – |
| Streptomycin 1 g/day | 54 | 53 | 7 (13%) | 33/40 (82.5%) |
| SP | 53 | 52 | 14 (27%) | 5/33 (15%) |

PAS administered in 4 oral doses of 5 g given from 8 a.m. to 8 p.m. Streptomycin given by intramuscular injection.

of combination chemotherapy to prevent the emergence of drug resistance.

*Discovering Isoniazid and Preventing the Development of Drug Resistance More Completely*

The second step towards the complete prevention of streptomycin resistance was made in 1951 with the discovery of the antituberculosis activity of isoniazid. The history of this discovery deserves to be remembered. Synthesized for their thesis in 1912 in Prague by Hans Meyer and Joseph Mally [16] as derivative of hydrazine ($NH_2$–$NH_2$), isoniazid was totally unknown to the pharmacopoeia for nearly 40 years. In 1945, the antituberculosis property of nicotinamide, a derivative of vitamin $B_3$, was serendipitously observed in humans [17] and then demonstrated in guinea pigs [18]. This observation prompted extensive testing of nicotinamide and its derivatives for their antituberculosis effects [19]. The investigations conducted independently by 3 pharmaceutical companies, Farbenfabriken Bayer [20], Hoffman-La Roche [21, 22] and Squibb Institute for Medical Research [23], led to the discovery of isoniazid as a potent antituberculosis agent. The first clinical trial began in 1951 at Sea View Hospital in Staten Island, N.Y., and the impressive results of it were reported to the public in 1952 [19].

By the spring of 1952, the BMRC set up a controlled clinical trial [24] comparing the activity of isoniazid 200 mg daily, in 2 tablets of 100 mg given 12-hourly, with that of the daily combination of streptomycin 1 g + PAS 20 g (SP). By August 1952, the results of the first 3 months of treatment could be analysed for 173 isoniazid-treated cases and 158 SP-treated cases. The administration of isoniazid alone was very effective but not more than that of the SP combination and was responsible for rapid emergence of drug resistance (fig. 1) associated with a lack of clinical and radiological progress. Such relatively disappointing

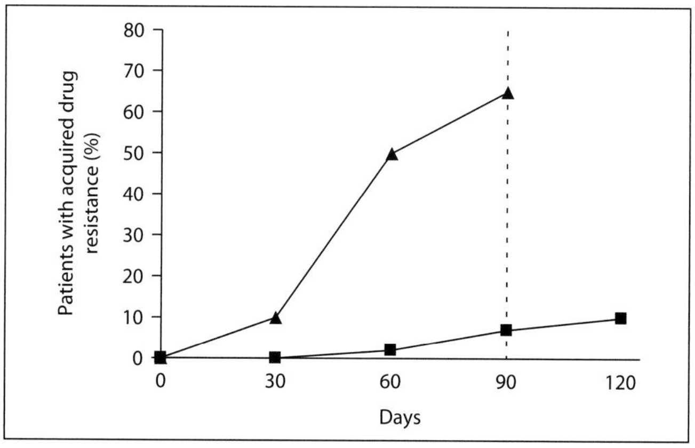


**Fig. 1.** Emergence of resistance to isoniazid (▲) in 173 patients treated with isoniazid alone and to streptomycin (■) in 158 patients treated with SP [24].

results led the tuberculosis chemotherapy trials committee of the BMRC to introduce a third treatment, streptomycin + isoniazid (SH), in the hope that the combination of the 2 most active drugs would prevent the emergence of resistance to isoniazid and to streptomycin. At the following 3 months' assessment [25], the proportion of patients bacteriologically negative was 67% for SH, 55% for SP and 37% for isoniazid and, as shown in table 2, the rate of acquired drug resistance was the lowest with SH treatment. The SH combination was therefore identified as the most active. However, as streptomycin needed to be administered by the intramuscular route and was not devoid of audiovestibular and renal toxicity, in September 1952 the BMRC started a new controlled clinical trial [26] comparing the activity of the combinations SH and PAS-isoniazid (PH), the latter having the great advantage of being totally oral and of very limited toxicity. Patients allocated to the SH treatment were subdivided into 2 subgroups, SH administered daily

**Table 2.** Results of the BMRC trial comparing isoniazid (H) alone, SP and SH against pulmonary tuberculosis [25]

| Drug regimen | Drug resistance in patients culture-positive with sensitivity tests | | | | | | | | | |
|---|---|---|---|---|---|---|---|---|---|---|
| | n | at 1 month | | | at 2 months | | | at 3 months | | |
| | | cult. + | R to H | R to S | cult. + | R to H | R to S | cult. + | R to H | R to S |
| H | 120 | 73 | 11% | – | 63 | 52% | – | 53 | 62% | – |
| SP | 102 | 47 | – | 2% | 31 | – | 3% | 17 | – | 5% |
| SH | 142 | 75 | 4% | 1% | 52 | 9% | 4% | 19 | 13% | 2% |

cult. + = Culture positive; R to H = with bacilli resistant to isoniazid; R to S = with bacilli resistant to streptomycin.

**Table 3.** Results of the BMRC trial comparing SH or PH against pulmonary tuberculosis [26]

| Drug regimen | Total incl. | Results of sputum cultures | | | | | | | |
|---|---|---|---|---|---|---|---|---|---|
| | | month 1 | | month 2 | | month 3 | | | |
| | | total | cult. – | total | cult. – | total | cult. – | cult. + | R to H |
| SH | 119 | 111 | 32% | 104 | 51% | 106 | 65% | 18 | 2 (11%) |
| $S_{2/7}H$ | 100 | | | | | | | 21 | 8 (38%) |
| $P_{20}H$ | 101 | 89 | 27% | 91 | 43% | 89 | 66% | 18 | 0 (0%) |
| $P_{10}H$ | 71 | | | | | | | 16 | 1 (6%) |

SH = daily streptomycin 1 g + daily isoniazid 200 mg; $S_{2/7}H$ = twice weekly streptomycin 1 g + daily isoniazid 200 mg; $P_{20}H$ = daily PAS 20 g + daily isoniazid 200 mg; $P_{10}H$ = daily PAS 10 g + daily isoniazid 200 mg; cult. – = culture negative; cult. + = culture positive; R to H = resistance to isoniazid.

and $S_{2/7}H$ with streptomycin administered twice weekly and isoniazid daily. Patients allocated to PH treatment were also subdivided into 2 subgroups, $P_{20}H$ administered daily with a 20-gram dose of PAS, and $P_{10}H$ administered daily with a 10-gram dose of PAS. Individual doses of streptomycin and isoniazid were 1 g and 200 mg, respectively. After 3 months of treatment (table 3), $P_{20}H$ and SH were clinically and bacteriologically equivalent. $P_{10}H$ appeared as effective as $P_{20}H$ whereas $S_{2/7}H$ was less effective than SH in preventing the development of isoniazid resistance. These preliminary findings were confirmed 2 years later [27] on a total of 241 patients treated for a period of 6 months. SH, $P_{20}H$ and $P_{10}H$ treatments equally prevented the development of bacterial resistance to isoniazid but not $S_{2/7}H$: 8 of the 9 positive cultures at 6 months were resistant to isoniazid. The conclusion was crystal clear: (1) streptomycin should be given daily, at least during the initial phase of treatment; (2) 10 g of PAS per day is as adequate as 20 g, and (3) because a small group of patients with PAS-resistant organisms was not protected from the risk of development of isoniazid resistance during treatment with PH, the logical next step was to give the 3 drugs together, at least during the initial phase of treatment. The remaining question was to determine the optimum duration of treatment to prevent disease reactivation.

*Preventing Relapse after Treatment Cessation*

The BMRC [28] enrolled 284 patients with cavitary pulmonary tuberculosis between January 1956 and January 1958 in a co-operative study. They received PH for durations of 6 months, 1, 2 or 3 years supplemented during the first 6 weeks with daily streptomycin. Because 8 of the first 13 patients randomized to the 6-month treatment relapsed in the 2.5-year period of subsequent observation, the 6-month course was quickly ruled inadequate. Among patients allocated to 1, 2 and 3 years of treatment, the relapse rates were 14 of 74 (19%), 1 of 42 (2%) and 0 of 29 (0%), respectively. It was therefore concluded that extending the course of treatment from 1 to 2 years was highly beneficial but extending it from 2 to 3 years brought little additional benefit. As a result,

**Table 4.** International investigation of the efficacy of chemotherapy [29]

| Patients | Number | Percent |
|---|---|---|
| Included[1] | 581 | 100 |
| Received the prescribed treatment | 317 | 54.6[2] |
| Did not receive the prescribed treatment | 196 | 33.7 |
| Dead | 10 | 1.8 |
| Lost to follow-up | 58 | 9.9 |

[1] With organisms fully susceptible to streptomycin, isoniazid and PAS.
[2] All cured.

the gold standard duration of treatment for tuberculosis was set at 18–24 months.

## Implementation of the 18-Month Standard Treatment of Tuberculosis

*Rate of Stable Culture Conversion*

At the end of the 1950s, a majority of tuberculosis experts were still convinced that cure or stable culture conversion of pulmonary tuberculosis could not be obtained with the standard treatment in some patients because of the 'extent and nature' of the lung disease. To address that issue, an international study involving 29 medical centres in 21 countries around the world was conducted between October 1960 and January 1962 under the auspices of the International Union against Tuberculosis [29]. Previously untreated patients with smear-positive, drug-susceptible, cavitary pulmonary tuberculosis were treated during the first 12 weeks with daily streptomycin 1 g, isoniazid 300 mg and PAS 12 g, and from the 13th to the 28th weeks with streptomycin 1 g 3 times a week and daily isoniazid and PAS as in the initial phase. Patients had to be kept in hospital for at least 28 weeks from the start of treatment, as this was the minimum rule at the time in industrialized countries. As shown in table 4, the results were unambiguous: among the 581 patients who had fully drug-susceptible organisms at treatment initiation, 317, i.e. 54.6%, received the prescribed drugs during the whole year of the study, and all of them responded favourably to the treatment, became and remained culture negative. Thus, the activity of the standard treatment of pulmonary tuberculosis was demonstrated all over the world. However, other findings of importance also emerged: only half of the patients received the prescribed treatment, one third did not receive it and 10% were lost to follow-up, illustrating the huge problem of physician and patient non-compliance.

**Table 5.** Results of 12 months of treatment at home or in a sanatorium with isoniazid and PAS in Madras [30]

| Patients | Location of treatment | |
|---|---|---|
| | home | sanatorium |
| Total | 82 (100) | 81 (100) |
| Cure | 67 (82) | 73 (90) |
| Failure | 13 (16) | 6 (7) |
| Death | 2 (2) | 2 (3) |

Figures are patient numbers, with percentages in parentheses.

*Ambulatory Treatment*

Before the antibiotic era, in industrialized countries, patients with tuberculosis were mainly hospitalized for prolonged periods of time in sanatoria, where the only treatments were long-term bed rest and the artificial pneumothorax. None of these were readily available in developing countries. Consequently, in 1955, the government of India, moved by the disproportionate numbers of patients with bacteriologically confirmed tuberculosis (estimated as at least 1.5 million relative to the 23,000 beds available), received support from the World Health Organization and BMRC to investigate home-based treatment for tuberculosis. The results of studies conducted by Wallace Fox [30] and colleagues at the Tuberculosis Chemotherapy Centre, Madras, are internationally known: home or ambulatory treatment was almost as effective as treatment in a sanatorium (table 5), provided that regular use of antibiotics is well organized and supervised by the health care team. Moreover, the family contacts of patients treated at home were not more likely to become infected than family members of hospitalized patients. Ambulatory treatment quickly became the rule, especially in developing countries. Unfortunately, the explicit condition set forth by Fox for the success of ambulatory treatment, i.e. the rigorous organization and supervision of antibiotic intake, was then and is still now so overlooked that the percentage of patients who do not take the prescribed treatment may exceed 50%.

*Intermittent Treatment*

To address the challenges of daily supervision of the antibiotic intake by patients treated at home, Fox [31] and colleagues in Madras conceived of intermittent administration of antibiotics. With 94% of culture conversions at 12 months, twice weekly SH proved at least as active as the 85% of culture conversions obtained with daily PH. The intermittent treatment was gradually adopted in many countries as an alternative to daily treatment, especially in cities where twice weekly access to health centres is relatively easy.

*Discovery of Ethambutol*

Ethambutol is another product of organic synthesis, discovered in 1961 through an extensive screening program at Lederle Laboratories. Ethambutol was reported to be 4 times as active as streptomycin against wild strains of *M. tuberculosis* and also to be active in vivo against strains resistant to streptomycin or isoniazid [32]. Having a predominantly bacteriostatic activity like PAS but being much better tolerated, ethambutol soon replaced PAS in the standard regimen.

## Towards the 6-Month Short-Course Chemotherapy for Tuberculosis

*Discovery of Rifampicin*

In 1957, a story similar to that of Albert Schatz and streptomycin took place in Italy. A *Streptomyces* strain, designated strain ME/83 and later named *Amycolatopsis mediterranei,* was isolated from a soil sample in the Lepetit Research Laboratories. From this strain, several compounds were isolated, and by reduction of one of these, namely rifamycin B, a promising compound was obtained, rifamycin SV. Although very active against *M. tuberculosis* in vitro, rifamycin SV was not orally bioavailable. Further chemical modifications led to a semisynthetic orally active substance, rifampicin [33]. When tested alone and in combination with isoniazid in a mouse model of tuberculosis [34], rifampicin exhibited

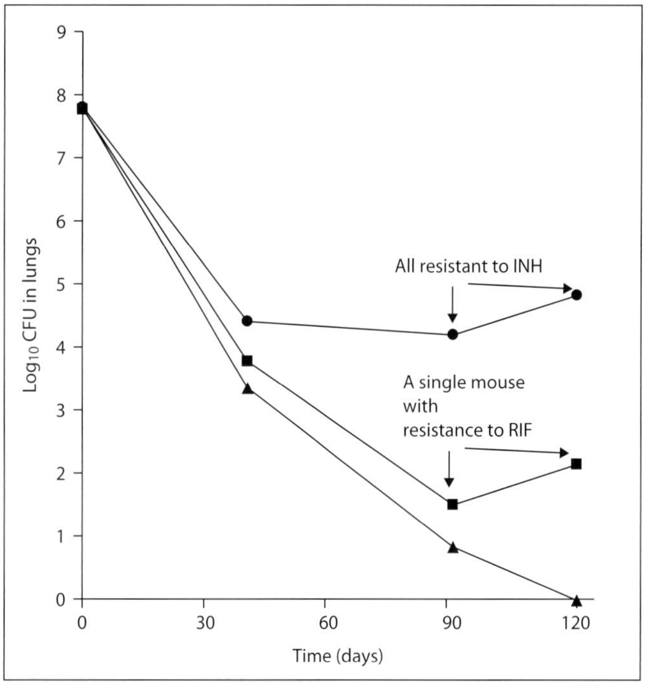


**Fig. 2.** Activity of rifampicin (RIF) and isoniazid (INH) alone or in combination in mice [34]. ● = Isoniazid 25 mg/kg; ■ = rifampicin 25 mg/kg; ▲ = isoniazid 25 mg/kg + rifampicin 25 mg/kg.

spectacular activity: mice treated with the combination of isoniazid 25 mg/kg and rifampicin 25 mg/kg all became culture negative by 120 days after treatment initiation (fig. 2), a phenomenon that had never been observed previously with any drug combination given at clinically relevant doses. For example, with the combination SH some mice remain lung culture positive with few colonies even after 12 months of daily therapy. The rapid culture conversion obtained in mice illustrated the potential of rifampicin to shorten the 18- to 24-month-long treatment for tuberculosis.

*Shortening the Duration of Standard Chemotherapy to 9 Months*

Numerous controlled clinical studies were initiated to assess the possibility to reduce the duration of treatment with rifampicin containing regimens. As all gave similar results, those obtained in the study conducted in the early 1970s by the British Thoracic and Tuberculosis Association [35] are given as an example in table 6. Followed with a relapse rate of 5%, the 6-month course of treatment was not optimal but a 9-month course of the rifampicin-isoniazid combination supplemented by an initial 2-month phase of streptomycin or ethambutol was as active as 18–24 months of the standard chemotherapy and was followed by no relapse. In a few

**Table 6.** Short-course chemotherapy with rifampicin in pulmonary tuberculosis [35]

| Condition on admission | Duration of treatment[1] months | Eligible | Died[2] | Emigrated or absconded | Remained | Relapse |
|---|---|---|---|---|---|---|
| No cavity or cavity <2 cm | 6 | 182 | 10 | 12 | 160 | 8 (5%) |
| | 12 | 181 | 7 | 19 | 155 | 2 (1%) |
| Cavity >2 cm | 9 | 153 | 8 | 10 | 135 | 0 |
| | 18 | 149 | 8 | 14 | 127 | 0[3] |

[1] With isoniazid and rifampicin + either streptomycin or ethambutol for the first 2 months of treatment; results obtained with streptomycin- or ethambutol-containing regimens were mixed because they were not different.
[2] Of other cause than tuberculosis.
[3] A single patient produced an isolated positive culture.

years, 9-month rifampicin-containing regimens replaced the 18-month standard treatment.

*Discovery and Rediscovery of Pyrazinamide*

The serendipitous observation of nicotinamide antituberculosis activity in humans [17], then confirmed in the guinea pig [18], resulted in extensive screening of nicotinic acid (niacin or vitamin $B_3$) derivatives by large pharmaceutical companies [19]. In 1948 it was observed that nicotinamide given as 0.5–0.75% in the diet (equivalent to 20–25 mg/kg/day) prevented the dissemination of tuberculosis in infected mice as effectively as 50 mg/kg of streptomycin given 4 times daily [36]. After several passages in mice treated with nicotinamide, there was evidence of development of resistance to nicotinamide, an indirect confirmation of its antituberculosis activity. In addition, the streptomycin-nicotinamide combination was more active than either drug alone [36]. Investigations of closely related derivatives identified pyrazinamide [37] as a candidate antituberculosis drug. Like isoniazid, pyrazinamide had been synthesized by Dalmer and Walter in 1936 (German patent 632257), long before its antituberculosis activity was recognized. Further animal studies [38] demonstrated that this compound was 3 times as effective as PAS or nicotinamide, but less effective than streptomycin. Despite its clinical activity [39], pyrazinamide was overshadowed by isoniazid and had only a marginal therapeutic role until it was literally rediscovered in 1972 by the East Africa and British Medical Research Councils [40]. In the pivotal clinical trial, patients with drug-susceptible pulmonary tuberculosis were randomized to one of four 6-month daily treatment groups, SH, SH + thiacetazone (SHT), SH + pyrazinamide (SHZ) and SH + rifampicin (SHR). Eighteen months of SHT, with daily streptomycin for the first 2 months, was a control regimen. On treatment completion of the 6-month regimens, only 2 patients, both treated with SH, were still culture positive. Relapses occurred during the ensuing 6 months in 18% of the 94 SH-treated patients, 21% of the 84 SHT-treated patients, 6% of the 88 SHZ-treated patients and 4% of the 99 SHR-treated patients, suggesting similar contributions of pyrazinamide and rifampicin [40]. This was confirmed by a second study conducted in Hong Kong that compared 9 months of SHZ and SHR [41].

**Table 7.** Relapse rate within 2 years of termination of rifampicin and pyrazinamide-containing treatment for pulmonary tuberculosis [42]

| Drug regimen | Total duration months | Cases | Relapses |
|---|---|---|---|
| 2SRHZ/4RH | 6 | 119 | 1 (0.8%) |
| 2RHZE/4RH | 6 | 127 | 3 (2.3%) |
| 2RHE/7RH | 9 | 127 | 2 (1.5%) |

S = Streptomycin 0.75 g 6 days a week; R = rifampicin 600 mg daily; H = isoniazid 300 mg daily; Z = pyrazinamide 2 g daily; E = ethambutol 25 mg/kg daily.

Combining both pyrazinamide and rifampicin was the next logical step. It resulted in the present 6-month short-course chemotherapy for tuberculosis the efficacy of which has been demonstrated around the world, as illustrated (table 7) by the findings of the British Thoracic Society [42]: 6 months of treatment with rifampicin + pyrazinamide-containing regimens were as effective as 9 months of treatment with either rifampicin- or pyrazinamide-containing regimens.

## References


1 Koch R: Die Aetiologie der Tuberkulose. Berl Klin Wochenschr 1882;19:221–230.
2 Avery OT, Dubos RJ: The specific action of a bacterial enzyme on pneumococci of type III. Science 1930;72B:151–152.
3 Domagk G: Ein Beitrag zur Chemotherapie der bakteriellen Infektionen. Dtsch Med Wochenschr 1935;61:250–253.
4 Domagk G, Behnisch R, Mietzsch F, Schmidt H: Über eine neue, gegen Tuberkelbazillen in vitro wirksame Verbindungsklasse. Naturwissenschaften 1946;33:1–4.
5 Dubos RJ: Bactericidal effect of an extract of a soil bacillus on Gram positive cocci. Proc Soc Exp Biol Med 1939;40:311–312.
6 Schatz A, Bugie E, Waksman S: Streptomycin, a substance exhibiting antibiotic activity against Gram-positive and Gram-negative bacteria. Proc Soc Exp Biol Med 1944;55:66–69.
7 Feldman WH, Hinshaw HC: Effects of streptomycin on experimental tuberculosis in guinea pigs. Proc Staff Meet Mayo Clin 1944;19:593–599.
8 Feldman WH, Hinshaw HC, Mann FC: Streptomycin in experimental tuberculosis. Am Rev Tuberc 1945;52:269–298.
9 Hinshaw HC, Feldman WH, Pfuetze KH: Treatment of tuberculosis with streptomycin: a summary of observations on one hundred cases, J Am Med Assoc 1946;132:778–782.
10 Medical Research Council investigation: Streptomycin treatment of pulmonary tuberculosis. Br Med J 1948;ii:769–782.
11 Hinshaw HC, Feldman WH: Evaluation of chemotherapeutic agents in clinical tuberculosis: a suggested procedure. Am Rev Tuberc 1944;50:202–213.
12 Lehmann J: Para-aminosalicylic acid in the treatment of tuberculosis. Lancet 1946;247:15–16.
13 Bernheim F: The effect of salicylate on the oxygen uptake of the tubercle bacillus. Science 1940;92:204.
14 Medical Research Council Investigation: Treatment of pulmonary tuberculosis with streptomycin and para-amino-salicylic acid. Br Med J 1950;ii:1073–1085.
15 Bignall JR, Clegg JW, Crofton JW, Douglas Smith BJ, Holt D, Mitchison DA, Armitage P: Intermittent dosage in the treatment of pulmonary tuberculosis with streptomycin. Br Med J 1950;i:1224–1230.
16 Meyer H, Mally J: Über Hydrazinderivate der Pyridincarbonsäuren. Monatsh Chem verw Teile anderer Wiss 1912;23:393–414.
17 Huant E: Note sur l'action de très fortes doses d'amide nicotinique dans les lésions bacillaires. Gaz Hôp 1945;16:259–260.
18 Chorine V: Action de l'amide nicotinique sur les bacilles du genre *Mycobacterium*. C R Acad Sci 1945:220:150–151.
19 Editorial: New drugs for tuberculosis. N Engl J Med 1952;246:797–799.
20 Domagk G, Offe HA, Siefken W: Ein weiterer Beitrag zur experimentellen Chemotherapie der Tuberkulose (Neoteben). Dtsch Med Wochenschr 1952;77:573–578.
21 Benson WM, Stefko PL, Roe MD: Pharmacologic and toxicologic observations on hydrazine derivatives of isonicotinic acid (Rimifon, Marsilid). Am Rev Tuberc 1952;65:376–391.
22 Fox HH: The chemical approach to the control of tuberculosis. Science 1952;116:129–134.
23 Bernstein J, Lott WA, Steinberg BA, Yale HL: Chemotherapy of experimental tuberculosis. V. Isonicotinic acid hydrazide (Nydrazid) and related compounds. Am Rev Tuberc 1952;65:357–364.
24 Medical Research Council: The treatment of pulmonary tuberculosis with isoniazid. Br Med J 1952;ii:735–746.
25 Medical Research Council: Isoniazid in the treatment of pulmonary tuberculosis. Br Med J 1953;i:521–536.
26 Medical Research Council: Isoniazid in combination with streptomycin or with PAS in the treatment of pulmonary tuberculosis. Br Med J 1953;ii:1005–1014.
27 Medical Research Council: Various combinations of isoniazid with streptomycin or with PAS in the treatment of pulmonary tuberculosis. Br Med J 1955;i:435–445.
28 Medical Research Council-Tuberculosis Chemotherapy Trials Committee: Long-term chemotherapy in the treatment of chronic pulmonary tuberculosis with cavitation. Tubercle 1962;43:201–267.
29 International Union against Tuberculosis: An international investigation of the efficacy of chemotherapy. Bull Int Union Tuberc 1964;34:79–191.
30 Fox W: Ambulatory chemotherapy in a developing country: clinical and epidemiological studies. Adv Tuberc Res 1963;12:28–149.
31 Fox W: Methods of chemotherapy in developing countries. Bull Int Union Tuberc 1966;337:249–260.
32 Wilkerson RG, Shepherd RG, Thomas DP, Baughn C: Stereospecificity in a new type of antituberculosis agent. J Am Chem Soc 1961;83:2212–2213.
33 Sensi P: History of development of rifampin. Rev Infect Dis 1983;5:S402–S406.
34 Grumbach F, Rist N: Activité antituberculeuse expérimentale de la rifampicine, dérivée de la rifamycine SV. Rev Tuberc Pneum 1967;31:749–762.
35 British Thoracic and Tuberculosis Association: Short-course chemotherapy in pulmonary tuberculosis: a controlled trial. Lancet 1976;ii:1102–1104.
36 McKensie D, Malone L, Kushner S, Oleson JJ, Subbarow Y: Effect of nicotinamide acid amide on experimental tuberculosis of white mice. J Lab Clin Med 1948;33:1249–1253.
37 Kushner S, Dalalian H, Sanjurjo H, Bach JL Jr, Safir SR, Smith VK Jr, Williams JH: Experimental chemotherapy of tuberculosis. II. The synthesis of pyrazinamides and related compounds. J Am Chem Soc 1952;74:3617–3621.
38 Malone L, Schurr A, Lindh H, McKenzie D, Kiser JS, Williams JH: The effect of pyrazinamide (Aldinamide) on experimental tuberculosis in mice. Am Rev Tuberc 1952;65:511–518.
39 Yeager RL, Munroe WGC, Dessau FI: Pyrazinamide (Aldinamide) in the treatment of pulmonary tuberculosis. Am Rev Tuberc 1952;65:523–534.
40 East African/British Medical Research Councils: Controlled clinical trial of short-course (6-month) regimens of chemotherapy for treatment of pulmonary tuberculosis. Lancet 1972;i:1079–1085.
41 Hong Kong Tuberculosis Treatment Services/British Medical Research Council: Controlled trial of 6- and 9-month regimens of daily and intermittent streptomycin plus isoniazid plus pyrazinamide for pulmonary tuberculosis in Hong Kong. Tubercle 1975;56:81–96.
42 British Thoracic Society: A controlled trial of 6 months' chemotherapy in pulmonary tuberculosis. Final report: results during the 36 months after the end of chemotherapy and beyond. Br J Dis Chest 1984;78:330–336.



Jacques Grosset
Department of Medicine
Johns Hopkins University School of Medicine
1550 Orleans Street, Baltimore, MD 21287 (USA)
Tel. +1 410 502 8234, E-Mail jgrosse4@jhmi.edu

## Chapter 2

Donald PR, van Helden PD (eds): Antituberculosis Chemotherapy.
Prog Respir Res. Basel, Karger, 2011, vol 40, pp 10–16

# Tuberculosis Treatment Trials Past and Present: Old and New Challenges

Andrew Nunn

MRC Clinical Trials Unit, London, UK

**Abstract**

The principles determining the conduct of clinical trials in tuberculosis (TB) have changed very little since the 1940s when the British Medical Research Council's streptomycin trial was conducted. Many of the challenges facing researchers remain the same, but the advent of highly effective treatments, under controlled conditions, has resulted in the need for much larger studies with non-inferiority designs. The intention-to-treat population is the right choice for superiority trials because it is conservative with respect to any differences that might exist between study arms; this is not however appropriate when the aim is to demonstrate that no difference exists as in a non-inferiority trial. End points used in the assessment of patient outcomes in drug-sensitive TB have evolved from mortality, clinical assessments and radiographic appearances in early trials to an almost exclusive emphasis on bacteriology. New challenges include the emergence of HIV co-infection, the need to distinguish reinfections from relapses, and the use of liquid culture medium with its increased sensitivity which may or may not be helpful for determining outcome. The requirements of regulators, particularly in relation to the classification of patients lost to follow-up after completing treatment, is a topic yet to be satisfactorily resolved.

Copyright © 2011 S. Karger AG, Basel

## Introduction

How much have the design and analysis of clinical trials in tuberculosis (TB) changed over the last 60 years? The short answer would seem to be not a great deal. The Medical Research Council's streptomycin trial published in 1948 was a landmark trial both with respect to the significance of its findings but also because it became a model trial in the way it was designed and conducted [1]. Its distinctive feature was the concealment of the randomization schedule which prevented any access to treatment allocation until a patient was determined to be eligible for enrolment. A few years after the publication of the streptomycin trial, Wallace Fox [2] wrote a paper describing recent developments in controlled trials in TB, elucidating principles which remain the foundation of well-conducted trials to this day. These include ethical considerations, design issues such as sample size and sections on the analysis of results [2]. The sound instruction and advice in Fox's review are as relevant today as they were 50 years ago.

Over the years there have been important advances in statistical methodology of clinical trials such as the introduction of time to event analyses, including the proportional hazards model. The need for large, simple, well-designed and carefully conducted trials, however, remains as does the challenge to ensure that results can be read, interpreted and accepted with confidence.

## Which Population Should We Be Using?

This is relevant both to the eligibility criteria and the data analysis. Eligibility criteria have implications for the external validity, or generalizability, of the results. The early TB treatment trials were extremely restrictive being limited to 'acute, progressive, bilateral pulmonary TB of presumably recent origin, bacteriologically proved, unsuitable for collapse therapy, age 15–30' [2]. Postrandomization exclusions should always be kept to a minimum, but may sometimes be unavoidable; an example of this is exclusion of patients having multidrug-resistant TB (MDR-TB) which cannot always be done before enrolment.

In the reports of the pivotal trials conducted by the British Medical Research Council (BMRC) throughout the 1970s and 1980s which led to the establishment of short-course chemotherapy, the primary analysis was consistently conducted on what would be described as the per-protocol or protocol-correct population (although not usually termed as such) with only an occasional intention-to-treat (ITT) analysis. Was this approach justified?

In an editorial published in the *British Journal of Cancer*, Lewis and Machin [3] addressed the question of when ITT analyses should be used and when they need to be interpreted with particular caution, making particular mention of non-inferiority trials. They cited the earliest reference to ITT being in the 1955 edition of Bradford Hill's *Principles of Medical Statistics* [4] although his earlier publications suggest he had been using this approach for some time before that.

Although the use of ITT is now enshrined as good practice by most researchers, it has given rise to considerable, and at times acrimonious, debate since the concept of a patient randomized to one treatment who then does not receive it, or worse still receives the alternative treatment, being analysed as though he had received his allocated treatment, seems hard to accept – especially if it fails to give the desired answer! There is probably a much better understanding and acceptance among the medical profession today as to why the ITT approach is less likely to be biased than analysing as treated, or per protocol. In simple terms it is understood to be a reflection of real life.

It is of interest that all 107 patients randomized in the streptomycin trial were included in the analysis although a careful reading of the first report would suggest that the ITT and per-protocol populations were in fact the same [1]. A high proportion of patients experienced toxic effects from the 2-gram dose of streptomycin; 36 of 55 on the treated arm reported giddiness in addition to other side effects but none of them stopped treatment. The very brief section on adverse events, less than half a page in a 14-page report, does not indicate whether any patients interrupted treatment, although a decision was made part way through the study to limit treatment to 4 months. The reporting of adverse events has become a much more important feature of trials in recent years, not least because of the need to identify suspected unexpected serious adverse reactions and their likely attribution.

In the long term 5-year follow-up of the streptomycin trial, all the patients were contacted or confirmed to have died [5]. This was the first attempt at contact since the publication of the initial report. Somewhat surprisingly Bradford Hill was not an author of that paper. It is notable that the status of the patients was given according to their initial study arm, even though several of the control, bed rest group had received anti-TB chemotherapy, monotherapy with streptomycin or para-aminosalicylic acid (PAS), or combined treatment with streptomycin and PAS. This was indeed a complete ITT analysis; no attempt was made to perform a per-protocol analysis of patients who had remained on their initial regimen.

So were the trials of short-course chemotherapy conducted by the BMRC in the 70s and 80s analysed inappropriately using per-protocol populations? In answering this question it is essential to recognize the distinction between superiority trials and non-inferiority trials. In most randomized clinical trials the objective is to demonstrate that one treatment is superior to another. There are occasions, however, when the aim is not to show the new drug or regimen is better but 'as good as' the control, i.e. non-inferior. Garratini and Bertele [6] have argued that all such trials are unethical since they serve only commercial interests and not the interests of the patients who are put at unnecessary risk. Whereas the authors were right to caution that such trials could be unethical, they were quite wrong to advocate that all such trials should be banned. Highly effective chemotherapy for TB has been available for many years both in the developed world [7] and in developing countries [8]. However, in both settings the long duration of chemotherapy required led to poor adherence and resulted in unsatisfactory outcomes. The advent of rifampicin raised the possibility that patients might be treated with much shorter but equally effective regimens.

In practice many regimens fall far short of their potential in field conditions, an observation made by Hill [9], who wrote 'at its best . . . a trial shows what can be accomplished with a medicine under careful observation and certain restricted conditions. The same results will not invariably or necessarily be observed when the medicine passes into general use'. However, even if standard treatment is highly effective, it must be desirable to minimize the duration of exposure to potentially toxic drugs along with the inconvenience and cost of having to take long courses of treatment.

The expression 'non-inferiority' was not used in the description of the design of the first short-course chemotherapy studies, neither were they described as equivalence trials. Writing many years later, in 1998, Röhmel [10] refers to a new phrase 'non-inferiority trial' having been coined. A subsequent methodological paper published by Kang and Cheng [11] in 2000 quotes an analysis by Dunnett and Gent [12] of data from a study assessing whether equivalent outcomes

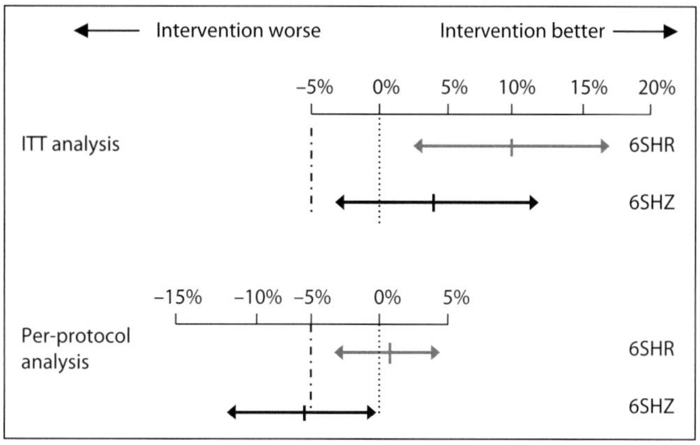


**Fig. 1.** Difference in relapse-free rates of 2STH/16TH and two 6-month regimens, 6SHR and 6SHZ (95% confidence intervals for difference). S = Streptomycin; H = isoniazid; R = rifampicin; Z = pyrazinamide; T = thiacetazone.

to those obtained by physicians could be obtained by nurse practitioners as measured by the quality of patient care.

How should the results of a non-inferiority trial be analysed? Neither ITT nor per-protocol analyses are ideal, the former because it tends to minimize differences, thereby increasing the likelihood of falsely declaring non-inferiority, and the latter because of the bias associated with excluding patients who, for example, have not completed treatment on account of being unable to tolerate it. The contrasting results using these two approaches are shown in figure 1, using a post hoc definition of non-inferiority of 5% with data from the 30-month follow-up of the first BMRC short-course trial [13] (an approach clearly unacceptable under normal circumstances). Using the ITT populations both the pyrazinamide regimen (6SHZ) and the rifampicin regimen (6SHR) would be considered non-inferior to the control, 2STH/16TH, the rifampicin regimen being significantly better. In contrast in the per-protocol analysis, whereas the rifampicin regimen is still seen to be non-inferior, the pyrazinamide regimen is significantly inferior to the control regimen. In line with the recommendations of the Committee for Proprietary Medicinal Products [14] which requires consistent findings from both the per-protocol and ITT analyses, only the rifampicin regimen could be considered non-inferior.

It also needs to be remembered that particular attention must be paid to the rigour with which non-inferiority trials are conducted; a poorly conducted trial can lead to a false conclusion of no difference when a difference exists, if for example an inadequate laboratory fails to detect all of the relapses.

## Selecting the Margin of Non-Inferiority

The rationale for the choice of Δ, the margin of non-inferiority, will depend on the circumstances. For a trial designed as a licensing application for a new regimen, both the Food and Drug Administration and the European Medicines Agency (EMEA) give clear criteria which need to be followed [15, 16]. In their document the EMEA refers to Committee for Medicinal Products for Human Use guidance [14] on the choice of a non-inferiority margin and the need to avoid biocreep, whereby incremental losses of efficacy occur from one trial to another due to acceptance of reduced levels of efficacy in the control regimen. The choice of Δ in the REMox trial, in which the duration of one regimen is shortened while substituting moxifloxacin for ethambutol, was determined in part on the basis of data from earlier trials of 4-month regimens in East Africa and Singapore which showed that reducing treatment from 6 to 4 months in a rifampicin-isoniazid-based regimen resulted in a 9–10% loss of efficacy [17].

In the trials conducted by the International Union against Tuberculosis and Lung Disease in recent years an arbitrary choice of Δ was based on a doubling of the expected failure/relapse rate [18]. This was a pragmatic decision since smaller margins would have resulted in unrealistically large sample sizes. A key assumption in the sample size calculation is the expected favourable outcome rates within the control and intervention regimens. Here again pragmatism can be a determining factor since an assumption of a reduced favourable response rate on the intervention arm rapidly inflates the total numbers required. If, for example, the failure/relapse rate in the control arm is considered to be 5% and Δ is also chosen to be 5%, a trial where the intervention is considered to be equally effective would require 400 patients per arm, using a one-sided 97.5% confidence interval and 90% power. If the failure/relapse rate in the intervention arm was, however, considered to be greater than 5%, say 6 or 7% whilst retaining the same 5% value for Δ, the numbers per arm increase to 683 or a staggering 1,315 per arm, respectively [17].

Do non-inferiority trials always need to be very large? Clearly the choice of Δ will be a critical determining factor. A margin of less than 10% may be regarded by some as being too strict although in the context of high bacteriological success rates in trials of regimens for patients with fully sensitive disease, a 10% margin would almost certainly be regarded as unacceptable. If the experimental treatment is expected to be more effective than the control, as could be the case in a non-inferiority trial assessing new treatments of MDR-

**Table 1.** Total number of patients required in superiority or non-inferiority design for trial of a new MDR-TB regimen

| Favourable response in control arm | Increased favourable response in intervention arm relative to the favourable response in the control arm | | | | |
|---|---|---|---|---|---|
| | superiority | | non-inferiority | | |
| | +10% | +15% | none | +10% | +15% |
| 65% | 920 | 396 | 958 | 220 | 132 |
| 70% | 824 | 348 | 884 | 196 | 114 |

Assuming 90% power and two-sided 5% significance level for superiority, one-sided 2.5% significance level and a margin of non-inferiority of 10% for non-inferiority.

TB, the total sample size is less than when it is assumed to be equally or less effective, as illustrated in table 1. Whereas 396 patients are required to demonstrate the superiority of an 80% favourable response over a 65% response, only 220 patients are needed to satisfy the prespecified requirements of non-inferiority if the intervention is considered to be only 10% superior in efficacy. Such an experimental regimen would be particularly attractive if given for a much reduced duration. It is also worth noting that a design in which patients are randomized in the ratio 2:1, for intervention to control, requires only a relatively small increase in the total number of patients required compared to equal allocation and represents an attractive option not only for patients, but also for researchers who would be able to obtain more data on risks associated with exposure to the new treatment.

In a paper addressing current issues in non-inferiority trials, Fleming [19] comments on the conditions under which active control non-inferiority trials provide a reliable assessment of efficacy of the new intervention. The control regimen should be substantially effective, precisely estimated with estimates of efficacy relevant to the setting of the trial, preferably from multiple well-controlled trials [19]. Each of these conditions can certainly be said to be met for drug-sensitive TB among those uninfected by HIV. The situation is very different for MDR-TB.

## Reinfection

A topic currently being debated is whether or not reinfected patients should or should not be considered unfavourable when assessing the efficacy of new regimens. The trials which formed the basis of today's regimens of short-course chemotherapy did not have the ability to differentiate between relapse and reinfection. However, reinfection is more likely to occur in patients co-infected with HIV who would have represented only a small proportion of the total at the time of the first short-course trials. Rates of reinfection as high as 50–80% have been reported in HIV-infected patients who have experienced a recurrence of disease [20, 21]. Should these patients be considered to have an unfavourable outcome?

Regulators, and some researchers, have taken a conservative approach on this issue and have said that a supportive comparison of relapse and reinfection rates should be provided. This is at least in part recognition of the fact that the available technology does not provide a 100% guarantee that a patient can be correctly classified. Although there may not be good reason to suppose that the experimental regimens will be effective against preventing reinfection with a strain different from that with which patients were originally infected, it would seem reasonable to perform a secondary analysis in which all recurrences are classified as unfavourable.

## Trial Duration

It has long been a matter for concern that the pivotal phase III trial takes a very long time in the drug development process. This is partly due to concerns to ensure that trials are conducted to the appropriate standard required for licensing studies resulting in longer periods of preparation and slower rates of recruitment than might occur in a different setting. However, a major factor in the time taken from the first patient randomized to locking of the trial database is the length of follow-up required. The early short-course trials conducted by the BMRC followed all patients for at least 2 years after completion of treatment. In some instances, such as the first East African trial, the most successful regimen was followed for a total of 54 months after treatment. Since then, 24 months have become the standard duration for follow-up after treatment. Is such a long duration necessary? An analysis of 15 trials conducted by the BMRC involving over 7,300 patients from African and Asian sites revealed that 78% of the recurrences occurred within 6 months and 90% within 12 months of stopping treatment [22].

A trial enrolling patients over 24 months, with 24 months of follow-up after the last patient allocated 6 months of treatment has completed treatment – as is currently recommended by the regulators [15] – plus a further 6 months to collect the last of the data would take 5 years from randomization to close-out. A way of shortening such a trial by 18 months would be to terminate the follow-up 12 months after the last patient had been randomized. In those circumstances 50% of patients would have 18–24 months of follow-up and only about 10% of the total relapses expected if all patients were followed for 24 months would be missed. It should be noted that these estimates were based on studies conducted before the onset of the HIV epidemic, and currently only limited data exist on the timing of relapse in HIV-infected patients.

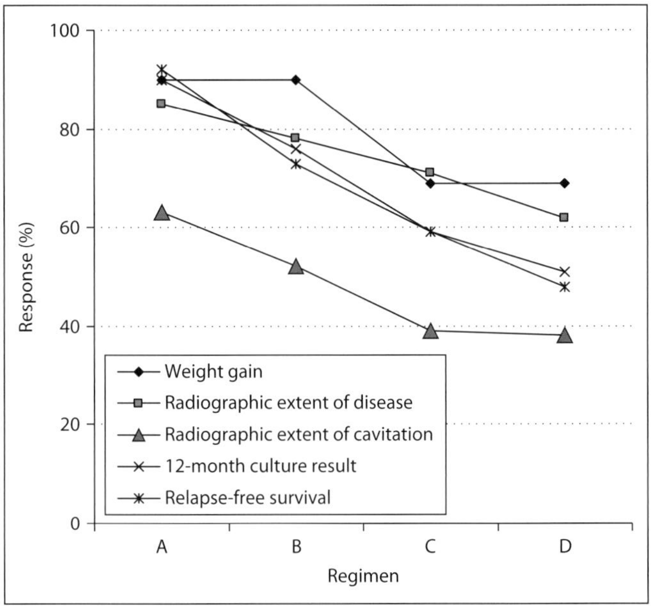


**Fig. 2.** Response in 5 different disease-related assessments in 4 regimens of anti-TB chemotherapy [24]. Regimen A = 3.9–5.5 mg/kg isoniazid + 0.2–0.3 mg/kg PAS daily in 2 doses (standard); B = 7.8–9.6 mg/kg isoniazid daily in 1 dose; C = 7.8–9.6 mg/kg isoniazid daily in 2 doses; D = 3.9–5.5 mg/kg isoniazid daily in 2 doses.

## End Points

End points in clinical trials have obviously changed since the streptomycin trial when preventing death was the primary objective. In the 1953 report of isoniazid in the treatment of TB there was a brief mention of mortality followed by an extensive clinical section addressing such issues as changes in general condition, weight, febrile state, raised erythrocyte sedimentation rate and radiographic appearance [23]. There followed a bacteriological section describing changes in smear, culture and sensitivity tests. By the 1960s, reports focussed more on bacteriological failure during treatment and subsequent relapse but continued to report on radiographic change during treatment. From the mid-1970s to the present day, the emphasis has been firmly on bacteriological failure and relapse with chest radiography relegated to baseline characteristics and its predictive impact in less effective regimens. Is it possible that in focussing almost exclusively on bacteriology we have lost some important aspects of the effectiveness of modern chemotherapeutic regimens?

The reports of the earlier trials were much more extensive than those available in today's journals with their strict limitation on space. Both Methods and Results sections have had to be severely curtailed to conform with editorial requirements. In contrast the Results section of the isoniazid trial referred to above ran to 16 pages, and the streptomycin trial gave illustrated pictures of individual radiographic changes.

An interesting example of how different measures of improvement related to each other in one of the Madras Tuberculosis Chemotherapy Centre trials comes from the 1960 publication of a study of 4 regimens involving isoniazid and PAS [24]. Figure 2 shows changes in weight, radiographic extent of disease, the disappearance of cavitation on radiographs, culture negativity at 12 months and relapse-free survival. There is a remarkable similarity in the relative responses in these 5 different markers across the 4 regimens.

There is much discussion regarding the need for surrogate markers to enable the shortening of regimens. It is clear in the above example that change in radiographic disease across the 4 regimens mirrored the differences in relapse-free survival. But are different markers of early response or long-term outcome also important because they inform on the speed with which patients become symptom free or the extent to which they achieve a return to normal activity in their quality of life?

In the Transkei study of TB pericarditis, 383 patients with constrictive pericarditis or pericardial effusion were randomized to receive prednisolone or placebo in addition to standard anti-TB treatment to assess the role of steroids in the management of their disease. In the long-term 10-year follow-up report, outcome data were obtained on 96% of the randomized patients [25]. There was a significant overall survival benefit to those receiving steroids (hazard ratio = 0.64, 95% confidence interval = 0.41–0.99). However, an equally important finding was the extent to which patients were able to return to normal activity. There was no evidence of benefit from the intervention in either series. Of those with constriction 69% who were allocated prednisolone and 67% allocated placebo were out and about, with or without some restriction of activity. The results for those with effusions were also very similar, namely 69 and 66%, respectively.

## The Primary End Point

If it is currently accepted that bacteriological end points are the best way of differentiating between regimens in a randomized controlled trial, how should departures from the protocol be handled in the ITT analysis? It seems reasonable to consider a change of regimen for any reason as being an unfavourable outcome, particularly a change for adverse drug reactions, but what of deaths and of losses to follow-up? Regulators would tend towards using a conservative classification but this may lead to difficulties in interpretation of those trials with long-term follow-up where losses to follow-up may exceed the true bacteriological failures or relapses. This was well illustrated in the Priftin trial: bacteriological relapses occurred in 5% of patients on the rifampicin-based regimen compared to 11% on the rifapentine-based regimen but approximately one third of patients were lost to follow-up and when this group combined with patients unassessable for other reasons was added to the bacteriological failures, the rates increased to over 50% [unpubl. data]. The true bacteriological relapses were greatly outnumbered by these other groups.

In a trial of a new antibiotic lasting no more than 2 weeks it is reasonable to expect no losses to follow-up and to classify any such patients as unfavourable. A very different situation pertains in TB trials where a key indicator of outcome is relapse during posttreatment follow-up. Losses during this phase are difficult to avoid, and classifying them as unfavourable could easily distort the results.

In the most recent published EMEA guidelines for the development of new agents no mention is made of how losses to follow-up should be classified but there is a statement about deaths indicating that it is acceptable to either count all deaths as failures or to count as failures all deaths excluding those that were clearly not related to *Mycobacterium tuberculosis* (e.g. deaths from trauma) [15]. The guidelines go on to say that early deaths under treatment (e.g. within the first 4 or 6 months) may be a particularly important end point in patients with MDR-TB due to the appreciable early mortality rate.

Discussions with regulators are ongoing at the time of writing as to how patients failing to complete treatment or lost during follow-up should be classified. One proposal is that all losses during treatment, including deaths from any cause, should be regarded as having an unfavourable outcome, the exception being defaulters who return for the final assessment who can then be classified. Losses during post-treatment follow-up will be considered unassessable unless there is any suggestion that they might be relapsing. The challenge to researchers is, as always, to minimize such losses to follow-up, thereby increasing confidence in the analysis of assessable cases. A consequence of inflating unfavourable rates in the control arm by inclusion of losses to follow-up is the need for even larger studies [17].

There are several features of long-term efficacy trials at the present time which are different from those conducted during the development of short-course chemotherapy. The HIV epidemic has had a dramatic impact on TB notification rates in sub-Saharan Africa with 70% or more of new cases being co-infected in some countries. This has also resulted in a considerable increase in reinfection rates during post-treatment follow-up. One of the unanswered questions is whether HIV-infected patients receiving appropriate anti-retroviral treatment can be effectively treated with the same regimens and for the same duration as uninfected patients. Most of the data currently available are from studies conducted at a time when few if any patients were receiving anti-retroviral treatment.

Two features of trials which have changed are the introduction of liquid culture media methods and, in some trials, a reduction in the intensity of the schedule for collection of sputum samples. Both of these changes may have implications for the assessment of end points. While the faster reporting of results using liquid media methods is beneficial, the greater sensitivity of detection may not be. This is partly on account of a greater likelihood of detecting non-tuberculous mycobacteria but also because a positive result detected by liquid media which would not have been detected using solid media may be of no clinical consequence. Isolated positive culture results in solid media studies are a recognized phenomenon; they are not always on account of laboratory or labelling errors but can arise from patients' lesions [26, 27]. Classifying isolated positive results as failures or relapses will distort or dilute findings – an increased risk in studies with limited follow-up bacteriology [28].

## Conclusion

The principles enunciated so clearly by Fox [2] have not changed over 60 years; what has changed is the environment in which trials are conducted. It required only 107 randomized patients to demonstrate the efficacy of streptomycin [1], and there were just over 150 patients per arm assessed in the first short-course trial. Today's trials commonly require at least 4–5 times more patients to demonstrate non-inferiority [17]. There is a pressing need for validated surrogate end points to reduce the number and size of long-term trials and shorten the approval process for new drug regimens. The need for long-term trials is unlikely to be eliminated completely, and the challenges addressed here will remain for some time to come.

## References


1 Medical Research Council: Streptomycin treatment of pulmonary tuberculosis: a Medical Research Council investigation. BMJl 1948;2:769.
2 Fox W: Recent developments in controlled trials in pulmonary tuberculosis. Br Med Bull 1954;10:108.
3 Lewis JA, Machin D: Intention to treat – who should use ITT? Br J Cancer 1993;68:647.
4 Hill AB: Principles of Medical Statistics, ed 6. London, The Lancet 1955.
5 Fox W, Sutherland I, Daniels M: A five-year assessment of patients in a controlled trial of streptomycin in pulmonary tuberculosis: report to the Tuberculosis Chemotherapy Trials Committee of the Medical Research Council. Q J Med 1954;23:347.
6 Garattini S, Bertele V: Non-inferiority trials are unethical because they disregard patients' interests. Lancet 2007;370:1875–1877.
7 Medical Research Council: Long-term chemotherapy in the treatment of chronic pulmonary tuberculosis with cavitation: a report to the Medical Research Council by their Tuberculosis Chemotherapy Trials Committee. Tubercle 1962;43:201–267.
8 East African/British Medical Research Council: Isoniazid with thiacetazone (thioacetazone) in the treatment of pulmonary tuberculosis in East Africa – third report of fifth investigation. Tubercle 1973;54:169–179.
9 Hill AB: Principles of Medical Statistics, ed 11. London, The Lancet 1984.
10 Rohmel J: Therapeutic equivalence investigations: statistical considerations. Stat Med 1998;17:1703–1714.
11 Kang SH, Chen JJ: An approximate unconditional test of non-inferiority between two proportions. Stat Med 2000;19:2089–2100.
12 Dunnett CW, Gent M: Significance testing to establish equivalence between treatments, with special reference to data in the form of 2 × 2 tables. Biometrics 1977;33:593–602.
13 East African/British Medical Research Councils: Controlled clinical trial of four short-course (6-month) regimens of chemotherapy for treatment of pulmonary tuberculosis: third report. Lancet 1974;304:237–240.
14 EMEA Committee for Medicinal Products for Human Use: Guideline on the choice of the non-inferiority margin. EMEA/CPMP/EWP/2158/99. London, July 2005.
15 EMEA Committee for Medicinal Products for Human Use: Addendum to the note for guidance on evaluation of medicinal products indicated for treatment of bacterial infections to specifically address the clinical development of new agents to treat disease due to *Mycobacterium tuberculosis*. EMEA/CPMP/EWP/14377/2008. London, January 2010.
16 FDA: Draft guidance for industry non-inferiority clinical trials. Rockville, March 2010.
17 Nunn AJ, Phillips PPJ, Gillespie SH: Design issues in pivotal drug trials for drug sensitive tuberculosis (TB). Tuberculosis 2008;88:S85–S92.
18 Jindani A, Nunn AJ, Enarson DA: Two 8-month regimens of chemotherapy for treatment of newly diagnosed pulmonary tuberculosis: international multicentre randomised trial. Lancet 2004;364:1244–1251.
19 Fleming TR: Current issues in non-inferiority trials. Stat Med 2008;27:317–332.
20 Crampin A, Mwaungulu JN, Mwaungulu FD, Mwafulirwa DT, Munthali K, Floyd S, Fine PEM, Glynn JR: Recurrent TB: relapse or reinfection? The effect of HIV in a general population cohort in Malawi. AIDS 2010;24:417.
21 Narayanan S, Swaminathan S, Supply P, Shanmugam S, Narendran G, Hari L, Ramachandran R, Locht C, Jawahar MS, Narayanan PR: Impact of HIV infection on the recurrence of tuberculosis in South India. J Infect Dis 2010;201:691–703.
22 Nunn AJ, Phillips PPJ, Mitchison DA: Timing of relapse in short-course chemotherapy trials for tuberculosis. Int J Tuberc Lung Dis 2010;14:241–242.
23 Medical Research Council: Isoniazid in the treatment of pulmonary tuberculosis: second report. BMJ 1953;521–536.
24 Tuberculosis Chemotherapy Centre Madras: A concurrent comparison of isoniazid plus PAS with three regimens of isoniazid alone in the domiciliary treatment of pulmonary tuberculosis in South India. Bull World Health Organ 1960;23:535–585.
25 Strang JIG, Nunn AJ, Johnson DA, Casbard A, Gibson DG, Girling DJ: Management of tuberculous constrictive pericarditis and tuberculous pericardial effusion in Transkei: results at 10 years follow-up. Q J Med 2004;97:525.
26 Burman WJ, Reves RR: Review of false positive cultures for *Mycobacterium tuberculosis* and recommendations for avoiding unnecessary treatment. Clin Infect Dis 2000;31:1390–1395.
27 Mitchison DA, Keyes AB, Edwards EA, Ayuma P, Byfield SP, Nunn AJ: Quality control in tuberculosis bacteriology. 2. The origin of isolated positive cultures from the sputum of patients in four studies of short course chemotherapy in Africa. Tubercle 1980;61:135.
28 Phillips P, Nunn A: Challenges of phase III study design for trials of new drug regimens for the treatment of TB. Future Med Chem 2010;2:1273–1282.



Prof. A.J. Nunn
MRC Clinical Trials Unit
Aviation House
125 Kingsway
London WC2B 6NH (UK)
Tel. +44 207 670 4703, E-Mail ajn@ctu.mrc.ac.uk

# Present Treatment

## Chapter 3

Donald PR, van Helden PD (eds): Antituberculosis Chemotherapy.
Prog Respir Res. Basel, Karger, 2011, vol 40, pp 18–24

# The Rifamycins: Renewed Interest in an Old Drug Class

William Burman[a] · Kelly E. Dooley[b] · Eric L. Nuermberger[b]

[a]Denver Public Health and University of Colorado School of Medicine, Denver, Colo., and [b]Johns Hopkins University School of Medicine, Baltimore, Md., USA

**Abstract**

There is renewed interest in the rifamycins, primarily from evidence that higher doses than have been previously used may allow a markedly shortened treatment of active and latent tuberculosis (TB). We review recent studies of the pharmacokinetics, pharmacodynamics and pharmacogenomics of rifampicin, rifapentine and rifabutin. The rifamycins have complex metabolic pathways and, therefore, have wide interpatient variability in drug exposure (10-fold or greater). Some of the reasons for the broad range in rifamycin exposure are now being elucidated: body weight, disease state, ingestion with food and polymorphisms in genes for drug transporter proteins. Children require 2- to 3-fold higher doses of rifampicin and rifapentine than adults do. Greater rifamycin exposure is closely correlated with bactericidal and sterilizing activities in the mouse model of TB treatment. The use of high-dose rifampicin and daily rifapentine allows treatment to be shortened to 3 months in the mouse model, and clinical trials are under way to evaluate these regimens in humans. Little is known about the relationship between rifamycin dose and toxicity, when daily dosing is used. New ways of using an old drug class – the rifamycins – may markedly improve TB treatment yet again.

Copyright © 2011 S. Karger AG, Basel

The rifamycin antibiotic class revolutionized tuberculosis (TB) treatment 30 years ago. The addition of rifampicin to isoniazid-based therapy allowed treatment duration to be cut in half, from 18 to 9 months, while decreasing the risk of treatment failure and acquired drug resistance. The 'short-course' regimen based on rifampicin became the basis for global TB control. Perhaps in part because of the magnitude of this accomplishment, there was little effort in the next 30 years to explore other ways of using the rifamycins.

The HIV pandemic re-ignited the TB epidemic and brought renewed interest and funding to TB research. However, the rifamycin class seemed to be of little interest in this new era of TB drug development. Rising rates of rifampicin resistance were reported from a number of places in the world. Drug-drug interactions with key classes of antiretroviral agents highlighted one of rifampicin's faults – its remarkable potency as an inducer of drug-metabolizing enzymes, thereby decreasing the concentrations and efficacy of a broad spectrum of drugs. Rifabutin was developed as a form of prophylaxis for disseminated *Mycobacterium avium* complex, but was soon supplanted by a more effective agent (azithromycin). Rifabutin was also shown to have problematic drug interactions, causing toxic concentrations of the drug (and its principal metabolite) when given with inhibitors of cytochrome P450-3A4 (CYP3A4). Finally, interest in rifapentine waned after regimens designed to take advantage of its long half-life did not perform as well as more frequently administered rifampicin-based regimens [1–3].

Ten years later, there has been a remarkable renaissance in interest in the rifamycins (table 1). Higher doses of rifampicin and higher and more frequently dosed rifapentine are being evaluated as interventions to shorten the treatment of drug-susceptible TB. Despite its problematic drug-drug interactions, rifabutin is being evaluated as a key element in the cotreatment of patients with HIV-related TB who have HIV strains resistant to the non-nucleoside reverse-transcriptase inhibitors (NNRTIs). Several rifamycin-based regimens are being evaluated as ways to markedly decrease the duration of treatment of latent TB infection.

**Table 1.** Current and planned clinical trials with rifampicin, rifapentine and rifabutin

| Rifamycin | Indication | Rationale |
|---|---|---|
| Rifampicin | Treatment of latent TB infection | 3- to 4-month regimen improves treatment completion and is better tolerated (compared to 9 months of isoniazid) |
| | Treatment shortening for active TB | Higher-dose rifampicin (>10 mg/kg) may allow treatment to be shortened to 4 months |
| Rifapentine | Treatment of latent TB infection | Highly intermittent (once weekly) rifapentine + isoniazid may both shorten and foster supervised therapy |
| | Treatment of latent TB infection | Daily rifapentine + isoniazid may allow treatment shortening to 1 month |
| | Treatment-shortening for active TB | Daily rifapentine-based therapy may allow treatment shortening to 3–4 months |
| Rifabutin | Treatment of latent TB | 3- to 4-month regimen may be efficacious while avoiding the drug interactions of rifampicin |
| | Treatment of active TB | Use of rifabutin may allow highly active TB treatment and use of antiretroviral drugs that have problematic drug interactions with rifampicin (e.g. the HIV-1 protease inhibitors) |

We review the basis for the renewed interest in the 3 rifamycins currently in clinical development – rifampicin, rifapentine and rifabutin – and then highlight areas in need of additional research. The pharmacokinetics of the rifamycins are being more carefully studied, including the pharmacogenomics of rifamycin metabolism. There is now greater understanding of the mechanisms of the many drug-drug interactions of the rifamycins. For the first time, the pharmacodynamics – the relationship between drug concentrations and treatment outcomes (efficacy and toxicity) – of the rifamycins is being rigorously evaluated.

## Updated Review of the Pharmacokinetics of the Rifamycins

Although rifamycins are one of the oldest classes of antimicrobials, many of the aspects of their complex pharmacokinetics have been elucidated only recently. Rifampicin and rifapentine are well absorbed from the gastrointestinal tract, whereas the bioavailability of rifabutin (approx. 20%) is substantially lower, perhaps due to the extent of metabolism in the gut wall [4]. Ingestion with food has relatively little effect on the absorption of rifampin and rifabutin, but a variety of types of food markedly increase the bioavailability of rifapentine and its principal, biologically active metabolite [5]. To enhance absorption, some clinical trials require that subjects take the study drug with food, but the magnitude of increase in oral bioavailability differs by food type, and it is not clear that this strategy will be feasible in the broad range of clinical settings in which tuberculosis treatment is given.

The hepatic metabolism of the rifamycins has been the focus of attention for many years. Rifampin and rifapentine are metabolized by esterases in hepatocytes to desacetyl derivatives, and both parent and metabolite are excreted into the bile and eliminated largely in the faeces. The metabolism of these two drugs is not mediated by cytochrome P450 enzymes, but their pharmacokinetics are complex, with drug metabolism and transport at the levels of the gut and liver each playing a role. The brush border membrane of enterocytes contains P-glycoprotein (PGP), an efflux transporter. Rifampicin both induces PGP activity and is a PGP substrate [6, 7]. Drug that escapes the PGP efflux pump and successfully enters the portal venous system may enter the hepatocyte via influx transporters, organic anionic transport proteins 1B1 and 1B3 (OATP1B1and OATP1B3) located in the basolateral membrane [8]. Once in the hepatocyte, rifamycins can be metabolized and/or pumped out via PGP into the biliary tract to be eliminated (or reabsorbed). Interestingly, rifampicin is not only a substrate of OATP1B1 and OATP1B3, but it also inhibits the OATP1B1- and OATP1B3-mediated uptake of drugs into the liver [9]. In addition, once rifampicin enters the hepatocyte, it may then interact with pregnane X receptor (PXR) leading to upregulation of multiple metabolizing enzymes and transporters.

To enter the systemic circulation, a drug must be absorbed, enter the portal system and pass through the liver without being metabolized or excreted. Rifamycins are subject to the 'first-pass effect' via the mechanisms described above, which reduce bioavailability. However, hepatic elimination of rifampicin, at least, is saturable, which results in non-linear increases in drug exposure with doses above 5–7.5 mg/kg. The use of rifampicin is further complicated by time-varying pharmacokinetics. After multiple oral or intravenous doses, there are substantial reductions in half-life regardless of the route of administration, suggesting auto-induction of hepatic metabolism and/or elimination [10]. Bioavailability of oral drug is diminished after multiple doses, pointing to induction of prehepatic metabolism or elimination. The mechanism by which rifampicin increases its own clearance after multiple doses is unclear, but may involve auto-induction of hepatic and gut metabolizing enzymes or PXR-mediated induction of PGP. Rifapentine may also induce its own elimination, leading to decreased parent drug and metabolite concentrations [11].

Given the complexity of rifamycin absorption, metabolism and elimination, it is not surprising that there are marked interpatient differences in drug exposure: 10-fold or greater differences in the maximal concentration and area under the curve (AUC) of rifampicin, rifapentine and rifabutin [12–14]. Rifampicin concentrations below recommended targets are common, with suboptimal levels seen in as many as 70–80% of TB patients in some populations [15, 16]. Factors associated with low rifamycin exposure include high or low body weight, unapproved formulation, HIV co-infection and male sex [12, 15]. Recent studies suggest that patients with active TB have lower rifampicin and rifapentine exposure than healthy controls [12, 17]. More work needs to be done to evaluate this association between disease state and rifamycin exposure. Possible explanations for lower exposure among patients with active TB include differences in absorption (perhaps related to the effects of companion drugs) or to effects of tuberculosis and/or related inflammation on rifamycin metabolism.

Pharmacogenomics may help explain the marked interpatient variability in rifamycin pharmacokinetics. Polymorphisms in the solute carrier organic anion transporter family, member 1B1 *(SLCO1B1)* gene that encodes the OATP1B1 transmembrane receptor affect rifampicin drug concentrations. Persons with the *SLCO1B1* rs11045819 gene mutation at exon 4 (variant name c463C→A) had 42% lower AUC and 34% lower maximal concentration values than those without it [12], and an rs4149032 C→T polymorphism was associated with 20 and 28% reductions in rifampicin bioavailability in heterozygotes and homozygotes, respectively [18].

Age-dependent changes in organ function and body composition affect drug absorption, distribution, metabolism and excretion. However, children were nearly completely left out of the series of clinical trials that led to current tuberculosis treatment regimens [19], and with 1 exception, drug doses recommended by the World Health Organization for the treatment of TB in children are the same as those in adults [20]. Only in the last few years has rifamycin exposure been carefully evaluated among children. Children with and without HIV co-infection who were receiving the 10 mg/kg dose of rifampicin recommended by the World Health Organization had mean 2-hour plasma concentrations of 3.9 and 4.8 mg/l, respectively [21], far below the recommended value of 8 mg/l for adults [22]. Children also have a higher oral clearance of rifapentine and lower drug exposures than adults [23]. Doses of rifampicin and rifapentine for young children need to be 2- to 3-fold higher than adult doses [21, 24].

Due to the lack of child-friendly formulations of the rifamycins, clinics use extemporaneous formulations to administer these drugs to children who cannot swallow a whole tablet (e.g. crushed tablets in a vehicle such as applesauce). Initial work with rifapentine suggests that administration in such an extemporaneous preparation is associated with significantly lower drug exposure [24]. Therefore, it is critical that future clinical trials of the rifamycins include children and that pharmacokinetics be assessed, including the effects of differences in drug formulation and administration.

## Pharmacodynamics of the Rifamycins

Given its use for over 30 years and in millions of TB patients, one would think that the standard dose of rifampicin (450 mg for weight ≤45 kg and 600 mg for weight >45 kg) was the result of careful dose comparisons. However, the standard rifampicin dose was based on the results of 2 relatively small clinical trials [25, 26]. Higher doses of rifampicin were evaluated, primarily in studies of highly intermittent dosing (once or twice weekly) and were abandoned because of increased risks of hypersensitivity (flu-like syndrome) [27]. Higher daily doses of rifampicin were used in small non-comparative studies, and appeared to be well tolerated and more efficacious than the standard dose [28]. Similarly, rifapentine was nearly abandoned when initial clinical trials showed insufficient efficacy of once weekly therapy dosing during the continuation phase of therapy of what may prove to be a low dose of the drug [1–3]. Much of the current interest in the rifamycins stems from a better understanding of rifamycin pharmacodynamics, coupled with research in the mouse model with higher doses of rifampicin and higher and more frequent doses of rifapentine.

Dose fractionation studies in an in vitro hollow-fibre system [29] and in mice [30] indicate that the bactericidal activity of rifampicin against *Mycobacterium tuberculosis* is most closely correlated with the ratio of AUC and minimal inhibitory concentration (MIC). Importantly, dose-ranging studies with both rifampicin and rifapentine in mice and humans have not found an AUC/MIC ceiling [30–34], indicating that the extent of bacterial killing by rifamycins is limited only by the dose. Therefore, it follows that the optimal rifamycin dose is the highest dose that is well tolerated and safe. However, currently recommended rifampicin doses are at the low end of the steep and deep rifamycin dose-response curve, as is evident from studies in mice and humans in which small reductions in dose change the bactericidal activity of rifampicin [25, 31, 34]. Indeed, the selection of the current dose of rifampicin was largely based on the minimum effective dose that could be implemented around the world at the lowest cost. As there is no satisfactory rationale for a 'maximum' dose of 600 mg, and rifampicin is decidedly less expensive than in the past, there is substantial current interest in optimizing its dose [35].

What impact could an increase in rifampicin doses have? Increasing the dose of rifampicin from 10 to 40 mg/kg in combination with standard doses of isoniazid and pyrazinamide in mice enables a reduction in the treatment duration needed to prevent relapse from 6 to 3 months in the mouse model [34]. The activity of rifampicin monotherapy in the first week of therapy in humans ('early bactericidal activity') shows a clear dose-response over the clinically feasible range of doses (5–20 mg/kg), with markedly greater activity from a 20 mg/kg dose [31, 32]. These findings in the mouse model and the initial experience with monotherapy are the basis for phase II trials of the tolerability and activity of higher doses of rifampicin in combination with other first-line drugs.

Rifapentine is more potent than rifampicin. In vitro, the MIC of rifapentine is 2–4 times lower than that of rifampicin [36]. Moreover, due primarily to its longer half-life, rifapentine attains higher serum exposures at a given dose in mice and humans compared to rifampicin [37, 38]. In mice receiving daily therapy with concomitant isoniazid and pyrazinamide, rifapentine is 4 times more active than rifampicin [34]. Initial studies in humans have shown that weekly doses up to 1,200 mg are well tolerated [39], and a phase IIB trial of daily rifapentine versus rifampicin (both at 8–12 mg/kg) is nearing completion.

A key aspect of using the mouse model of TB treatment in the design of clinical trials is to assure comparable drug exposure in mouse and man. Without assessment of pharmacokinetics of the rifamycins, it may be difficult to interpret the results of clinical trials. Rifamycin pharmacokinetics in uninfected mice and in healthy human volunteers are very similar [37, 38]. However, it is becoming increasingly clear that TB patients often have lower rifampicin and rifapentine exposures than do mice and healthy volunteers [12, 38, 40, 41]. On one hand, this may lead to concerns that the treatment-shortening potential of higher-dose rifampicin or rifapentine in humans may be less than that predicted in mice. On the other hand, it is reasonable to expect that, on the linear portion of the dose-response curve, a similarly proportionate increase in rifamycin exposure in mice and in TB patients should result in similarly proportionate increases in bactericidal activity. Clearly, assessment of rifamycin pharmacokinetics needs to be a routine part of phase II and III trials to assure optimal drug exposures in the greatest number of subjects.

There are few data linking rifamycin exposures directly to clinical outcomes, making it impossible to establish rifamycin AUC/MIC targets necessary for optimal treatment outcomes. In a single-arm study of a twice weekly rifabutin-based regimen in patients with HIV-associated TB, subjects with failure or relapse with acquired rifamycin resistance had lower rifabutin $AUC_{0-24}$ values compared to those without acquired rifamycin resistance failure or relapse [14]. After adjustment for rifabutin AUC, a lower isoniazid AUC was also associated with acquired rifamycin resistance failure or relapse. In a randomized trial of continuation phase therapy with either twice weekly rifampicin-isoniazid or once weekly rifapentine-isoniazid, rifamycin exposure was not associated with outcome, whereas low isoniazid exposure was associated with failure or relapse in the once-weekly rifapentine-isoniazid group [42].

While these data clearly associate low drug exposures with poor clinical outcome, they also illustrate the difficulty of isolating a single drug effect in the context of combination therapy. Moreover, the lack of rifamycin MIC data prevented a more rigorous assessment of the association between AUC/MIC and outcome. Finally, it is noteworthy that these pharmacokinetic substudies sought to identify drug exposures associated with poor outcomes after treatment with conventional 6-month 'short-course' regimens. If shorter treatment durations are entertained, higher rifamycin exposures will need to be achieved. In the absence of feasible and economical methods for therapeutic drug monitoring or identification of patients with genetic polymorphisms associated with low rifamycin exposures, the rifamycin dose will need to be increased for all patients.

Clearly, the most common impediment to increasing the dose of any therapeutic agent is drug-associated toxicity. However, little is known about the pharmacodynamics of rifamycin toxicity. As described above, early studies established that higher doses of rifampicin (up to 1,800 mg), given once weekly, resulted in a higher prevalence of antibodies directed at rifampicin and higher rates of flu-like syndrome [27]. Yet, no such association has been made with higher daily doses of rifampicin. In initial trials, once weekly administration of rifapentine was not associated with the flu-like syndrome [1, 2, 39]. Whereas asymptomatic elevations of conjugated bilirubin and induction of hepatic metabolic enzymes are dose dependent [43], it remains unknown whether unusual but serious adverse effects, such as drug-related liver injury, are related to rifamycin dose/exposure. Dose escalation of rifabutin is more likely to be associated with serious toxicity. A clinical syndrome of uveitis, myalgias and/or neutropenia is clearly associated with high-dose rifabutin or, more commonly, administration of rifabutin with CYP3A inhibitors (clarithromycin, HIV-1 protease inhibitors) that markedly increase rifabutin exposure.

### Updated Review of Drug Interactions with the Rifamycins

Rifampicin is the most drug interaction-prone agent known to man. Rifampicin has a high affinity for PXR, and binding PXR unleashes a cascade of intracellular events that culminates in the upregulation of multiple nuclear gene targets including CYP450 enzymes, phase II drug-metabolizing enzymes, UDP glucurosyltransferases and drug transporters such as PGP. Induction of metabolizing enzymes and upregulation of transporters by rifampicin (or rifapentine) can result in complex, and sometimes unexpected, drug-drug interactions, both with other TB drugs and with drugs used for other indications. A major question regarding rifamycin drug interactions is whether the magnitude of the effects on other drugs will be greater with higher and more frequent doses of rifampicin and rifapentine.

Cotreatment of TB and HIV is particularly nettlesome owing to rifamycin-related drug-drug interactions, pill burden and overlapping toxicities. Since protease inhibitors and NNRTIs are metabolized by CYP3A4, induction of CYP3A4 by rifampicin can lead to reduced serum concentrations of antiretroviral drugs with risk for treatment failure or emergence of resistance to them [44]. However, the cotreatment regimen of rifampicin-based TB treatment and efavirenz-based antiretroviral therapy is safe and efficacious [45].

For those patients with contraindications to or resistance to NNRTIs who require protease-inhibitor-based antiretroviral therapy, however, there are major uncertainties about the optimal cotreatment regimen. Rifampicin co-administration results in dramatic decreases in the serum concentrations of the protease inhibitors. This effect can be overcome by higher doses of the pharmacokinetic enhancer ritonavir, but regimens of rifampicin with a ritonavir-boosted protease inhibitor cause high rates of hepatotoxicity in healthy volunteers, and there are limited data on the safety and efficacy of this combination in patients with HIV-related TB. Rifabutin has little effect on serum concentrations of current protease inhibitors, and substitution of rifabutin for rifampicin is a reasonable option for HIV/TB co-infected patients. However, the optimal dose of rifabutin for use with protease inhibitors is not known, and rifabutin is not available in areas with the highest burden of HIV-related TB.

Use of integrase inhibitors rather than protease inhibitors for treatment of patients who require antiretroviral drugs and a rifampicin-containing TB regimen but have NNRTI resistance is one potential strategy for treating co-infected patients. However, integrase inhibitors, such as raltegravir, are metabolized by UDP glucuronosyltransferase 1A1 subtype enzymes, and rifampicin induces them. Raltegravir concentrations are diminished when it is co-administered with rifampicin, but the clinical implications of these reductions are unclear. A clinical trial is under way to evaluate HIV viral suppression in patients taking rifampicin together with raltegravir at 1 of 2 doses.

### Implications for Clinical Trials and Clinical Practice

Recent studies on the pharmacokinetics, pharmacodynamics and pharmacogenomics of the rifamycins have several implications for clinical practice and the design of clinical trials. The large interpatient variance in rifamycin exposure is likely to affect both efficacy and toxicity. In particular, patients at the lower end of the distribution of drug exposure are probably at an increased risk of treatment failure and relapse. Therefore, it makes sense to try to minimize, to the extent possible, the interpatient variance in rifamycin exposure. The association between body weight and rifampicin exposure argues for weight-based dosing of the rifamycins to a greater extent than has been used to this point. For example, current guidelines for rifampicin dosing recommend only 2 doses (450 and 600 mg) despite a large range of body weights among adults being treated for active TB [46]. The use of qualified combination formulations of first-line TB drugs is one way to achieve better weight-based dosing, while maintaining simple dosing instructions for TB control programmes.

The genetic control of rifamycin exposure has possible ramifications for clinical trials. As pharmacogenomic relationships are identified, it will be critical to characterize the distribution of key genetic polymorphisms in different patient populations. An initial study suggested that *SLCO1B* polymorphisms associated with low rifampicin AUC are more common among patients of African descent, perhaps offering some explanation for the worse clinical outcomes among African patients in several recent clinical trials [12]. Despite the challenges in doing so, it is important that host genomics be incorporated in TB clinical trials. Second, if pharmacogenomic relationships of sufficient magnitude are identified, it may be possible to customize rifamycin dosing, as genetic testing becomes cheaper and point-of-care testing methods are developed.

There is clearly much more work that needs to be done to optimize the use of rifamycins among children and persons with HIV co-infection. Age-specific dosing recommendations are only just now being developed and need to be fully validated, including among infants. Child-friendly dose sizes and formulations with proven bioavailability are needed. Among patients with HIV co-infection, there is a growing need for a regimen that can be used for patients who cannot tolerate NNRTIs or who have infection with NNRTI-resistant viral strains.

A more basic lesson from the recent work with the rifamycins is the importance of more fully exploring broader ranges of doses and dosing frequencies, both in the mouse model of treatment and in phase II trials, before selecting dosing schemes to be evaluated in phase III trials. New methodologies are needed to accelerate progress in this area. The end point commonly used in phase IIB trials – 2-month sputum culture status – requires large sample sizes (75–225 per arm, depending on assumptions) [47]. Better knowledge of key pharmacodynamic parameters of the rifamycins and the use of a continuous outcome measure with a wide dynamic range (rather than the dichotomous outcome of culture status at 2 months) could allow phase IIB trials to be performed with much smaller sample sizes, thus fostering the assessment of a broader range of doses and dosing frequencies.

## References


1 Benator D, Bhattacharya M, Bozeman L, Burman W, Cantazaro A, Chaisson R, Gordin F, Horsburgh CR, Horton J, Khan A, Lahart C, Metchock B, Pachucki C, Stanton L, Vernon A, Villarino ME, Wang YC, Weiner M, Weis S, Tuberculosis Trials Consortium: Rifapentine and isoniazid once a week versus rifampicin and isoniazid twice a week for treatment of drug-susceptible pulmonary tuberculosis in HIV-negative patients: a randomised clinical trial. Lancet 2002;360:528–534.

2 Tam CM, Chan SL, Lam CW, Leung CC, Kam KM, Morris JS, Mitchison DA: Rifapentine and isoniazid in the continuation phase of treating pulmonary tuberculosis: initial report. Am J Respir Crit Care Med 1998;157:1726–1733.

3 Vernon A, Burman W, Benator D, Khan A, Bozeman L: Relapse with rifamycin mono-resistant tuberculosis in HIV-infected patients treated with supervised once-weekly rifapentine and isoniazid. Lancet 1999;353:1843–1847.

4 Burman WJ, Gallicano K, Peloquin C. Comparative pharmacokinetics and pharmacodynamics of the rifamycin antibacterials. Clin Pharmacokinet 2001;40:327–341.

5 Zvada SP, van der Walt JS, Smith PJ, Fourie PB, Roscigno G, Mitchison D, Simonsson US, McIlleron HM: Effects of four different meal types on the population pharmacokinetics of single-dose rifapentine in healthy male volunteers. Antimicrob Agents Chemother 2010;54:3390–3394.

6 Fromm MF, Kauffmann HM, Fritz P, Burk O, Kroemer HK, Warzok RW, Eichelbaum M, Siegmund W, Schrenk D: The effect of rifampin treatment on intestinal expression of human MRP transporters. Am J Pathol 2000;157:1575–1580.

7 Hartkoorn RC, Chandler B, Owen A, Ward SA, Bertel Squire S, Back DJ, Khoo SH: Differential drug susceptibility of intracellular and extracellular tuberculosis, and the impact of P-glycoprotein. Tuberculosis (Edinb) 2007;87:248–255.

8 Vavricka SR, Van Montfoort J, Ha HR, Meier PJ, Fattinger K: Interactions of rifamycin SV and rifampicin with organic anion uptake systems of human liver. Hepatology 2002;36:164–172.

9 Smith NF, Figg WD, Sparreboom A: Role of the liver-specific transporters OATP1B1 and OATP1B3 in governing drug elimination. Expert Opin Drug Metab Toxicol 2005;1:429–445.

10 Loos U, Musch E, Jensen JC, Mikus G, Schwabe JK, Eichelbaum M: Pharmacokinetics of oral and intravenous rifampicin during chronic administration. Klin Wochenschr 1985;63:1205–1211.

11 Dooley K, Flexner C, Hackman J, Peloquin CA, Nuermberger E, Chaisson RE, Dorman SE: Repeated administration of high-dose intermittent rifapentine reduces rifapentine and moxifloxacin plasma concentrations. Antimicrob Agents Chemother 2008;52:4037–4042.

12 Weiner M, Peloquin C, Burman W, Luo CC, Engle M, Prihoda TJ, MacKenzie WR, Bliven-Sizemore E, Johnson JL, Vernon A: Effects of tuberculosis, race, and human gene *SLCO1B1* polymorphisms on rifampin concentrations. Antimicrob Agents Chemother 2010;54:4192–4200.

13 Weiner M, Bock N, Peloquin CA, Burman WJ, Khan A, Vernon A, Zhao Z, Weis S, Sterling TR, Hayden K, Goldberg S: Pharmacokinetics of rifapentine at 600, 900, and 1,200 mg during once-weekly tuberculosis therapy. Am J Respir Crit Care Med 2004;169:1191–1197.

14 Weiner M, Benator D, Burman W, Peloquin C, Khan A, Vernon A, Jones B, Silva-Trigo C, Zhao Z, Hodge T, Tuberculosis Trials Consortium: The association between acquired rifamycin resistance and the pharmacokinetics of rifabutin and isoniazid among patients with tuberculosis and HIV. Clin Infect Dis 2005;40:1481–1491.

15 McIlleron H, Wash P, Burger A, Norman J, Folb PI, Smith P: Determinants of rifampin, isoniazid, pyrazinamide, and ethambutol pharmacokinetics in a cohort of tuberculosis patients. Antimicrob Agents Chemother 2006;50:1170–1177.
16 Tappero JW, Bradford WZ, Agerton TB, Hopewell P, Reingold AL, Lockman S, Oyewo A, Talbot EA, Kenyon TA, Moeti TL, Moffat HJ, Peloquin CA: Serum concentrations of antimycobacterial drugs in patients with pulmonary tuberculosis in Botswana. Clin Infect Dis 2005;41:461–469.
17 Peloquin D, Weiner M, Engle M, Johnson J, Nsubuga P, Bliven E, Padayatchi N, Mthethwa T, MacKenzie W: Pharmacokinetics of rifapentine in TB patients receiving 600 mg daily. 3rd Int Workshop Clin Pharmacol Tuberculosis Drugs, Boston, 2010.
18 Chiqutsa E, Visser M, Egan D, Holford N, Smith P, Owen A, McIlleron H: Population pharmacokinetics of rifampicin in South African tuberculosis patients and the influence of drug transporter polymorphisms. 3rd Int Workshop Clin Pharmacol Tuberculosis Drugs, Boston, 2010.
19 Burman WJ, Cotton MF, Gibb DM, Walker AS, Vernon AA, Donald PR: Ensuring the involvement of children in the evaluation of new tuberculosis treatment regimens. PLoS Med 2008;5:e176.
20 Treatment of tuberculosis: guidelines for national programmes, ed 3. Geneva, World Health Organization, 2003.
21 Schaaf HS, Willemse M, Cilliers K, Labadarios D, Maritz JS, Hussey GD, McIlleron H, Smith P, Donald PR: Rifampin pharmacokinetics in children, with and without human immunodeficiency virus infection, hospitalized for the management of severe forms of tuberculosis. BMC Med 2009;7:19.
22 Peloquin CA: Using therapeutic drug monitoring to dose the antimycobacterial drugs. Clin Chest Med 1997;18:79–87.
23 Blake MJ, Abdel-Rahman SM, Jacobs RF, Lowery NK, Sterling TR, Kearns GL: Pharmacokinetics of rifapentine in children. Pediatr Infect Dis J 2006;25:405–409.
24 Weiner M, Wing D, Burman W, Peloquin C, Engle M, Prihoda T, MacKenzie W, Bliven E, Benator D, Weis S, Sterling T, Villarino E: Rifapentine pharmacokinetics in children and adults receiving once-weekly rifapentine and isoniazid for the treatment of latent tuberculosis infection. 39th World Conf Lung Health, Paris, October 2008.
25 Long MW, Snider DEJ, Farer LS: US Public Health Service trial of three rifampin-isoniazid regimens in treatment of pulmonary tuberculosis. Am Rev Respir Dis 1979;119:879–894.
26 Jeanes CWL, Jessamine AG, Eidus L: Treatment of chronic drug-resistant pulmonary tuberculosis with rifampin and ethambutol. Can Med Assoc J 1972;106:884–888.
27 Grosset J, Leventis S. Adverse effects of rifampin. Rev Infect Dis 1983;5(suppl 3):S440–S445.
28 Kreis B, Pretet S, Birenbaum J, Guibout P, Hazeman JJ, Orin E, Perdrizet S, Weil J: Two three-month treatment regimens for pulmonary tuberculosis. Bull Int Union Against Tuberc 1976;51:71–75.
29 Gumbo T, Louie A, Deziel MR, Liu W, Parsons LM, Salfinger M, Drusano GL: Concentration-dependent *Mycobacterium tuberculosis* killing and prevention of resistance by rifampin. Antimicrob Agents Chemother 2007;51:3781–3788.
30 Jayaram R, Gaonkar S, Kaur P, Suresh BL, Mahesh BN, Jayashree R, Nandi V, Bharat S, Shandil RK, Kantharaj E, Balasubramanian V: Pharmacokinetics-pharmacodynamics of rifampin in an aerosol infection model of tuberculosis. Antimicrob Agents Chemother 2003;47:2118–2124.
31 Jindani A, Baer VR, Edwards EA, Mitchison DA: The early bactericidal activity of drugs in patients with pulmonary tuberculosis. Am Rev Respir Dis 1980;121:939–949.
32 Diacon AH, Patientia RF, Venter A, van Helden PD, Smith PJ, McIlleron H, Maritz JS, Donald PR: Early bactericidal activity of high-dose rifampin in patients with pulmonary tuberculosis evidenced by positive sputum smears. Antimicrob Agents Chemother 2007;51:2994–2996.
33 Sirgel FA, Fourie PB, Donald PR, Padayatchi N, Rustomjee R, Levin J, Roscigno G, Norman J, McIlleron H, Mitchison DA: The early bactericidal activities of rifampin and rifapentine in pulmonary tuberculosis. Am J Respir Crit Care Med 2005;172:128–135.
34 Grosset J, Rosenthal I, Zhang E, Nuermberger E: Dose-ranging comparison of rifampin and rifapentine in combination with isoniazid and pyrazinamide in the mouse model of tuberculosis. 48th Annu Intersci Conf Antimicrob Agents Chemother, Washington, 2008.
35 Peloquin C: What is the 'right' dose of rifampin? Int J Tuberc Lung Dis 2003;7:3–5.
36 Heifets LB, Lindhom-Levy P, Flory MA: Bactericidal activity in vitro of various rifamycins against *Mycobacterium avium* and *Mycobacterium tuberculosis*. Am Rev Respir Dis 1990;141:626–630.
37 Rosenthal IM, Zhang M, Williams KN, Peloquin CA, Tyagi S, Vernon AA, Bishai WR, Chaisson RE, Grosset JH, Nuermberger EL: Daily dosing of rifapentine cures tuberculosis in three months or less in the murine model. PLoS Med 2007;4:e344.
38 Langdon G, Wilkins J, McFadyen L, McIlleron H, Smith P, Simonsson US: Population pharmacokinetics of rifapentine and its primary desacetyl metabolite in South African tuberculosis patients. Antimicrob Agents Chemother 2005;49:4429–4436.
39 Bock NN, Sterling TR, Hamilton CD, Pachucki C, Wang YC, Conwell DS, Mosher A, Samuels M, Vernon A: A prospective, randomized, double-blind study of the tolerability of rifapentine 600, 900 and 1,200 mg plus isoniazid in the continuation phase of tuberculosis treatment. Am J Respir Crit Care Med 2002;165:1526–1530.
40 Rosenthal IM, Williams K, Tyagi S, Peloquin CA, Vernon AA, Bishai WR, Grosset JH, Nuermberger EL: Potent twice-weekly rifapentine-containing regimens in murine tuberculosis. Am J Respir Crit Care Med 2006;174:94–101.
41 Wilkins JJ, Savic RM, Karlsson MO, Langdon G, McIlleron H, Pillai G, Smith PJ, Simonsson US: Population pharmacokinetics of rifampin in pulmonary tuberculosis patients, including a semi-mechanistic model to describe variable absorption. Antimicrob Agents Chemother 2008;52:2138–2148.
42 Weiner M, Burman W, Vernon A, Benator D, Peloquin CA, Khan A, Weis S, King B, Shah N, Hodge T: Low isoniazid concentrations and outcome of tuberculosis treatment with once-weekly isoniazid and rifapentine. Am J Respir Crit Care Med 2003;167:1341–1347.
43 Saukkonen JJ, Cohn DL, Jasmer RM, Schenker S, Jereb JA, Nolan CM, Peloquin CA, Gordin FM, Nunes D, Strader DB, Bernardo J, Venkataramanan R, Sterling TR: An official ATS statement: hepatotoxicity of antituberculosis therapy. Am J Respir Crit Care Med 2006;174:935–952.
44 Burman WJ, Gallicano K, Peloquin C: Therapeutic implications of drug interactions in the treatment of HIV-related tuberculosis. Clin Infect Dis 1999;28:419–430.
45 Boulle A, Van Cutsem G, Cohen K, Hilderbrand K, Mathee S, Abrahams M, Goemaere E, Coetzee D, Maartens G: Outcomes of nevirapine- and efavirenz-based antiretroviral therapy when coadministered with rifampicin-based antitubercular therapy. JAMA 2008;300:530–539.
46 Blumberg HM, Burman WJ, Chaisson RE, Daley CL, Etkind SC, Friedman LN, Fujiwara P, Grzemska M, Hopewell PC, Iseman MD, Jasmer RM, Koppaka V, Menzies RI, O'Brien RJ, Reves RR, Reichman LB, Simone PM, Starke JR, Vernon AA: American Thoracic Society/Centers for Disease Control and Prevention/Infectious Diseases Society of America: treatment of tuberculosis. Am J Respir Crit Care Med 2003;167:603–662.
47 Burman WJ, Goldberg S, Johnson JL, Muzanye G, Engle M, Mosher AW, Choudhri S, Daley CL, Munsiff SS, Zhao Z, Vernon A, Chaisson RE: Moxifloxacin versus ethambutol in the first 2 months of treatment for pulmonary tuberculosis. Am J Respir Crit Care Med 2006;174:331–338.

William Burman, MD
Denver Public Health
605 Bannock Street
Denver, CO 80204 (USA)
Tel. +1 303 602 8723, E-Mail bburman@dhha.org

## Chapter 4

Donald PR, van Helden PD (eds): Antituberculosis Chemotherapy.
Prog Respir Res. Basel, Karger, 2011, vol 40, pp 25–31

# Isoniazid Pharmacokinetics and Efficacy in Adults and Children

Peter R. Donald · H. Simon Schaaf

Department of Paediatrics and Child Health and Desmond Tutu TB Centre, Faculty of Health Sciences, Stellenbosch University and Tygerberg Children's Hospital, Tygerberg, South Africa

**Abstract**

Isoniazid (INH), nearly 60 years after its discovery, remains an essential drug in tuberculosis regimens. Recent studies confirm its excellent bactericidal activity; the rapid killing of approximately 90% of bacilli in microscopy smear-positive sputum within 48 h explains its great efficacy in preventing drug resistance in companion drugs. Studies of the pharmacokinetics and pharmacodynamics of INH suggest that INH dosages giving serum concentrations 2 h after dosing of 3 μg/ml will suffice for the killing of fully drug-sensitive *Mycobacterium tuberculosis* isolates; concentrations of 5 μg/ml will aid the suppression of a significant proportion of isolates resistant to lower INH concentrations. Hepatotoxicity is one of the most important complications of INH therapy; increases in the values of the hepatic enzymes aspartate aminotransferase and alanine aminotransferase have been shown to be more common in slow acetylators of INH than in faster acetylators of INH. N-acetyltransferase genotyping may make it possible to treat slow acetylators with lower doses of INH and thus achieve optimal efficacy without increasing the risk of hepatotoxicity. Recent studies suggest that children under the age of approximately 10 years should receive INH doses of 10–15 mg/kg to reach serum concentrations equivalent to those of adults receiving 4–6 mg/kg INH.

Copyright © 2011 S. Karger AG, Basel

## Introduction

Nearly 60 years after its discovery, isoniazid (INH) is still designated as an essential antituberculosis agent by the World Health Organization (WHO) [1]. It is the most bactericidal antituberculosis agent in routine use, has good pharmacokinetics, a wide therapeutic margin and is relatively cheap; finally, it is the most effective agent for preventing the development of resistance in companion agents. Despite being the oldest member of current 'first-line' regimens, new information continues to emerge regarding the actions and pharmacokinetics of INH which help to place policies regarding dosing and regimens on a more rational footing.

## The Actions of Isoniazid and Isoniazid Resistance

Early observations of the loss of acid fastness and catalase peroxidase activity in many resistant mycobacteria following exposure to INH suggested that the cell wall was the target for the action of INH and that catalase peroxidase was associated with the actions of INH; it is now clear that INH is a prodrug needing a *katG* gene product, catalase peroxidase, for activation; the activated INH targets the NADH-dependent enoyl-acyl carrier protein reductase coded for by the *inhA* promoter region that is responsible for the synthesis of long fatty acyl chains of mycolic acids [2, 3].

It is also of clinical relevance that recent studies have shown that *inhA* promoter mutations are also associated with high-level ethionamide (ETH) resistance [4], but low-level INH resistance, whereas *katG* mutations will leave susceptibility to ETH unchanged, but will often, but not always, be associated with high-level INH resistance. Another perspective with regard to these findings is that INH can, potentially, inhibit a certain proportion of its own resistant mutants. This was shown in a neglected series of publications from Madras (now Chennai), India, between 1960 and 1964 that described the use of INH monotherapy for the treatment of pulmonary tuberculosis [5, 6]. INH was given in 3 doses starting with 200 mg, given as 100 mg twice daily, 200 mg twice daily and finally

400 mg once daily. These regimens were compared to a control regimen of INH and para-aminosalicylic acid. Patients were phenotyped as slow or rapid acetylators of INH, and INH serum concentrations were determined in a majority of patients. The proportion of patients achieving bacterial quiescence after a year in each treatment group fell from 72 and 66% amongst the slow and fast acetylators of INH receiving INH 400 mg once daily to 48 and 44% amongst the slow and fast acetylators receiving INH 100 mg twice daily. Although the differences in the slow and fast acetylators of INH in the individual INH monotherapy groups were not significant, there is a clear gradation across the range of dosages with the slower acetylators faring better in each instance. Almost without exception the cause of treatment failure was the emergence of INH resistance. Therapeutic efficacy improved above a critical peak concentration of approximately 3 μg/ml, but increasing the maximal concentration ($C_{max}$) to more than approximately 5 μg/ml brought no further benefit; the success of INH monotherapy was considered to be due to suppression of INH-resistant mutants [6]. The success of the regimen of 400 mg INH daily was associated with the higher peak INH serum concentrations rather than the period when a minimal concentration was maintained. From this point much emphasis in the tuberculosis literature tended to be placed upon once-a-day treatment, and peak concentrations were emphasized rather than time above a particular concentration.

This information may permit the tailoring of therapy for INH and multidrug resistance with high-dose INH (sufficient to give a $C_{max}$ of approx. 5 μg/ml) combined with ETH. Resistant strains with an *inhA* mutation will have a minimal inhibitory concentration (MIC) in the range of 0.1–0.2 μg/ml in liquid medium. Recent data from experimental animals [7] and clinical experience suggest that high-dose INH does have detectable efficacy in many cases [8]. When 45 INH-resistant isolates from South African children were evaluated recently, an *inhA* promoter mutation was found in 15 (33%), and 12 of 14 (86%) of these isolates were also ETH resistant; of these 15 isolates, 14 (93%) had low or intermediate-level resistance (MIC in liquid media 0.1–0.2 μg/ml); of the 21 isolates with a *katG* mutation, 16 (76%) had an MIC of 0.2 μg/ml and 5 (24%) one of 5 μg/ml [9]. Although mutations in the *katG* and *inhA* genes are responsible for the majority of INH resistance, mutations of the *aphC, kasA* and *ndh* genes may also be associated with INH resistance. An evaluation of the Genotype® MTBDRplus (Hain Lifescience, Nehren, Germany) assay in a high tuberculosis incidence area of the Western Cape Province of South Africa found 54% of INH monoresistant and 38% of multidrug-resistant *Mycobacterium tuberculosis* strains to have an *inhA* mutation, but these proportions will vary in different communities [10].

INH monoresistance is usually considered to have little influence on the outcome of multidrug short-course treatment. However, a recent systematic review and meta-analysis concluded that the results of retreatment regimens in cohorts of patients with pretreatment INH resistance are unsatisfactory, particularly under programme conditions in middle- and low-income countries [11]. When INH resistance is suspected, intermittent treatment should be avoided in the intensive phase of any retreatment regimen that should include at least 4 effective drugs and be followed by a continuation phase with at least 3 effective drugs, including pyrazinamide, if this can be tolerated for a long period. Concern has also been voiced that the expanded use of INH for preventive treatment may lead to increased levels of INH resistance [12]. The recent introduction of a rapid PCR-based line probe mutation analysis (Genotype MTBDRplus test) will expedite the detection of rifampicin resistance and the commonest forms of INH resistance, and assist clinicians to construct appropriate regimens for the treatment of patients with INH monoresistance and so limit the further expansion of drug resistance.

### The Pharmacokinetics and Pharmacodynamics of Isoniazid

INH is easily absorbed from the gastrointestinal tract but is subject to first-pass metabolism, especially in faster acetylators; peak serum concentrations of INH in faster acetylators are significantly lower following oral dosing in comparison to intravenous administration of the drug. A significant proportion of this first-pass effect can be attributed to N-acetyltransferase 2 (NAT2) situated in the mucosa of the gut cells, in addition to the liver, although much smaller amounts of NAT2 have also been found in a number of other sites [13]. INH is subject to very little protein binding, distributes readily to the total body water compartment, crosses membranes with ease and penetrates into most body tissues and organ systems including the cerebrospinal fluid.

Acetylation is the most important pathway for INH metabolism and is dependent upon polymorphic arylamine NAT2; individuals may be homozygous fast, heterozygous fast or homozygous slow acetylators of INH; acetyl-INH is biotransformed to isonicotinic acid and monoacetyl hydrazine, and monoacetyl hydrazine is in turn acetylated to diacetylhydrazine. Faster acetylators acetylate both INH and monoacetylhydrazine to a far greater extent than slow acetylators

[14]. Small amounts of hydrazine, hydrazones with pyruvic and ketoglutaric acid, ammonia and isonicotinylhydrazide are also produced. Early studies of the pharmacokinetics of INH depended upon phenotypification of individuals into fast or slow acetylators or eliminators of INH, and although there was an awareness of the probable existence of a group of even faster acetylators of INH [14] these could not be differentiated with certainty. More recently it has proved possible to identify significant phenotypic differences between the 3 NAT2 genotypes [15]. At an INH dose of 10 mg/kg, the area under the curve (AUC) over 0–6 h after dose was 31.12 mg/h/l in homozygous slow acetylators of INH, compared to 7.73 mg/h/l (24.8%) for homozygous fast acetylators; at a lower INH dose of 5 mg/kg, the respective exposures are 14.18 and 2.31 mg/h/l (16.3%). It is a tribute to the wide therapeutic margin of INH that these significant differences in exposure to INH were seldom reflected in clinical trials in the past with the exception of once weekly intermittent therapy [16]. The spread of human immunodeficiency virus (HIV) has again highlighted the vulnerability of fast acetylators of INH with the occurrence of relapse in HIV-infected patients with pulmonary tuberculosis treated with once weekly INH and rifapentine [17]. Failure or relapse was associated with fast NAT2 genotypes causing more rapid excretion of INH with consequently a low AUC [18]; moreover in the face of HIV-associated pulmonary tuberculosis, twice weekly regimens have also proved inadequate, and importantly failure and relapse were also often associated with the development of rifamycin monoresistance [19]. The important protective role of INH was again emphasized in another recent study of thrice weekly regimens amongst HIV-infected patients in India when acquired rifampicin resistance was strongly associated with pre-existing INH resistance [20].

Studies of the early bactericidal activity (EBA) of INH have also provided more clarity as to the relationship between the pharmacokinetics and pharmacodynamics of INH. During the first such study, which measured the fall in viable colony-forming units (CFU) per millilitre of sputum of *M. tuberculosis* per day, INH was shown to have the highest bactericidal activity of any of the drugs, or combinations of drugs evaluated [21]. This was particularly evident during the first 2 days of treatment. A subsequent study confirmed that a 90% fall in the number of viable CFU present in sputum occurred during the first 2 days of treatment with INH [22]. This study also illustrated the very wide therapeutic margin of INH with some activity detectable at a total dose as low as 18 mg, but reaching a maximum at approximately 300 mg. A consequence of this might be that, even when fixed-dose combination formulations of antituberculosis agents, frequently containing only 75 mg of INH in each tablet, are used, patients who choose to take only 1 or 2 tablets may still be exposed to sufficient INH to promote the emergence of INH resistance as the concentrations of the companion drugs may be too low to have any protective effect.

Further EBA studies explored the relationship between the EBA of INH and INH serum concentrations and the NAT2 genotype [23, 24]. In these studies the mean maximum EBA over days 0–2 of INH was a daily fall per millilitre of sputum in viable CFU of *M. tuberculosis* of 0.569 $\log_{10}$ and the $EBA_{90}$ (90% of the mean maximum EBA) was 0.512. The mean 2-hour INH serum concentration associated with this EBA was 2.19 (SE 0.68) µg/ml and the $AUC_{0-\infty}$ 10.52 (SE 3.69) µg/ml/h. These results provide backing for the suggestion, based on considerable experience in healthy volunteers and tuberculosis patients, that 2-hour INH concentrations of 3–5 µg/ml should be aimed at [25].

Thus it appears that a daily INH dosage delivering a 2-hour postdose serum concentration of approximately 3 µg/ml, which will be fairly close to $C_{max}$, will suffice to ensure optimal killing of fully INH drug-susceptible bacilli in pulmonary tuberculosis patients; also, in the light of the discussion above, a 2-hour concentration of 5 µg/ml could be looked upon as a mutant prevention concentration likely to inhibit the multiplication of a significant proportion of INH-resistant mutants; exposure to higher 2-hour INH concentrations is unlikely to bring any additional benefit. These concentrations could be reached in homozygous slow acetylators following an INH dose of 3 mg/kg body weight, but 6 mg/kg for heterozygous fast acetylators and at least 10 mg/kg for homozygous fast acetylators. Using these criteria it should thus be possible to personalize INH dosages in those circumstances where the NAT2 genotype can be determined, thus maximizing efficacy and minimizing INH toxicity. One recent suggestion is that homozygous slow acetylators of INH should receive an INH dose of 2.5 mg/kg, heterozygous fast acetylators 5 mg/kg and homozygous fast acetylators 7.5 mg/kg [26]; in another assessment of Japanese volunteers, the optimal INH dose for individuals with a homozygous fast acetylator genotype was calculated as 430 mg or 7.2 mg/kg [27].

## The Dosage of Isoniazid in Children

When INH was first introduced, considerably higher doses of INH were used by many experienced clinicians in children than in adults, and there was frequent comment that children did not appear to experience undue toxicity despite these higher doses. Nonetheless the WHO, until recently,

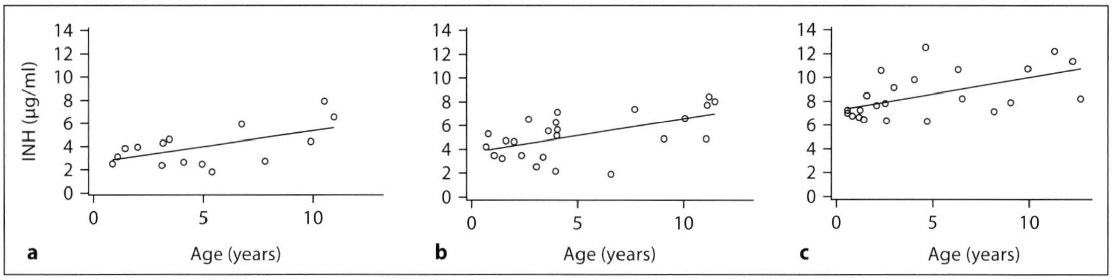


**Fig. 1.** INH serum concentrations in young children 2 h after an INH dose of 10 mg/kg in relation to age and NAT2 genotype. **a** Homozygous fast acetylators of INH. Mean concentration 2.54 µg/ml. **b** Heterozygous fast acetylators of INH. Mean concentration 3.738 µg/ml. **c** Homozygous slow acetylators of INH. Mean concentration 7.28 µg/ml.

**Table 1.** The serum concentrations of INH in adults and children of a similar genetic background receiving an INH dose of 10 mg/kg [15, 29]

| NAT2 genotype | Adults | Children | Elimination rate constant K, n/h | | $AUC_{0-5}$, µg/ml/h | | Mean INH 2-hour concentration, µg/ml | |
|---|---|---|---|---|---|---|---|---|
| | | | adults | children | adults | children | adults | children |
| SS | 21 (35%) | 25 (39%) | 0.19 | 0.25 | 24.9 | 18.4 | 10.9 | 8.6 |
| FS | 27 (45%) | 24 (38%) | 0.43 | 0.51 | 15.3 | 8.2 | 8.7 | 5.1 |
| FF | 12 (20%) | 15 (23%) | 0.68 | 0.65 | 8.1 | 5.4 | 6.0 | 4.0 |

FF = Homozygous NAT2 fast acetylators; FS = heterozygous NAT2 fast acetylators; SS = homozygous NAT2 slow acetylators.

recommended an INH dose of 5 mg/kg for both adults and children [28]. Recent experience, discussed above, has confirmed that 2-hour postdose INH serum concentrations of 3–5 µg/ml are desirable for optimal INH efficacy. Table 1 gives pharmacokinetic details of children and adults from the Western Cape Province of South Africa, both receiving an INH dose of 10 mg/kg, and it is clear that the exposure of the children to INH is significantly less than that of adults and that, even at a dose of 10 mg/kg, there will be a proportion of homozygous rapid acetylators of INH who do not reach the suggested criteria [29]. Age also plays a role [30], and figure 1 illustrates the combined effects of NAT2 genotype and increasing age of these children on the INH serum concentrations 2 hours after receiving and INH dosage of 10mg/kg. Similar conclusions have been reached by others who found that, while children aged 8–13 years reached mean INH concentrations above 3 µg/ml 2 h after dosing, children aged 1–8 years did not, and it was suggested that children 0–5 years of age required an INH dose of 8–10 mg/kg, those aged 6–9 years 7–8 mg/kg and those aged 10–14 years 5–6 mg/kg [31]. Other researchers concluded that children who were slow acetylators should receive an INH dose of 4.2 mg/kg, but that fast acetylators needed a higher dose of 10.3 mg/kg to achieve the same exposure to INH [32]. The danger of uniform recommendations for all populations and age groups is illustrated by a group of 10 Indian children aged 6–12 years, who were most likely slow acetylators of INH and amongst whom the mean $C_{max}$ after an INH dose of 5 mg/kg was 4.75 µg/ml (SEM ±0.31) [33]. This suggests that in somewhat older children who are homozygous slow acetylators of INH, a dose of 5 mg/kg may be adequate.

The most recent recommendations by the WHO recognize the influence of both age and genetic diversity with regard to INH metabolism, and an INH dose ranging from 10 to 15 mg/kg (maximum 300 mg) is recommended for use in children [34]. This new recommendation, however, does not specify the upper age limit of children who should receive the higher dose, and we suggest that the higher dose should be used in children less than 10 years of age.

## Isoniazid Toxicity

*Hepatotoxicity*

When the danger of hepatotoxicity due to INH was first recognized, there was great interest in the influence of the NAT2 phenotype on susceptibility to INH antituberculosis drug-induced hepatotoxicity, and the subject generated considerable controversy. The fact that fast acetylators of INH generate more acetylhydrazine suggested that they might be more susceptible to antituberculosis drug-induced hepatotoxicity; however, although fast acetylators generate more acetyl-INH, they eliminate it (by the same process of acetylation) equally rapidly. NAT2 genotyping has now confirmed that the serum levels of hepatic transaminases, aspartate aminotransferase and alanine aminotransferase, in homozygous slow acetylators of INH are much more likely to rise than in fast (homo- or heterozygous) acetylators [35, 36]. Whether this translates into susceptibility to hepatotoxicity leading to overt jaundice and liver failure remains uncertain. However, assuming that a rise in aspartate and alanine aminotransferase values does indicate a degree of hepatotoxicity, using NAT2 genotyping, when available, to personalize INH doses will potentially maximize INH efficacy and minimize toxicity [26, 27].

The potential danger of INH-associated hepatotoxicity is emphasized by recent reports of severe hepatotoxicity occurring in the USA in adults, but also in children, necessitating liver transplantation in some instances [37, 38]. It is suggested that patients with HIV infection, chronic liver disease, pregnant women or women who have given birth, the elderly and those who abuse alcohol should be considered for baseline liver function tests. It is emphasized that a common fault was the continuation of INH in the face of symptoms suggestive of hepatotoxicity.

### Peripheral Neuropathy and Vitamin $B_6$ (Pyridoxine) Supplementation

Shortly after INH had been introduced, it was noted that peripheral neuropathy developed in some patients, and it was particularly frequent in those receiving higher INH doses. It was also noted that INH increased the urinary excretion of vitamin $B_6$ and that vitamin $B_6$ supplementation could prevent peripheral neuropathy and that peripheral neuropathy was more common amongst slow acetylators of INH.

These observations led to recommendations that malnourished patients receiving INH should also receive vitamin $B_6$ supplementation to prevent peripheral neuropathy. The situation is further complicated amongst patients receiving antiretroviral agents because stavudine, and other nucleoside reverse-transcriptase inhibitors, may also cause peripheral neuropathy. The fourth edition of the WHO *Treatment of Tuberculosis Guidelines* [1] recommends that pregnant women and individuals who are HIV-infected, or have diabetes, chronic liver disease or renal failure should receive supplementation with 10 mg/day of pyridoxine together with their anituberculosis treatment.

Amongst children receiving INH the occurrence of peripheral neuropathy is unusual even in conditions of poverty and malnutrition, and the need for vitamin $B_6$ supplementation is contested [39, 40]. A recent study evaluated serum plasma pyridoxal-5-phosphate (PLP) concentrations in a group of young children with serious forms of tuberculosis receiving INH-containing regimens [41]. Amongst 19 HIV-infected children and 33 HIV-uninfected children, mean PLP concentrations 1 month after commencing treatment were 8.32 (SD 6.57) and 11.28 (SD 5.20) ng/ml ($p = 0.11$), respectively, but following routine multivitamin supplementation 6.75 (SD 2.71) and 14.76 (SD 7.96) ng/ml ($p < 0.001$) after 4 months of treatment. Serum PLP concentrations were also related to serum C-reactive protein concentrations that were initially raised in both the HIV-infected and HIV-uninfected children, but at 4 months after starting treatment those in the HIV-infected children were still raised, whilst those in the HIV-uninfected children had normalized. No relationship was found in this study between PLP concentrations and INH dosage or NAT2 genotype. As vitamin $B_6$ has a number of other functions important for immunity, supplementation of HIV-infected children receiving INH would seem necessary, while the necessity of supplementing HIV-uninfected children receiving antituberculosis chemotherapy remains uncertain.

### Acknowledgements

This review was supported in part by a grant from the WHO as part of the Better Medicines for Children project. P.R.D. and H.S.S. are supported by the National Research Foundation of South Africa.

## References


1 World Health Organization: Treatment of Tuberculosis: Guidelines, ed 4. WHO/HTM/TB/2009.420. Geneva, WHO, 2010.

2 Zhang Y, Heym B, Allen B, Young D, Cole S: The catalase-peroxidase gene and isoniazid resistance of *Mycobacterium tuberculosis.* Nature 1992;358:591–593.

3 Banerjee A, Dubnau E, Quemard A, Balasubramanian V, Um KS, Wilson T, Collins D, de Lisle G, Jacobs WR: *inhA,* a gene encoding a target for isoniazid and ethionamide in *Mycobacterium tuberculosis.* Science 1994;263:227–230.

4 Morlock GP, Metchock, Sikes D, Crawford JT, Cooksey RC: *ethA, inhA,* and *katG* loci of ethionamide-resistant clinical *Mycobacterium tuberculosis* isolates. Antimicrob Agents Chemother 2003;47:3799–3805.

5 Selkon JB, Fox W, Gangadharam PRJ, Ramachandran K, Ramakrishnan CV, Velu S: Rate of inactivation of isoniazid in South Indian patients with pulmonary tuberculosis. 2. Clinical implications in the treatment of pulmonary tuberculosis either alone or in combination with PAS. Bull World Health Org 1961;25:779–792.

6 Mitchison DA: Plasma concentrations of isoniazid in the treatment of tuberculosis; in Davies DS, Prichard BNC (eds): Biological Effects of Drugs in Relation to Their Plasma Concentration. Oxford, British Pharmacological Society, Macmillan, 1973, pp 169–182.

7 Cynamon MH, Zhang Y, Harpster T, Cheng S, De Stefano MS: High-dose isoniazid therapy for isoniazid resistant murine *Mycobacterium tuberculosis* infection. Antimicrob Agents Chemother 1999;43:2922–2924.

8 Katiyar SK, Bihari S, Prakash S, Mamtani M, Kulkarni HA: A randomized controlled trial of high-dose isoniazid adjuvant therapy for multidrug-resistant tuberculosis. Int J Tuberc Lung Dis 2008;12:139–145.

9 Schaaf HS, Victor TC, Venter A, Brittle W, Jordaan AM, Hesseling AC, Marais BJ, van Helden PD, Donald PR: Ethionamide cross- and co-resistance in children with isoniazid-resistant tuberculosis. Int J Tuberc Lung Dis 2009;13:1155–1159.

10 Barnard M, Albert H, Coetzee G, O'Brien R, Bosman ME: Rapid molecular screening for multidrug-resistant tuberculosis in a high-volume public health laboratory in South Africa. Am J Respir Crit Care Med 2008;77:787–782.

11 Menzies D, Benedetti A, Paydar A, Royce S, Madhukar P, Burman W, Vernon A, Lienhardt C: Standardized treatment of active tuberculosis in patients with previous treatment and/or with mono-resistance to isoniazid: a systematic review and meta-analysis. PLoS Med 2009;6:e1000150.

12 Cohen T, Lipsitch M, Walensky RP, Murray M: Beneficial and perverse effects of isoniazid preventive therapy for latent tuberculosis infection in HIV tuberculosis coinfected populations. Proc Natl Acad Sci USA 2006;103:7042–7047.

13 Husain A, Zhang X, Doll MA, States C, Barker DF, Hein DW: Identification of N-acetyltransferase (NAT2) transcription start sites and quantification of NAT2 mRNA in human tissues. Drug Metab Dispos 2007;35:721–727.

14 Ellard GA: Variations between individuals and populations in the acetylation of isoniazid and its significance for the treatment of pulmonary tuberculosis. Clin Pharmacol Ther 1976;19:610–625.

15 Parkin DP, Vandenplas S, Botha FJ, Vandenplas ML, Seifart HI, van Helden PD, van der Walt BJ, Donald PR, van Jaarsveld PP: Trimodality of isoniazid elimination: phenotype and genotype in patients with tuberculosis. Am J Respir Crit Care Med 1997;155:1717–1722.

16 Ellard G: The potential clinical significance of isoniazid acetylator phenotype in the treatment of pulmonary tuberculosis. Tubercle 1984;65:211–227.

17 Vernon A, Burman W, Benator D, Khan A, Bozeman L: Relapse with rifamycin mono-resistant tuberculosis in HIV-infected patients treated with supervised once weekly rifapentine and isoniazid. Lancet 1999;353:1843–1847.

18 Weiner M, Burman W, Vernon A, Benator D, Peloquin CA, Khan A, Weis S, King B, Shah N, Hodge T, Tuberculosis Trials Consortium: Low isoniazid concentrations and outcome of tuberculosis treatment with once weekly isoniazid and rifapentine. Am J Respir Crit Care Med 2003;167:1341–1347.

19 Burman W, Benator D, Vernon A, Khan A, Jones B, Silva C, Lahart C, Weis S, King B, Mangura B, Weiner M, El-Sadr W, Tuberculosis Trials Consortium: Acquired rifamycin resistance with twice-weekly treatment of HIV-related tuberculosis. Am J Respir Crit Care Med 2006;173:350–356.

20 Swaminathan S, Narendran G, Venkatesan P, Iliayas S, Santhanakrishnan R, Menon PA, et al. Efficacy of 6-month versus 9-month intermittent treatment regimen in HIV-infected patients with tuberculosis. Am J Respir Crit Care 2010;181:743–751.

21 Jindani A, Aber VR, Edwards EA, Mitchison DA: The early bactericidal activity of drugs in patients with pulmonary tuberculosis. Am Rev Respir Dis 1980;121:939–949.

22 Donald PR, Sirgel FA, Botha FJH, Seifart HI, Parkin DP, Vandenplas ML, van de Wal BW, Maritz JS, Mitchison DA: The early bactericidal activity of isoniazid related to its dose size in pulmonary tuberculosis. Am J Respir Crit Care Med 1997;156:895–900.

23 Donald PR, Sirgel FA, Venter A, Parkin DP, Seifart HI, van de Wal BW, Werely C, van Helden PD, Maritz JS: The influence of human N-acetyltransferase genotype on the early bactericidal activity of isoniazid. Clin Infect Dis 2004;39:1425–1430.

24 Donald PR, Parkin DP, Seifart HI, Schaaf HS, van Helden PD, Werely CJ, Sirgel FA, Venter A, Maritz JS: The influence of dose and N-acetyltransferase-2 (NAT2) genotype and phenotype on the pharmacokinetics and pharmacodynamics of isoniazid. Eur J Clin Pharmacol 2007;63:633–639.

25 Peloquin CA: Therapeutic drug monitoring: principles and applications in mycobacterial infections. Drug Ther 1992;22:31–36.

26 Kinzig-Schippers M, Tomalik-Scharte D, Jetter A, Scheidel B, Jakob V, Rodamer M, Cascorbi I, Doroshyenko O, Sörgel F, Fuhr U: Should we use N-acetyltransferase type 2 genotyping to personalize isoniazid doses? Antimicrob Agents Chemother 2005;49:1733–1738.

27 Kubota R, Ohno M, Hasunuma T, Iijima H, Azuma J: Dose-escalation study of isoniazid in healthy volunteers with rapid acetylator genotype of arylamine N-acetyltransferase 2. Eur J Clin Pharmacol 2007;63:927–933

28 World Health Organization: Treatment of Tuberculosis: Guidelines for National Programmes. WHO/CDS/TB/2003.313. Geneva, WHO, 2003.

29 Schaaf HS, Parkin DP, Seifart HI, Werely CJ, Hesseling PB, van Helden PD, Maritz JS, Donald PR: Isoniazid pharmacokinetics in children treated for respiratory tuberculosis. Arch Dis Child 2005;90:614–618.

30 Maritz JS, Parkin DP, Donald PR, Schaaf HS, Seifart HI, Werele C: The association of age and elimination of isoniazid: an example of median regression with heteroscedasticity. S Afr Stat J 2003;37:191–202.

31 Thee S, Detjen AA, Wahn U, Magdorf K: Isoniazid pharmacokinetic studies of the 1960s: considering a higher isoniazid dose in childhood tuberculosis. Scand J Infect Dis 2010;42:294–298.

32 Rey E, Pons G, Crémier O, Vauzelle-Kervroëdan F, Pariente-Khayat A, d'Athis P, Badoual J, Olive G, Gendrel D: Isoniazid dose adjustment in a pediatric population. Ther Drug Monitor 1998;20:50–55.

33 Roy V, Tekur U, Chopra K: Pharmacokinetics of isoniazid in pulmonary tuberculosis – a comparative study at two dose levels. Indian Pediatr 1996;33:287–291.

34 World Health Organization: Dosing instructions for the use of currently available fixed-dose combination TB medicines for children. Geneva, WHO, 2009. http://www.who.int/tb/challenges/interim_paediatric_fdc_dosing_instructions_sept09.pdf (accessed October 8, 2010).

35 Possuelo LG, Castelan JA, de Brito TC, Ribeiro AW, Cafrune PI, Picon PD, Santos AR, Teixeira RL, Gregianini TS, Hutz MH, Rossetti ML, Zaha A: Association of N-acetyltransferase 2 profile and anti-TB drug-induced hepatotoxicity in patients from Southern Brazil. Eur J Clin Pharmacol 2008;64:673–681.

36 Higuchi N, Tahara N, Yanagihara K, Fukushima K, Suyama N, Inoue Y, Miyazaki Y, Kobayashi T, Yoshiura K, Niikawa N, Wen CY, Isomoto H, Shikuwa S, Omagari K, Mizuta Y, Kohno S, Tsukamoto K: *NAT2*6A*, a haplotype of the N-acetyltransferase 2 gene, is an important biomarker for risk of anti-tuberculosis drug-induced hepatotoxicity in Japanese patients with tuberculosis. World J Gastroenterol 2007;13:6003–6008.

37 Wu SS, Chao CS, Vargas JH, Sharp HL, Martín MG, McDiarmid SV, Sinatra FR, Ament ME: Isoniazid related hepatic failure in children: a survey of liver transplantation centers. Transplantation 2007;84:173–179.

38 Harrington T, Manangan L, Jereb J, Navin T, Powell K: Severe isoniazid-associated liver injuries among persons being treated for latent tuberculosis infection – United States, 2004–2008. MMWR 2010;59:224–229.

39 Mbala L, Matendo R, Nkailu R: Is vitamin $B_6$ supplementation of isoniazid therapy useful in childhood tuberculosis? Trop Doctor 1998;28:28:103–104.

40 Rasul CH, Das SC: Vitamin $B_6$ supplementation with isoniazid therapy. Trop Doctor 2000;30:55–56.

41 Cilliers K, Labadarios D, Schaaf HS, Willemse M, Maritz JS, Werely CJ, Hussey G, Donald PR: Pyridoxal-5-phosphate concentrations in children receiving tuberculosis chemotherapy including isoniazid. Acta Paediatr 2010;99:705–710.

Prof. P.R. Donald
Paediatrics and Child Health
Stellenbosch University
PO Box 19063, Tygerberg 7505 (South Africa)
Tel. +27 21 9389 592, E-Mail prd@sun.ac.za

Donald PR, van Helden PD (eds): Antituberculosis Chemotherapy.
Prog Respir Res. Basel, Karger, 2011, vol 40, pp 32–43

# Recent Developments in the Study of Pyrazinamide: An Update

Denis A. Mitchison[a] · Ying Zhang[b]

[a]Centre for Infection, St. George's, University of London, London, UK; [b]W. Harry Feinstone Department of Molecular Microbiology and Immunology, Bloomberg School of Public Health, Johns Hopkins University, Baltimore, Md., USA

## Abstract

Pyrazinamide (PZA) is an unusual antituberculosis drug because its bactericidal activity increases as bacterial metabolism decreases, for instance in models of bacterial persistence, from the action of energy inhibitors, during hypoxic incubation and at low incubation temperatures. These characteristics make PZA particularly effective in killing persistent bacteria that other antibacterials fail to kill, and so make it an essential drug to be included in any current or new drug combination. This behaviour is explained by the Zhang model of PZA in which PZA is first deaminated to the active form of the drug pyrazinoic acid (POA) which enters the cell by passive pH-dependent diffusion but can only leave through an inefficient efflux pump which requires energy. If insufficient energy is available to drive its efflux, POA accumulates within the cell and is lethal. Weak acids, iron, oxidative stress, UV and DNA damage also increase PZA activity. Resistance to PZA is almost always due to mutations that occur widely distributed within the *pncA* gene that codes for pyrazinamidase involved in the conversion of the prodrug PZA to POA. We suggest increasing the cut-off concentration defining resistance in pH 6.0 medium and the use of the Brander test with high concentrations of nicotinamide in medium at normal pH for phenotype-based PZA susceptibility testing. Sequencing of *pncA* for mutations represents a rapid molecular test for detecting PZA resistance and avoids the problem of conventional phenotype-based PZA susceptibility testing.

Copyright © 2011 S. Karger AG, Basel

Pyrazinamide (PZA) is a critical frontline tuberculosis (TB) drug that plays a unique role in shortening the treatment period from 9 to 6 months [1–3]. The inclusion of PZA with isoniazid and rifampicin (RIF) forms the basis for our current short-course chemotherapy. The experimental basis for this was elegantly demonstrated first in the 1950s by McCune et al. [4] and McCune and Tompsett [5] in a mouse model of TB infection. This powerful sterilizing activity is due to PZA killing a population of persister tubercle bacilli that are not killed by other drugs [6]. More recent efforts to find optimal drug combinations with new drug candidates for shortening TB treatment in the mouse model suggest that PZA is the only drug that cannot be replaced without compromising treatment efficacy [7–9]. PZA is an intriguing, unconventional and paradoxical drug. Despite its powerful in vivo sterilizing activity demonstrated both in the animal model [4, 5] and in humans in shortening TB chemotherapy [6], PZA has no activity in vitro under normal culture conditions at neutral pH [10], but is active only at an acid pH (e.g. pH 5.5) in vitro [11]. Furthermore, unlike most other TB drugs such as isoniazid and RIF, the bactericidal activity of PZA increases with low metabolic activity. PZA only kills *Mycobacterium tuberculosis* slowly in vitro at acid pH [12], and a minimum inhibitory concentration (MIC) below the peak concentration found in patients is only obtained when it acts against bacilli with low metabolism. PZA therefore has a high sterilizing activity against a persisting bacterial population in an acidic environment [13, 14], which is responsible for its ability to shorten TB therapy. Despite its use since 1952, and despite its importance as an irreplaceable frontline agent in shortening TB therapy, the mode of action of PZA is the least understood of all TB drugs [15]. Progress has been made in our understanding of PZA in recent years. Much of the historical and clinical aspects of PZA were covered in our previous review article published in 2003 [15] and will not be detailed here. This article will mainly focus on new developments in PZA since then while retaining the basic important information.

## Mechanisms of Pyrazinamide Action

The mode of action of PZA is unusual and has puzzled investigators for decades since its discovery in 1952. The main reason is that PZA is very different from common antibiotics that are primarily active against growing bacteria, since PZA has low activity against growing tubercle bacilli and is primarily active against non-growing persisters. PZA, a nicotinamide analogue, is a prodrug that is converted to the active form pyrazinoic acid (POA) by the pyrazinamidase (PZase)/nicotinamidase encoded by the *pncA* gene in *M. tuberculosis* [16]. The purified recombinant *M. tuberculosis* PncA is an $Mn^{2+}$- and $Fe^{2+}$-containing enzyme that is a monomer with specific activity of 82 μm/min/mg with PZA as a substrate [17]. The mechanism of PZA conversion to POA has recently been suggested to be similar to that of the nitrilase superfamily in which the nucleophilic attack by an active-site cysteine generates a tetrahedral intermediate that collapses with the loss of ammonia and subsequent hydrolysis of the thioester bond by water [18, 19].

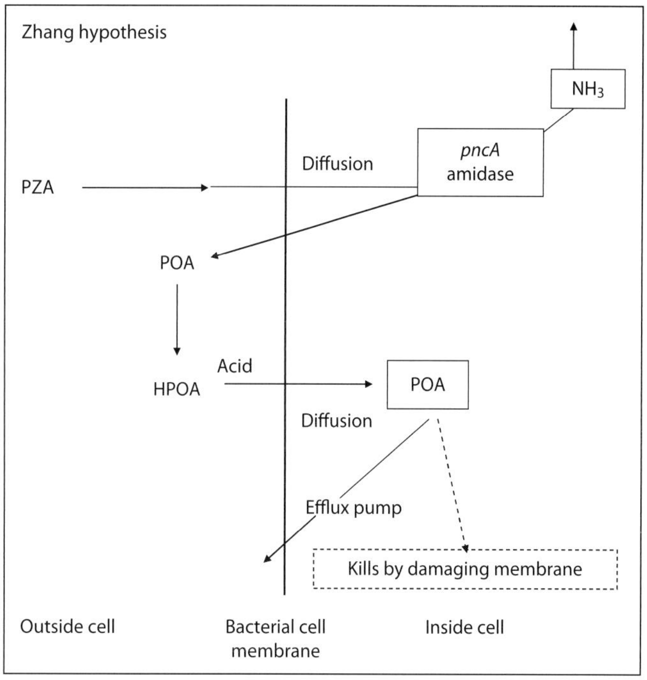


**Fig. 1.** Zhang hypothesis for the mode of action of PZA. The vertical line represents the cell membrane with the cytoplasm to the right and the cell exterior to the left. At the top, PZA enters the cell by passive diffusion and is deaminated to POA and ammonia ($NH_3$). The protonated POA (HPOA) can enter the cell in a pH-dependent manner by passive diffusion but it can only be excreted by an inefficient efflux pump that requires energy. POA accumulating within the cell probably kills by acidification and membrane damage.

*The Zhang Model*

Based on our studies [16, 20–22], we proposed the following model for the mode of action of PZA (fig. 1) [15, 22]. PZA enters bacilli through passive diffusion and is converted into POA (a moderately strong acid with a $pK_a$ of 2.9) by the cytoplasmic PZase encoded by *pncA*. POA then gets out of the cell through passive diffusion and a deficient efflux mechanism in *M. tuberculosis* [20]. Once POA is outside the cell, if the extracellular pH is acidic (e.g. pH 5.5), a small proportion of POA will become uncharged protonated acid HPOA, which readily permeates through the membrane. The acid-facilitated POA influx can overcome the weak deficient POA efflux, which causes accumulation of POA in *M. tuberculosis* cells at acid pH over time [20]. The HPOA brings protons into the cell, and this could eventually cause cytoplasmic acidification so that vital enzymes could be inhibited. In addition, POA could de-energize the membrane by collapsing proton motive force and affect membrane transport inhibiting protein and RNA synthesis [22]. At neutral or alkaline pH, there is little POA found in tubercle bacilli [20], because over 99.9% of POA will be in a charged anion form [21], does not get into cells easily and remains outside the cells [20]. This observation explains why PZA is active at acidic pH but not at neutral pH [11] and also explains the correlation between the MIC of PZA and acidic pH values, which can be expressed by the Henderson-Hasselbalch equation (table 2) [21]. It is worth noting that acid pH not only allows the active form of PZA, POA, to re-enter and accumulate in the bacilli [20], but also decreases the membrane potential and inhibits bacterial metabolism. The unique activity of PZA against *M. tuberculosis* appears to be at least partly due to a deficient POA efflux mechanism [20] that is unable to counteract the effect of acid-facilitated POA influx, which could cause increased accumulation of POA to sufficiently high concentrations to inhibit as yet unknown cellular targets and eventual acidification of the cytoplasm, de-energized membrane and cell death, especially in non-growing persisters with low metabolism at acid pH.

A modification to this hypothesis has been suggested by Mitchison (fig. 2), who proposes that ammonia produced by deamination of PZA would be converted to ammonium ion immediately on contact with cell water and combine with POA to form ammonium pyrazinoate, which could diffuse easily out of the bacterial cell. In an acid environment outside the cell, it would dissociate and form HPOA that

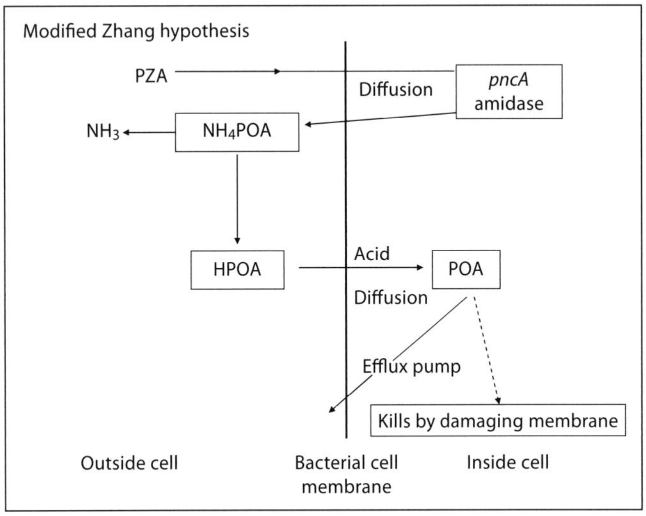


**Fig. 2.** Zhang hypothesis with suggested Mitchison modification. In this, the PZA is deaminated and converted to ammonium pyrazinoate ($NH_4POA$). The HPOA is then absorbed by passive diffusion into the cell and accumulates under acid pH.

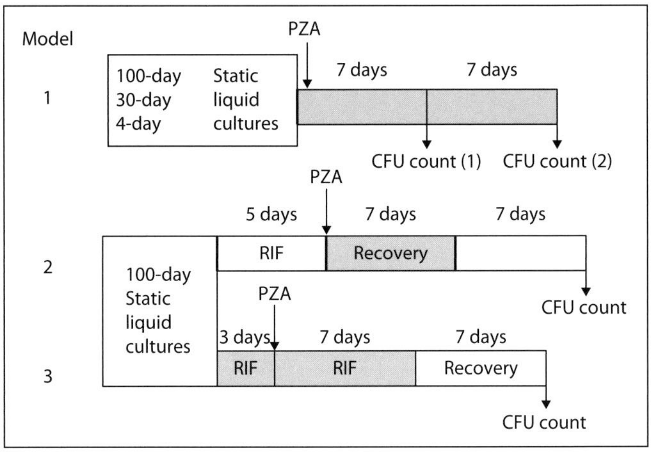


**Fig. 3.** The Hu/Coates models. In model 1, either 100-day or 30-day static liquid cultures or 4-day log phase cultures were exposed to PZA in acid medium and CFU counts were done after 7 and 14 days. Only 100-day-old static cultures were used in models 2 and 3. In model 2, such a culture was incubated in liquid medium containing RIF. PZA was added on day 5 to the RIF-tolerant organisms which were allowed to recover before CFU counting. In model 3, PZA was added while the organisms were exposed to RIF. Shaded boxes have culture medium at pH 5.5. Reproduced with permission from the *International Journal of Tuberculosis and Lung Disease* [24].

would diffuse passively into the cell (fig. 2). There is as yet no experimental evidence for this modification. The reason for this modification is that POA when first produced by deamination has to be excreted from the cell with fair efficiency so that its pH dependency on reabsorption is demonstrable. However, when reabsorbed, it is not easily excreted leading eventually to cell death [20, 23]. The two mechanisms imply differences in speeds of excretion. The proposed modification does not change the overall conclusion and prediction of the model.

*Predictions from the Model*

Various conclusions stem from these hypotheses concerning the bactericidal activity of PZA.

1 Activity is strongly related to the pH of the micro-environment of the bacilli, with activity increasing with acidity. This mechanism was demonstrated by the early studies at Cornell University [11].

2 As diffusion of POA into the cell occurs passively but its removal requires energy to run the efflux pump, bactericidal activity is greatest when bacterial energy sources are at their lowest. This conclusion was first demonstrated by the finding that old cultures were more susceptible to PZA than young actively growing cultures [21]. The specificity of this action on persisters was then demonstrated using the Hu/Coates models of persisters [24] and with work that showed increased bactericidal activity when low metabolic activity was produced, for instance by energy inhibitors [22, 25], by anaerobic conditions [26] and when incubation temperatures were reduced from 37°C to within the range of 15–25°C [23].

## Pyrazinamide Activity in Persister Models

*Hu/Coates Models*

Hu/Coates models explore the action of drugs on persisters and therefore substantiate the hypothesis that PZA has unusual activity against this bacterial subpopulation (fig. 3). The results obtained with them are therefore crucial to the overall thesis concerning the bacillary populations against which it is most effective. In model 1, cultures of *M. tuberculosis* incubated without shaking and with caps screwed on for periods of up to 100 days were sampled, PZA added and bactericidal activity measured (fig. 4). It is evident that as the duration of previous incubation and starvation increased from 4 days (log phase) to 30 days and then 100 days, the bactericidal activity of PZA increased. The 100-day cultures used in models 2 and 3 contained a bacterial subpopulation that was initially highly tolerant of 100 mg/l RIF and also incapable of growing on solid medium. After selection of this

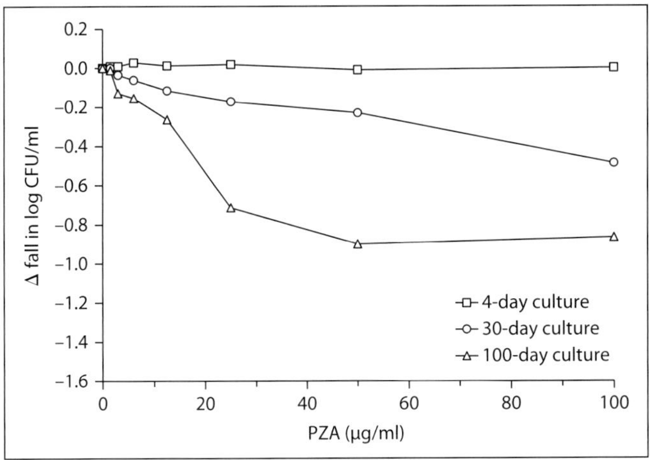


**Fig. 4.** The results of CFU counts after 7 days in model 1. While the counts on the log phase 4-day culture were hardly altered, those on the 30-day static culture were reduced and those on the 100-day culture were reduced even further. Reproduced with permission from the *International Journal of Tuberculosis and Lung Disease* [24].

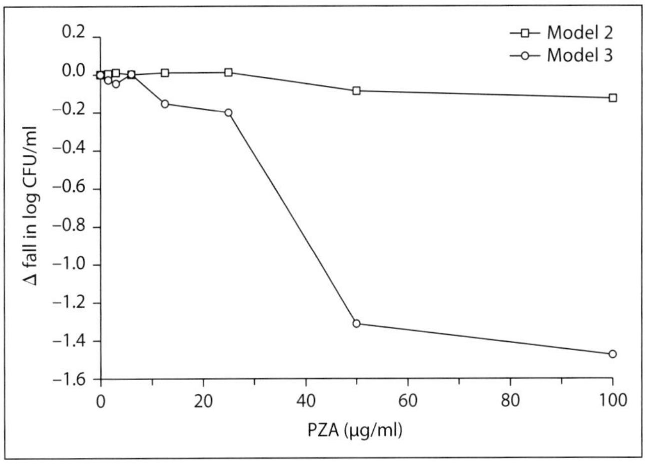


**Fig. 5.** The results of the CFU counts in models 2 and 3. In model 2, the organisms were actively recovering from exposure to RIF and as they had high metabolism were hardly killed by PZA. In model 3, counts were done on the tolerant fraction during selection by RIF, and appreciable killing occurred. Reproduced with permission from the *International Journal of Tuberculosis and Lung Disease* [24].

population by subculture in RIF-containing liquid medium, both of these characteristics returned to the normal pattern of susceptibility to RIF and ability to grow on solid medium during culture for 7 days in RIF-free liquid medium. In model 2, the cultures were sampled immediately after selection of the RIF-tolerant population when regrowth was occurring and bacterial metabolism high. PZA had little bactericidal activity against these actively growing bacilli (fig. 5). In model 3, the cultures are sampled at 3 days after inoculation into RIF-containing liquid medium when growth and metabolism of the subpopulation would be expected to be minimal. PZA was highly bactericidal against this population (fig. 5). The action of PZA in these 3 models demonstrates that PZA is most bactericidal when cultures of *M. tuberculosis* are the most static.

*Starvation*

We tested the effect of starvation in PBS buffer on PZA activity against *M. tuberculosis* bacilli. Indeed, we found that starvation decreased membrane potential and enhanced PZA activity, especially for old bacilli [26]. In addition, it is worth noting that *M. tuberculosis* starved in PBS had an increased expression of *pncA* [27], which is expected to increase PncA enzyme levels needed for conversion of PZA to the active form POA, and may also contribute to increased killing of tubercle bacilli by PZA under starvation conditions.

*Energy Inhibitors*

Since PZA depletes the membrane potential in *M. tuberculosis* [22], we reasoned that energy inhibitors could enhance PZA activity. Indeed, we found that the activity of PZA was significantly enhanced by energy inhibitors such as dicyclohexylcarbodiimide (DCCD, an F1F0-ATPase inhibitor), rotenone (NADH dehydrogenase I-complex I inhibitor) and azide (cytochrome c oxidase inhibitor) (fig. 6a) [22], and also carbonylcyanide-*m*-chlorophenylhydrazone, dinitrophenol, valinomycin and cyanide [25]. The subsequent observation in 2005 that diarylquinoline, an inhibitor of F1F0-ATPase, could synergize with PZA [28], a finding just like DCCD synergy with PZA we had shown earlier in 2003 [22], is also consistent with our model of PZA. These energy inhibitors deplete membrane energy, which renders tubercle bacilli more susceptible to the energy-depleting action of POA. This effect of energy inhibitors on enhancing PZA activity is specific to PZA, as they did not enhance the activity of other control drugs like isoniazid or RIF [25].

*Anaerobic and Hypoxic Conditions*

PZA activity is significantly enhanced under hypoxic or anaerobic conditions compared with atmospheric conditions with ambient oxygen (fig. 7) [26]. Under microaerophilic or anaerobic conditions, bacteria produce less energy (ATP and membrane potential) due to less efficient nitrate or fumarate electron acceptor usage, compared with

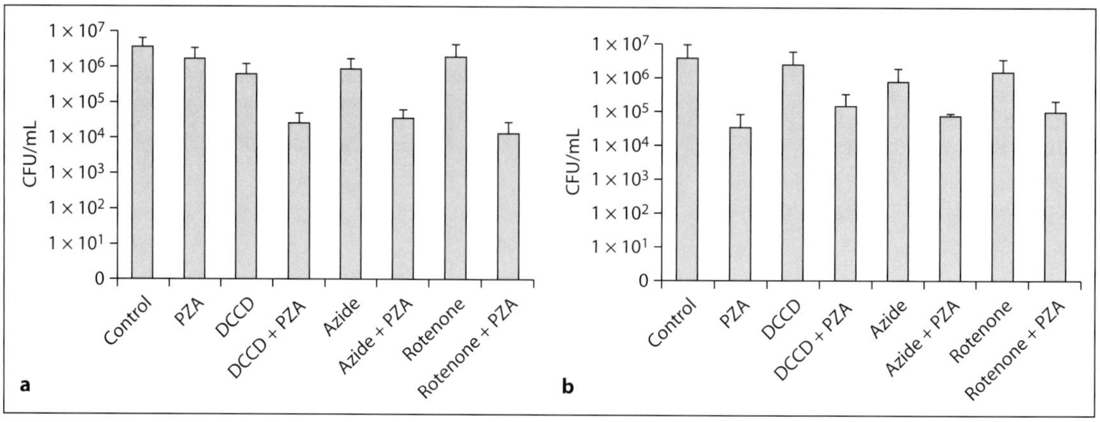


**Fig. 6.** Effect of energy inhibitors and PZA activity under aerobic and anaerobic conditions. *M. tuberculosis* H37Ra cells were treated with PZA (100 μg/ml), DCCD (1 mM), azide (0.1 mM) and rotenone (4 μM) under aerobic (**a**) and anaerobic conditions (**b**) for 5 days at pH 5.0 prior to CFU determination on 7H11 plates. Modified from Wade and Zhang [26].

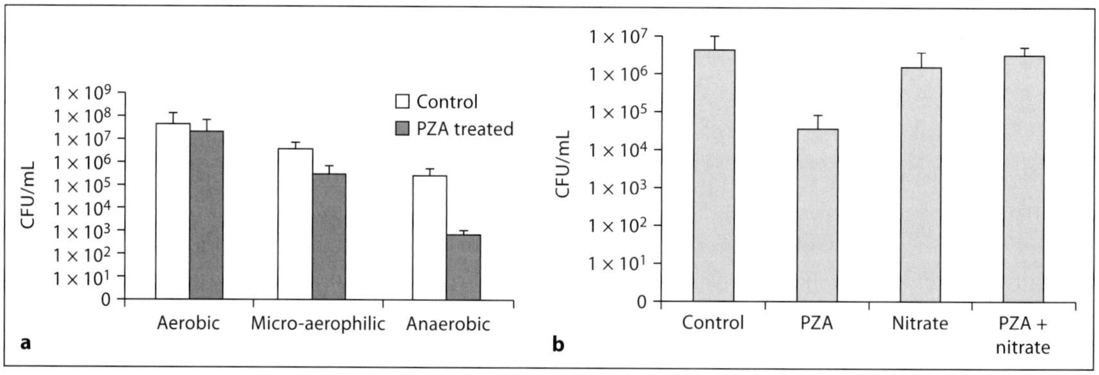


**Fig. 7.** Effect of aeration and nitrate on PZA activity against *M. tuberculosis*. Error bars represent standard deviations. Modified from Wade and Zhang [26]. **a** *M. tuberculosis* H37Ra cells from a 7-day-old culture were treated with PZA (100 μg/ml) under aerobic, micro-aerophilic or anaerobic conditions for 5 days at pH 5.0 prior to CFU determination on 7H11 plates. **b** The effect of nitrate on PZA activity under anaerobic conditions was assessed using *M. tuberculosis* H37Ra cells treated with PZA (100 μg/ml) and nitrate (10 mM) under anaerobic conditions for 5 days at pH 5.0 prior to CFU determination on 7H11 plates.

respiration with oxygen at aerobic conditions, which produces more energy using oxygen as electron acceptor. The preferential activity of PZA against tubercle bacilli under hypoxic or anaerobic conditions is presumably due to low energy production under such conditions so that the bacilli are more prone to the energy-depleting effect of PZA. By contrast, supplementation of alternative electron donor nitrate to supply energy under anaerobic conditions antagonized PZA activity (fig. 7b) [26]. While the energy inhibitors rotenone and azide still enhanced PZA activity under anaerobic conditions [26], DCCD which enhanced PZA activity under aerobic ambient oxygen conditions [22] failed to do so under anaerobic conditions (fig. 6b) [26]. It is worth noting that PZA acts differently from a general weak acid effect, since although energy inhibitors such as DCCD, rotenone or azide could increase the activity of both PZA and other weak acids, weak acids have no activity under anaerobic conditions where PZA had increased activity for *M. tuberculosis* [26, 29].

*Effects of Different Incubation Temperatures*

When the incubation temperature is in the range a little below 28°C, cultures of *M. tuberculosis* survive and must therefore metabolize, but do not multiply [30]. They would be expected to have low energy requirements decreasing as the temperature dropped towards 8°C when active

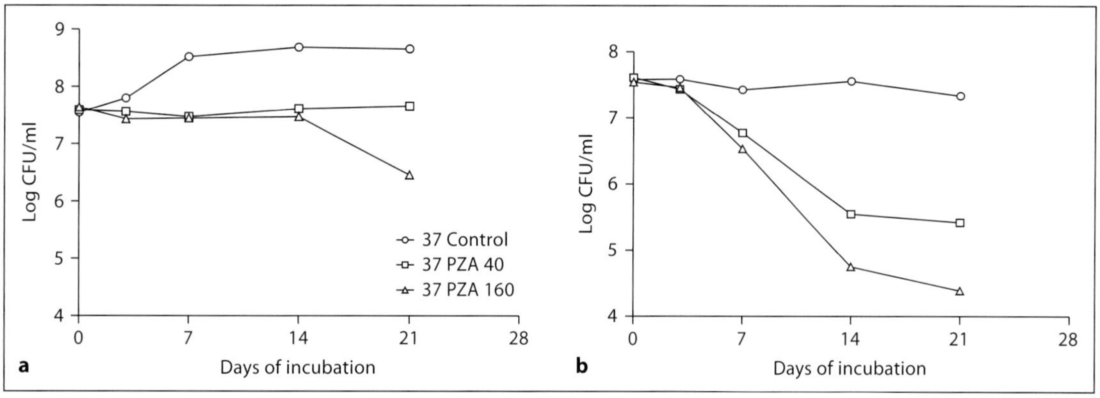


**Fig. 8.** Survival curves for 30-day static cultures of *M. tuberculosis* exposed to PZA at 40 or 160 μg/ml for 21 days at temperatures of 37°C (**a**) or at 22°C (**b**). Modified from Coleman et al. [30].

metabolism is minimal. When incubation temperatures were reduced from 37°C (fig. 8a) to 22°C (fig. 8b), there was a considerable increase in the bactericidal activity of PZA (fig. 8).

### Conditions That Affect PZA Activity Other than Those That Slow Bacterial Metabolism

*Certain Weak Acids Enhance PZA Activity*

Also predicted from our model, weak acids, which disrupt membrane energy, could enhance the activity of PZA. We have shown that weak acids including benzoic acid (2 mM), propyl hydroxybenzoic acid (1 mM) and sorbic acid (1 mM) could indeed enhance PZA activity in vitro [23, 29]. However, the weak acid enhancement of PZA activity is mainly seen for old bacilli and is generally not as effective as energy inhibitors, which could be a reflection of an additive effect between weak acids and PZA rather than a synergistic effect between energy inhibitors and PZA. However, some weak acids such as lactic acid and $C_{10}$ fatty acid had no effect on enhancing PZA activity [23]. Common clinically used weak acids aspirin and ibuprofen enhanced the activity of PZA in the mouse model of TB infection [31].

*Effects of Iron, Oxidative Stress and DNA Damage on PZA Activity*

The separation of PZA activity in vitro and in vivo prompted us to examine the effect of iron, which could potentially be elevated in local inflammatory lesions, on PZA activity in vitro. We found that iron enhanced PZA and POA activity against *M. tuberculosis* [32]. Other metal ions such as $Mg^{2+}$, $Ca^{2+}$ and $Zn^{2+}$ did not enhance the activity of PZA or POA [32]. Iron is known to enhance oxidative stress by producing reactive oxygen species, which can damage DNA and the membrane causing inhibition of cell division, a condition that allows PZA to act more effectively. Alternatively, iron has been shown to enhance the activity of PncA [17], which in turn results in increased PZA conversion to the active form POA, causing more effective killing. Sodium nitroprusside (1 mM), a reactive nitrogen nitric oxide producer, enhanced PZA activity (100 μg/ml) against old but not young cultures [25]. However, other oxidative stress agents such as menadione and hydrogen peroxide did not significantly enhance PZA activity. UV light, which is known to damage DNA and membranes causing inhibition of cell division and depleting membrane energy, respectively, has been shown to enhance the activity of PZA against *M. tuberculosis* [25, 29]. Since iron, UV and acid stress all cause oxidative damage to DNA, it is quite likely that oxidative damage may be related to PZA action. It is possible that DNA damage leads to growth inhibition or cell stasis, which could then potentiate PZA activity, but the detailed mechanisms remain to be determined.

*Effect of Mutations in Energy Production and NAD Pathways on PZA Susceptibility*

Based on the model of PZA [22], we predicted that energy production defects either due to chemical energy inhibitors or genetic mutations will lead to increased susceptibility to PZA. Indeed, this has proven to be true in the case of the diarylquinoline and PZA synergy reported subsequently [28, 33]. Furthermore, we found that *M. tuberculosis* mutants defective in energy production (made available by Tuberculosis Animal Research and Gene Evaluation Task

**Table 1.** PZA susceptibility of *M. tuberculosis* mutants with defect in energy metabolism

| Strain | Gene/function | MIC (at pH 5.5) µg/ml |
|---|---|---|
| CDC1551 | wild type | 25–50 |
| MT3240 | *nuoH*, NADH dehydrogenase | 10 |
| MT3246 | *nuoN*, NADH dehydrogenase | 10 |
| MT2968 | *fdhF*, formate dehydrogenase α-subunit | 10 |
| MT1199 | *narH*, nitrate reductase β-subunit | 10 |
| MT1372 | *pncB1*, nicotinate phosphoribosyltransferase | 10 |
| MT2345 | *yjcE*, Na/H exchanger | 10 |
| MT1058 | *kdpA*, potassium-transporting ATPase | 10 |
| MT48 | transcription regulator MarR family | 25–50 |
| MT3006 | ATP-binding protein | 25–50 |
| MT3981 | putative ATPase | 25–50 |

Force, Johns Hopkins University), had higher PZA susceptibility (MIC = 10 µg/ml) than the wild-type strain (MIC = 50 µg/ml; table 1) [S. Denken and Y. Zhang, unpubl. data]. These mutants include mutations in NADH dehydrogenase subunits H and N *(nuoH, nuoN)*, nitrate reductase *narH*, formate dehydrogenase *fdhF*, *kdpA* (potassium transport ATPase) and *yjcE* ($Na^+/H^+$ exchanger) involved in potassium and sodium ion transport, and *pncB1* (Rv1330c) involved in NAD recycling. NADH dehydrogenase *nuoH* and *nuoN* mutants, nitrate reductase *narH* mutant and formate dehydrogenase *fdhF* mutant, involved in energy production under anaerobic conditions, were also highly susceptible to PZA with a 5-fold reduction in MIC from 50 µg/ml in the parent strain to 10 µg/ml in the mutants. It is of interest to note that mutation in *pncB1*, involved in NAD recycling and energy metabolism, is also more susceptible to PZA. The observation that mutation in *kdpA* and *yjcE,* involved in potassium and sodium ion transport, respectively, caused higher susceptibility to PZA suggests that potassium and sodium ion homeostasis involved in pH regulation may be important for PZA action. However, mutations in transcription regulator *marR,* MT3006 (ATP-binding protein) and MT3981 (putative ATPase) did not have a significant effect on PZA susceptibility. The above findings are consistent with our current model of PZA [15, 22] and confirm that energy production pathways are important for PZA action. It is unlikely that all the above diverse energy production enzymes whose mutations cause increased PZA susceptibility represent targets of POA. It is more likely as we predicted in our model of PZA that since POA disrupts membrane energy [22], any defect in energy production pathways or ion homeostasis could enhance PZA activity as we have shown previously [22, 25].

Overall, PZA is a peculiar TB drug whose activity is influenced not only by concentration, but is also increased by local acid pH [11, 20], by a low metabolic state of the bacilli and by other factors such as hypoxia and iron concentration. Of particular importance, factors that reduce the metabolic activity of bacilli tend to enhance the activity of PZA, and PZA activity is increased when bacterial metabolic activity is decreased.

## Target of Pyrazinamide

There is controversy about the target of PZA. This has been suggested to be fatty acid synthase I (Fas-I) in a study using *Mycobacterium smegmatis* and 5-Cl-PZA [34]. However, no mutations in Fas-I have been found in PZA-resistant *M. tuberculosis* strains. The proposition that Fas-I is the target of PZA in *M. tuberculosis* was questioned by Boshoff et al. [35] who showed that Fas-I is the target of 5-Cl-PZA but not of PZA. In fact, recent studies have shown that 5-Cl-PZA and PZA act very differently in that 5-Cl-PZA is converted by PzaA, a second PZase enzyme not related to PncA, to less active 5-Cl-POA [36] and is not converted by PncA, the enzyme involved in PZA conversion to POA [37]. Overexpression of Fas-I (target of 5-Cl-PZA) and PzaA (involved in inactivating 5-Cl-PZA) caused 5-Cl-PZA resistance in *M. smegmatis.* However, overexpression of Fas-I in *M. tuberculosis* was toxic. In contrast, overexpression of PzaA in *M. smegmatis* caused increased PZA susceptibility. In addition, the study aimed at identifying the target of PZA using a transposon mutagenesis approach to isolate mutants resistant to POA and 5-Cl-PZA was unsuccessful. The studies on Fas-I as a possible target of PZA in cell-free assays or in whole cells are not convincing as extremely high concentrations of PZA or POA above the physiological concentrations were used [38, 39]. The fact that no POA-resistant mutants can be isolated in vitro [40] makes the identification of a PZA target difficult. Clinical isolates of *M. tuberculosis* resistant to PZA are susceptible to POA [40]. It is unclear whether the inability to obtain a POA-resistant mutant is because the target mutant is non-viable or because POA affects many targets in the cell so that no mutant can be isolated. Our current model (fig. 1) can best explain the various unusual features of PZA, including the requirement of acid pH for drug activity [20], relationship between pH and PZA MIC [21], preferential activity against old non-growing bacilli over growing bacilli [21], unique susceptibility of PZA against *M. tuberculosis* [20], higher activity of PZA under hypoxic and anaerobic conditions than in normoxia [26], enhancement of PZA activity by energy inhibitors [22, 25], UV [25] and iron [32] and weak acid enhancement of PZA activity [25]. Other models including the Fas-I target model cannot explain all these unusual features. However, the real targets of POA remain to be identified.

## Pyrazinamide Resistance

*Mechanism of Resistance*

PZA-resistant *M. tuberculosis* strains lose PZase/nicotinamidase activity [41]; this monomeric enzyme appears to contain manganese and ferrous iron at a 1:1 ratio [17]. There is a good correlation between loss of PZase activity and PZA resistance in *M. tuberculosis* [41–43]. Mutations in the *pncA* gene encoding nicotinamidase/PZase are the major mechanism of PZA resistance [16, 40]. The nature of the identified *pncA* mutations is largely missense mutations causing amino acid substitutions, and in some cases nucleotide insertions or deletions, nonsense mutations in the *pncA* structural gene or in the putative promoter region of *pncA* (e.g. at –11 position) [40, 44]. The *pncA* mutations are highly diverse and scattered along the gene [40]. The diverse nature of *pncA* mutations is unique to PZA resistance and is not understood. The role of various *pncA* mutations in affecting PncA enzyme activity and contributing to PZA resistance was evaluated recently by expressing the mutant PncA enzymes and assessing their enzyme activity [45]. It was found that mutations causing varying PncA enzyme activities in general correlated with the level of PZA resistance, but were not sufficient to explain a high variability of PZA resistance levels [45]. The authors suggested that complementary mechanisms for PZA resistance with mutations in *pncA* might play a role [45]. However, inaccurate PZA susceptibility testing may underlie some of the discrepancies between PZase activity and levels of PZA resistance. It would be of interest to validate the proposal of complementary mechanisms of PZA resistance with *pncA* mutations by transformation studies with the mutant PncA with varying enzyme activity in the background of a null PZase *M. tuberculosis* background.

Despite the highly diverse and scattered distribution of *pncA* mutations, there is some degree of clustering in 3 regions of the PncA, 3–17, 61–85 and 132–142 [40]. These regions happen to contain catalytic sites and metal-binding sites of the PZase enzyme [18, 46]. The crystal structure of *Pyrococcus horikoshii* PncA (37% identity with *M. tuberculosis* PncA) has provided some insight into how *pncA* mutations in *M. tuberculosis* might cause PZA resistance [46]. The 3 regions where *pncA* mutations appear to cluster correspond to 3 of the 4 loops that contribute to the scaffold of the active site. Mutations at C138, D8, K96, D49, H51 and H71 modify the active site triad and metal-binding site. Residues F13, L19, H57 (position of characteristic mutation of H57D in *M. bovis*), W68, G97, Y103, I113, A134 and H137 line up the active site, and mutations at these positions are also predicted to cause loss of enzyme activity. Mutations at Q10, D12, S104 and T142 are predicted to disrupt hydrogen-bonding interactions between the side chain and main chain atoms. Loss of PZase activity due to mutations at other sites can be attributed to potential perturbation of the active site or disruption of the protein core. These predictions need to be confirmed when the structure of the *M. tuberculosis* PncA is determined. Recently, the crystal structure of *M. tuberculosis* PncA was solved (http://www.ncbi.nlm.nih.gov/Structure/mmdb/mmdbsrv.cgi?uid = 80790). The wild-type *M. tuberculosis* PncA structure was found to be a monomer that contains manganous and ferrous ions. It would be of interest to determine how diverse mutant PncAs affect PZA activation and cause PZA resistance.

Most PZA-resistant *M. tuberculosis* strains (up to 97%) can be accounted for by mutations in *pncA* [15, 47]. However, a few PZA-resistant strains do not have *pncA* mutations; one such type is PZase negative with high levels of resistance [48–50], indicating that mutations in an undefined *pncA* regulatory gene may be involved in PZA resistance. Another type of such strains has low-level PZA resistance and positive PZase activity, presumably due to alternative mechanisms of resistance. We have found a few such strains, i.e. DHM444 [40], 9739 [48] with low-level PZA resistance (MIC = 200–300 μg/ml with resistance cut-off of 100 μg/ml PZA). The mechanism of resistance in such strains remains to be determined. The clinical significance of the rare low-level PZA-resistant strains is unclear.

*PZA Susceptibility Testing*

Although PZA is a critical drug for the treatment of TB, PZA susceptibility testing is not commonly performed due to various problems [15, 51], such as requirement of an acid pH which could inhibit the growth of some clinical isolates, and an inoculum effect that can inadvertently neutralize medium pH caused by higher inocula [21]. Therefore, most drug resistance surveys do not have information on PZA resistance. The current PZA susceptibility testing in BACTEC 460 or

**Table 2.** Relationship between medium pH and PZA MIC

| pH | PZA MIC, μg/ml |
|---|---|
| 4.5 | 5 |
| 5.0 | 16 |
| 5.5 | 50 |
| 5.6 | 63 |
| 5.8 | 100 |
| 6.0 | 156 |
| 6.6 | 625 |
| 6.8 | 992 |
| 7.0 | 1,563 |

The PZA MICs were theoretical values calculated using the Henderson-Hasselbalch equation based on PZA MIC being 50 μg/ml at pH 5.5. Adapted from Zhang et al. [21].

MGIT 960 uses a slightly acidic pH 6.0 and the MIC cut-off for resistance of 100 μg/ml (Becton Dickinson). However, PZA concentration of 100 μg/ml at pH 6.0 as a resistance cut-off seems a bit too low, which can cause a false resistance problem [52]. Based on the Henderson-Hasselbalch equation, the MIC for PZA at pH 6.0 should be about 150–200 μg/ml instead of 100 μg/ml (table 2) [21]. It may be safe to increase the PZA resistance cut-off to 200–300 μg/ml. In fact, Heifets [53] suggested the use of 300 μg/ml PZA as resistance cut-off. Unlike drug susceptibility testing for other TB drugs, the levels of PZA resistance are difficult to determine because of the problem with PZA susceptibility testing. Due to the problems of phenotype-based PZA susceptibility testing, sequencing of the *pncA* gene instead of phenotype testing has been suggested for more rapid and reliable detection of PZA resistance [54] (see below).

A method is under development [Coleman and Mitchison, in preparation] in which the test *M. tuberculosis* strain is inoculated onto Lowenstein-Jensen medium slopes buffered at pH 6.0 and containing a range of PZA concentrations. These are then left at room temperature protected from light for 14 days and then incubated at 37°C. PZA is actively bactericidal during the incubation at room temperature, which results in better separation of sensitive and resistant strains by a concentration of 150 or 200 μg/ml PZA, a concentration that agrees well with the prediction from the Henderson-Hasselbalch equation (table 2) [21]. All resistant strains tested have MICs well above 200 μg/ml PZA. This test is too time-consuming for routine use but is probably more accurate than other methods, and above all, this finding is consistent with our model that PZA is more active when bacterial metabolism is reduced.

*Nicotinamide Test*

Since our review that emphasized the need to evaluate the use of nicotinamide at neutral pH as a surrogate for PZA susceptibility testing [55] was published in 2003 [15], new recently published studies suggest that nicotinamide at 500 μg/ml at neutral pH provides a useful susceptibility testing for PZA [56, 57]. This nicotinamide-based test at neutral pH was recently used together with a nitrate reductase assay [56, 58] and a malachite green microtube assay for PZA susceptibility testing with good results [56–58]. Both the nitrate reductase and malachite green microtube assays showed sensitivities of 93.75% and specificities of 97.67% [58]. The nicotinamide-based colorimetric assays appear to be promising and inexpensive alternatives for detection of PZA resistance in resource-limiting countries. More studies are needed to evaluate these inexpensive assays with nicotinamide at neutral pH for the detection of PZA resistance in larger sample sizes.

However, like any culture-based drug susceptibility test, phenotype-based susceptibility testing with PZA or nicotinamide is very time-consuming due to the slow growth of mycobacteria. Similarly, although the Wayne PZase test has been used as a correlate of PZA susceptibility [42, 43], it generally has less sensitivity for detection of PZA resistance compared with the gold standard BACTEC 460, MGIT 960 or sequencing of the *pncA* gene [59] and has the same drawback of culture-based drug susceptibility testing as it requires culture. Since most PZA-resistant strains have *pncA* mutations, identification of *pncA* mutations by molecular methods such as DNA sequencing, line probe assay [60] and micro-array [61, 62] has been used for detection of PZA resistance. Because sequencing has become more affordable, it may now be economical to use *pncA* sequencing as a rapid molecular test for detecting PZA resistance in the clinic laboratories. Indeed, there is recent interest to offer *pncA* sequencing as a clinical diagnostic test of PZA resistance at Mayo Clinic [N. Wengenack, pers. commun.].

*Frequency of PZA Resistance in Multidrug Resistance Disease*

It is worth noting that PZA resistance in multidrug-resistant (MDR) TB seems to be quite high, ranging from 49% in Thailand [59], 50% in Central Africa [63], 52% in South Africa [64], 53% in Japan [65], to up to 85% in India [47]. Rapid detection of PZA resistance in MDR-TB may be important for devising appropriate treatment for such patients. Future studies are needed to determine the role of PZA resistance in the treatment outcome of MDR-TB patients.

### Future Perspectives and Implications of Pyrazinamide for New Persister Drug Development

PZA is an important frontline drug that plays a unique role in our fight against TB. The increasing emergence and outbreaks of MDR and extensively drug-resistant TB calls for urgent development of new drugs [66, 67]. It is increasingly recognized that the new drugs should not only be active for drug-resistant TB, but also more importantly should shorten the current 6-month therapy [68–71]. Developing new drugs that have activity for persister TB bacteria is critical for shortening TB therapy. Although there are currently several drug candidates in clinical development [71, 72], none can replace PZA, and all the drug candidates, including the highly potent TMC207, will have to be used with PZA since any drug combination without PZA is invariably inferior in animal studies [7, 8, 28, 73]. PZA is a prototype antipersister drug that plays an irreplaceable role in any new drug combination. Indeed, in a recent study on the sterilizing activities of new drug regimens in the mouse model, all regimens contained PZA [74]. Improved understanding of how PZA works is important for the design of new drugs that further shorten the therapy. In addition, there is interest to improve PZA activity by adding agents like weak acids such as aspirin and ibuprofen to enhance PZA activity [31]. Since *M. tuberculosis* does not develop resistance to POA (the active form of PZA) [40], there is also interest to use POA nanoparticle delivery to the lung for improved treatment of MDR/extensively drug-resistant TB and drug-susceptible TB [75].

### Acknowledgements

The PZA work in the Zhang laboratory was largely supported by NIH grant R01AI44063. We apologize to our colleagues whose work could not be cited due to space limitations. The work reported by Mitchison was supported by a grant from Tibotec Pharmaceuticals.

### References

1 British Thoracic and Tuberculosis Association: Short-course chemotherapy in pulmonary tuberculosis. Lancet 1976;ii:1102–1104.

2 British Thoracic Association: A controlled trial of six months chemotherapy in pulmonary tuberculosis. Second report: results during the 24 months after the end of chemotherapy. Am Rev Respir Dis 1982;126:460–462.

3 Fox W, Ellard GA, Mitchison DA: Studies on the treatment of tuberculosis undertaken by the British Medical Research Council tuberculosis units, 1946–1986, with relevant subsequent publications. Int J Tuberc Lung Dis 1999;3:S231–S279.

4 McCune RM Jr, McDermott W, Tompsett R: The fate of *Mycobacterium tuberculosis* in mouse tissues as determined by the microbial enumeration technique. II. The conversion of tuberculous infection to the latent state by the administration of pyrazinamide and a companion drug. J Exp Med 1956;104:763–802.

5 McCune RM Jr, Tompsett R: Fate of *Mycobacterium tuberculosis* in mouse tissues as determined by the microbial enumeration technique. I. The persistence of drug-susceptible tubercle bacilli in the tissues despite prolonged antimicrobial therapy. J Exp Med 1956;104:737–762.

6 Mitchison DA: The action of antituberculosis drugs in short course chemotherapy. Tubercle 1985;66:219–225.

7 Nuermberger E, Tyagi S, Tasneen R, Williams KN, Almeida D, Rosenthal I, Grosset JH: Powerful bactericidal and sterilizing activity of a regimen containing pa-824, moxifloxacin, and pyrazinamide in a murine model of tuberculosis. Antimicrob Agents Chemother 2008;52:1522–1524.

8 Rosenthal IM, Zhang M, Williams KN, Peloquin CA, Tyagi S, Vernon AA, Bishai WR, Chaisson RE, Grosset JH, Nuermberger EL: Daily dosing of rifapentine cures tuberculosis in three months or less in the murine model. PLoS Med 2007;4:e344.

9 Veziris N, Ibrahim M, Lounis N, Chauffour A, Truffot-Pernot C, Andries K, Jarlier V: A once-weekly R207910-containing regimen exceeds activity of the standard daily regimen in murine tuberculosis. Am J Respir Crit Care Med 2009;179:75–79.

10 Tarshis MS, Weed WA Jr: Lack of significant in vitro sensitivity of *Mycobacterium tuberculosis* to pyrazinamide on three different solid media. Am Rev Tuberculosis 1953;67:391–395.

11 McDermott W, Tompsett R: Activation of pyrazinamide and nicotinamide in acidic environment in vitro. Am Rev Tuberculosis 1954;70:748–754.

12 Heifets LB, Lindholm-Levy PJ: Is pyrazinamide bactericidal against *Mycobacterium tuberculosis?* Am Rev Respir Dis 1990;141:250–252.

13 McCune RM, Feldmann FM, Lambert HP, McDermott W: Microbial persistence. I. The capacity of tubercle bacilli to survive sterilization in mouse tissues. J Exp Med 1966;123:445–468.

14 McCune RM, Feldmann FM, McDermott W: Microbial persistence. II. Characteristics of the sterile state of tubercle bacilli. J Exp Med 1966;123:469–486.

15 Zhang Y, Mitchison D: The curious characteristics of pyrazinamide: a review. Int J Tuberc Lung Dis 2003;7:6–21.

16 Scorpio A, Zhang Y: Mutations in *pncA*, a gene encoding pyrazinamidase/nicotinamidase, cause resistance to the antituberculous drug pyrazinamide in tubercle bacillus. Nat Med 1996;2:662–667.

17 Zhang H, Deng JY, Bi LJ, Zhou YF, Zhang ZP, Zhang CG, Zhang Y, Zhang XE: Characterization of *Mycobacterium tuberculosis* nicotinamidase/pyrazinamidase. FEBS J 2008;275:753–762.

18 Fyfe PK, Rao VA, Zemla A, Cameron S, Hunter WN: Specificity and mechanism of *Acinetobacter baumanii* nicotinamidase: implications for activation of the front-line tuberculosis drug pyrazinamide. Angew Chem Int Ed Engl 2009;48:9176–9179.

19 Seiner DR, Hegde SS, Blanchard JS: Kinetics and inhibition of nicotinamidase from *Mycobacterium tuberculosis*. Biochemistry 2010, E-pub ahead of print.

20 Zhang Y, Scorpio A, Nikaido H, Sun Z: Role of acid pH and deficient efflux of pyrazinoic acid in unique susceptibility of *Mycobacterium tuberculosis* to pyrazinamide. J Bacteriol 1999;181:2044–2049.

21 Zhang Y, Permar S, Sun Z: Conditions that may affect the results of susceptibility testing of *Mycobacterium tuberculosis* to pyrazinamide. J Med Microbiol 2002;51:42–49.

22 Zhang Y, Wade MM, Scorpio A, Zhang H, Sun Z: Mode of action of pyrazinamide: disruption of *Mycobacterium tuberculosis* membrane transport and energetics by pyrazinoic acid. J Antimicrob Chemother 2003;52:790–795.

23 Huang Q, Chen ZF, Li YY, Zhang Y, Ren Y, Fu Z, Xu SQ: Nutrient-starved incubation conditions enhance pyrazinamide activity against *Mycobacterium tuberculosis*. Chemotherapy 2007;53:338–343.

24 Hu Y, Coates AR, Mitchison DA: Sterilising action of pyrazinamide in models of dormant and rifampicin-tolerant *Mycobacterium tuberculosis*. Int J Tuberc Lung Dis 2006;10:317–322.

25 Wade MM, Zhang Y: Effects of weak acids, UV and proton motive force inhibitors on pyrazinamide activity against *Mycobacterium tuberculosis* in vitro. J Antimicrob Chemother 2006;58:936–941.

26 Wade MM, Zhang Y: Anaerobic incubation conditions enhance pyrazinamide activity against *Mycobacterium tuberculosis*. J Med Microbiol 2004;53:769–773.

27 Betts J, Lukey P, Robb L, McAdam R, Duncan K: Evaluation of a nutrient starvation model of *Mycobacterium tuberculosis* persistence by gene and protein expression profiling. Mol Microbiol 2002;43:717–731.

28 Andries K, Verhasselt P, Guillemont J, Gohlmann H, Neefs J, Winkler H, Van Gestel J, Timmerman P, Zhu M, Lee E, Williams P, de Chaffoy D, Huitric E, Hoffner S, Cambau E, Truffot-Pernot C, Lounis N, Jarlier V: A diarylquinoline drug active on the ATP synthase of *Mycobacterium tuberculosis*. Science 2005;307:223–227.

29 Gu P, Constantino L, Zhang Y: Enhancement of the antituberculosis activity of weak acids by inhibitors of energy metabolism but not by anaerobiosis suggests that weak acids act differently from the front-line tuberculosis drug pyrazinamide. J Med Microbiol 2008;57:1129–1134.

30 Coleman D, Waddell S, Mitchison DA: Effects of low incubation temperatures on the bactericidal activity of anti-tuberculosis drugs. J Antimicrob Chemother 2011;66:146–150.

31 Byrne ST, Denkin SM, Zhang Y: Aspirin and ibuprofen enhance pyrazinamide treatment of murine tuberculosis. J Antimicrob Chemother 2007;59:313–316.

32 Somoskovi A, Wade MM, Sun Z, Zhang Y: Iron enhances the antituberculous activity of pyrazinamide. J Antimicrob Chemother 2004;53:192–196.

33 Ibrahim M, Andries K, Lounis N, Chauffour A, Truffot-Pernot C, Jarlier V, Veziris N: Synergistic activity of R207910 combined with pyrazinamide against murine tuberculosis. Antimicrob Agents Chemother 2007;51:1011–1015.

34 Zimhony O, Cox JS, Welch JT, Vilcheze C, Jacobs WR Jr: Pyrazinamide inhibits the eukaryotic-like fatty acid synthetase I (FasI) of *Mycobacterium tuberculosis*. Nat Med 2000;6:1043–1047.

35 Boshoff HI, Mizrahi V, Barry CE 3rd: Effects of pyrazinamide on fatty acid synthesis by whole mycobacterial cells and purified fatty acid synthase I. J Bacteriol 2002;184:2167–2172.

36 Cynamon MH, Speirs RJ, Welch JT: In vitro antimycobacterial activity of 5-chloropyrazinamide. Antimicrob Agents Chemother 1998;42:462–463.

37 Baughn AD, Deng J, Vilcheze C, Riestra A, Welch JT, Jacobs WR Jr, Zimhony O: Mutually exclusive genotypes for pyrazinamide and 5-chloropyrazinamide resistance reveal a potential resistance proofing strategy. Antimicrob Agents Chemother 2010;54:5323–5328.

38 Ngo SC, Zimhony O, Chung WJ, Sayahi H, Jacobs WR Jr, Welch JT: Inhibition of isolated *Mycobacterium tuberculosis* fatty acid synthase I by pyrazinamide analogs. Antimicrob Agents Chemother 2007;51:2430–2435.

39 Zimhony O, Vilcheze C, Arai M, Welch JT, Jacobs WR Jr: Pyrazinoic acid and its n-propyl ester inhibit fatty acid synthase type I in replicating tubercle bacilli. Antimicrob Agents Chemother 2007;51:752–754.

40 Scorpio A, Lindholm-Levy P, Heifets L, Gilman R, Siddiqi S, Cynamon M, Zhang Y: Characterization of *pncA* mutations in pyrazinamide-resistant *Mycobacterium tuberculosis*. Antimicrob Agents Chemother 1997;41:540–543.

41 Konno K, Feldmann FM, McDermott W: Pyrazinamide susceptibility and amidase activity of tubercle bacilli. Am Rev Respir Dis 1967;95:461–469.

42 McClatchy JK, Tsang AY, Cernich MS: Use of pyrazinamidase activity on *Mycobacterium tuberculosis* as a rapid method for determination of pyrazinamide susceptibility. Antimicrob Agents Chemother 1981;20:556–557.

43 Trivedi SS, Desai SG: Pyrazinamidase activity of *Mycobacterium tuberculosis* – a test of sensitivity to pyrazinamide. Tubercle 1987;68:221–224.

44 Zhang Y, Telenti A: Genetics of drug resistance in *Mycobacterium tuberculosis;* in Hatfull G, Jacobs WR (eds): Molecular Genetics of Mycobacteria. Washington, ASM Press, 2000, pp 235–254.

45 Sheen P, Ferrer P, Gilman RH, Lopez-Llano J, Fuentes P, Valencia E, Zimic MJ: Effect of pyrazinamidase activity on pyrazinamide resistance in *Mycobacterium tuberculosis*. Tuberculosis (Edinb) 2009;89:109–113.

46 Du X, Wang W, Kim R, Yakota H, Nguyen H, Kim SH: Crystal structure and mechanism of catalysis of a pyrazinamidase from *Pyrococcus horikoshii*. Biochemistry 2001;40:14166–14172.

47 Shenai S, Rodrigues C, Sadani M, Sukhadia N, Mehta A: Comparison of phenotypic and genotypic methods for pyrazinamide susceptibility testing. Indian J Tuberculosis 2009;56:82–90.

48 Cheng SJ, Thibert L, Sanchez T, Heifets L, Zhang Y: *pncA* mutations as a major mechanism of pyrazinamide resistance in *Mycobacterium tuberculosis:* spread of a monoresistant strain in Quebec, Canada. Antimicrob Agents Chemother 2000;44:528–532.

49 Lemaitre N, Sougakoff W, Truffot-Pernot C, Jarlier V: Characterization of new mutations in pyrazinamide-resistant strains of *Mycobacterium tuberculosis* and identification of conserved regions important for the catalytic activity of the pyrazinamidase PncA. Antimicrob Agents Chemother 1999;43:1761–1763.

50 Marttila HJ, Marjamaki M, Vyshnevskaya E, Vyshnevskiy BI, Otten TF, Vasilyef AV, Viljanen MK: *pncA* mutations in pyrazinamide-resistant *Mycobacterium tuberculosis* isolates from northwestern russia. Antimicrob Agents Chemother 1999;43:1764–1766.

51 Hewlett D Jr, Horn DL, Alfalla C: Drug-resistant tuberculosis: inconsistent results of pyrazinamide susceptibility testing. JAMA 1995;273:916–917.

52 Pandey S, Newton S, Upton A, Roberts S, Drinkovic D: Characterisation of *pncA* mutations in clinical *Mycobacterium tuberculosis* isolates in New Zealand. Pathology 2009;41:582–584.

53 Heifets L: Susceptibility testing of *Mycobacterium tuberculosis* to pyrazinamide. J Med Microbiol 2002;51:11–12.

54 Dormandy J, Somoskovi A, Kreiswirth BN, Driscoll JR, Ashkin D, Salfinger M: Discrepant results between pyrazinamide susceptibility testing by the reference BACTEC 460TB method and *pncA* DNA sequencing in patients infected with multidrug-resistant W-Beijing *Mycobacterium tuberculosis* strains. Chest 2007;131:497–501.

55 Brander E: A simple way of detecting pyrazinamide resistance. Tubercle 1972;53:128–131.

56 Martin A, Cubillos-Ruiz A, Von Groll A, Del Portillo P, Portaels F, Palomino JC: Nitrate reductase assay for the rapid detection of pyrazinamide resistance in *Mycobacterium tuberculosis* using nicotinamide. J Antimicrob Chemother 2008;61:123–127.

57 Martin A, Takiff H, Vandamme P, Swings J, Palomino JC, Portaels F: A new rapid and simple colorimetric method to detect pyrazinamide resistance in *Mycobacterium tuberculosis* using nicotinamide. J Antimicrob Chemother 2006;58:327–331.

58 Mirabal NC, Yzquierdo SL, Lemus D, Madruga M, Milian Y, Echemendia M, Takiff H, Martin A, Van der Stuyf P, Palomino JC, Montoro E: Evaluation of colorimetric methods using nicotinamide for rapid detection of pyrazinamide resistance in *Mycobacterium tuberculosis*. J Clin Microbiol 2010;48:2729–2733.

59 Jonmalung J, Prammananan T, Leechawengwongs M, Chaiprasert A: Surveillance of pyrazinamide susceptibility among multidrug-resistant *Mycobacterium tuberculosis* isolates from Siriraj Hospital, Thailand. BMC Microbiol 2010;10:223.

60 Sekiguchi J, Nakamura T, Miyoshi-Akiyama T, Kirikae F, Kobayashi I, Augustynowicz-Kopec E, Zwolska Z, Morita K, Suetake T, Yoshida H, Kato S, Mori T, Kirikae T: Development and evaluation of a line probe assay for rapid identification of *pncA* mutations in pyrazinamide-resistant *Mycobacterium tuberculosis* strains. J Clin Microbiol 2007;45:2802–2807.

61 Wade MM, Volokhov D, Peredelchuk M, Chizhikov V, Zhang Y: Accurate mapping of mutations of pyrazinamide-resistant *Mycobacterium tuberculosis* strains with a scanning-frame oligonucleotide microarray. Diagn Microbiol Infect Dis 2004;49:89–97.
62 Denkin S, Volokhov D, Chizhikov V, Zhang Y: Microarray-based *pncA* genotyping of pyrazinamide-resistant strains of *Mycobacterium tuberculosis.* J Med Microbiol 2005;54:1127–1131.
63 Minime-Lingoupou F, Pierre-Audigier C, Kassa-Kelembho E, Barilone N, Zandanga G, Rauzier J, Cadet-Daniel V, Le Faou A, Gicquel B: Rapid identification of multidrug-resistant tuberculosis isolates in treatment failure or relapse patients in Bangui, Central African Republic. Int J Tuberc Lung Dis 2010;14:782–785.
64 Mphahlele M, Syre H, Valvatne H, Stavrum R, Mannsaker T, Muthivhi T, Weyer K, Fourie PB, Grewal HM: Pyrazinamide resistance among South African multidrug-resistant *Mycobacterium tuberculosis* isolates. J Clin Microbiol 2008;46:3459–3464.
65 Ando H, Mitarai S, Kondo Y, Suetake T, Sekiguchi JI, Kato S, Mori T, Kirikae T: Pyrazinamide resistance in multidrug-resistant *Mycobacterium tuberculosis* isolates in Japan. Clin Microbiol Infect 2010;16:1164–1168.
66 WHO: Anti-tuberculosis drug resistance in the world, report No 4. Geneva, WHO, 2008.
67 WHO: XDR-TB, extensively drug-resistant tuberculosis. 2006. http://www.who.int/tb/xdr/en/index.html.
68 GATB: Tuberculosis. Scientific blueprint for tuberculosis drug development. Tuberculosis (Edinb) 2001;81(suppl 1):1–52.
69 Mitchison D: The search for new sterilizing anti-tuberculosis drugs. Front Biosci 2004;9:1059–1072.
70 Zhang Y: The magic bullets and tuberculosis drug targets. Annu Rev Pharmacol Toxicol 2005;45:529–564.
71 Yew WW, Cynamon M, Zhang Y: Emerging drugs for the treatment of tuberculosis. Expert Opin Emerg Drugs 2011;16:1–21.
72 Nuermberger EL, Spigelman MK, Yew WW: Current development and future prospects in chemotherapy of tuberculosis. Respirology 2010;15:764–778.
73 Tasneen R, Tyagi S, Williams K, Grosset J, Nuermberger E: Enhanced bactericidal activity of rifampin and/or pyrazinamide when combined with PA-824 in a murine model of tuberculosis. Antimicrob Agents Chemother 2008;52:3664–3668.
74 Andries K, Gevers T, Lounis N: Bactericidal potencies of new regimens are not predictive of their sterilizing potencies in a murine model of tuberculosis. Antimicrob Agents Chemother 2010;54:4540–4544.
75 Mitchison DA, Fourie PB: The near future: Improving the activity of rifamycins and pyrazinamide. Tuberculosis (Edinb) 2010;90:177–181.

Ying Zhang
W. Harry Feinstone Department of Molecular Microbiology and Immunology
Bloomberg School of Public Health, Johns Hopkins University
Baltimore, MD 21205 (USA)
Tel. +1 410 614 2975, E-Mail yzhang@jhsph.edu

Chapter 6

Donald PR, van Helden PD (eds): Antituberculosis Chemotherapy.
Prog Respir Res. Basel, Karger, 2011, vol 40, pp 44–50

# Experience with Phase III Clinical Trials of Antituberculosis Drugs and Regimens: Conclusions and Lessons for the Future

Amina Jindani

Division of Clinical Science, St. George's, University of London, London, UK

**Abstract**

Phase III clinical trials of new drugs and regimens for tuberculosis treatment are essential for determining efficacy, including cure and relapse rates. Regulations governing the conduct of clinical trials are increasing in rigour and complexity, resulting in exponential and restrictive increases in costs and making it very difficult for academic institutions to conduct appropriately powered trials. In recent years, a number of 'for-profit' organizations have become established that claim capacity to conduct every aspect of a trial from feasibility studies to complete trial management. Engaging the services of such organizations increases trial costs. Financial demands of participating centres also continue to increase as they undertake trial activities as a means of fund-raising for their organizations. Increasing the complexity of regulations poses extra demands on potential research centres, limiting the number able to participate and, consequently, reducing the availability of therapeutic options for patients in resource-poor countries. The trend of increasing regulation, complex record keeping and increases in costs complicates the execution of phase III trials, slows efficient patient enrolment and delays the completion of essential trials of new drugs and regimens.

Copyright © 2011 S. Karger AG, Basel

Of all stages in drug development, from discovery to marketing, the phase III clinical trial is the critical determinant of long-term safety, efficacy and marketability of the drug. This is especially so in tuberculosis where the efficacy of tuberculosis drugs and regimens is finally assessed on relapse rates after completing treatment. Further, tuberculosis treatment requires the combination of more than one drug at any one time as monotherapy quickly results in resistance to the drug given. Thus, even if a drug is safe and efficacious, its marketability is determined by the fact that it must be given in combination with drugs which are also safe and efficacious and with which there are no interactions that will reduce the efficacy of any one of those drugs. These considerations, combined with the fact that tuberculosis is a disease of poverty, resulted in a lack of interest by pharmaceutical companies and low investment in drug discovery. Thus, the last drug to be brought into use specifically for tuberculosis was rifampicin which was marketed some 40 years ago.

Once the sterilizing efficacy of rifampicin and pyrazinamide had been demonstrated in a series of rigorously conducted phase III clinical trials [1], the treatment of tuberculosis was reduced to a 6-month regimen of almost 100% efficacy and a cost of approximately USD 20. As sanatoria closed, and treatment became completely ambulatory, tuberculosis eradication appeared to be an achievable goal. This may also have contributed to the lack of investment in further drug development.

Sadly, this fairy tale has not had a 'happy ever after' ending. The current incidence and prevalence of tuberculosis, in the 22 high-burden countries, have overwhelmed National Tuberculosis Control Programmes (NTPs), and it is estimated that 1 person dies of tuberculosis every 20 s.

With this in mind, in September 2009, 189 nations adopted the UN Millennium Declaration [2], one of the targets (6c.9) of which is to halt and begin to reverse the tuberculosis incidence by 2015. This is to be achieved through the development of a number of new tools including new drugs and drug regimens capable of reducing the treatment from 6 months to 1 month or less. Since then, several academic organizations and pharmaceutical companies have engaged in the search for new, effective drugs, and the drug development pipeline currently has a number of extremely promising candidates [3].

However, from the time of discovery of the rifamycins to the present, the drug development process has undergone significant changes all purporting to ensure the safety of participants in the 4 clinical phases of drug development. These changes have not only lengthened the time taken to bring a drug to market, they have also hugely increased costs and complexity for drug development as well as clinical trials.

## Previous Experience

Since the publication of the randomized controlled trial (RCT) of streptomycin [4], RCTs have become the gold standard for the clinical evaluation of single drugs and regimens.

Early trials were carried out by the US Veterans Administration, the US Public Health Services and later by the British Medical Research Council (BMRC) [1]. It was these BMRC trials that led to the abandonment of monotherapy, establishment of ambulatory treatment, definition of the initial intensive phase and, most significantly, reduction of treatment duration from 18 to 6 months.

The current 6-month regimen for tuberculosis treatment was developed through a series of phase III RCTs conducted by many academic institutions. These trials were carried out without formal consent from the patients who were invited to participate (and could refuse); trials were completed expeditiously and results published in peer-reviewed journals. Results were made available to agencies responsible for establishing treatment guidelines for tuberculosis, such as the World Health Organization (WHO) and NTPs of individual countries, and treatment changes were made based on trial results.

In the case of the BMRC trials, patients were always followed up until sputum culture remained negative for a period of 2 years following treatment cessation. Those who relapsed were retreated until they became culture negative again. Thus, good clinical practice (GCP) was the cornerstone of these trials.

The first short-course chemotherapy trial [5] was carried out in 42 centres in Kenya, Uganda, Tanzania and Zambia. At that time, the only requirement was that patients agree to remain in hospital for 6 months and return for monthly assessments for another 2 years. The retention rate, of a sample size exceeding 1,000 patients scattered over 4 countries in Africa, was 85%. This was all the more surprising because the retention rate was after treatment when patients were fully recovered and had no need to attend for further examination. Subsequent trials showed similar high post-treatment retention rates [Andrew Nunn, pers. commun.]. If patients decided to leave hospital earlier, arrangements could very often be made for them to receive the remainder of their treatment as outpatients and be supervised by a responsible person. This was the birth of the directly observed treatment which is advocated by the WHO and widely practised by NTPs.

Over the years, the WHO-recommended treatment regimens have changed based on published phase III trials. The first WHO guidelines, recommending short-course treatment, were published in 1993 [6]. Based on results of clinical trials which are not referenced, the guidelines recommend treatments for different categories of case definitions. For category I, new cases of smear-positive pulmonary tuberculosis and other severe forms, 2 regimens are recommended, both with a 2-month initial intensive phase of isoniazid, rifampicin, pyrazinamide and ethambutol or streptomycin. In the continuation phase, the recommendation was either isoniazid and rifampcin for 4 months (2HRZE/4HR) or isoniazid and ethambutol for 6 months (2HRZE/6HE). This recommendation continued through the second (1997) [7] and third editions (2003) [8]. However, the most recent guidelines (2010) [9], recommend phasing out the 8-month regimen based on robust evidence from a phase III RCT published in 2004 [10].

It is worth considering the procedures that led to the publication of this phase III multicentre, clinical RCT which resulted in a pivotal change in the WHO guidelines. The writing of the protocol, design, printing and despatch of the case-reporting forms, procurement and supply of the trial drugs, randomization schedules, recruitment and training of participating centres, establishment of the electronic database and data entry, site visits and trial monitoring, organization of meetings of the oversight committees and fund-raising were all carried out by 1 person. The only task not performed by the same individual was the analyses of the outcomes. The trial was conceived in 1997, patient enrolment began in March 1998 and the results were published in October 2004 [11]. The total number of patients enrolled was 1,355 in 6 centres. The total cost incurred was approximately USD 300,000.

None of the participating centres had any previous experience of carrying out clinical RCTs. However, several have since participated in other trials. Ethics committees, which were absent then (approval for participation was given by the Ministry of Health and Directors of the NTPs), have since been established in the countries involved in the trial. Visits to the laboratories, by a senior technologist, resulted in improvement of laboratory practices.

In contrast, a second multicentre clinical RCT [11], conceived in 2004, has evolved at a different pace. In this trial there has been no multitasking by 1 person. All the trial co-applicants had input into protocol development. The case-reporting forms were designed by the trial manager, the database was developed by an information technology group and the packing and despatching of drugs by several institutions. Approval had to be obtained from a total of 18 ethics and regulatory bodies from the 5 participating countries. In the case of the South African Medicines Control Council, approval was obtained 14 months after protocol submission. In the case of the Medicines Control Authority of Zimbabwe, this process took 20 months. As a result, although approval for funding, by the donor, was received in 2006, the first patient was not enrolled until August 15, 2008. As at August 15, 2010, of the total sample size of 1,100, 560 patients (51%) have been enrolled. Because of delays in starting patient enrolment, significant amounts of one of the investigational medical products were time expired and had to be replaced at considerable cost. The total approved budget was EUR 4,251,990. Delays in obtaining approvals and in starting patient enrolment have resulted in a financial deficit, and it has become necessary to request an additional amount of EUR 896,979 in order to complete the trial. The estimated date of publication of outcomes is during the first quarter of 2013. Thus, in the space of a decade, time to carry out clinical trials has lengthened significantly and costs have soared.

## Current Situation

Nowadays, each trial must provide written approval from the appropriate ethic and regulatory bodies before starting patient enrolment. The regulations are reviewed periodically and continue to increase in number and complexity. Increasingly the process of drug development is far lengthier, complicated and very highly regulated and, consequently, so expensive that applications for funding for RCTs are frequently rejected as 'not competitive'.

Increasing complexity of regulations is such that academic institutions are discouraged from undertaking them. This has led to the establishment of 'for-profit' organizations that can carry out all the functions of an academic institution but at a substantial cost. Thus, over a period of several years, clinical trials have been transformed from an academic exercise to a multimillion dollar industry. Even the vocabulary has changed with 'vendors' of services offering their 'products' ranging from protocol development to the completion of the trial. The participating patients are 'clients'. The 'products' on offer are as follows:

*Feasibility Studies*
It has always been the case that, before centres are invited to participate, they are able to meet certain criteria which would include their ability to recruit sufficient numbers of patients and manage them for the full period of the trial. However, the process of deciding whether a centre could participate was usually rather informal. The head of the centre would express a wish to participate and claimed to have sufficient numbers of patients in the particular disease group to make the participation worthwhile. This process has now become more formalized and, before a centre can be considered for participation, a feasibility study must be undertaken to assess the centre's capability and capacity to participate. This includes evidence of previous experience, ability to enrol, treat, document and follow up significant numbers of patients for a period of, at least, 1 year. Since the process can be lengthy and complicated, there are now organizations that carry out a formal and structured evaluation of each site. The final report comes with a substantial bill.

*Obtaining Necessary Approvals*
Since the streptomycin trial [4] in 1944 until almost the end of the last millennium, there were no ethics or regulatory bodies in countries where such trials were being conducted. Indeed, any regulatory oversight in the countries of the agencies (academic or pharmaceutical) that were conducting trials tended to be rather perfunctory. Inevitably, there were trials being carried out which would never have been approved by today's rigorous standards. The need for oversight became necessary, and, gradually, each country established its own ethics and regulatory bodies with, often, their own requirements.

Such oversight, however necessary, can only be efficient if protocols are reviewed within a few weeks of submission. As mentioned earlier, substantial delays can lead to substantial increases in costs and delays in publishing trial outcomes. Further, any amendment to the protocol, however trivial, must be resubmitted to all the ethics committees of the participating countries leading to further delays in implementing the amendments.

*Good Clinical Practice*
In 1997, the GCP guidelines for Japan, the USA and Europe were amalgamated within the International Conference on Harmonization of Technical Requirements for Registration of Pharmaceuticals for Human Use. The guideline E6 [12] is that which provides International Conference on Harmonization definitions of GCP. Although these regulations apply only to trials for licensing a drug, donor agencies now require they are applied to all clinical trials which they fund. Although some funding bodies may have their own GCP guidelines, it is the International Conference on Harmonization GCP guidelines that are most applied.

It is now mandatory for all medical and paramedical staff involved in a trial to be in possession of a certificate showing that they have been trained in GCP. Because of constantly increasing guidelines, this training has to be renewed every 2 years.

This has seen the establishment of 'limited companies', sometimes limited to one person, to provide such training for a per-capita fee. Usually, training involves no more than the repetition of the guidelines and provision of links to a number of relevant web sites. Since GCP guidelines are available in only 2 European languages, many countries with a high tuberculosis burden are hampered in their efforts to participate in clinical trials.

*Recruitment and Retention of Patients*
In order to be able to enrol as many patients as possible, in as short a time as possible, it is no longer sufficient to wait for patients to present at hospitals and clinics. Increasing use is made of social media to raise awareness, in the general public, of the existence of a trial. These include not only poster campaigns and advertisements in the local press, but also the Internet and its facilities such as 'facebook', 'twitter' and 'blogging'. Local media and activist groups must also be kept informed as their help may be required to increase patient recruitment and locate lost ones. While some of such facilities can be found in larger cities, they are non-existent in rural areas. Centres, where such technology is lacking, would not readily be considered for participation in a trial. In the case of tuberculosis, since most trials are carried out in centres where such facilities are absent, this deficiency puts them at a disadvantage when being considered for participation.

*Drug Distributing and Packaging*
In the early BMRC tuberculosis trials, which were carried out in Africa, India, Hong Kong and Czechoslovakia, drugs for the trial were sent in bulk and dispensed by trial nurses, according to the trial doctor's prescription. No import licenses were required and drugs were stored in a cupboard in the clinic. Currently, in order to import drugs, laws governing the importation of drugs must be complied with. If the experimental drug is not licensed in that country, special permission has to be sought and a plethora of documents supplied to the appropriate authorities.

In a multicentre trial, each country has regulations with relevant documentation to complete in order to import the drugs. If a smooth transit through customs is not obtained, drugs may be held up for many weeks, disrupting the distribution cold chain and compromising their quality. Drugs for export have to be packed in a way that guarantees their quality in climate extremes. Once imported, storage conditions must be suitable. Thus, the whole supply chain must be regulated in a way which may not be possible in many resource-poor countries.

For the purposes of a clinical trial, each drug has to be packaged and labelled appropriately. While this is a reasonable requirement, in a multi-arm trial the work involved, especially when the quantities prescribed are according to different weight bands, is very time consuming and, indeed, beyond the capacity of most dispensing pharmacies. In a double-blind, placebo-controlled trial, it is quite impossible for the site pharmacy/dispensary to perform this task. Instead, this task has to be performed by organizations which sell this 'product' at a significant cost.

*Informed Consent Process*
Because of documented failures to obtain consent from patients before subjecting them to experimental procedures, patient consent must be documented. Over a period of time, this process has become increasingly complex. It is no longer considered sufficient to inform a patient of the existence of a trial and invite his/her participation. There must be an information sheet describing the trial to the patients as well as the risks and benefits to them from their participation. This sheet, which could run into more than 20 pages, must be translated into the native language of the patient and then translated back into the original language to show that nothing has been lost in translation! The patient information sheet for a phase III trial [11] was found to be too long by the ethics body of one country and too short in another country! In some centres, patients are asked to listen to an audiotape (and, perhaps, watch a videotape) explaining the trial. Patients are then asked to undergo a written examination to evaluate their degree of comprehension of trial procedures and their participation in the trial. A member of the family, or an 'independent' person, is also put through this

process. In spite of these requirements, studies have shown that trial subjects may have little understanding of the procedures to which they are to be subjected [13].

*Site Management*
This can no longer be left to the principal investigator and staff at the site because they cannot be trusted to remain unbiased when reviewing trial patients and also to complete case-reporting forms without tampering with the data. There are now organizations that offer this 'product' for a fee.

*Trial Monitoring*
It is no longer acceptable for trial monitoring to be carried out by the trial management team at the site. Monitoring must be conducted by an independent person or body. There are now many contract research organizations (CROs) that perform this function.

*The Time and Cost of Phase III Trials*
While these regulations may ensure the safety of the patients in the trial (although in the case of one well-documented clinical trial [14], the regulations completely failed to do so), there may be serious detractors to clinical groups, and, as a result, patients may well be denied best treatment.

For instance the time to develop a new drug in 1960 was 8 years. In 1991, this amount had almost doubled to 15.3 years [15]. As a result, costs to drug development have increased exponentially which, in turn, increases the cost at which the drug is marketed. This prevents health services from purchasing a drug which could result in higher cure rates and denies patients a better standard of care.

*Equipoise*
Before undertaking a clinical trial, investigators are supposed to be in equipoise as to the eventual outcome of the trial. If, however, they are not required to be involved in any aspect of trial conduct, this could disadvantage the patients as CROs are not concerned with equipoise. They simply carry out the trial according to the protocol which has been supplied to them and for financial benefit.

*Capacity Building*
The most serious disadvantage is capacity building in centres not familiar with carrying out RCTs and, as a result, loss of potential sites and of trial subjects in those sites. Because regulations governing the conduct of clinical trials are rigorous and onerous, trials can be conducted only in centres with an established track record of conducting trials successfully. In failing to go to less experienced centres, the overall capacity for clinical trials is reduced with a concomitant failure to achieve adequately powered trials in a reasonable time.

*Patient Care*
It is generally acknowledged that patients participating in a clinical trial receive a better standard of care than those not in a trial. Trial patients not only receive best available treatment and follow-up, adverse events are rapidly recognized and treated, leading to better survival and an improved quality of life. This is denied to patients whose health care facility is unable to participate in RCTs. This is particularly true of tuberculosis where patients are not supervised to the same extent and not followed up after treatment has been completed. Lack of adequate supervision results in a failure to recognize treatment failures and relapses as soon as they occur and may result in the emergence of drug resistance.

## Discussion

The current treatment of tuberculosis consists of 4 drugs for the first 2 months followed by 2 drugs for another 4 months. Sputum examinations show that culture conversion is almost complete at the end of the first 2 months. However, there is then a long 4-month period during which the more persistent bacilli in the original bacterial population have to be eliminated. Thus, while drugs can be assessed for their bactericidal action during the first 2 months by the speed with which they eliminate viable bacilli from sputum, relapse is the only way of measuring the final success of treatment. But because of low relapse rates of the standard regimen [10], a comparison of relapse rates is statistically inefficient requiring large numbers of patients to show a significant difference. Moreover, the sterilizing activity measured by relapse rates often arranges drugs and regimens in a different order from that following bactericidal activity studies [16]. The order obtained in animal studies may be different in humans, and several phase III trials are required to establish the place of a sterilizing combination.

The early BMRC clinical trials of tuberculosis were pivotal to advances in the treatment of tuberculosis [1], and, while all the regulations encountered today were absent, it was the rule that patients in the trials were followed up until they were cured. The question has to be posed whether, had these regulations been in existence, these trials would have been conducted at all and whether there would be a 6-month regimen with an almost 100% cure rate.

Trials which ignored patient safety have been well documented, and there is no dispute that, in any trial, the safety of the patients is paramount and overrides any other consideration. Much needed guidelines have been established, and all trials must have oversight committees that ensure that considerations of patient safety are maintained throughout the trial and, where feasible, after the trial is completed and the results published. But has the process gone too far? Is there now a danger that the regulations are so demanding that it has become more difficult and more expensive for phase III trials to be carried out by academic groups? Certainly, more physicians say that they no longer conduct clinical trials because the regulations are too onerous.

As more drugs in the pipeline come to clinical testing [3], phase III trials will continue to be essential to identify safe and effective tuberculosis treatments. However, as competition for the same trial sites increases, capacity must continue to be built by conducting trials in sites less familiar with RCTs. It is only by participating in such trials that site weaknesses can be identified and strengthened.

As the physician pool of trialists decreases, the number of CROs that carry out clinical trials is increasing. A search of the website of the Association of the British Pharmaceutical Industry lists hundreds in the UK alone. Increasingly, CROs are being employed to carry out RCTs by pharmaceutical companies and some academic institutions as well. Of all the organizations offering a specific 'product' for RCTs, CROs have been the most successful in launching their services and, as a result, are financially very successful. For example, in 2003, the gross earnings of Quintiles were 2.04 billion dollars [15]. Moreover, since all the regulations are drawn up to ensure patient safety, are the CROs fit for purpose and can they be held liable for serious adverse events? This question arose in the phase I trial, approved by the UK regulatory body Medicines and Healthcare Products Regulatory Agency, of an immunomodulatory drug, TGN1412, manufactured by Boehringer-Ingelheim and developed by Tegenero Immuno Therapeutics. The CRO, Parexel, was contracted to carry out the trial. When a serious adverse event occurred, which eventually led to the loss of fingers and toes in 6 previously healthy young men, the CRO denied liability on the grounds that they followed the protocol. The product-developing company denied responsibility and went into liquidation, thereby avoiding having to pay compensation to the men [14]. While regulations cannot prevent such occurrences, they can increasingly make clinical trials more difficult and more expensive to conduct.

There is another concerning factor increasing trial costs and that is the financial demands of the cooperating clinical centres which have risen substantially over the last few years. It used to be the case that clinical centres were often prepared to participate in the trial without payment or for only minimal help with extra tests involved, but it is now becoming more usual to demand the total cost of the treatment of the patients, salaries for staff already employed and also many of the other costs of the centre that is doing the work. Thus, clinical trials are required to finance a substantial proportion of the cost necessary to upgrade the clinical efficacy and tuberculosis service in resource-poor countries. This problem becomes more acute as the management and running of such a study increase in complexity so that there are fewer and fewer centres capable of undertaking GCP-compliant RCTs. If these financial demands are not contained to a reasonable level, the pool of trial centres will be limited, and patients, particularly in resource-poor countries, will be deprived of better care and best practice.

Yet another downside to the commercialization of phase III trials is that, not infrequently, aspiring doctors and nurses can carry out limited specialized investigations within the trial as the thesis for a Masters or PhD degree. These candidates may then continue down this career path and undertake further phase III trials. If the trials are conducted by CROs, there is no scope for such activity, and the pool of trialists will continue to decrease.

Finally, results of phase III clinical trials of tuberculosis appear regularly in the medical journals. If increasing regulations continue to increase the length of trial duration, by the time they come to publication, it may well be that the results are superseded by other trials and become irrelevant. Timely completion and publications of clinical trials are, therefore, of the greatest importance.

## Conclusions

In the development of drugs for tuberculosis, while early phase trials, such as pharmacokinetic, early bactericidal activity and toxicity studies, can give an indication of the safety and bactericidal ability of the drug with smaller patient numbers, the ability of a regimen to cure tuberculosis and prevent relapse can only be assessed in phase III trials of the efficacy of treatment regimens. Thus, there will always be a need for such trials.

Phase III trials in tuberculosis typically have a sample size of over 1,000 patients. Since it would be impossible to enrol this number of patients in one centre in a short period of time, such trials are always multicentre trials and in several different countries with a high burden of disease. Continuing increases in regulations result in concomitant increases in trial costs and, by excluding centres that are not trained to be GCP compliant, they reduce the available pool of potential trial candidates and deny the patients best care.

The trend of increasing regulation is a significant discouragement to academic institutions from undertaking phase III trials. This is leading to increasing commercialization of phase III RCTs, thereby increasing costs without a concomitant increase in patient protection. There is no doubt that, when it comes to trials using human subjects, the highest standards, both ethical and regulatory, must be applied. The question now is: do they really protect the patients or, rather, do they protect the trialists? Further, have they gone too far, and are these very strict conditions leading to the ultimate demise of clinical trials? The Millennium Development Goals for tuberculosis are not being met [17] and great care must be taken that these regulations do not lead to loss of much needed clinical trials if these goals are to be met.

## References


1 Fox W, Ellard GA, Mitchison DA: Studies on the treatment of tuberculosis undertaken by the British Medical Research Council Tuberculosis Units, 1946–1986, with relevant publications. Int J Tuberc Lung Dis 1999;3:S231–S279.
2 http://www.undp.org/mdg/basics.shtml.
3 http://www.newtbdrugs.org/pipeline.php.
4 Medical Research Council: Streptomycin treatment of pulmonary tuberculosis. BMJ 1948;ii:769–782.
5 East African/British Medical Research Council: Results at 5 years of a controlled comparison of a 6-month and a standard 18-month regimen of chemotherapy for pulmonary tuberculosis. Am Rev Respir Dis 1977;116:3–8.
6 World Health Organization: Treatment of Tuberculosis: Guidelines for National Programmes. Geneva, WHO, 1993.
7 World Health Organization: Treatment of Tuberculosis: Guidelines for National Programmes, ed 2. Geneva, WHO, 1997.
8 World Health Oganization: Treatment of Tuberculosis: Guidelines for National Programmes, ed 3. Geneva, WHO, 2003.
9 World Health Organization: Treatment of Tuberculosis: Guidelines, ed 4. Geneva, WHO, 2010.
10 Jindani A, Nunn AJ, Enarson DA: Two 8-month regimens of chemotherapy for treatment of newly diagnosed pulmonary tuberculosis: international multicentre randomised trial. Lancet 2004;364:1244–1251
11 Jindani A, Nunn AJ, Mitchison DA, Harrison T, Hatherill M, Charalambous S, Mungofa S, Zizhou S, van Dijk J: An international multicentre controlled clinical trial to evaluate high dose rifapentine and a quinolone in the treatment of pulmonary tuberculosis (rifaquin). Ongoing.
12 http://www.ich.org/LOB/media/MEDIA482.pdf.
13 Krosin MT, Klitzman R. Levin B, Cheng J, Ranney ML: Problems in comprehension of informed consent in rural and peri-urban Mali, West Africa. Clin Trials 2006;3:306–313.
14 Tegenero files for bankruptcy. Biotechnol Law Rep 2006;25:408.
15 Kittredge C: A shrinking target. Scientist 2005;19:46–49.
16 Koen A, Gevers T, Lounis N: Bactericidal potencies of new regimens are not predictive for their sterilizing potencies in a murine model of tuberculosis. Antimicrob Agents Chemother 2010;51:1011–1015.
17 United Nations Millennium Development Goals Report. 2010.



Amina Jindani, MD, FRCP
Division of Clinical Science
St. George's, University of London
Cranmer Terrace, London SW17 0RE (UK)
Tel. + 44 20 8725 2810, E-Mail ajindani@sgul.ac.uk

Chapter 7
Donald PR, van Helden PD (eds): Antituberculosis Chemotherapy.
Prog Respir Res. Basel, Karger, 2011, vol 40, pp 51–60

# Fluoroquinolones in the Management of Tuberculosis

Kasha P. Singh[a] · Stephen H. Gillespie[b]

[a]Department of Infection, University College London, London, and [b]School of Medicine, University of St. Andrews, St. Andrews, UK

**Abstract**

Fluoroquinolones (FQs) have been demonstrated to have excellent activity against *Mycobacterium tuberculosis* in vitro and in mouse models. This combined with their pharmacokinetic profiles make them attractive agents for the treatment of tuberculosis. Several mouse models have suggested that substitution of FQ for ethambutol or isoniazid might allow treatment duration to be shortened to 4 months. Phase III pivotal trials are under way to test regimens built on moxifloxacin or gatifloxacin, and the results of these studies are eagerly awaited. Until the results of pivotal studies are available, patients with fully susceptible disease should not be treated with FQs. FQs have an important role to play in the management of patients with drug toxicity and multiple drug resistance and form part of treatment recommendations by national and international bodies. Nevertheless, well-controlled clinical trials of the role of FQs are still required. Resistance to FQs is a growing concern due to the increasing frequency with which resistant strains are being reported.

Copyright © 2011 S. Karger AG, Basel

Fluoroquinolones (FQs) are the newest agents to be introduced into use for the treatment of tuberculosis (TB). They have many characteristics that make them ideal antimycobacterial agents, with a unique mechanism of action and no cross-resistance or antagonism with other antimycobacterial drugs. They exhibit excellent oral bioavailability, and once daily dosing is possible for most FQs. Preclinical and early clinical studies have shown excellent activity against *Mycobacterium tuberculosis*. Phase III trials are in progress to assess their ability to enable treatment shortening for drug-susceptible TB. In the meantime they have firmly established themselves for use in TB treatment in cases of drug intolerance and drug-resistant disease. Undoubtedly important for TB, their optimal role in management is under debate.

## Development and Structure

FQs are a group of synthetic antimicrobial agents characterized by the addition of a fluorine molecule at position 6 of the basic 4-quinolone bicyclic ring structure. They target bacterial type II DNA topo-isomerases, known as DNA gyrase [1]. The addition of a fluorine molecule to the quinolone ring structure led to an increase in potency and spectrum of activity. In addition to Gram-negative activity, newer agents are active against Gram-positive and atypical organisms as well as anaerobes. Further chemical modification of the FQ nucleus has also resulted in compounds with clinically significant activity against mycobacteria including *M. tuberculosis* [2]. Antimycobacterial activity does not appear to be associated with any structural change; however, the addition of a methoxyl group at the C8 position does appear to be an important feature of agents with anti-TB activity and is found in moxifloxacin, gatifloxacin and the new FQ DC-159a [3, 4].

Other FQs with significant anti-TB activity include sparfloxacin, sitafloxacin, clinafloxacin, ciprofloxacin, ofloxacin and levofloxacin (the optically active L-isomer of ofloxacin). Of these the first 3 are no longer available due to toxicity concerns and will not be covered in this review. Ciprofloxacin is not recommended for use in the treatment of TB due to inadequate activity in clinical studies [5].

**Table 1.** Selected studies of FQ in vitro activity against *M. tuberculosis* isolates

| Agent | Strains n | Selection | Range mg/l | $MIC_{90}$ mg/l | Method used | Reference |
|---|---|---|---|---|---|---|
| Ciprofloxacin | 206 | mixed | ≤0.125–16 | 1 | agar dilution | Ruiz-Serrano et al. [6], 2000 |
| | 22 | rifampicin-susceptible | | 0.78 | agar/broth dilution | Blower and Chou [7], 2004 |
| | 18 | | <0.25–1 | 0.5 | proportion | Gillespie and Billington [8], 1999 |
| Ofloxacin | 206 | mixed | ≤0.125–16 | 1 | agar dilution | Ruiz-Serrano et al. [6], 2000 |
| Levofloxacin | 22 | rifampicin-susceptible | | 0.39 | agar dilution | Blower and Chou [7], 2004 |
| | 206 | mixed | ≤0.125–8 | 0.5 | agar dilution | Ruiz-Serrano et al. [6], 2000 |
| | 19 | | 0.25–0.5 | >0.25 | proportion | Gillespie and Billington [8], 1999 |
| | 21 | DS | 0.25–1 | 0.5 | agar dilution | Disratthakit and Doi [4], 2010 |
| | 243 | mixed | | 0.5 | agar dilution | Rodriguez et al. [9], 2001 |
| | 10 | | 0.5–1.0 | 0.5 | agar/broth dilution | Peloquin et al. [10], 2008 |
| Gatifloxacin | 22 | rifampicin-susceptible | | 0.78 | agar dilution | Blower and Chou [7], 2004 |
| | 21 | DS | 0.06–0.25 | 0.25 | agar dilution | Disratthakit and Doi [4], 2010 |
| | 243 | mixed | | 0.25 | agar dilution | Rodriguez et al. [9], 2001 |
| | 10 | | 0.1–0.2 | 0.2 | agar/broth dilution | Peloquin et al. [10], 2008 |
| Moxifloxacin | 19 | | 0.06–0.25 | 0.25 | proportion | Gillespie and Billington [8], 1999 |
| | 21 | DS | 0.125–0.5 | 0.25 | agar dilution | Disratthakit and Doi [4], 2010 |
| | 243 | mixed | | 0.5 | agar dilution | Rodriguez et al. [9], 2001 |
| | 73 | mixed | | 1.0 | BACTEC MGIT 960 | Rodrigues et al. [11], 2008 |
| | 9 | | 0.5 | 0.5 | agar/broth dilution | Peloquin et al. [10], 2008 |
| DC-159a | 21 | DS | 0.03–0.125 | 0.06 | agar dilution | Disratthakit and Doi [4], 2010 |
| | 11 | QR-MDR (levofloxacin MIC ≥2) | 0.125–0.5 | 0.5 | agar dilution | Disratthakit and Doi [4], 2010 |

DS = Drug-susceptible; QR = quinolone-resistant.

## Activity against Tuberculosis

### *In vitro Studies*

Multiple studies have been published demonstrating the in vitro activity of FQs against TB. Most strains are inhibited by concentrations of between 0.5 and 1 mg/l of ofloxacin and ciprofloxacin whilst the minimal inhibitory concentrations (MICs) of moxifloxacin, gatifloxacin and levofloxacin are <0.5 mg/l in most studies (table 1). The activity of the new broad-spectrum 8-methoxy-FQ DC-159a may be even greater, with a recent study demonstrating an MIC of 0.06 mg/l against drug-susceptible isolates as well as against levofloxacin-resistant strains of multidrug-resistant TB (MDR-TB) [4].

Classic in vitro susceptibility testing in nutrient media is probably not an accurate representation of the conditions in which organisms will come into contact with antimicrobials. *M. tuberculosis* is often found intracellularly within the mononuclear phagocyte, and FQ accumulation inside macrophages may be an important factor in their antimycobacterial activity [12, 13].

### *Animal Studies*

Clinical trials of shortened therapy for TB using FQs have their basis in a series of murine experiments. In a mouse model of an ofloxacin-containing regimen (2 months ofloxacin, ethionamide, amikacin and pyrazinamide followed by 10 months ethionamide and ofloxacin), ofloxacin was replaced by moxifloxacin or levofloxacin [14]. Only the 6-month control regimen led to culture-negative mouse spleens and lungs at 6 months of treatment; however, from month 9 onward all organs of mice treated with the moxifloxacin-containing regimen were culture negative. In contrast most organs from mice treated with the ofloxacin-containing regimen continued to be culture positive whilst results for levofloxacin were between

**Table 2.** Pharmacokinetic characteristics of selected FQs

| Drug | Oral bioavailability % | Plasma protein binding % | Plasma half-life h | $C_{max}$ mg/l | AUC mg/l•h | AUC/MIC (approx.) |
|---|---|---|---|---|---|---|
| Ciprofloxacin (500 mg)[1] | 70–80 | 20–30 | 5.0 | 2.1 | 11.6 | 11.6–23.2 |
| Ofloxacin (400 mg)[1] | 95–100 | 25 | 5.7 | 4.4 | 36.8 | 36.8 |
| Levofloxacin (1,000 mg)[2] | 95–100 | 30–40 | 7.4 | 15.55 | | 188 |
| Moxifloxacin (400 mg)[2, 3] | 90–95 | 40–42 | 6.5 | 6.13 (400) | 35 | 70–140[3]<br>59.35[2] |
| Gatifloxacin[2] | | 30–50 | 5.0 | 4.75 (400) | | 180 |

$C_{max}$ = Maximum concentration, dose given in parentheses; AUC = area under the curve.
[1] From Wise and Honeybourne [19], 1999.
[2] From Peloquin et al. [10], 2008.
[3] Summary of product characteristics.

those for ofloxacin and those for moxifloxacin-containing regimens.

Moxifloxacin substituted for ethambutol or isoniazid in combination with rifampicin, pyrazinamide and isoniazid/ethambutol, respectively, demonstrated a more rapid rate of killing in mouse models [15]. In a study of combination therapy for 3, 4, 5 or 6 months, no relapse was observed amongst mice treated for at least 4 months with rifampicin, moxifloxacin and pyrazinamide, whereas mice treated with rifampicin, isoniazid and pyrazinamide required 6 months of therapy to achieve 'no relapse'. For mice treated with rifampicin, moxifloxacin and pyrazinamide, a similar efficacy was found irrespective of the duration of pyrazinamide treatment [16].

The combination of gatifloxacin and rifampicin has also been evaluated in the mouse model with promising results [17]. Recent results from animal models also indicate that the potential for shortening therapy with moxifloxacin may be greatly enhanced by combination with novel agents such as the new nitroimidazo-oxazine PA-824 [18].

*Activity in Humans*

The pharmacokinetic properties of newer FQ agents favour their activity in humans (table 2) [10, 13, 19, 20]. Once or twice daily dosing is possible and agents exhibit high oral bioavailability and low protein binding. Maximum concentrations are generally achieved within 1–2 h and exceed the MIC at doses that are well tolerated. Importantly for the treatment of TB, the FQs are widely distributed around the body and particularly accumulate in lung tissue. They are concentrated in macrophages and other phagocytic cells, bronchial mucosa and epithelial lining fluid where levels are higher than those found in serum.

In a recent study assessing the pharmacokinetics of levofloxacin, moxifloxacin and gatifloxacin in Brazilian patients, levofloxacin at a dose of 1,000 mg/day displayed the most favourable profile with the highest maximum plasma concentrations, largest volume of distribution and longest elimination half-life [10].

The efficacy of FQs against TB has been demonstrated to correlate with the area under the curve/MIC parameter [13, 21], although it is debated as to whether this is a reflection of concentration-dependent killing (as it is in their activity against other bacteria) or due to their postantibiotic effect on *M. tuberculosis* [22].

Studies of early/extended bactericidal activity (in which the candidate drug is given alone for a period of between 48 h and 14 days and the log fall in bacterial count in sputum is measured) demonstrate that ofloxacin [23] gatifloxacin and moxifloxacin have significant activity in patients with smear-positive pulmonary TB [8, 23–26]. The degree of activity, as assessed by these studies, was less than that of isoniazid and greater than that of rifampicin. These results prompted the formation of clinical development consortia for both agents. A comparable early bactericidal activity is seen with levofloxacin when given at the higher dose of 1,000 mg/day [26].

## Clinical Trials

On the basis of preclinical and early bactericidal activity studies, combinations including moxifloxacin and gatifloxacin have been tested in phase IIb clinical studies to assess

**Table 3.** Early bactericidal activity (EBA) studies of FQs in the treatment of drug-susceptible TB

| | Ofloxacin 800 mg | Levofloxacin 1,000 mg | Gatifloxacin 400 mg | Moxifloxacin 400 mg | Isoniazid 300 mg |
|---|---|---|---|---|---|
| EBA (0–2) log CFU/ml/day | | | | | |
| Gosling et al. [25], 2003 | | | | 0.53 | 0.77 |
| Johnson et al. [26], 2006 | | 0.45 | 0.35 | 0.33 | 0.67 |
| Sirgel et al. [23], 2000 | 0.27 | | | | |
| Extended EBA (2–5, odds ratio 2–7) | | | | | rifampicin 600 mg |
| Sirgel et al. [23], 2000 | 0.20 | | | | 0.24 |
| Pletz et al. [24], 2004 | | | | 0.27 | – |
| Johnson et al. [26], 2006 | | 0.18 | 0.17 | 0.17 | – |

their potential to shorten the duration of treatment for patients with drug-susceptible TB (table 3).

Ofloxacin substitution in a shortened regimen was assessed in a large study in India. Although the results were promising in general, interpretation was difficult due to the absence of a control arm and the inclusion of patients with variable resistance patterns [27].

Other phase II studies have used the interim measure of culture-negative sputum at 8 weeks of treatment as a primary outcome. In the first of these, a 6-month control group was compared with 3 experimental arms in which ethambutol was substituted for ofloxacin, moxifloxacin or gatifloxacin [28]. Moxifloxacin substitution appeared superior during the early phase of treatment as measured by a fall in colony counts, and improved killing in the later phase was found for both moxifloxacin and gatifloxacin. Substitution of ofloxacin had no effect. The differences in the proportion of patients who were culture negative at 8 weeks just failed to achieve statistical significance.

Moxifloxacin substituted for ethambutol in the 6-month standard treatment (in combination with rifampicin, isoniazid and pyrazinamide) did lead to a significantly greater proportion of patients with culture-negative sputum at 8 weeks in 1 of 2 subsequent phase II studies of this regimen [29]. In both studies a significantly greater proportion of patients in the moxifloxacin-containing regimen had negative sputum cultures at weeks 4 and 6 of treatment [30].

Substitution of moxifloxacin for isoniazid was tested in an international trial with no significant difference found in negative sputum culture at 8 weeks (99/164 in the moxifloxacin arm vs. 90/164, $p = 0.97$) [31]. The interpretation of this study was handicapped by the difference in sputum conversion rate on liquid media between African and non-African sites [32].

Ultimately the role of novel agents must be defined in phase III controlled trials. Three phase III trials are currently under way to evaluate moxifloxacin and gatifloxacin for a role in treatment shortening for drug-sensitive TB (table 4). The gatifloxacin (OFLOTUB) study has now completed recruitment with patients due to complete post-treatment follow-up in April 2011 [33]. The REMox study, assessing two possible moxifloxacin substitution arms (one for ethambutol and the other for isoniazid) is due to complete recruitment in December 2011 [34]. These pivotal studies will provide a definitive answer regarding the use of FQs in the treatment of new cases of TB, but unless and until these data are presented to regulatory agencies these drugs remain an unlicensed and currently unproven therapy for TB.

## Other Clinical Studies and Series

Despite data from controlled trials still pending, it is a reflection of the dearth of tolerable and effective agents for TB that FQs have already become established in two circumstances: management of drug-resistant disease and cases of drug intolerance and suspected or potential toxicity. Numerous publications have reported their use worldwide, and they are recommended in treatment guidelines including American Thoracic Society and WHO guidelines [35–37].

### *Drug Intolerance*

FQs are frequently substituted for other drugs in the treatment for drug-sensitive TB in cases of drug intolerance or toxicity occurring during standard therapy. Hepatitis is the most common serious adverse event during treatment for TB with current standard therapy. A number of reports

**Table 4.** Phase II and III studies of ofloxacin, moxifloxacin, gatifloxacin and levofloxacin

| | Study design, population and location | Regimens | Outcomes assessed and results |
|---|---|---|---|
| *Phase II* | | | |
| TRC [27], 2002 | Prospective, randomized<br>416 with drug-susceptible and drug-resistant pulmonary TB<br>India | (1) 3HRZO, 3HRZO b.w.<br>(2) 3HRZO, 1HR b.w.<br>(3) 3HRZO, 2HR b.w.,<br>(4) 2HRZO, 2HR b.w.<br>No control arm | Treatment failure/relapse in 18/469<br>(113 excluded due to limited compliance) |
| Burman et al. [30], 2006 (study 27) | Prospective, randomized<br>336 with smear-positive TB<br>Multisite (63% African sites) | (1) HRZE 5 vs. 3 days/week (after 2-week daily therapy)<br>(2) HRZM 5 vs. 3 days/week | Negative sputum culture at completion of 8-week treatment in<br>98/138 vs. 99/139 (p = 0.97) |
| Rustomjee et al. [28], 2008 | Prospective, randomized<br>217 newly diagnosed sputum smear-positive TB cases<br>South Africa | (1) 2RHZE, 4HR<br>(2) 2RHZG, 4HR<br>(3) 2RHZM, 4HR<br>(4) 2RHZO, 4HR | Significant and similar acceleration of bacillary elimination during the late phase with G/M<br>(p = 0.002) |
| Conde et al. [29], 2009 (JHU study) | Prospective, double-blind, randomized<br>170 newly diagnosed sputum smear-positive TB cases<br>Brazil | HRZEMpl. (85)<br>HRZMEpl. (85)<br>Both 5 days/week for 8 weeks | Negative sputum culture at completion of 8-week treatment in 45/72 vs. 59/74 (p = 0.03) |
| Dorman et al. [31], 2009 (study 28) | Prospective, randomized double-blind<br>433 newly diagnosed sputum smear-positive TB cases<br>Multicentre, international | (1) RZEMHpl.<br>(2) RZEHMpl.<br>Both 5 days/week for 8 weeks | Negative sputum culture at completion of 8-week treatment in 99/164 vs. 90/164 (p = 0.37) |
| *Phase III* | | | |
| Gatifloxacin in short-course therapy OFLOTUB [33] | Prospective, randomized, open-label, non-inferiority<br>5 centres in Africa | (1) 2RHZE, 2GHR<br>(2) 2RHZG, 4HR | Recruitment complete, results awaited |
| REMox TB [34] | Prospective, randomized double-blind, non-inferiority<br>Multicentre, international | (1) 2RZHEMpl., 2RHMpl.2RH<br>(2) 2RZMHEpl., 2RHM2Rpl.Hpl.<br>(3) 2RZMEHpl., 2RMHpl.2Rpl. Hpl. | Recruiting |
| Moxifloxacin and rifapentine shortened therapy 'Rifaquin' | Prospective, randomized, open-label, non-inferiority<br>African centres<br>Sputum smear positive, newly diagnosed | (1) 2EMRZ/2M2P2<br>(2) 2EMRZ/4M1P1<br>(3) 2EHRZ/4HR | Recruiting |

H = Isoniazid; R = rifampicin; P = rifapentine; Z = pyrazinamide; O = ofloxacin; M = moxifloxacin; L = levofloxacin; G = gatifloxacin; pl. = placebo. Dosing is daily unless otherwise stated; b.w. = biweekly.

describe case series of patients successfully treated with FQ-containing regimens after hepatotoxicity due to treatment for TB [38, 39]. Whilst FQ treatment in various combinations is well tolerated in those who have experienced drug toxicity during treatment for TB, with results from phase III studies pending clinicians faced with building regimens in this context will need to base their choices on extrapolations from early-phase clinical studies in susceptible disease. It is important to note that although generally perceived as 'liver friendly', hepatic impairment is listed in product information for both moxifloxacin and levofloxacin and fulminant hepatitis was added as 'very rare' to the label for moxifloxacin in 2007 [40, 41]. The results from phase III studies will help to define relative rates of hepatotoxicity with different regimens more accurately.

*Treatment of MDR-TB and Extensively Drug-Resistant TB*
FQs and injectable agents are the mainstay of therapy for MDR-TB and are used in combination with companion drugs of lesser activity [37]. Randomized controlled phase III studies of FQ use have never been performed in MDR-TB, and the construction of treatment regimens is based on basic principles and extrapolation from available evidence. A large number of studies have reported the use of FQs in the treatment of MDR-TB [36, 42]. It is difficult to synthesize these data as they are a mix of retrospective reviews, small-scale anecdotal reports and prospective case series. The interpretation of results is complicated by the diversity of patients selected for study, their susceptibility patterns, differences in the degree of clinical information and varying regimens chosen and inconsistent comparators. For example some studies report an FQ arm that contains patients treated with different quinolones.

Despite this, some trends emerge including that during treatment for MDR-TB patients have a better outcome when an FQ is included in the treatment and that the outcome may be better when a newer FQ is used [42, 43]. Promising evidence that FQs may also enable shortened treatment for MDR-TB has recently been published in a prospective observational study in which remarkable success for a gatifloxacin-containing regimen for MDR-TB was demonstrated [44]. The regimen required a minimum of 9 months of treatment with gatifloxacin, clofazimine, ethambutol and pyrazinamide throughout the treatment period supplemented by prothionamide, kanamycin and high-dose isoniazid during an intensive phase of a minimum of 4 months and gave a relapse-free cure rate of 87.9% (95% confidence interval, 0.26–0.59). The difference in the frequency of failures from those on the ofloxacin-containing regimens was highly significant.

In extensively drug-resistant TB, defined as TB with resistance to at least rifampicin, isoniazid, any member of the quinolone family and at least one of the injectable agents kanamycin, capreomycin or amikacin, a meta-analysis of 13 observational studies (560 patients) found more favourable treatment outcomes in studies in which a higher proportion of patients received a later-generation FQ [45]. These results suggest that the addition of later-generation FQs to extensively drug-resistant TB regimens may improve treatment outcomes and should be systematically evaluated in well-designed clinical studies.

*Preventative Therapy after MDR-TB Exposure*
A combination of FQ and pyrazinamide as preventative therapy for use in those exposed to MDR-TB has been suggested [46, 47]; however, problems with tolerability have been reported in patients receiving levofloxacin plus pyrazinamide with events including rash, nausea and asymptomatic hepatitis [48]. No clinical evidence exists for these options, and we would advocate great care in implementation of these strategies, with intensive monitoring for the presence of active disease and potential for the development of further resistance with effective monotherapy.

## Resistance

Resistance to FQs emerges through the acquisition of point mutations in chromosomal genes. The rate of spontaneous FQ-resistant mutants is 1 in $10^{-7}$ to $10^{-8}$ mutants/cell division [49]. In the presence of subtherapeutic drug levels, these mutants are selected at a greater rate and may become dominant.

A mutation in the gene *gyrA* encoding the 'A' subunit of the drug target (DNA gyrase) is the most frequently detected change amongst drug-resistant isolates. Mutations are found in a conserved region of the gene, the quinolone resistance-determining region or QRDR (320 bp) analogous to FQ resistance in other bacteria [49, 50]. The most commonly described mutations in clinical and laboratory-selected isolates of *M. tuberculosis* occur at positions Ala-90 and Asp-94. Other mutations include codons 74, 83, 87 and 91 [49–52]. Mutation at codon 95 is considered to be a polymorphism not involved in resistance [53]. A region of the *gyrB* gene has also been recognized as a QRDR; however, *gyrB* mutations appear to be much rarer amongst clinical isolates. Recent work has shown that these residues are located in the 'quinolone binding pocket' with amino acid changes leading to modification of the pocket geometry [54].

The proportion of FQ-resistant strains of *M. tuberculosis* with mutations detected in the QRDR, as well as the particular mutations detected, varies significantly amongst published studies. This may be related to selection bias, the molecular detection methodology used or the existence of other mechanisms of resistance such as decreased cell wall permeability to drug, drug efflux pump activity or others. Geographical or strain variation have also been suggested as possible factors. In general it appears that resistance in strains with QRDR mutations is higher than in those strains without QRDR mutations.

Cross-resistance has been detected between FQ agents in some studies but is not uniform [50, 52]. It is widely recognized that strains tested to be resistant to ofloxacin may in some cases be successfully treated with more potent agents such as moxifloxacin or gatifloxacin; however, the molecular basis for this is not understood. Attempts have been made to evaluate the possible correlation between specific gene mutations and the level of in vitro resistance to different FQs based on their MIC but this remains unclear [52, 55]. In a recent murine study, the MIC of ofloxacin and moxifloxacin to *M. tuberculosis* strains containing various mutations was determined and found to vary. Moxifloxacin was used with some success to treat strains with the lowest MIC at suitable doses; however, this was not effective against the strain with the highest MIC (4 μg/ml) [56].

It has been suggested that FQ resistance involves 'stepwise' accumulation of mutations which would then be associated with increasing MIC and resistance to more potent agents [49, 57, 58]; however, this has not been confirmed in other studies with only a handful of strains having multiple mutations detected and the correlation with levels of susceptibility and to different agents being inconsistent [59].

FQ-resistant TB is currently recognized primarily in patients who already have MDR-TB and is likely a result of injudicious use of FQs in the management of MDR-TB. Poor adherence or inappropriate prescription of MDR-TB treatment regimens may lead to inadequate 'protection' of the FQs, with strains resistant to FQs being selected out, particularly given the low activity of companion drugs.

Additionally, although the superiority of other agents over ofloxacin is increasingly acknowledged, ofloxacin is still widely used including in TB programmes in countries including India, South Africa and Lesotho. It is possible that properties of newer FQs including chemical stability, pharmacokinetics and activity against TB may reduce the selection of resistant mutants relative to older agents [37, 60]. Cross-resistance raises concern that profligate use of less effective agents may compromise the potential of newer FQs in TB treatment.

Studies show that the risk of resistance may vary with drug dose exposure [61]. It has been suggested that a 'mutant prevention concentration' can be defined at which the selection of resistant mutants during treatment is suppressed [62]. This concept has been investigated extensively in a wide spectrum of bacterial species including mycobacteria for a range of FQs [63–65] (table 2). The likelihood of development of resistance to each medication is reflected in the comparison between the mutant prevention concentration and the drug levels in serum/tissue at normal dosing. This comparison shows the lowest ratio for earlier-generation FQs suggesting a greater likelihood of the generation of resistance during use of these agents. Earlier-generation FQs are less active and achieve lower effective concentrations at the site of infection with the result that for part of the day the FQ concentration may fall below the mutant prevention concentration allowing mutants to emerge rapidly. As noted for other mycobacterial species, sub-MIC concentrations of FQs may increase the rate of mutation of *M. tuberculosis*, potentially threatening the accelerated generation of additional resistance [66].

Resistance amongst non-MDR-TB strains may also be related to use of FQs for indications other than TB including respiratory infections. The development of FQ resistance in *M. tuberculosis* has been documented to occur after as little as 13 day's treatment with FQ monotherapy (in the case of unsuspected TB) [67]. Studies show that FQ prescription is frequent in areas of high TB incidence for a variety of indications and that it is not uncommon for patients subsequently diagnosed with TB to have been prescribed FQ [68]. Initial treatment with an FQ was, until recently, recommended as part of WHO guidelines for undiagnosed respiratory symptoms as part of the diagnostic/management algorithm for TB until recently and remains widely practiced [69]. Whilst multiple anecdotal reports and ecological data exist to illustrate that FQ use may result in increased FQ-resistant TB and diagnostic delay, case-control studies have shown conflicting results [70–73].

Calls have been made for FQs to be reserved for use in TB [73] or even only for MDR-TB [74] because of the risks of increasing resistance, diagnostic delay and partial treatment and consequent morbidity and potential for increased transmission. However, given the many drugs of this class available and their widespread use worldwide for a variety of indications, as well as the existence of cross-resistance between agents, a general restriction may be unrealistic and restriction of only some agents may be ineffective.

If FQs prove successful in treatment shortening for TB, further questions will remain regarding their optimal role in therapy, in particular whether their increased use in first-line treatment for TB may compromise a role in resistant disease. Overall rates of primary resistance against FQs may be increasing and whilst calls for the restriction of availability are being made, given the uncertainties around the issues of cross-resistance and the significance of the development of resistance during treatment for other indications, it is not clear how widespread measures controlling use would have an impact on resistance.

## Safety

FQs are generally well tolerated and in the treatment of TB have been found to be associated with lower overall rates of adverse events and drug cessation compared to other regimens including first-line drugs [75, 76]. Current clinical trials will provide further useful evidence about how the incidence of adverse events including hepatotoxicity compares with standard therapy. Furthermore, many antibiotics in the class have been extensively trialled for a diversity of bacterial indications, and the safety profile of currently marketed compounds is comprehensively understood. Substantive postmarketing surveillance programmes are also in place. Whilst some agents have been withdrawn from the market for safety reasons, many of these problems have been resolved in the development of newer agents, particularly where these have been related to specific structural features (e.g. phototoxicity).

Gatifloxacin has been withdrawn from the market in some countries because of concerns about dysglycaemia [76, 77]; however, it is still available in many parts of the world and being evaluated for use in shortened TB regimens. The antimycobacterial potency of this drug and its availability in generic form make it an attractive agent for resource-poor settings in which the problem of TB is most significant.

American Thoracic Society treatment guidelines favour levofloxacin amongst FQ antibiotics for TB because of greater clinical experience with this older agent. However, with results soon to be available for phase III studies of the use of moxifloxacin and gatifloxacin in TB, improved data for the extended duration and in combinations required for TB will soon be available on which to base treatment decisions.

## Fluoroquinolones in Development for Tuberculosis

DC-159a is a new 8-methoxy-FQ. In vitro studies indicate significant activity against drug-susceptible TB as well as against strains of MDR-TB resistant to levofloxacin [4]. Novel mutations have been found in strains resistant to DC-159a [78]. In murine studies it displays a pharmacokinetic profile similar to moxifloxacin with greater activity during both initial and continuation phases of treatment [79]. Further studies are eagerly anticipated.

## The Future of Fluoroquinolones

It is clear that FQs have a role in TB treatment especially in the context of drug toxicity and resistance. Should the trials currently under way demonstrate that FQ-containing regimens can shorten treatment duration, they may play a role in the first-line management of susceptible disease. Until the results of these pivotal trials are known, patients with fully susceptible disease should not be treated with FQ-containing regimens.

## References


1 Hooper DC: Mechanisms of action of antimicrobials: focus on fluoroquinolones. Clin Infect Dis 2001;32(suppl 1):S9–S15.

2 Gillespie SH, Kennedy N: Fluoroquinolones: a new treatment for tuberculosis? Int J Tuberc Lung Dis 1998;2:265–271.

3 Aubry A, Pan XS, Fisher LM, Jarlier V, Cambau E: *Mycobacterium tuberculosis* DNA gyrase: interaction with quinolones and correlation with antimycobacterial drug activity. Antimicrob Agents Chemother 2004;48:1281–1288.

4 Disratthakit A, Doi N: In vitro activities of DC-159a, a novel fluoroquinolone, against *Mycobacterium* species. Antimicrob Agents Chemother 2010;54:2684–2686.

5 Ziganshina LE, Squire SB: Fluoroquinolones for treating tuberculosis. Cochrane Database Syst Rev 2008;1:CD004795.

6 Ruiz-Serrano MJ, Alcala L, Martinez L, Diaz M, Marin M, Gonzalez-Abad MJ, Bouza E: In vitro activities of six fluoroquinolones against 250 clinical isolates of *Mycobacterium tuberculosis* susceptible or resistant to first-line antituberculosis drugs. Antimicrob Agents Chemother 2000;44:2567–2568.

7 Blower SM, Chou T: Modeling the emergence of the 'hot zones': tuberculosis and the amplification dynamics of drug resistance. Nat Med 2004;10:1111–1116.

8 Gillespie SH, Billington O: Activity of moxifloxacin against mycobacteria. J Antimicrob Chemother 1999;44:393–395.

9 Rodriguez JC, Ruiz M, Climent A, Royo G: In vitro activity of four fluoroquinolones against *Mycobacterium tuberculosis*. Int J Antimicrob Agents 2001;17:229–231.

10 Peloquin CA, Hadad DJ, Molino LP, Palaci M, Boom WH, Dietze R, Johnson JL: Population pharmacokinetics of levofloxacin, gatifloxacin, and moxifloxacin in adults with pulmonary tuberculosis. Antimicrob Agents Chemother 2008;52:852–857.

11 Rodrigues C, Jani J, Shenai S, Thakkar P, Siddiqi S, Mehta A: Drug susceptibility testing of *Mycobacterium tuberculosis* against second-line drugs using the Bactec MGIT 960 system. Int J Tuberc Lung Dis 2008;12:1449–1455.

12 Duman N, Cevikbas A, Johansson C: The effects of rifampicin and fluoroquinolones on tubercle bacilli within human macrophages. Int J Antimicrob Agents 2004;23:84–87.

13 Shandil RK, Jayaram R, Kaur P, Gaonkar S, Suresh BL, Mahesh BN, Jayashree R, Nandi V, Bharath S, Balasubramanian V: Moxifloxacin, ofloxacin, sparfloxacin, and ciprofloxacin against *Mycobacterium tuberculosis:* evaluation of in vitro and pharmacodynamic indices that best predict in vivo efficacy. Antimicrob Agents Chemother 2007;51:576–582.
14 Veziris N, Truffot-Pernot C, Aubry A, Jarlier V, Lounis N: Fluoroquinolone-containing third-line regimen against *Mycobacterium tuberculosis* in vivo. Antimicrob Agents Chemother 2003;47:3117–3122.
15 Nuermberger EL, Yoshimatsu T, Tyagi S, O'Brien RJ, Vernon AN, Chaisson RE, Bishai WR, Grosset JH: Moxifloxacin-containing regimen greatly reduces time to culture conversion in murine tuberculosis. Am J Respir Crit Care Med 2004;169:421–426.
16 Nuermberger EL, Yoshimatsu T, Tyagi S, Williams K, Rosenthal I, O'Brien RJ, Vernon AA, Chaisson RE, Bishai WR, Grosset JH: Moxifloxacin-containing regimens of reduced duration produce a stable cure in murine tuberculosis. Am J Respir Crit Care Med 2004;170:1131–1134.
17 Cynamon M, Sklaney MR, Shoen C: Gatifloxacin in combination with rifampicin in a murine tuberculosis model. J Antimicrob Chemother 2007;60:429–432.
18 Nuermberger E, Tyagi S, Tasneen R, Williams KN, Almeida D, Rosenthal I, Grosset JH: Powerful bactericidal and sterilizing activity of a regimen containing PA-824, moxifloxacin, and pyrazinamide in a murine model of tuberculosis. Antimicrob Agents Chemother 2008;52:1522–1524.
19 Wise R, Honeybourne D: Pharmacokinetics and pharmacodynamics of fluoroquinolones in the respiratory tract. Eur Respir J 1999;14:221–229.
20 Zhanel GG, Noreddin AM: Pharmacokinetics and pharmacodynamics of the new fluoroquinolones: focus on respiratory infections. Curr Opin Pharmacol 2001;1:459–463.
21 Gumbo T, Louie A, Deziel MR, Parsons LM, Salfinger M, Drusano GL: Selection of a moxifloxacin dose that suppresses drug resistance in *Mycobacterium tuberculosis,* by use of an in vitro pharmacodynamic infection model and mathematical modeling. J Infect Dis 2004;190:1642–1651.
22 Berning SE: The role of fluoroquinolones in tuberculosis today. Drugs 2001;61:9–18.
23 Sirgel FA, Donald PR, Odhiambo J, Githui W, Umapathy KC, Paramasivan CN, Tam CM, Kam KM, Lam CW, Sole KM, Mitchison DA: A multicentre study of the early bactericidal activity of anti-tuberculosis drugs. J Antimicrob Chemother 2000;45:859–870.
24 Pletz MW, De RA, Roth A, Neumann KH, Mauch H, Lode H: Early bactericidal activity of moxifloxacin in treatment of pulmonary tuberculosis: a prospective, randomized study. Antimicrob Agents Chemother 2004;48:780–782.
25 Gosling RD, Uiso LO, Sam NE, Bongard E, Kanduma EG, Nyindo M, Morris RW, Gillespie SH: The bactericidal activity of moxifloxacin in patients with pulmonary tuberculosis. Am J Respir Crit Care Med 2003;168:1342–1345.
26 Johnson JL, Hadad DJ, Boom WH, Daley CL, Peloquin CA, Eisenach KD, Jankus DD, Debanne SM, Charlebois ED, Maciel E, et al: Early and extended early bactericidal activity of levofloxacin, gatifloxacin and moxifloxacin in pulmonary tuberculosis. Int J Tuberc Lung Dis 2006;10:605–612.
27 Centre TR: Shortening short course chemotherapy: a randomised clinical trial for treatment of smear positive pulmonary tuberculosis with regimens using ofloxacin in the intensive phase. Indian J Tuberculosis 2002;49:12.
28 Rustomjee R, Lienhardt C, Kanyok T, Davies GR, Levin J, Mthiyane T, Reddy C, Sturm AW, Sirgel FA, Allen J, et al: A phase II study of the sterilising activities of ofloxacin, gatifloxacin and moxifloxacin in pulmonary tuberculosis. Int J Tuberc Lung Dis 2008;12:128–138.
29 Conde MB, Efron A, Loredo C, De Souza GR, Graca NP, Cezar MC, Ram M, Chaudhary MA, Bishai WR, Kritski AL, Chaisson RE: Moxifloxacin versus ethambutol in the initial treatment of tuberculosis: a double-blind, randomised, controlled phase II trial. Lancet 2009;373:1183–1189.
30 Burman WJ, Goldberg S, Johnson JL, Muzanye G, Engle M, Mosher AW, Choudhri S, Daley CL, Munsiff SS, Zhao Z, et al: Moxifloxacin versus ethambutol in the first 2 months of treatment for pulmonary tuberculosis. Am J Respir Crit Care Med 2006;174:331–338.
31 Dorman SE, Johnson JL, Goldberg S, Muzanye G, Padayatchi N, Bozeman L, Heilig CM, Bernardo J, Choudhri S, Grosset JH, et al: Substitution of moxifloxacin for isoniazid during intensive phase treatment of pulmonary tuberculosis. Am J Respir Crit Care Med 2009;180:273–280.
32 MacKenzie WR, Heilig CM, Bozeman L, Johnson JL, Muzanye G, Dunbar D, Jost KC Jr, Diem L, Metchock B, Eisenach K, et al: Geographic differences in time to culture conversion in liquid media: Tuberculosis Trials Consortium study 28. Culture conversion is delayed in Africa. PLoS One 2011;6:e18358.
33 A controlled trial of a 4-month quinolone-containing regimen for the treatment of pulmonary tuberculosis. http://clinicaltrials.gov/ct2/show/NCT00216385?term=gatifloxacin±tuberculosis&rank=2.
34 Controlled comparison of two moxifloxacin containing treatment shortening regimens in pulmonary tuberculosis (REMox TB). http://clinicaltrials.gov/ct2/show/NCT00864383?term=moxifloxacin±tuberculosis&rank=1.
35 Blumberg HM, Burman WJ, Chaisson RE, Daley CL, Etkind SC, Friedman LN, Fujiwara P, Grzemska M, Hopewell PC, Iseman MD, et al: American Thoracic Society/Centers for Disease Control and Prevention/Infectious Diseases Society of America: treatment of tuberculosis. Am J Respir Crit Care Med 2003;167:603–662.
36 Moadebi S, Harder CK, Fitzgerald MJ, Elwood KR, Marra F: Fluoroquinolones for the treatment of pulmonary tuberculosis. Drugs 2007;67:2077–2099.
37 WHO: Guidelines for the programmatic management of drug-resistant tuberculosis: emergency update. Geneva, WHO, 2008.
38 Szklo A, Mello FC, Guerra RL, Dorman SE, Muzy-de-Souza GR, Conde MB: Alternative anti-tuberculosis regimen including ofloxacin for the treatment of patients with hepatic injury. Int J Tuberc Lung Dis 2007;11:775–780.
39 Ho CC, Chen YC, Hu FC, Yu CJ, Yang PC, Luh KT: Safety of fluoroquinolone use in patients with hepatotoxicity induced by anti-tuberculosis regimens. Clin Infect Dis 2009;48:1526–1533.
40 Summary of product characteristics Avelox 400 mg. http://www.medicines.org.uk/emc/medicine/11841.
41 Summary of product characteristics Tavanic 500 mg tablets. http://www.medicines.ie/document.aspx?documentId=5377.
42 Johnston JC, Shahidi NC, Sadatsafavi M, Fitzgerald JM: Treatment outcomes of multidrug-resistant tuberculosis: a systematic review and meta-analysis. PLoS One 2009;4:e6914.
43 Yew WW, Chan CK, Leung CC, Chau CH, Tam CM, Wong PC, Lee J: Comparative roles of levofloxacin and ofloxacin in the treatment of multidrug-resistant tuberculosis: preliminary results of a retrospective study from Hong Kong. Chest 2003;124:1476–1481.
44 Van Deun A, Maug AK, Salim MA, Das PK, Sarker MR, Daru P, Rieder HL: Short, highly effective, and inexpensive standardized treatment of multidrug-resistant tuberculosis. Am J Respir Crit Care Med 2010;182:684–692.
45 Jacobson KR, Tierney DB, Jeon CY, Mitnick CD, Murray MB: Treatment outcomes among patients with extensively drug-resistant tuberculosis: systematic review and meta-analysis. Clin Infect Dis 2010;51:6–14.
46 Cain KP, Nelson LJ, Cegielski JP: Global policies and practices for managing persons exposed to multidrug-resistant tuberculosis. Int J Tuberc Lung Dis 2010;14:269–274.
47 Management of persons exposed to multidrug-resistant tuberculosis. MMWR Morb Mortal Wkly Rep 1992;41:61–71.
48 Papastavros T, Dolovich LR, Holbrook A, Whitehead L, Loeb M: Adverse events associated with pyrazinamide and levofloxacin in the treatment of latent multidrug-resistant tuberculosis. CMAJ 2002;167:131–136.
49 Takiff HE, Salazar L, Guerrero C, Philipp W, Huang WM, Kreiswirth B, Cole ST, Jacobs WR Jr, Telenti A: Cloning and nucleotide sequence of *Mycobacterium tuberculosis gyrA* and *gyrB* genes and detection of quinolone resistance mutations. Antimicrob Agents Chemother 1994;38:773–780.

50 Alangaden GJ, Manavathu EK, Vakulenko SB, Zvonok NM, Lerner SA: Characterization of fluoroquinolone-resistant mutant strains of *Mycobacterium tuberculosis* selected in the laboratory and isolated from patients. Antimicrob Agents Chemother 1995;39:1700–1703.
51 Cheng AF, Yew WW, Chan EW, Chin ML, Hui MM, Chan RC: Multiplex PCR amplimer conformation analysis for rapid detection of gyrA mutations in fluoroquinolone-resistant *Mycobacterium tuberculosis* clinical isolates. Antimicrob Agents Chemother 2004;48:596–601.
52 Von Groll A, Martin A, Jureen P, Hoffner S, Vandamme P, Portaels F, Palomino JC, da Silva PA: Fluoroquinolone resistance in *Mycobacterium tuberculosis* and mutations in gyrA and gyrB. Antimicrob Agents Chemother 2009;53:4498–4500.
53 Sreevatsan S, Pan X, Stockbauer KE, Connell ND, Kreiswirth BN, Whittam TS, Musser JM: Restricted structural gene polymorphism in the *Mycobacterium tuberculosis* complex indicates evolutionarily recent global dissemination. Proc Natl Acad Sci USA 1997;94:9869–9874.
54 Piton J, Petrella S, Delarue M, Andre-Leroux G, Jarlier V, Aubry A, Mayer C: Structural insights into the quinolone resistance mechanism of *Mycobacterium tuberculosis* DNA gyrase. PLoS One 2010;:e12245.
55 Cui Z, Wang J, Lu J, Huang X, Hu Z: Association of mutation patterns in *gyrA/B* genes and ofloxacin resistance levels in *Mycobacterium tuberculosis* isolates from East China in 2009. BMC Infect Dis 2011;11:78.
56 Poissy J, Aubry A, Fernandez C, Lott MC, Chauffour A, Jarlier V, Farinotti R, Veziris N: Should moxifloxacin be used for the treatment of extensively drug-resistant tuberculosis? An answer from a murine model. Antimicrob Agents Chemother 2010;54:4765–4771.
57 Kocagoz T, Hackbarth CJ, Unsal I, Rosenberg EY, Nikaido H, Chambers HF: Gyrase mutations in laboratory-selected, fluoroquinolone-resistant mutants of *Mycobacterium tuberculosis* H37Ra. Antimicrob Agents Chemother 1996;40:1768–1774.
58 Kam KM, Yip CW, Cheung TL, Tang HS, Leung OC, Chan MY: Stepwise decrease in moxifloxacin susceptibility amongst clinical isolates of multidrug-resistant *Mycobacterium tuberculosis:* correlation with ofloxacin susceptibility. Microb Drug Resist 2006;12:7–11.
59 Aubry A, Veziris N, Cambau E, Truffot-Pernot C, Jarlier V, Fisher LM: Novel gyrase mutations in quinolone-resistant and -hypersusceptible clinical isolates of *Mycobacterium tuberculosis:* functional analysis of mutant enzymes. Antimicrob Agents Chemother 2006;50:104–112.
60 Somasundaram S, Paramasivan NC: Susceptibility of *Mycobacterium tuberculosis* strains to gatifloxacin and moxifloxacin by different methods. Chemotherapy 2006;52:190–195.
61 Zhou J, Dong Y, Zhao X, Lee S, Amin A, Ramaswamy S, Domagala J, Musser JM, Drlica K: Selection of antibiotic-resistant bacterial mutants: allelic diversity among fluoroquinolone-resistant mutations. J Infect Dis 2000;182:517–525.
62 Zhao X, Drlica K: Restricting the selection of antibiotic-resistant mutants: a general strategy derived from fluoroquinolone studies. Clin Infect Dis 2001;suppl 3:S147–S156.
63 Dong Y, Zhao X, Kreiswirth BN, Drlica K: Mutant prevention concentration as a measure of antibiotic potency: studies with clinical isolates of *Mycobacterium tuberculosis.* Antimicrob Agents Chemother 2000;44:2581–2584.
64 Blondeau JM, Zhao X, Hansen G, Drlica K: Mutant prevention concentrations of fluoroquinolones for clinical isolates of *Streptococcus pneumoniae.* Antimicrob Agents Chemother 2001;45:433–438.
65 Sindelar G, Zhao X, Liew A, Dong Y, Lu T, Zhou J, Domagala J, Drlica K: Mutant prevention concentration as a measure of fluoroquinolone potency against mycobacteria. Antimicrob Agents Chemother 2000;44:3337–3343.
66 Gillespie SH, Basu S, Dickens AL, O'Sullivan DM, McHugh TD: Effect of subinhibitory concentrations of ciprofloxacin on *Mycobacterium fortuitum* mutation rates. J Antimicrob Chemother 2005;56:344–348.
67 Ginsburg AS, Grosset JH, Bishai WR: Fluoroquinolones, tuberculosis, and resistance. Lancet Infect Dis 2003;3:432–442.
68 Van den Boogaard J, Semvua HH, Boeree MJ, Aarnoutse RE, Kibiki GS: Sale of fluoroquinolones in northern Tanzania: a potential threat for fluoroquinolone use in tuberculosis treatment. J Antimicrob Chemother 2010;65:145–147.
69 Sterling TR: The WHO/IUATLD diagnostic algorithm for tuberculosis and empiric fluoroquinolone use: potential pitfalls. Int J Tuberc Lung Dis 2004;8:1396–1400.
70 Long R, Chong H, Hoeppner V, Shanmuganathan H, Kowalewska-Grochowska K, Shandro C, Manfreda J, Senthilselvan A, Elzainy A, Marrie T: Empirical treatment of community-acquired pneumonia and the development of fluoroquinolone-resistant tuberculosis. Clin Infect Dis 2009;48:1354–1360.
71 Devasia RA, Blackman A, Gebretsadik T, Griffin M, Shintani A, May C, Smith T, Hooper N, Maruri F, Warkentin J, et al: Fluoroquinolone resistance in *Mycobacterium tuberculosis:* the effect of duration and timing of fluoroquinolone exposure. Am J Respir Crit Care Med 2009;180:365–370.
72 Chen TC, Lu PL, Lin CY, Lin WR, Chen YH: Fluoroquinolones are associated with delayed treatment and resistance in tuberculosis: a systematic review and meta-analysis. Int J Infect Dis 2011;15:e211–216.
73 Chiang CY: State of the art series on drug-resistant tuberculosis: it's time to protect fluoroquinolones. Int J Tuberc Lung Dis 2009;13:1319.
74 Cox H, Ford N, Keshavjee S, McDermid C, von Schoen-Angerer T, Mitnick C, Goemaere E: Rational use of moxifloxacin for tuberculosis treatment. Lancet Infect Dis 2011;11:259–260.
75 Marra F, Marra CA, Moadebi S, Shi P, Elwood RK, Stark G, Fitzgerald JM: Levofloxacin treatment of active tuberculosis and the risk of adverse events. Chest 2005;128:1406–1413.
76 Chan ED, Laurel V, Strand MJ, Chan JF, Huynh ML, Goble M, Iseman MD: Treatment and outcome analysis of 205 patients with multidrug-resistant tuberculosis. Am J Respir Crit Care Med 2004;169:1103–1109.
77 Park-Wyllie LY, Juurlink DN, Kopp A, Shah BR, Stukel TA, Stumpo C, Dresser L, Low DE, Mamdani MM: Outpatient gatifloxacin therapy and dysglycemia in older adults. N Engl J Med 2006;354:1352–1361.
78 Sekiguchi JI, Disratthakit A, Maeda S, Doi N: Characteristic resistance mechanism of DC-159a, a new respiratory quinolone, in *Mycobacterium tuberculosis.* Antimicrob Agents Chemother 2011, E-pub ahead of print.
79 Ahmad Z, Minkowski A, Peloquin CA, Williams KN, Mdluli KE, Grosset JH, Nuermberger EL: Activity of the fluoroquinolone DC-159a in the initial and continuation phases of treatment of murine tuberculosis. Antimicrob Agents Chemother 2011;55:1781–1783.



Dr. Stephen H. Gillespie, MB, BCh, BAO, MD, DSc, FRCP (Edin), FRCPath, Sir James Black Professor of Medicine
School of Medicine, University of St. Andrews, North Haugh
St. Andrews KY16 9TF (UK)
Tel. +44 13 3446 1871, E-Mail shg3@st-andrews.ac.uk

Donald PR, van Helden PD (eds): Antituberculosis Chemotherapy.
Prog Respir Res. Basel, Karger, 2011, vol 40, pp 61–72

# Current Standard Treatment

Andrew A. Vernon

Division of TB Elimination, NCHHSTP, OID, Centers for Disease Control and Prevention, Atlanta, Ga., USA

**Abstract**

Therapy of tuberculosis has been hailed as one of the great achievements of the mid-20th century. The remarkable efficacy of short-course chemotherapy (SCC) as developed by the British Medical Research Council and others is now well established. However, problems of long duration, complexity, toxicity, failure of intermittency to succeed in important subpopulations, and pharmacokinetic variability persist. Some of the evidence for the success of SCC is presented, as are some of the reasons why alternatives are being sought.
Copyright © 2011 S. Karger AG, Basel

Therapy of tuberculosis (TB) has been hailed as one of the great achievements of the mid-20th century; the remarkable series of clinical trials carried out by the British Medical Research Council (BMRC) and their colleagues in Africa, India, Hong Kong and Singapore represent one of the major accomplishments of modern medicine [1]. These trials, in conjunction with related trials carried out by many others, have defined standard TB short-course chemotherapy (SCC) for the past 30 years. Nearly 2 decades ago, TB treatment with SCC was hailed as one of the most cost-effective public health interventions available: 'These very low costs translate into costs per DALY saved of about USD 1 to USD 3, making chemotherapy for tuberculosis one of the most cost-effective of all interventions' [2]. Thirteen years later, despite a 5- to 20-fold increase in costs, it could still be asserted that, with application of the World Health Organization's directly observed treatment short-course (DOTS) strategy [3], 'short-course chemotherapy for the treatment of infectious and noninfectious TB patients is highly cost-effective for the control of either epidemic or endemic TB. When a new treatment program is compared with a previous program, DOTS often saves money as well as preventing cases and deaths '[4]. The budget in 2009 for first-line anti-TB drugs in the national programmes of the 22 high-burden countries designated by the World Health Organization is a median of only USD 33 per patient (range USD 18–308) and increased only 20% over the prior 7 years [5]. This standard 6-month regimen [consisting of 2 months of isoniazid, rifampicin and pyrazinamide (±ethambutol or streptomycin), followed by 4 months of isoniazid and rifampicin, administered either daily or thrice weekly] has been shown to be universally effective, with virtually no failures during therapy and a low rate (1–3%) of relapse after completion of therapy. With such an exceptionally effective and affordable treatment, one may legitimately wonder why the disease remains a major problem, responsible still for over 1.5 million deaths and over 9 million new cases worldwide each year. However, despite the continuing longevity of this intervention, it is uncertain for a variety of reasons whether it will remain the mainstay of successful TB control programmes. These reasons include:

1 requirement for long duration (6–9 months) of a complex regimen employing 3–5 different medications, and consequent susceptibility of the regimen to failures of adherence ('default'), entailing risks of clinical and microbiological failure, relapse and acquisition of new drug resistance;
2 persistent and problematic toxicity of some member drugs within the regimen;
3 relative weakness of intermittent regimens, especially among persons with HIV-associated TB, limiting the

ability of programmes to render this approach more cost-friendly when combined with supervision of therapy;
4 wide variation in individual pharmacokinetics of member drugs, resulting probably in the unpredictable inadequacy of therapy in some patients.

## Establishment and Efficacy of Short-Course Chemotherapy, the Current Standard of Care

SCC was developed as a result of the global effort in the period 1945–1990 to develop regimens for the treatment of TB. The history of this effort is well portrayed in multiple texts [6]. The leaders in this effort were the senior scientists directing the studies and clinical trials of the BMRC (table 1), including particularly Wallace Fox and Denis Mitchison [1]. The first modern randomized clinical trial was that conducted to evaluate the impact of streptomycin (alone) in the treatment of pulmonary TB [7]. That trial demonstrated that use of streptomycin had a substantial impact upon short-term morbidity and mortality; follow-up studies revealed that long-term mortality was affected very little, due to the acquisition of resistance to streptomycin by the large majority of those receiving it [8, 9]. Thus, it became almost immediately evident that single-drug therapy was unlikely to be effective in the long-term management of TB. Multidrug therapy, composed of streptomycin and para-aminosalicylic acid, was tested shortly thereafter and shown to be considerably more effective, despite the relative weakness of para-aminosalicylic acid [10]. With the advent of isoniazid in the early 1950s, multiple drug therapy combining isoniazid, para-aminosalicylic acid and streptomycin was rapidly shown to be even more successful, and became the standard of care for a decade [11].

The role of adherence was recognized in the 1950s by MRC investigators [12], who subsequently conducted their trials with supervised administration of medication. They also demonstrated that therapies shown to be effective in clinical trials would achieve less dramatic rates of success when applied in programmatic settings [13]. Additional drugs became available over the next 20 years. Rifamycins proved to be the major addition to this group of agents; in combination with isoniazid, rifampicin shortened the period of therapy required to achieve a nearly relapse-free cure from 18–24 months to 6–9 months. Ethambutol offered further protection against drug resistance and had the advantage of being orally active; it was used with, or in place of, streptomycin when isoniazid or rifampicin were lost to drug resistance, as much because of its relative freedom from toxicity as because of its potency, which was relatively low. Pyrazinamide, a drug which appeared to possess remarkable sterilizing ability in animal models and in humans [14], had been early disfavoured after its use at high doses (approx. 50 mg/kg) had resulted in deaths from liver toxicity [15]. Its re-introduction at lower doses (25–40 mg/kg) limited its toxicity while preserving much of its remarkable sterilizing potency [16], and the addition of 2 months of pyrazinamide to the combination of isoniazid and rifampicin permitted the shortening of the total therapy duration from 9 to 6 months [1, 17, 18]. Finally, this same group of gifted investigators demonstrated in Hong Kong and Singapore that TB could be cured with largely similar rates of success using intermittent drug administration, an advance that rendered such therapies more accessible to the developing world [1].

Table 1 shows the results of the MRC trials that were pivotal in the development of what is now standard SCC for drug-sensitive pulmonary TB.

With all of these regimens, failure during therapy became rare. It should be remembered that the MRC was working to define a regimen that would be effective for developing countries. The initial high costs of the newer drugs led them to explore regimens that limited the use of these drugs. This also diminished their interest in exploration of higher doses of rifampicin, despite some early indications that higher doses might be more effective [19].

These trials established that regimens with 6 months of isoniazid and rifampicin in combination with an initial 2 months of pyrazinamide were highly efficacious; there were rarely failures during therapy when treating susceptible organisms, and relapse rates after treatment were only 1–3% when therapy was administered daily. Moreover, relapse rates in regimens administered thrice weekly were equivalent. These MRC trials demonstrated the association between cavitation and/or extent of disease and risk of eventual relapse [20]. Comparisons of findings in East/Central Africa and in Hong Kong demonstrated that different geographic populations can differ substantially in response to TB therapy, even when rates of cavitation, extent of disease and 2-month sputum conversion are considered (table 2). While these data come from different trials and are thus subject to intertrial variability, recent data from the Tuberculosis Trials Consortium comparing responses in patients in North America and Africa have also reflected potential geographic differences in response to TB therapy [29], as have results of a trial of treatment shortening reported by Johnson et al.

**Table 1.** Two-month and 2-year outcomes of selected arms in MRC TB trials, Africa and Hong Kong [1]

| Study | Year begun | Regimen | Dosing rhythm days/week | Duration months | n | 2 months sputum culture negative % | 2-year relapse rate, % |
|---|---|---|---|---|---|---|---|
| E/CA1 | 1970 | 6SHR | 7/7 | 6 | 152 | 69 | 3 |
| | | 6SHZ | 7/7 | 6 | 153 | 66 | 8 |
| | | 6SH | 7/7 | 6 | 112 | 49 | 29 |
| E/CA2 | 1972 | 6SHR | 7/7 | 6 | 171 | 70 | 2 |
| | | 6HR | 7/7 | 6 | 164 | 64 | 7 |
| | | 2SHRZ/4TH | 7/7 | 6 | 179 | 83 | 7 |
| E/CA4 | 1976 | 2SHRZ/2HR | 7/7 | 4 | 104 | 85 | 11 |
| | | 2SHRZ/2HRZ | 7/7 | 4 | 104 | 85 | 16 |
| E/CA5 | 1978 | 2SHRZ/4HR | 7/7 | 6 | 166 | 84 | 3 |
| | | 2SHRZ/4HZ | 7/7 | 6 | 164 | 84 | 8 |
| | | 2SHRZ/4H | 7/7 | 6 | 156 | 84 | 10 |
| | | 2SHRZ/6H | 7/7 | 8 | 123 | 84 | 3% |
| S1 | 1970 | 2SHRZ/4HR | 7/7 | 6 | 80 | 98 | 2 |
| | | 2SHRZ/4HRZ | 7/7 | 6 | 78 | 98 | 0 |
| HK3 | 1977 | $6(HRZS)_3$ | 3/7 | 6 | 151 | 90 | 1 |
| | | $6(HRZE)_3$ | 3/7 | 6 | 160 | 90 | 2 |
| | | 6HRZE | 7/7 | 6 | 163 | 94 | 1 |
| HK4 | 1979 | $6(HRZS)_3$ – 2 months Z | 3/7 | 6 | 220 | 91 | 3 |
| | | $6(HRZS)_3$ – 4 months Z | 3/7 | 6 | 205 | 91 | 5 |
| | | $6(HRZS)_3$ – 6 months Z | 3/7 | 6 | 208 | 91 | 3 |
| | | $6(HRZ)_3$ – 6 months Z | 3/7 | 6 | 199 | 88 | 6 (+2% failure)[a] |

E/CA1, 2, 4, 5 = First, second, fourth, fifth East/Central Africa trials; S1 = first Singapore trial; HK3, 4 = third, fourth Hong Kong trials.
H = Isoniazid; R = rifampicin; Z = pyrazinamide; S = streptomycin; T = thiacetazone; E = ethambutol; $(HRZE)_3$ = HRZE thrice weekly.
[a] Bacteriological failure occurred only in this group.

[30] from Uganda, the Philippines and Brazil. Studies of persons with silico-TB in Hong Kong provided one of the earliest indications that persons with immune deficits might require therapy for longer than the 6-month period of the short-course regimen (table 3) [1, 31].

A large number of trials were conducted by groups other than the BMRC, and these trials served often to confirm or extend the findings of MRC work (table 4). Unique among the contributions of these other trials were investigations of twice weekly regimens.

Hypotheses concerning the biology of the tubercle bacillus were developed during these same years, based largely upon quantitative bacteriological investigations conducted in parallel with the MRC trials. The leading model, conceptualized by Professor Denis Mitchison, envisions several differing populations of bacilli within a diseased host: one

**Table 2.** Comparison of similar regimens in MRC's East/Central Africa and Hong Kong trials

| 6-month regimen | Study site | Patients assessed for relapse n | Moderate/ extensive cavitation % | Moderate/ extensive disease % | Culture negative at 2 months % | 2-year rate of relapse % |
|---|---|---|---|---|---|---|
| 6SHR | East Africa 2 [21, 22] | 171 | 73 | 78 | 70 | 2 |
| | Hong Kong 2 [23, 24] | 143 | 40 | 49 | 88 | 6 |
| 6SHZ | East Africa 1 [25, 26] | 153 | 82 | 84 | 66 | 8 |
| | Hong Kong 1 [27, 28] | 60 | 40 | 57 | 77 | 18 |
| 2SHRZ/4(SHZ)$_2$ | East Africa 2 [21, 22] | 159 | 80 | 82 | 80 | 4 |
| | Hong Kong 2 [23, 24] | 87 | 40 | 49 | 95 | 7 |

For study details, see footnote to table 1.

**Table 3.** Comparison of 2 regimen durations in patients with silico-TB in Hong Kong

| Regimen and duration | Patients n | Duration of therapy months | Culture negative at 2 months % | 3-year rate of relapse % | 5-year rate of relapse % |
|---|---|---|---|---|---|
| 6(SHRZ)$_3$ | 49 | 6 months | 80 | 22 | 33 |
| 8(SHRZ)$_3$ | 50 | 8 months | 80 | 7 | 11 |

For study details, see footnote to table 1.

population undergoes relatively rapid replication, a second replicates and metabolizes more slowly in acidic microenvironments, and a third manifests only intermittent and rare periods of metabolism and multiplication [42]. The several 'first-line' drugs are hypothesized to act preferentially on different populations: isoniazid is thought to be quickly lethal for rapidly replicating bacilli, pyrazinamide is lethal for more slowly replicating bacilli in acidic microenvironments [43], while rifampicin kills populations of relatively dormant bacilli [44]. These differing effects are well demonstrated in early bactericidal activity studies, first developed by Jindani and Mitchison [45, 46]. Over the first 2 days there is a rapid early 'kill' attributed to isoniazid; this drug plays another important role in protecting against the development of resistance to companion drugs. Discussions about 'sterilizing activity' (the ability to prevent relapse after treatment) remain confusing, as noted by Davies recently [47]. Regimens with a high 2-month sputum conversion rate (later proposed as an indicator of 'sterilizing activity' [48]) may still relapse substantially, as illustrated by the 4th African and 1st Singapore trials of 4-month therapy [1].

Only relatively modest advances in therapy of drug-sensitive TB have been made in the past 25 years. Some of these merit comment, but none has led to a fundamental change in the standard regimen for drug-susceptible TB. Among the advances achieved in this domain are (1) the development of rifabutin [49, 50], a drug initially but mostly incorrectly thought to possess activity against rifampicin-resistant bacilli, and now especially useful when induction of cytochrome P450 enzymes must be minimized (e.g. with concurrent use of HIV protease inhibitors) [51], and (2) the identification of a role for newer fluoroquinolones in the treatment of drug-sensitive TB [52], when isoniazid cannot be used. In addition, (3) the emerging problem of HIV-associated TB has identified points of relative weakness in this standard regimen, and these are now open to correction. Advances in the approaches used in the clinical development of new drugs have hinged upon the improved understanding of the response of drug-sensitive TB to this standard regimen as well.

Rifabutin was for some years a more costly rifamycin than rifampicin, useful primarily in the treatment of *Mycobacterium avium intracellulare* infections in persons

**Table 4.** Two-month and 2-year outcomes for selected non-MRC TB trials

| Study | Year begun | Regimen | Dosing rhythm days/week | Duration months | n | 2 months sputum culture negative % | 2-year relapse rate % |
|---|---|---|---|---|---|---|---|
| BTA1 [32] | 1972 | HRS/E | 7/7 | 6 (0–2 cm cavity) | 160 | n.r. | 5 |
| | | HRS/E | 7/7 | 12 (0–2 cm cavity) | 155 | n.r. | 2 |
| | | HRS/E | 7/7 | 9 (>2 cm cavity) | 135 | n.r. | 0 |
| | | HRS/E | 7/7 | 18 (>2 cm cavity) | 127 | n.r. | 0 |
| BTA2 [17] | 1979 | 2HRZS/HR | 7/7 | 6 | 125 | 77 | 1 |
| | | 2HRZE/HR | 7/7 | 6 | 132 | 77 | 2 |
| | | 2HRE/HR | 7/7 | 9 | 136 | 64 | 1 |
| Poland [33, 34] | 1974 | 6HRE | 7/7 | 6 | 87 | 63 | 13 |
| | | $2HRE/4(HR)_2$ | 7/7→2/7 | 6 | 86 | 69 | 18 |
| | | $2HRE/4(HRE)_1$ | 7/7→1/7 | 6 | 83 | 66 | 22 |
| | | $2HRE/4(HRE)_2$ | 7/7→2/7 | 6 | 84 | 75 | 8 |
| Poland [35] | 1977 | $2HRZS/4(HR)_2$ | 7/7→2/7 | 6 | 85 | 91 | 0 |
| Poland [35, 36] | 1980 | $2HRZS/4(HR)_2$ | 7/7→2/7 | 6 | 56 | 74 | 2 |
| | | $2HRZ/4(HR)_2$ | 7/7→2/7 | 6 | 116 | 85 | 4 |
| Arkansas [37] | 1976 | $1HR/8(HR)_2$ | 7/7→2/7 | 9 | 1028 | 93 S–<br>68 S+ | 2.8 F<br>2.1 R |
| PHS19 [38] | 1970 | 5HR/12HE: R450 | 7/7 | 5→7–12 | 105 | ~60 | 5.7 F<br>1.6 R |
| | | 5HR/12HE: R600 | 7/7 | 5→7–12 | 224 | ~70 | 0.4 F<br>1.4 R |
| | | 5HR/12HE: R750 | 7/7 | 5→7–12 | 223 | ~75 | 1.8 F<br>0.0 R |
| PHS20 [39] | 1975 | 6HR→9HE | 7/7 | 6→9 | 192 | n.r. | 2 |
| | | 6HR | 7/7 | 6 | 187 | n.r. | 9 |
| PHS21 [18] | 1981 | 2HRZ(E)/4HR | 7/7 | 6 | 385 | 74 | 5 |
| | | 9HR | 7/7 | 9 | 231 | 67 | 3 |
| PHS22 [40] | 1995 | $2HRZE\text{-}S/4(HR)_2$ | var.→2/7 | 6 | 440 | 82 | 6 |
| | | $2HRZE\text{-}S/4(HP)_1$ | var.→1/7 | 6 | 455 | 77 | 10 |
| Denver [41] | 1981 | ½HRZE/1½<br>$(HRZE)_2/4(HR)_2$ | 7/7→2/7 | 6 | 125 | 75 | 2 |

BTA1, 2 = First, second British Thoracic Association trials; PHS19, 20, 21, 22 = US Public Health Service Trials 19–22; var. = variable [PHS22 allowed daily (47%), thrice weekly (3%) or twice weekly (50%) intensive phases with standard therapy, prior to enrollment at completion of intensive phase]; S = sputum; n.r. = not reported; n = number enrolled or assessed for relapse; F = failure during therapy; R = relapse after therapy. Outcomes include failures and relapses, based on radiometric liquid culture. ½HRZE/1½ $(HRZE)_2/4(HR)_2$ = 0.5 months HRZE, followed by 1.5 months HRZE twice weekly, then 4 months HR twice weekly. For other explanations, see also footnote to table 1.

**Table 5.** Stratified estimates of failure, relapse and acquired drug resistance in randomized controlled trials of new cases of pulmonary TB (from Menzies et al. [55])

| Outcome | Feature | Events/participants | Pooled event rate across all trials |
|---|---|---|---|
| Failure | rifampicin 1–2 months | 94/4,133 | 1.8 (0.2–3.3) |
| | rifampicin 3–5 months | 16/2,508 | 0.3 (0–0.6) |
| | rifampicin 6–7 months | 150/10,060 | 0.4 (0.1–0.7) |
| | rifampicin ≥8 months | 10/1,384 | 0.2 (0–0.6) |
| Relapse | rifampicin 1–2 months | 367/3,349 | 16.0 (11.1–20.9) |
| | rifampicin 3–5 months | 185/2,389 | 7.1 (4.5–9.7) |
| | rifampicin 6–7 months | 364/8,639 | 3.8 (2.9–4.7) |
| | rifampicin ≥8 months | 14/1,181 | 1.0 (0.2–1.7) |
| Acquired drug resistance | rifampicin 1–2 months | 41/2,847 | 0.8 (0–1.6) |
| | rifampicin 3–5 months | 10/1,932 | 0.3 (0–0.6) |
| | rifampicin 6–7 months | 60/7,180 | 0.4 (0.1–0.7) |
| | rifampicin ≥8 months | 6/1,249 | 0.2 (0–0.5) |

Figures in parentheses indicate 95% confidence intervals.

with HIV/AIDS. A 2007 Cochrane Review by Davies et al. [53] concluded that replacement of rifampicin by rifabutin for first-line treatment of TB was not supported by the current evidence, and that HIV-positive people with TB, the group most likely to benefit from the rifabutin use, were underrepresented in trials to date. Rifabutin is no longer on patent; in 2009, the Clinton Foundation announced an agreement with Pfizer which will make the drug available in low-resource settings at a cost of 1 USD per 150-mg dose, or USD 90 for a full treatment course in persons receiving concurrent anti-HIV therapy with ritonavir-boosted HIV protease inhibitors [54]. This use of rifabutin would reduce the cost of the boosted protease inhibitor antiretroviral therapy, with resultant overall cost savings in the treatment of both diseases; as a result, the World Health Organization has now added rifabutin to its list of 'essential medicines'.

It is apparent that all of these regimens contain at least 4 months of rifampicin. A superb recent systematic review and meta-analysis by Menzies et al. [55], evaluating clinical trial data involving new cases of pulmonary TB in non-HIV-infected persons, concluded that regimens containing shorter durations of rifampicin have significantly worse outcomes (more failure, relapse and acquired drug resistance) than those with longer durations of rifampicin treatment (table 5). This key role of the rifamycin component of SCC was demonstrated more dramatically in the Union's Study A reported by Jindani et al. [56]. In that study, continuation phases of 6HE (isoniazid-ethambutol) and 4HR (isoniazid-rifampicin) followed daily or thrice weekly induction with 2HRZE(isoniazid-rifampicin-pyrazinamide-ethambutol); the 6HE arms experienced 10–14% unfavourable outcomes, compared to 5% in the 4HR arm.

The same review of Menzies et al. [55] presented worrisome evidence that the earlier assumption, based on MRC data [57], that baseline isoniazid resistance could be adequately treated with standard SCC might not be entirely correct. Menzies et al. found significantly higher rates of failure, relapse and acquired drug resistance among trial participants who entered with baseline isoniazid resistance (table 6), suggesting that isoniazid resistance might merit the label of 'gateway to multidrug resistance'.

The Menzies group performed a similar review of trials involving HIV-associated TB and found non-significantly increased rates of failure and relapse (but not death) among such patients treated for shorter periods with rifampicin (table 7) [58]. The group reported that intermittent therapy during the intensive phase of treatment was associated with

**Table 6.** Stratified estimates of failure, relapse and acquired drug resistance in randomized controlled trials of new cases of pulmonary TB (from Menzies et al. [55])

| Outcome | Feature | Events/participants | Pooled event rate across all trials |
|---|---|---|---|
| Failure | drug sensitive | 120/14,900 | 0.3 (0.1–0.4) |
| | isoniazid resistance | 25/477 | 2.8 (0.7 to 5.0) |
| Relapse | drug sensitive | 684/13,302 | 3.7 (2.8–4.7) |
| | isoniazid resistance | 60/403 | 11.4 (6.5–16.2) |
| Acquired drug resistance | drug sensitive | 70/12,256 | 0.3 (0.1–0.4) |
| | isoniazid resistance | 13/380 | 2.4 (0.5–4.4) |

Figures in parentheses indicate 95% confidence intervals.

**Table 7.** Stratified estimates of failure, relapse and death in randomized controlled trials of new cases of pulmonary TB in persons co-infected with HIV (from Khan et al. [58])

| Outcome | Feature | Events/participants | Pooled event rate across all trials |
|---|---|---|---|
| Failure | rifampicin 2 months | 27/872 | 2.9 (1.0–4.8) |
| | rifampicin 6 months | 45/1,377 | 2.6 (1.1–4.1) |
| | rifampicin ≥8 months | 14/441 | 1.9 (0–4.0) |
| Relapse | rifampicin 2 months | 40/258 | 10.8 (0–25.1) |
| | rifampicin 6 months | 100/730 | 9.8 (0–19.8) |
| | rifampicin ≥8 months | 20/314 | 3.3 (0–9.0) |
| Death during treatment | rifampicin 2 months | 205/1,077 | 16.6 (10.2–22.9) |
| | rifampicin 6 months | 196/1,573 | 10.5 (6.8–14.3) |
| | rifampicin ≥8 months | 60/501 | 11.7 (5.9–18.4) |

Figures in parentheses indicate 95% confidence intervals.

significantly higher rates of failure and relapse (table 8); this was not seen in the review of largely HIV-negative persons with TB [55]. The NYC TB Program reported that the nature of the intensive phase regimen had a significant impact upon the frequency of relapse and of acquired rifamycin resistance among patients with HIV-TB [59]. They found a 6- to 7-fold increase in the risk of relapse and of acquired rifamycin resistance among patients who received intermittent therapy during the intensive phase. However, they did not report an association of shorter rifampicin or treatment duration with relapse or acquired rifamycin resistance.

The TB Trials Consortium Study 22 assessed once weekly therapy with isoniazid and rifapentine in the continuation phase, and early reported that acquired rifamycin resistance developed frequently among persons with HIV-TB receiving the once weekly regimen; risk was concentrated among those with more advanced HIV disease [60]. A similar finding occurred in TB Trials Consortium Study 23, which assessed an intermittent rifabutin-based regimen suitable for co-administration with antiretroviral therapy; in that study, relapse with acquired rifamycin monoresistance was associated with initial CD4 cell count below 100/mm$^3$, and

**Table 8.** Pooled estimates of outcomes stratified by schedule of treatment administration during the initial intensive phase (first 8 weeks) in randomized controlled trials of new cases of pulmonary TB in persons co-infected with HIV (from Khan et al. [58])

| Outcome | Feature | Events/participants | Pooled event rate across all trials |
|---|---|---|---|
| Failure | daily | 74/2,531 | 2.5 (1.5–3.5) |
| | thrice weekly | 12/163 | 5.3 (0.4–10.2) |
| Relapse | daily | 142/1,241 | 6.7 (0.6–12.8) |
| | thrice weekly | 18/65 | 28.1 (0–69.5) |
| Death during treatment | daily | 430/2,957 | 11.9 (8.5–15.3) |
| | thrice weekly | 31/194 | 14.3 (4.8–23.9) |

Figures in parentheses indicate 95% confidence intervals.

was encountered more frequently among patients receiving highly intermittent (twice weekly) intensive-phase therapy [61]. Swaminathan et al. [62] in Chennai compared 6 versus 9 months of therapy with India's standard thrice weekly regimen [$2(HRZE)_3$ $4(HR)_3$ vs. $2(HRZE)_3$ $7(HR)_3$] in persons with HIV-TB. They reported high rates of acquired rifamycin resistance among failures in both arms, and reported higher rates of bacteriological recurrence in the 6-month arm.

Risk factors for relapse with standard SCC have been evaluated within a number of clinical trials. In these studies, certain factors have been consistently shown to influence treatment outcomes. Those shown in table 9 include the best established of these [66].

## Intermittency: Efficient and Cost-Effective, or Not?

Mitchison and colleagues considered early the possibility that TB therapy might be effective when administered intermittently. An early (and unsuccessful) effort investigated whether intermittent administration might diminish the rate at which streptomycin resistance was acquired during monotherapy [67]. Intermittent administration remained attractive in the early years of TB chemotherapy due to the high cost of the new agents such as rifampicin. Later, the great difficulties encountered in supervising therapy for the extended periods required even by 'short-course' regimens rendered the concept appealing. Mitchison's group reported on bacteriological findings which might support the use of intermittent regimens, in particular the existence of a lag in active culture growth between withdrawal of drug and resumption of bacillary multiplication, called the postantibiotic effect [68–70]. This effect suggested that intermittent regimens might be equally effective as daily regimens. Considerable effort has been devoted to the demonstration of the efficacy of intermittent regimens (see Hong Kong thrice weekly trials in table 1, and Polish, Study 22 and Denver twice weekly trials in table 4), which performed adequately in non-immunosuppressed patients. Intermittent regimens remain highly attractive for programmatic reasons, making supervision of therapy considerably more practicable. However, as noted earlier, substantial evidence now supports the view that increasing intermittency during the intensive phase is disadvantageous to persons at high risk for relapse, especially those who are immunosuppressed. The Hong Kong TB programme reviewed over 12,000 patients and performed a nested case-control study using a conditional logistic regression model to assess factors influencing the risk of relapse. They found a significant increase in risk with the thrice-weekly-throughout regimen compared to the daily regimen [71]. Moreover, a growing body of experimental literature suggests that maintenance of higher and consistent drug levels through more frequent administration and/or higher dosing of some anti-TB drugs can lead to more rapid cure [72].

## Supervision of Therapy: Does DOT Matter?

In most areas of the globe, the elements of current standard treatment include attention to supervision of therapy. In the USA, many programmes support DOT for most or all patients.

**Table 9.** Factors predictive of relapse in TB treatment trials of current SCC

| Authors | Year | Trial site/population | Factors significantly associated with relapse |
|---|---|---|---|
| Aber and Nunn [20] | 1978 | East Africa<br>Hong Kong | 2- to 3-month sputum culture<br>Pretreatment cavitation<br>Residual cavitation<br>2-month smear<br>Residual extent of disease on CXR<br>Months of treatment |
| Zierski et al. [34] | 1980 | Poland | Extensive disease on CXR<br>Large or persistent cavities<br>Heavy growth on pretreatment sputum cultures<br>Slow sputum conversion<br>Heavy use of alcohol<br>Concomitant disease |
| Johnson et al. [63] | 1997 | Uganda/HIV positive | (Thiacetazone regimen)<br>Age 30 or greater<br>Irregular compliance |
| Tam et al. [64] | 2002 | Hong Kong/<br>HIV negative | Once weekly therapy<br>Male sex |
| TB Trials Consortium [42] | 2002 | North America/<br>HIV negative | 2-month sputum culture<br>Baseline cavitation on CXR<br>Underweight<br>Bilateral disease on CXR<br>Non-Hispanic white race |
| Hoechst Marion Roussel [65] | 2002 | South Africa,<br>North America/<br>HIV negative | Male sex<br>2-month sputum culture<br>Adherence in intensive phase |

CXR = Chest X-ray.

Internationally, supervision of therapy is one of the elements of the DOTS approach. The Global Stop TB Strategy's first principal component calls for strengthening of the third element of DOTS, 'standardized treatment, with supervision and patient support', as 1 of 5 lines of action to pursue:

> Supervised treatment, which may have to include direct observation of therapy (DOT), helps patients to take their drugs regularly and complete treatment, thus achieving cure and preventing the development of drug resistance. Supervision must be carried out in a context-specific and patient-sensitive manner, and is meant to ensure adherence on the part both of providers (in giving proper care and support) and of patients (in taking regular treatment). Depending on the local conditions, supervision may be undertaken at a health facility, in the workplace, in the community or at home. It should be provided by a treatment partner or treatment supporter who is acceptable to the patient and is trained and supervised by health services. [3]

The concept of direct supervision of ambulatory therapy was championed by Wallace Fox of the BMRC [73]. There has been considerable debate over the use of DOT since then [74]. Strong and enthusiastic endorsements of DOT have come from multiple experiences in the USA [75–78]. It is particularly thought to be important when intermittent treatment regimens are employed, since each individual dose represents a larger proportion of the total medication received. Studies in international settings have had variable results. Some studies have demonstrated utility for DOT, especially when implemented as part of an overall case management strategy [79, 80]. Some studies with negative findings have been criticized for poor implementation of DOT [81] or for poor representation of the universe of TB patients [82]. Other studies of DOT have demonstrated substantial cost-effectiveness in both low- and high-resource settings [83, 84]. One of the obvious advantages of DOT is that it provides a self-apparent measure (the number of doses taken) of the adequacy of the treatment course, which otherwise is often only approximated by the duration of the treatment period or the consumption of the full complement of medications over an unspecified time period. It is also notable that virtually every trial of standard therapy has employed some form of supervision of therapy; generalization of trial results to the unsupervised circumstance is thus of uncertain validity.

## Conclusion

The great success of the current standard SCC for TB is evident from many trials and from its programmatic history. Some of its limitations, and thus some of the justification for efforts to identify new and improved therapies, are also evident. A remarkable combination of intelligence, creativity, diligence and luck supported the development of SCC. The same factors are needed in our search for improvements.

## References


1 Fox W, Ellard GA, Mitchison DA: Studies on the treatment of tuberculosis undertaken by the British Medical Research Council Tuberculosis Units, 1946–1986, with relevant subsequent publications. Int J Tuberc Lung Dis 1999;3:S231–S279.

2 World Bank: World Development Report 1993. Investing in Health. Oxford, Oxford University Press, 1993.

3 World Health Organization and Stop TB Partnership: The Stop TB Strategy: Building on and Enhancing DOTS to Meet the TB-Related Millennium Development Goals. WHO/HTM/TB/2006.368. Geneva, WHO, 2006, pp 9–11.

4 Dye C, Floyd K: Tuberculosis; in Jamison DT, Breman JG, Measham AR, et al (eds): Disease Control Priorities in Developing Countries, ed 2. New York, Oxford University Press, 2006, pp 289–312.

5 World Health Organization: Global Tuberculosis Control: Epidemiology, Strategy, Financing. WHO/HTM/TB/2009.411. Geneva, WHO, 2009, p 72.

6 Iseman MD: A Clinician's Guide to Tuberculosis. Philadelphia, Lippincott Williams and Wilkins, 2000, chapt 1.

7 Medical Research Council: Streptomycin treatment of pulmonary tuberculosis. Br Med J 1948;ii:769–782.

8 Crofton J, Mitchison DA: Streptomycin resistance in pulmonary tuberculosis. Br Med J 1948;ii:1009–1015.

9 Fox W, Sutherland I, Daniels M: A five-year assessment of patients in a controlled trial of streptomycin in pulmonary tuberculosis. Q J Med 1954;23:47–366.

10 Medical Research Council: Treatment of pulmonary tuberculosis with streptomycin and para-amino-salicylic acid. Br Med J 1950;ii:1073–1085.

11 Ferebee SH, Mount FW: Chemotherapy of tuberculosis, progress and promise. Publ Hlth Reports 1957;72:413–420.

12 Fox W: The problem of self-administration of drugs: with particular reference to pulmonary tuberculosis. Br Med J 1964;i:135–142.

13 Kent PW, Fox W, Miller AB, Nunn AJ, Tall R, Mitchison DA: The therapy of pulmonary tuberculosis in Kenya: a comparison of the results achieved in controlled clinical trials with those achieved by the routine treatment services. Tubercle 1970;51:24–38.

14 Yeager RL, Munroe WGC, Dessau FI: Pyrazinamide (Aldinamide) in the treatment of pulmonary tuberculosis. Am Rev Tuberc 1952;65:523–546.

15 McDermott W, Ormond L, Muschenheim C, Deuschle K, McCune RM, Tompsett R: Pyrazinamide-isoniazid in tuberculosis. Am Rev Tuberc 1954;69:319–333.

16 Hepatic toxicity of pyrazinamide used with isoniazid in tuberculous patients. A United States Public Health Service Tuberculosis Therapy Trial. Am Rev Respir Dis 1959;80:371–387.

17 British Thoracic Association: A controlled trial of six months chemotherapy in pulmonary tuberculosis. Second report: results during the 24 months after the end of chemotherapy. Am Rev Respir Dis 1982;126:460.

18 Combs DL, O'Brien RJ, Geiter LJ: USPHS Tuberculosis Short-Course Trial 21: effectiveness, toxicity and acceptability. The report of final results. Ann Intern Med 1990;112:397–406.

19 Kreis B, Pretet S, Birenbaum J, Guibout P, Hazeman JJ, Orin E, Perdrizet S, Weil J: Two three-month treatment regimens for pulmonary tuberculosis. Bull Int Union Tuberc 1976;51:71–75.

20 Aber VR, Nunn AJ: Factors affecting relapse following short-course chemotherapy. Bull Int Union Tuberc 1978;53:260–264.

21 East African/British Medical Research Councils: Controlled clinical trial of 4 short course (6-month) regimens of chemotherapy for treatment of pulmonary tuberculosis. Second East African/British Medical Research Council Study. Lancet 1974;ii:1100–1106.

22 East African/British Medical Research Councils: Controlled clinical trial of 4 short course (6-month) regimens of chemotherapy for treatment of pulmonary tuberculosis. Second report. Second East African/British Medical Research Council Study. Am Rev Respir Dis 1976;114:471–475.

23 Hong Kong Chest Service/British Medical Research Council: Controlled trial of 6-month and 8-month regimens in the treatment of pulmonary tuberculosis. First report. Am Rev Respir Dis 1978;118:219–227.

24 Hong Kong Chest Service/British Medical Research Council: Controlled trial of 6-month and 8-month regimens in the treatment of pulmonary tuberculosis. The results up to 24 months. Tubercle 1979;60:201–210.

25 East African/British Medical Research Councils: Controlled clinical trial of 4 short course (6-month) regimens of chemotherapy for treatment of pulmonary tuberculosis. Second Report. Lancet 1973;i:1332–1338.

26 East African/British Medical Research Councils: Controlled clinical trial of 4 short course (6-month) regimens of chemotherapy for treatment of pulmonary tuberculosis. Third report. Lancet 1974;i:237–240.

27 Hong Kong Tuberculosis Treatment Services/British Medical Research Council: Controlled trial of 6- and 9-month regimens of daily and intermittent streptomycin plus isoniazid plus pyrazinamide for pulmonary tuberculosis in Hong Kong. Tubercle 1975;56:81–96.

28 Hong Kong Tuberculosis Treatment Services/British Medical Research Council: Controlled trial of 6- and 9-month regimens of daily and intermittent streptomycin plus isoniazid plus pyrazinamide for pulmonary tuberculosis in Hong Kong. The results up to 30 months. Am Rev Respir Dis 1977;115:727–734.

29 MacKenzie WR, Heilig CM, Bozeman L, Johnson JL, Muzanye G, et al: Geographic differences in time to culture conversion in liquid media: Tuberculosis Trials Consortium Study 28. Culture conversion is delayed in Africa. PloS One 2011;6:e18358.

30 Johnson JL, Hadad DJ, Dietze R, Maciel EL, Sewali B, Gitta P, Okwera A, Mugerwa RD, Alcaneses MR, Quelapio MI, Tupasi TE, Horter L, Debanne SM, Eisenach KD, Boom WH: Shortening treatment in adults with noncavitary tuberculosis and 2-month culture conversion. Am J Respir Crit Care Med 2009;180:558–563.

31 Hong Kong Chest Service/Tuberculosis Research Centre, Madras/British Medical Research Council: A controlled clinical comparison of 6 and 8 months of antituberculosis chemotherapy in the treatment of patients with silicotuberculosis in Hong Kong. Am Rev Respir Dis 1991;143:262–267.
32 British Thoracic Society: A controlled trial of 6 months' chemotherapy in pulmonary tuberculosis. Final report: results during the 36 months after the end of chemotherapy and beyond. Br J Dis Chest 1984;78:330.
33 Zierski M, Bek E, Long MW, Snider DE Jr: Short-course (6-month) cooperative tuberculosis study in Poland: results 18 months after completion of treatment. Am Rev Respir Dis 1980;122:879–889.
34 Zierski M, Bek E, Long MW, Snider DE Jr: Short-course (6-month) cooperative tuberculosis study in Poland: results 30 months after completion of treatment. Am Rev Respir Dis 1981;124:249–251.
35 Snider DE Jr, Rogowski J, Zierski M, Bek E, Long MW: Successful intermittent treatment of smear-positive pulmonary tuberculosis in six months: a cooperative study in Poland. Am Rev Respir Dis 1982;125:265–267.
36 Snider E, Graczyk J, Bek E, Rogowski J: Supervised six-month treatment of newly diagnosed pulmonary tuberculosis using isoniazid, rifampin and pyrazinamide with and without streptomycin. Am Rev Respir Dis 1984;130:1091–1094.
37 Dutt AK, Moers D, Stead WW: Short-course chemotherapy for tuberculosis with mainly twice weekly isoniazid and rifampin. Community physicians' seven-year experience with mainly outpatients. Am J Med 1984;77:233–242.
38 Long MW, Snider DE, Farer LS: US Public Health Service cooperative trial of three rifampin-isoniazid regimens in treatment of pulmonary tuberculosis. Am Rev Respir Dis 1979;119:879.
39 Snider DE, Long ML, Cross FS, Farer LS: Six months isoniazid-rifampin therapy for pulmonary tuberculosis. Report of a United States Public Health Service cooperative trial. Am Rev Respir Dis 1984;129:573–579.
40 Benator D, Bhattacharya M, Bozeman L, Burman W, Catanzaro A, Chaisson R, Gordin F, Horsburgh CR, Horton J, Khan A, et al, Tuberculosis Trials Consortium: Rifapentine and isoniazid once a week versus rifampicin and isoniazid twice a week for treatment of drug-susceptible pulmonary tuberculosis in HIV-negative persons: a randomized clinical trial. Lancet 2002;360:528–534.
41 Cohn DL, Catlin BJ, Peterson KL, Judson FN, Sbarbaro JA: A 62-dose, 6-month therapy for pulmonary and extrapulmonary tuberculosis: a twice weekly, directly observed and cost-effective regimen. Ann Intern Med 1990;112:407–415.
42 Mitchison DA: Basic mechanisms of chemotherapy. Chest 1979;76(suppl):771–781.
43 McDermott W, Tompsett R: Activation of pyrazinamide and nicotinamide in acidic environment in vitro. Am Rev Tuberc 1954;70:748–754.
44 Mitchison DA: Role of individual drugs in the chemotherapy of tuberculosis. Int J Tuberc Lung Dis 2000;4:796–806.
45 Jindani A, Aber VR, Edwards EA, Mitchison DA: The early bactericidal activity of drugs in patients with pulmonary tuberculosis. Am Rev Respir Dis 1980;121:939–949.
46 Jindani A, Doré CJ, Mitchison DA: Bactericidal and sterilizing activities of antituberculosis drugs during the first 14 days. Am J Respir Crit Care Med 2003;167:1348–1354.
47 Davies GR: Early clinical development of anti-tuberculosis drugs: science, statistics and sterilizing activity. Tuberculosis 2010;90:171–176.
48 Mitchison DA: Assessment of new sterilizing drugs for treating pulmonary tuberculosis by culture at 2 months. Am Rev Respir Dis 1993;147:1062–1063.
49 McGregor MM, Olliaro P, Wolmarans L, Mabuza B, Bredell M, Felten MK, Fourie PB: Efficacy and safety of rifabutin in the treatment of patients with newly diagnosed pulmonary tuberculosis. Am J Respir Crit Care Med 1996;154:1462–1467.
50 Burman W, Benator D, Vernon A, Khan A, Jones B, Silva C, Lahart C, Weis S, King B, Mangura B, Weiner M, El-Sadr W, Tuberculosis Trials Consortium: Acquired rifamycin resistance with twice-weekly treatment of HIV-related tuberculosis. Am J Respir Crit Care Med 2006;173:350–356.
51 CDC: Managing drug interactions in the treatment of HIV-related tuberculosis. 2007. http://www.cdc.gov/tb/TB_HIV_Drugs/default.htm.
52 Goldberg S, LoBue P: Pulmonary tuberculosis: focus on the fluoroquinolones. Clin Med Insights Ther 2010;2:341–352
53 Davies G, Cerri S, Richeldi L: Rifabutin for treating pulmonary tuberculosis. Cochrane Database Syst Rev 2007;4:CD005159.
54 http://www.clintonfoundation.org/news/news-media/press-release-president-clinton-pfizer-and-mylan-announce-new-agreements-to-lower-prices-of-medicines-for-patients-with-drug-resistant-hiv-in-developing-countries (accessed June 23, 2011).
55 Menzies D, Benedetti A, Paydar A, Martin I, Royce S, et al: Effect of duration and intermittency of rifampin on tuberculosis treatment outcomes: a systematic review and meta-analysis. PLoS Med 2009;6:e1000146.
56 Jindani A, Nunn AJ, Enarson DA. Two 8-month regimens of chemotherapy for treatment of newly diagnosed pulmonary tuberculosis: international multicentre randomised trial. Lancet 2004;364:1244–1251.
57 Mitchison DA, Nunn AJ: Influence of initial drug resistance on the response to short-course chemotherapy of pulmonary tuberculosis. Am Rev Respir Dis 1986;133:423–430.
58 Khan FA, Minion J, Pai M, Royce S, Burman W, Harries AD, Menzies D: Treatment of active tuberculosis in HIV-coinfected patients: a systematic review and meta-analysis. Clin Infect Dis 2010;50:1288–1299.
59 Li J, Munsiff SS, Driver CR, Sackoff J: Relapse and acquired rifampin resistance in HIV-infected patients with tuberculosis treated with rifampin- or rifabutin-based regimens in New York City, 1997–2000. Clin Infect Dis 2005;41:83–91.
60 Vernon A, Burman W, Benator D, Khan A, Bozeman L: Relapse with rifamycin mono-resistant tuberculosis in HIV-infected patients treated with supervised once-weekly rifapentine and isoniazid. Lancet 1999;353:1843–1847.
61 Burman W, Benator D, Vernon A, Khan A, Jones B, Silva C, Lahart C, Weis S, King B, Mangura B, Weiner M, El-Sadr W, Tuberculosis Trials Consortium: Acquired rifamycin resistance with twice-weekly treatment of HIV-related tuberculosis. Am J Respir Crit Care Med 2006;173:350–356.
62 Swaminathan S, Narendran G, Venkatesan P, Iliayas S, Santhanakrishnan R, Menon PA, Padmapriyadarsini C, Ramachandran R, Chinnaiyan P, Suhadev M, Sakthivel R, Narayanan PR: Efficacy of a 6-month versus 9-month intermittent treatment regimen in HIV-infected patients with tuberculosis: a randomized clinical trial. Am J Respir Crit Care Med 2010;181:743–751.
63 Johnson JL, Okwera A, Vjecha MJ, Byekwaso F, Nakibali J, Nyole S, Milberg J, Aisu T, Whalen CC, Mugerwa RD, et al: Risk factors for relapse in human immunodeficiency virus type 1 infected adults with pulmonary tuberculosis. Int J Tuberc Lung Dis 1997;1:446–453.
64 Tam CM, Chan SL, Kam KM, Goodall RL, Mitchison DA: Rifapentine and isoniazid in the continuation phase of a 6-month regimen. Final report at 5 years: prognostic value of various measures. Int J Tuberc Lung Dis 2002;6:3–10.
65 Package insert, rifapentine (Priftin). Kansas City, Hoechst Marion Roussel (now Aventis), 1998.
66 Vernon AA, Iademarco MI: In the treatment of tuberculosis, you get what you pay for. . .. Am J Respir Crit Care Med 2004;170:1040.
67 Bignall JR, Clegg JW, Crofton JW, Douglas Smith BJ, Holt HD, Mitchison DA, Armitage P: Intermittent dosage in the treatment of pulmonary tuberculosis with streptomycin: a report to the Streptomycin in Tuberculosis Committee of the Medical Research Council. Br Med J 1950;i:1224–1230.
68 Dickinson JM, Mitchison DA: In vitro and in vivo studies to assess the suitability of antituberculous drugs for use in intermittent chemotherapy regimens. Tubercle 1968;49(suppl):66–70.
69 Dickinson JM, Ellard GA, Mitchison DA: Suitability of isoniazid and ethambutol for intermittent administration in the treatment of tuberculosis. Tubercle 1968;49:351–366.
70 Dickinson JM, Mitchison DA: Suitability of rifampicin for intermittent administration in the treatment of tuberculosis. Tubercle 1970;51:82–94.
71 Chang KC, Leung CC, Yew WW, Ho SC, Tam CM: A nested case-control study on treatment-related risk factors for early relapse of tuberculosis. Am J Respir Crit Care Med 2004;170:1124–1130.

72 Rosenthal IM, Zhang M, Williams KN, Peloquin CA, Tyagi S, et al: Daily dosing of rifapentine cures tuberculosis in three months or less in the murine model. PLoS Med 2007;4:e344.
73 Fox W: The chemotherapy of pulmonary tuberculosis: a review. Chest 1979;76(suppl):785–796.
74 Bayer R, Wilkinson D: Directly observed therapy for tuberculosis: history of an idea. Lancet 1995;345:1545–1548.
75 Weis SE, Slocum PC, Blais FX, et al: The effect of directly observed therapy on the rates of drug resistance and relapse in tuberculosis. N Engl J Med 1994;330:1179–1184.
76 Frieden TR, Fujiwara PI, Washko RM, Hamburg MA: Tuberculosis in New York City – turning the tide. N Engl J Med 1995;333:229–233.
77 Chaulk CP, Moore-Rice K, Rizzo R, Chaisson RE: Eleven years of community-based directly observed therapy for tuberculosis. JAMA 1995;274:945–951.
78 Jasmer RM, Seaman CB, Gonzalez LC, Kawamura M, Osmond DH: Tuberculosis treatment outcomes: directly observed therapy compared with self administered therapy. Am J Respir Crit Care Med 2004;170:561–566.
79 Newell JN, Baral SC, Pande SB, Bam DS, Malla P: Family-member DOTS and community DOTS for tuberculosis control in Nepal: a cluster-randomised controlled trial. Lancet 2006;367:903–909.
80 Thiam S, LeFevre AM, Hane F, Ndiaye A, Ba F, Fielding KL, Ndir M, Lienhardt C: Effectiveness of a strategy to improve adherence to tuberculosis treatment in a resource-poor setting: a cluster randomized controlled trial. JAMA 2007;297:380–386.
81 Walley JD, Khan MA, Newell JN, Khan MH: Effectiveness of the direct observation component of DOTS for tuberculosis: a randomised controlled trial in Pakistan. Lancet 2001;357:664–669.
82 Zwarenstein M, Schoeman JH, Vundule C, Lombard CJ, Tatley M: Randomised controlled trial of self-supervised and directly observed treatment of tuberculosis. Lancet 1998;352:1340–1343.
83 Floyd K, Wilkinson D, Gilks C: Comparison of cost effectiveness of directly observed treatment (DOT) and conventionally delivered treatment for tuberculosis: experience from rural South Africa. BMJ 1997;315:1407–1411.
84 Burman WJ, Dalton CB, Cohn DL, Butler JR, Reves RR: A cost effectiveness analysis of directly observed therapy vs self-administered therapy for treatment of tuberculosis. Chest 1997;112:63–70.

Andrew A. Vernon, MD, MHS
Chief, Clinical Research Branch, Division of TB Elimination, NCHHSTP, OID
Centers for Disease Control and Prevention
1600 Clifton Road NE, Atlanta, GA 30333 (USA)
Tel. +1 404 639 5341, E-Mail anv3@cdc.gov

Donald PR, van Helden PD (eds): Antituberculosis Chemotherapy.
Prog Respir Res. Basel, Karger, 2011, vol 40, pp 73–80

# Tuberculosis Recurrence: Exogenous or Endogenous?

Monique Williams · Borna Müller · Pieter Uys · Thomas C. Victor · Robin M. Warren · Nicolaas C. Gey van Pittius

DST/NRF Centre of Excellence for Biomedical TB Research/MRC Centre for Molecular and Cellular Biology, Division of Molecular Biology and Human Genetics, Faculty of Health Science, Stellenbosch University, Tygerberg, South Africa

### Abstract

With the advent of molecular epidemiology, perhaps the most significant finding has been that a recurrent episode of tuberculosis (TB) can occur by exogenous reinfection. This raises several questions: Does prior infection confer protective immunity? Do mixed infections occur, and does exogenous reinfection play a significant role in high-incidence settings, where individuals could be exposed to multiple infecting doses during their lifetime? Combining data from the literature with a simple mathematical model we illustrate that while disease due to exogenous reinfection after cure constitutes a significant proportion of recurrent TB, it represents a very small portion of the total number of TB cases. Although the true contribution of exogenous reinfection cannot be quantified, its association with recurrence serves as a barometer of its contribution to disease progression in previously untreated individuals. One of the most important functions of any new antituberculosis drug is the ability to prevent endogenous reactivation of disease. Molecular epidemiology now enables us to differentiate endogenous reactivation and exogenous reinfection. In this paper we discuss the clinical relevance of exogenous reinfection, questions surrounding its role in TB disease and its importance in the accurate evaluation of new drugs.

Copyright © 2011 S. Karger AG, Basel

## The Natural History of *Mycobacterium tuberculosis* Infection

Infection with *Mycobacterium tuberculosis*, the causative agent of tuberculosis, can either lead to rapid progression to clinical TB disease, known as primary disease in a previously uninfected individual, result in a latent infection or be cleared by the host. Latent TB is clinically defined as the absence of symptoms in an individual who is infected by *M. tuberculosis*, demonstrable by a significant immune response to *M. tuberculosis* antigens. The exact physiological state of the bacilli during latency is controversial [1]. One hypothesis is that bacteria enter a dormant state of non-replicating persistence, which is recalcitrant to killing by antimicrobials targeting active metabolism [2]. These organisms are thought to persist for the lifetime of the host and to resume replication when the immune system is compromised resulting in reactivation of disease. However, the ability of isoniazid monotherapy for 9 months to prevent the progression of individuals to disease suggests that some replication must occur, either at a constant low level or as sporadic bursts, since isoniazid is effective only against replicating organisms [3].

The risk of developing active tuberculosis after infection is highest within the first 2 years and is calculated to be approximately 5%, with a lifetime risk of developing active disease of around 10%. However, this value changes considerably once immunocompromising factors are added; thus, for example, the proportion of people with HIV infection who develop TB each year is estimated to be between 5 and 15%. This means that an individual co-infected with HIV and *M. tuberculosis* has a 50–60% lifetime risk of developing TB instead of the 10% amongst HIV-uninfected individuals. It is estimated that around 50% of the population of sub-Saharan Africa and 33% of the world's population are latently infected with *M. tuberculosis*. Furthermore, in sub-Saharan Africa it is estimated that around 22.4 million people are infected with HIV (around 66% of the global total). This constitutes a huge pool for potential endogenous reactivation events, specifically in sub-Saharan Africa.

## Postprimary Tuberculosis: Endogenous Reactivation or Exogenous Reinfection

The contribution of endogenous reactivation and exogenous reinfection to TB disease has been debated for many years. In the 1960s, after comparing the rate of infection of individuals exposed to different levels of TB present in different settings, Stead [4] proposed the unitary concept of pathogenesis. This theory states that TB always begins with primary infection, and subsequent episodes of active TB are due to reactivation of these dormant bacilli [4]. Canetti et al. [5] challenged this theory by demonstrating that inoculating guinea pigs with material from primary complexes from infected individuals did not cause disease in the majority of cases, suggesting that they no longer contained viable bacilli. They also argued that the presence of resistant strains in elderly patients who were initially infected before these resistant strains emerged was indicative of exogenous reinfection. The argument that exogenous reinfection occurs is supported by the concept that once individuals become infected with TB, they do not stop inhaling bacilli present in their environment, and may therefore be exposed to several infecting doses within their lifetime. It should be noted that the risk of inhaling the bacillus is not the same as establishing an infection and that our current diagnostic tools (tuberculin skin testing and γ-interferon release assays) are unable to accurately quantify repeated *M. tuberculosis* infection. A simple probability argument which models this situation shows that repeated exposure to an infecting dose is likely, particularly in high-incidence settings.

The risk of being exposed to a reinfecting dose is given by the (combinatorial) probability formula:

$$_nP_k = n^k p^k e^{-np}/k!$$

where $_nP_k$ is the probability that a particular individual will experience exactly k exposure events during a stay of n years (n may be fractional) in a setting where the annual risk of infection is p. Figure 1 and table 1 show the probability that an individual will experience a specified number of exposure events at various periods in a setting where the annual risk of infection is 5%. Age here is intended to mean the period spent in that setting and not necessarily the biological age of the person. This demonstrates that the risk of being exposed to exactly 1 infecting dose increases as age increases, and then eventually decreases. The decrease occurs because the risk of more than 1 potential infection event becomes more pronounced. Thus, by the age of 20 years the risk of exposure to 1 infecting dose is about 0.37, decreasing to 0.27 by the age of 40 years. Moreover, by the age of 40 the risk of experiencing 3 infections will have increased to about 0.18. By the age of 50 years a person will have almost certainly experienced at least 1 exposure (risk = 0.92) event. The probability formula does not take into account whether or not an infection event confers some degree of resistance to a further infection event, but simply quantifies the risk of exposure and potential infection. In addition, it should be noted that infection or subsequent reinfection does not imply a consequential episode of disease.

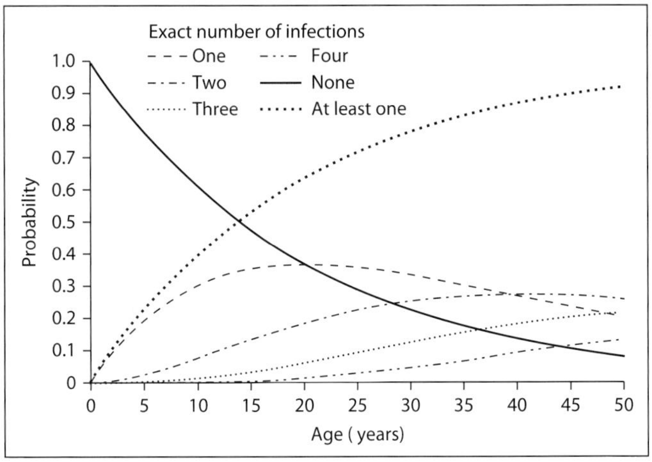


**Fig. 1.** The probability of experiencing a specified number of infection events for various periods spent in a setting where the annual risk of infection is 5%.

**Table 1.** The probability of experiencing 0, 1 or >1 infection event for various periods spent in a setting where the ARI is 5%

| Age | No infections | 1 infection | >1 infection |
|---|---|---|---|
| 10 years | 0.60 | 0.32 | 0.08 |
| 20 years | 0.36 | 0.38 | 0.26 |
| 30 years | 0.21 | 0.34 | 0.45 |
| 40 years | 0.13 | 0.27 | 0.60 |
| 50 years | 0.08 | 0.20 | 0.72 |

## Recurrent Tuberculosis

Recurrent TB is defined as TB which has re-occurred after a patient has previously had a diagnosis of TB and completed a full course of treatment. Recurrent TB can be either confirmed bacteriologically (positive smears for acid-fast bacilli and/or positive cultures for *M. tuberculosis*) or be diagnosed according to clinical and/or radiographic criteria.

The mechanisms underlying recurrence were only identified with the development of methodologies which allowed the differentiation of *M. tuberculosis* strains, which led to the birth of the science of molecular epidemiology.

## Differentiation of *M. tuberculosis* Strains

Classical epidemiology continues to provide extremely valuable insights into the epidemiology of TB. However, the analytical methods in use are unable to differentiate strains of *M. tuberculosis* causing disease. In the absence of this knowledge, it is not possible to track the movement of a specific *M. tuberculosis* strain through space and time within an epidemiological setting. The discovery of mycobacteriophages, which specifically infect certain strains of *M. tuberculosis* revolutionized epidemiological studies as these strain-specific properties enabled the classification of strains into distinct phage types; thus, it became possible to describe the strains causing disease in different episodes. Relapse was confirmed in patients whose sputum samples from different episodes showed strains with the same phage type [6]. Conversely, reinfection was defined in patients whose sputum specimens showed strains with different phage types [6]. However, the utility of this method was severely hampered by the discriminatory power of phage typing, which was only able to classify strains into 1 of 5 phage types. Despite these limitations this methodology challenged perceptions that recurrence occurred primarily through endogenous reactivation.

To date numerous genotyping methods have been developed, each with its own level of discrimination and applicability to answer epidemiological and clinical questions; 3 are internationally standardized. The most widely used genotyping method is spoligotyping, which allows the genetic classification of strains according to the number of direct variable repeat sequences present in the direct repeat region of the *M. tuberculosis* chromosome [7]. Strains are grouped into evolutionary lineages according to the presence of defined spoligotype signatures [8]. Currently, 22 lineages have been described, the Beijing lineage being most frequently reported followed by the Latin-American-Mediterranean lineage [9].

The internationally standardized IS*6110* DNA fingerprinting is based on quantification of the number of IS*6110* elements located within a strain's chromosome and their position relative to a specific endonuclease restriction site (*Pvu*II), which determines the physical size of the fragment when electrophoretically fractionated in an agarose gel [10]. This method is widely accepted as the 'gold standard' but has proved cumbersome, requiring growth of bacilli, DNA extraction, Southern blotting and hybridization, and therefore cannot be used in a 'real-time' manner to investigate epidemiological events. Despite this limitation, IS*6110* DNA fingerprinting remains the most informative method for the classification of clinical strains of *M. tuberculosis*. In an attempt to overcome these limitations, a PCR-based method, which amplifies mycobacterial interspersed repetitive unit/variable number tandem repeat (MIRU-VNTR) sequences, has been developed [11]. This method has a number of different formats with the 15 MIRU-VNTR combinations being proposed as the new standard for molecular epidemiology. In certain settings, this method has proved more informative than IS*6110* DNA fingerprinting in that a more precise correlation between genotype and epidemiological contact was observed [12]. However, the suitability of this method to define the epidemiology of TB in high-incidence settings has recently been challenged by the observed discordance between the definition of a strain by the MIRU-VNTR typing method compared to the IS*6110* DNA fingerprinting method [13].

Molecular epidemiological calculations, using either of the above genotyping methods, are based on the assumption that the genomes of *M. tuberculosis* strains are in constant flux and thus strains which show identical genotypes (within a defined geographical region) reflect a recent epidemiological event as insufficient time has lapsed for mutation/change to have occurred. Conversely, strains that show different genotypes imply that sufficient time has lapsed and thus these cases are thought to be epidemiologically unrelated. These definitions allow TB cases to be grouped into two categories: clustered cases (identical genotypes representing recent transmission) and unique cases (non-identical genotypes representing either reactivation, infection outside of the study site or failure to identify the index case) [14]. Applying these relatively simple definitions it was possible to infer the mechanism leading to recurrent TB by comparing the genotypes of strains isolated from an individual during different episodes of disease. As with phage typing, endogenous reactivation was defined when the isolates from each episode show the same genotype, and exogenous reinfection was inferred when the strains from each episode show different genotypes [15]. However, these definitions have certain caveats. Firstly, it is important to compare at least 2 isolates from each episode to exclude the chance of laboratory cross-contamination. Secondly, the genotypic difference between the 2 isolates needs to be sufficient in order to exclude evolution of the genome during infection and/or disease. Thirdly, strains cultured from different episodes which show identical genotypes may be incorrectly interpreted as reflecting endogenous reactivation rather than exogenous reinfection with a circulating strain.

The most significant limitation of the above methodology remains the sensitivity of the respective methods for detecting the presence of different strains within a single sputum specimen. In the absence of such tools it is impossible to exclude recurrence through endogenous reactivation of an already present, but underlying strain of *Mtb* (not detected by the genotyping method in use). To address this limitation, allele-specific PCR-based methods have been developed to detect sequences unique to a lineage of strains [16]. These methods are able to detect underlying strains in a ratio of >1:100; however, this methodology is limited in its ability to detect the presence of 2 unrelated strains from the same lineage. This leads to an underestimation of the presence of underlying strains.

## Molecular Epidemiology: Challenging the Dogma

The molecular classification of *M. tuberculosis* strains has provided novel insights into disease epidemiology by challenging classical epidemiological dogma, demonstrating the complexity of the population structure of *M. tuberculosis* strains and identifying laboratory cross-contamination [17]. Perhaps the most significant finding has been the demonstration that a recurrent episode of TB, after cure from a previous episode, can occur by exogenous reinfection [15]. This mechanism of recurrence is now widely accepted and has been documented in numerous settings irrespective of the incidence of TB disease [18, 19]. These findings challenge the concept that prior disease confers a significant level of protective immunity on people who have recovered from an episode of TB, and implies that a TB vaccine would need to stimulate immunity better than natural immunity. In addition, defining the mechanism of recurrence is of major importance in developing protocols for the assessment of relapse rates during the evaluation of new drugs. The inclusion of molecular genotyping methods within a clinical trial's protocol will enable a more accurate evaluation of the therapeutic effect of anti-TB drugs and should be a prerequisite for all trials.

## The Clinical Relevance of Exogenous Reinfection

A recent review of the literature on exogenous reinfection has questioned whether reinfection has important implications for TB control [18]. The authors conclude that recurrence due to exogenous reinfection has no significant implications for TB control programmes in most settings, with the exception of an extremely high TB incidence and HIV co-infection. This view is supported by a simple mathematical model (fig. 2) which estimates that exogenous reinfection contributes to only a minor proportion of the entire epidemic. In this model it is estimated that in South Africa 63% of new TB cases are cured by standardized first-line TB treatment. Five percent of cured cases are expected to experience a recurrent episode. Using the formula proposed by Wang et al. [21], the proportion of recurrence cases due to reinfection = $-29.7 + 36.8 \times \log(\text{incidence})$, it is estimated that 80% of these recurrent cases will result from exogenous reinfection. Of the 37% of patients who were not cured by standardized first-line treatment and it is expected that at least 50% will die or self-cure. Molecular epidemiology suggests that only 11% of those who present with a recurrent episode (without prior cure) will be exogenously reinfected. Thus, only 4.5% of new TB cases will experience a recurrent episode through exogenous reinfection. This translates to 3.6% of the total case load (new and retreatment cases).The model was calculated using WHO data for South Africa, a high-incidence setting.

Recurrent TB due to exogenous reinfection therefore serves as a surrogate of infection pressure [23], demonstrating that individuals within a community may be repeatedly infected. However, our knowledge of how exogenous reinfection contributes to primary/secondary TB is curtailed by our inability to genotype the infecting strain(s) in the absence of disease. Evidence for exogenous reinfection driving primary/secondary TB stems from mathematical models which predict the number of infections that may occur in an individual as a function of age and annual risk of infection (fig. 1). This model is supported by autopsy studies which have demonstrated the presence of different strains causing disease in different anatomical sites within a patient's lung [24]. In addition, analysis of sputum specimens using highly sensitive PCR-based techniques suggests that mixed infection may be frequent in high-incidence settings, although the clinical relevance of mixed infection remains unknown. It is unlikely that a mixed infection would influence treatment outcome if both strains are susceptible to the treatment regimen being given [25]. However, underlying drug-resistant strains may be masked by drug-susceptible strains, thereby obscuring a diagnosis of drug resistance according to the 1% proportion method. A recent study confirmed that a mixed infection at diagnosis could mask the presence of a drug-resistant *M. tuberculosis* population in a sputum culture [26]. Subsequent treatment for drug-susceptible TB

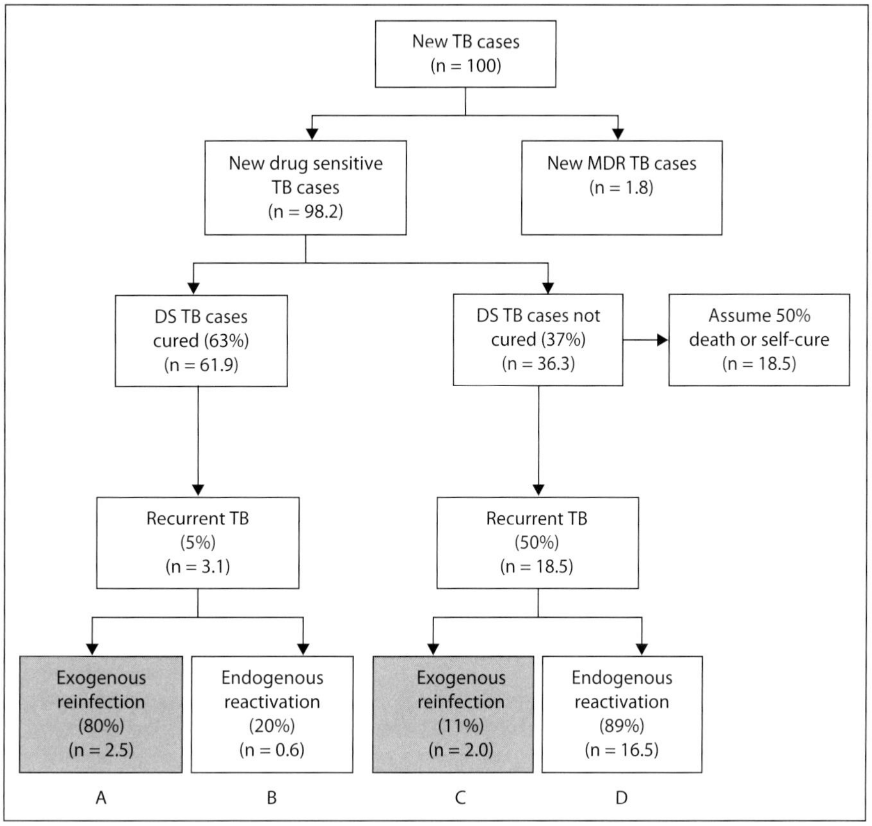


**Fig. 2.** Mathematical model which estimates the proportion of new drug-sensitive (DS) TB cases which experience recurrent disease due to exogenous reinfection and endogenous reactivation; MDR = multidrug-resistant. The numbers of cases in the various categories were calculated using WHO data [20] for South Africa, a high-incidence setting. Boxes A, B: calculated according to Wang et al. [21]; boxes C, D: calculated according to Verver et al. [22].

would lead to the emergence of drug resistance as a result of the preferential killing of the drug-susceptible population. This contrasts significantly with the clinical interpretation, which would suggest acquisition of resistance during treatment. Drug-resistant TB may therefore emerge in a patient by 1 of 4 documented mechanisms, namely primary infection, acquisition, mixed infection or exogenous reinfection.

People who have been successfully cured of a first episode of TB disease have an elevated risk of a further episode due to exogenous reinfection [22]. It is not yet clear why this is the case, although several possibilities are proposed. Firstly, the first episode of disease could deplete the immune cells to such an extent that the patient remains susceptible for an extended period following cure of the first episode [27]. Secondly, the individual could be genetically or immunologically susceptible to disease progression [28]. Thirdly, the patient could live in an environment that exposes him/her to greater risk of exogenous reinfection or under conditions that compromise his/her immune system. Lastly, it is also possible that a prior disease episode causes some damage to the lungs that renders the person more likely to progress to disease following reinfection. In contrast, recurrence after default occurs primarily through endogenous reactivation (fig. 2, boxes C and D), demonstrating that adequate sterilization was not achieved in these patients [22], and thereby highlighting the importance of treatment adherence. Only a few reports describe exogenous reinfection occurring during treatment [26, 29], and this is mainly associated with nosocomial transmission of drug-resistant TB.

The observation that the risk of exogenous reinfection is higher in previously treated TB cases than new cases raises important concerns around the management of patients who have completed treatment for a prior episode [22]. Greater vigilance is therefore necessary to monitor patients over extended periods following treatment completion. This is of particular importance in clinical trials investigating the sterilizing efficacy of new drugs. Furthermore, a recent study has highlighted the importance of follow-up of patients co-infected with HIV as such patients show a significantly higher risk of developing a subsequent episode through exogenous reinfection [30]. The association between exogenous reinfection and drug-resistant TB in HIV co-infected patients probably reflects nosocomial transmission through nosocomial exposure of patients with HIV and patients with drug-resistant TB [31]. Thus, it is essential to limit the risk of exposure to infectious sources (community and/or

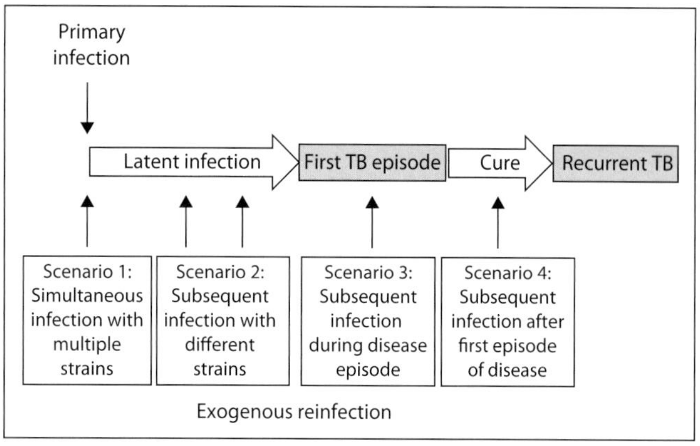


**Fig. 3.** Possible exogenous reinfection events during latent infection, treatment of TB and after cure of an episode of TB [19].

nosocomial). This can be achieved by implementation of infection control programmes in hospitals and clinics, while rapid and early diagnosis and case holding will limit community transmission.

## Outstanding Knowledge

Exogenous reinfection may occur at different time points relative to a primary infection or an episode of TB disease (fig. 3), and from an immunological perspective, at least 4 scenarios may be differentiated: (1) reinfections shortly after or concurrently with a primary infection, (2) at a later stage, after the primary infection has been contained by the host immune system, (3) during an episode of TB disease or (4) after a primary episode of TB disease has been cured. Whether these different scenarios affect progression to or recurrence of TB disease is currently unknown. For example, it is not clear if multiple exposure to the same source of TB infection, e.g. through continuous contact with a TB patient in the same household, or exposure to multiple TB sources (scenario 1) affects disease progression compared to infections established by a single exposure to TB. Estimates for the minimum amount of bacteria required to establish a primary TB infection range from a single bacterium upward [19].

While molecular epidemiology has demonstrated the importance of reinfection and mixed infections in TB high-incidence settings, little is known about the interrelationship between primary and recurrent infections with *M. tuberculosis*, including the immunological consequences and interplay between different bacterial populations within a host. A recent study in mice described trafficking of secondary infecting strains of *M. tuberculosis* to granulomas previously established during a primary infection [32]. The molecular mechanism that underlies this surprising observation as well as its role in TB disease are yet to be elucidated, and highlights our limited knowledge of how strain populations within the host interact. Questions arising from this observation are whether a successfully contained primary infection alters the containment of subsequent infections (scenario 2), or conversely whether reinfection can in fact trigger reactivation of a primary infection and facilitate progression to disease.

The surprisingly frequent presence of mixed infections with distinct strains of *M. tuberculosis* in high-TB-incidence populations has important implications for TB diagnosis. For example, it is unclear how well the populations in the human lung are represented in cultures of human sputum samples, and it has been demonstrated that the process of bacterial culture can skew the percentage distribution of multiple strains and affect the detection of such mixed infections [33]. Genotyping of *M. tuberculosis* isolates from lesions of resected lung tissue revealed that the population within the lung of an individual infected with a single strain is heterogeneous, since isolates from different lesions harboured different resistance mutations [34]. This suggests that the acquisition of mutations at different locations within the lung is a dynamic process, which may be influenced by the micro-environment of the bacteria and may arise due to differential exposure to different drugs or differing drug concentrations. Of interest, strains isolated from the sputum of these patients were not representative of all populations present within the lung, supporting the idea that drug susceptibility testing done on sputum may not always be a true reflection of the resistance profile of strains present in the lungs. It has been demonstrated that the fitness cost of rifampicin resistance in *M. tuberculosis* is determined both by the specific mutation, the strain background and the acquisition of compensatory mutations [35], suggesting that these factors may influence the detection of strains in patient samples.

Advances in comparative genomics and molecular epidemiology have enabled the study of host and pathogen factors which may contribute to the TB epidemic. In a cosmopolitan environment, mycobacterial lineages are more likely to spread in sympatric patient populations, suggesting that certain strains may be adapted to particular populations [36] or even host genetic backgrounds. Certain lineages also show increased pathogenicity [37], and are associated with altered disease presentation and progression [38]. These observations raise the question of how successive infections with different circulating strains may influence disease progression, and whether infection with a particular strain/lineage would better protect an individual against subsequent infections. These questions however are difficult to study due to our limited understanding of the host immune response at various stages of *M. tuberculosis* infection and TB disease.

## Conclusion

Exogenous reinfection is a widely accepted epidemiological phenomenon. Therefore, molecular strain typing is essential to accurately evaluate TB control programmes, treatment regimens, including clinical drug trials, and to categorize patients in studies aimed at identifying biomarkers to predict treatment outcome. The selection of the genotyping tool used to accurately define the mechanism of recurrence will be dependent on the population structure of *M. tuberculosis* in the study setting. Spoligotyping will provide sufficient discriminatory power in settings where the genetic diversity of *M. tuberculosis* strains is high [39]. In contrast, MIRU-VNTR typing and IS*6110* DNA fingerprinting provide the highest discriminatory resolution and should be used in settings where the genetic diversity of *M. tuberculosis* strains is low. Most importantly, such studies should endeavour to collect multiple specimens from each episode of disease to validate the definition of recurrence.

## References


1 Ehlers S: Lazy, dynamic or minimally recrudescent? On the elusive nature and location of the mycobacterium responsible for latent tuberculosis. Infection 2009;37:87–95.

2 Wayne LG, Sohaskey CD: Nonreplicating persistence of *Mycobacterium tuberculosis*. Annu Rev Microbiol 2001;55:139–163.

3 Diel R, Nienhaus A, Schaberg T: Cost-effectiveness of isoniazid chemoprevention in close contacts. Eur Respir J 2005;26:465–473.

4 Stead WW: Pathogenesis of a first episode of chronic pulmonary tuberculosis in man: recrudescence of residuals of the primary infection or exogenous reinfection? Am Rev Respir Dis 1967;95:729–745.

5 Canetti G, Sutherland I, Svandova E. Endogenous reactivation and exogenous reinfection: their relative importance with regard to the development of non-primary tuberculosis. Bull Int Union Tuberc 1972;47:116–134.

6 Raleigh JW, Wichelhausen R: Exogenous reinfection with *Mycobacterium tuberculosis* confirmed by phage typing. Am Rev Respir Dis 1973;108:639–642.

7 Kamerbeek J, Schouls L, Kolk A, van Agterveld M, van Soolingen D, Kuijper S, Bunschoten A, Molhuizen H, Shaw R, Goyal M, van Embden J: Simultaneous detection and strain differentiation of *Mycobacterium tuberculosis* for diagnosis and epidemiology. J Clin Microbiol 1997;35:907–914.

8 Streicher EM, Victor TC, van der Spuy G, Sola C, Rastogi N, van Helden PD, Warren RM: Spoligotype signatures in the *Mycobacterium tuberculosis* complex. J Clin Microbiol 2007;45:237–240.

9 Brudey K, Driscoll JR, Rigouts L, Prodinger WM, Gori A, Al Hajoj SA, Allix C, Aristimuno L, Arora J, Baumanis V, Binder L, Cafrune P, Cataldi A, Cheong S, Diel R, Ellermeier C, Evans JT, Fauville-Dufaux M, Ferdinand S, Garcia de Viedma D, Garzelli C, Gazzola L, Gomes HM, Gutierrez MC, Hawkey PM, van Helden PD, Kadival GV, Kreiswirth BN, Kremer K, Kubin M, Kulkarni SP, Liens B, Lillebaek T, Ly HM, Martin C, Martin C, Mokrousov I, Narvskaia O, Ngeow YF, Naumann L, Niemann S, Parwati I, Rahim MZ, Rasolofo-Razanamparany V, Rasolonavalona T, Rossetti ML, Rusch-Gerdes S, Sajduda A, Samper S, Shemyakin I, Singh UB, Somoskovi A, Skuce R, van Soolingen D, Streicher EM, Suffys PN, Tortoli E, Tracevska T, Vincent V, Victor TC, Warren R, Yap SF, Zaman K, Portaels F, Rastogi N, Sola C: *Mycobacterium tuberculosis* complex genetic diversity: mining the fourth international spoligotyping database (SpolDB4) for classification, population genetics and epidemiology. BMC Microbiol 2006;6:23.

10 Van Embden JD, Cave MD, Crawford JT, Dale JW, Eisenach KD, Gicquel B, Hermans P, Martin C, McAdam R, Shinnick TM: Strain identification of *Mycobacterium tuberculosis* by DNA fingerprinting: recommendations for a standardized methodology. J Clin Microbiol 1993;31:406–409.

11 Oelemann MC, Diel R, Vatin V, Haas W, Rusch-Gerdes S, Locht C, Niemann S, Supply P: Assessment of an optimized mycobacterial interspersed repetitive-unit-variable-number tandem-repeat typing system combined with spoligotyping for population-based molecular epidemiology studies of tuberculosis. J Clin Microbiol 2007;45:691–697.

12 Allix-Beguec C, Fauville-Dufaux M, Supply P: Three-year population-based evaluation of standardized mycobacterial interspersed repetitive-unit-variable-number tandem-repeat typing of *Mycobacterium tuberculosis*. J Clin Microbiol 2008;46:1398–1406.

13 Hanekom M, van der Spuy GD, Gey van Pittius NC, McEvoy CR, Hoek KG, Ndabambi SL, Jordaan AM, Victor TC, van Helden PD, Warren RM: Discordance between mycobacterial interspersed repetitive-unit-variable-number tandem-repeat typing and IS*6110* restriction fragment length polymorphism genotyping for analysis of *Mycobacterium tuberculosis* Beijing strains in a setting of high incidence of tuberculosis. J Clin Microbiol 2008;46:3338–3345.

14 Small PM, Hopewell PC, Singh SP, Paz A, Parsonnet J, Ruston DC, Schecter GF, Daley CL, Schoolnik GK: The epidemiology of tuberculosis in San Francisco: a population-based study using conventional and molecular methods. N Engl J Med 1994;330:1703–1709.

15 Van Rie A, Warren R, Richardson M, Victor TC, Gie RP, Enarson DA, Beyers N, van Helden PD: Exogenous reinfection as a cause of recurrent tuberculosis after curative treatment. N Engl J Med 1999;341:1174–1179.

16 Warren RM, Victor TC, Streicher EM, Richardson M, Beyers N, van Pittius NC, van Helden PD: Patients with active tuberculosis often have different strains in the same sputum specimen. Am J Respir Crit Care Med 2004;169:610–614.

17 Mathema B, Kurepina N, Bifani P, Kreiswirth B: Molecular epidemiology of tuberculosis: current insights. Clin Microbiol Rev 2006;19:658–684.

18 Lambert ML, Hasker E, van Deun A, Roberfroid D, Boelaert M, van der Stuyft P: Recurrence in tuberculosis: relapse or reinfection? Lancet Infect Dis 2003;3:282–287.

19 Chiang CY, Riley LW: Exogenous reinfection in tuberculosis. Lancet Infect Dis 2005;5:629–636.

20 WHO-IUTALD Global Project on anti-tuberculosis drug resistance surveillance: anti-tuberculosis drug resistance in the world (report No 4). http://www.who.int/tb/publications/2008/drs_report4_26feb08.pdf (accessed April 30, 2008).
21 Wang JY, Lee LN, Lai HC, Hsu HL, Liaw YS, Hsueh PR, Yang PC: Prediction of the tuberculosis reinfection proportion from the local incidence. J Infect Dis 2007;196:281–288.
22 Verver S, Warren RM, Beyers N, Richardson M, van der Spuy GD, Borgdorff MW, Enarson DA, Behr MA, van Helden PD: Rate of reinfection tuberculosis after successful treatment is higher than rate of new tuberculosis. Am J Respir Crit Care Med 2005;171:1430–1435.
23 Fine PE, Small PM: Exogenous reinfection in tuberculosis. N Engl J Med 1999;34:1226–1227.
24 Du Plessis DG, Warren R, Richardson M, Joubert JJ, van Helden PD: Demonstration of reinfection and reactivation in HIV-negative autopsied cases of secondary tuberculosis: multilesional genotyping of *Mycobacterium tuberculosis* utilizing IS6110 and other repetitive element-based DNA fingerprinting. Tuberculosis (Edinb ) 2001;81:211–220.
25 Behr MA: Tuberculosis due to multiple strains: a concern for the patient? A concern for tuberculosis control? Am J Respir Crit Care Med 2004;169:554–555.
26 Van Rie A, Victor TC, Richardson M, Johnson R, van der Spuy GD, Murray EJ, Beyers N, Gey van Pittius NC, van Helden PD, Warren RM: Reinfection and mixed infection cause changing *Mycobacterium tuberculosis* drug-resistance patterns. Am J Respir Crit Care Med 2005;172:636–642.
27 Ellner JJ: Immunoregulation in TB: observations and implications. Clin Transl Sci 2010;3:23–28.
28 Yim JJ, Selvaraj P: Genetic susceptibility in tuberculosis. Respirology 2010;15:241–256.
29 Kruuner A, Pehme L, Ghebremichael S, Koivula T, Hoffner SE, Mikelsaar M: Use of molecular techniques to distinguish between treatment failure and exogenous reinfection with *Mycobacterium tuberculosis*. Clin Infect Dis 2002;35:146–155.
30 Narayanan S, Swaminathan S, Supply P, Shanmugam S, Narendran G, Hari L, Ramachandran R, Locht C, Jawahar MS, Narayanan PR: Impact of HIV infection on the recurrence of tuberculosis in South India. J Infect Dis 2010;201:691–703.
31 Chaisson RE, Churchyard GJ: Recurrent tuberculosis: relapse, reinfection, and HIV. J Infect Dis 2010;201:653–655.
32 Cosma CL, Humbert O, Sherman DR, Ramakrishnan L: Trafficking of superinfecting *Mycobacterium* organisms into established granulomas occurs in mammals and is independent of the Erp and ESX-1 mycobacterial virulence loci. J Infect Dis 2008;198:1851–1855.
33 Martin A, Herranz M, Ruiz Serrano MJ, Bouza E, Garcia de Viedma D: The clonal composition of *Mycobacterium tuberculosis* in clinical specimens could be modified by culture. Tuberculosis (Edinb ) 2010;90:201–207.
34 Kaplan G, Post FA, Moreira AL, Wainwright H, Kreiswirth BN, Tanverdi M, Mathema B, Ramaswamy SV, Walther G, Steyn LM, Barry CE III, Bekker LG: *Mycobacterium tuberculosis* growth at the cavity surface: a microenvironment with failed immunity. Infect Immun 2003;71:7099–7108.
35 Gagneux S, Long CD, Small PM, Van T, Schoolnik GK, Bohannan BJ: The competitive cost of antibiotic resistance in *Mycobacterium tuberculosis*. Science 2006;312:1944–1946.
36 Gagneux S, de Riemer K, Van T, Kato-Maeda M, de Jong BC, Narayanan S, Nicol M, Niemann S, Kremer K, Gutierrez MC, Hilty M, Hopewell PC, Small PM: Variable host-pathogen compatibility in *Mycobacterium tuberculosis*. Proc Natl Acad Sci USA 2006;103, 2869–2873
37 Van der Spuy GD, Kremer K, Ndabambi SL, Beyers N, Dunbar R, Marais BJ, van Helden PD, Warren RM: Changing *Mycobacterium tuberculosis* population highlights clade-specific pathogenic characteristics. Tuberculosis (Edinb) 2009;89:120–125.
38 Thwaites G, Caws M, Chau TT, D'Sa A, Lan NT, Huyen MN, Gagneux S, Anh PT, Tho DQ, Torok E, Nhu NT, Duyen NT, Duy PM, Richenberg J, Simmons C, Hien TT, Farrar J: Relationship between *Mycobacterium tuberculosis* genotype and the clinical phenotype of pulmonary and meningeal tuberculosis. J Clin Microbiol 2008;46:1363–1368.
39 Warren RM, Streicher EM, Charalambous S, Churchyard G, van der Spuy GD, Grant AD, van Helden PD, Victor TC: Use of spoligotyping for accurate classification of recurrent tuberculosis. J Clin Microbiol 2002;40:3851–3853.

Robin M. Warren, PhD, DST/NRF
Centre of Excellence in Biomedical Tuberculosis Research/MRC Centre for Molecular and Cellular Biology
Department of Medical Biochemistry, Faculty of Health Sciences
Stellenbosch University, PO Box 19063, Tygerberg 7505 (South Africa)
E-Mail rw1@sun.ac.za

Chapter 10

Donald PR, van Helden PD (eds): Antituberculosis Chemotherapy.
Prog Respir Res. Basel, Karger, 2011, vol 40, pp 81–95

# Second-Line Antituberculosis Drugs: Current Knowledge, Recent Research Findings and Controversies

H. Simon Schaaf[a,b] · James A. Seddon[a,c] · Jose A. Caminero[d,e]

[a]Department of Paediatrics and Child Health, Desmond Tutu TB Centre, Faculty of Health Sciences, Stellenbosch University, and [b]Tygerberg Children's Hospital, Tygerberg, South Africa; [c]London School of Hygiene and Tropical Medicine, London, UK; [d]Department of Pneumology. University Hospital of Gran Canaria Dr. Negrin, Las Palmas, Spain; [e]International Union against Tuberculosis and Lung Disease, Paris, France

**Abstract**

The treatment of drug-resistant tuberculosis (TB) necessitates the use of drugs that are poorly understood, less efficacious and often associated with more adverse effects than those used to treat drug-susceptible TB. Many of these second-line compounds were discovered over 50 years ago and were soon superseded by more effective and better tolerated drugs. However, in treating drug-resistant TB, we must re-evaluate these drugs as the available armamentarium of drugs is so limited. New medications, as well as established medications not previously used against TB, need to also be considered. As diagnostic techniques improve and more cases of drug-resistant TB are diagnosed, clinicians must be familiar with these second-line drugs to enable them to successfully manage patients. This article reviews the literature, often limited and sometimes elderly, regarding the second-line drugs. It also examines recent research findings and identifies areas of controversy and discussion. It comments on the laboratory, pharmacokinetic and pharmacodynamic properties of the drugs as well as discussing adverse effects.

Copyright © 2011 S. Karger AG, Basel

Multidrug-resistant (MDR) and, more recently, extensively drug-resistant (XDR) tuberculosis (TB) has necessitated the use of second-line anti-TB agents. Worldwide, 440,000 new cases of MDR-TB were estimated to have occurred in 2008, 5.4% of which were XDR-TB cases [1]. The majority of these patients are not diagnosed, and only a small proportion is treated with appropriate second-line anti-TB regimens. There is currently a strong move to roll out diagnostic facilities to identify MDR-TB cases in high TB burden countries with limited resources. However, if the diagnosis of MDR-TB is improved, treatment must be available, and for treatment to be available, it is imperative that there should be a good knowledge of the agents used. Therefore this overview does not discuss treatment options for MDR/XDR-TB but rather presents the individual agents or drug groups that are used as second-line drugs with the emphasis on recent findings and controversies.

The World Health Organization (WHO) divides the agents for MDR/XDR-TB treatment into 5 major groups (table 1) [2]. Although the current WHO guidelines classify the injectable agents as group 2 and the fluoroquinolones as group 3, there are good reasons to argue that, due to the efficacy of the agents, the severity of adverse effects and also cost, the fluoroquinolones should rather be group 2 and the injectables group 3 [3]. In this overview we will discuss only second-line agents excluding the fluoroquinolones, as these are discussed in a separate paper (i.e. we will discuss groups 2, 4 and 5). A summary is provided in table 2.

## The Injectable Antituberculosis Agents: Aminoglycosides and Cyclic Polypeptides

The current WHO group 2 agents include streptomycin, kanamycin, amikacin and capreomycin (viomycin, another cyclic polypeptide, is not currently included) [2]. In many regions with MDR-TB, resistance surveillance shows high rates (>50%) of streptomycin resistance, precluding its use in routine MDR-TB management. For this reason kanamycin

**Table 1.** Anti-TB drug groups for the treatment of drug-resistant TB [2]

| Group | Group name | Drugs | Abbreviations |
|---|---|---|---|
| 1 | First-line oral agents | Isoniazid<br>Rifampicin<br>Ethambutol<br>Pyrazinamide<br>Rifabutin | H<br>R<br>E<br>Z<br>Rfb |
| 2 | Injectable agents | Kanamycin<br>Amikacin<br>Capreomycin<br>Streptomycin | Km<br>Am<br>Cm<br>S |
| 3 | Fluoroquinolones | Moxifloxacin<br>Levofloxacin<br>Ofloxacin | Mfx<br>Lfx<br>Ofx |
| 4 | Oral bacteriostatic second-line agents | Ethionamide<br>Prothionamide<br>Cycloserine<br>Terizidone<br>Para-aminosalicylic acid | Eto<br>Pto<br>Cs<br>Trd<br>PAS |
| 5 | Agents with unclear efficacy | Clofazimine<br>Linezolid<br>Amoxicillin-clavulanic acid<br>Thiacetazone<br>Imipenem/cilastatin<br>High-dose isoniazid<br>Clarithromycin | Cfz<br>Lzd<br>Amx/Clv<br>Thz<br>Imp/Cln<br>High-dose H<br>Clr |

or amikacin is preferred in MDR-TB treatment and, because there is a high cross-resistance rate between amikacin and kanamycin, if drug susceptibility testing (DST) shows resistance to one of these drugs, capreomycin is recommended (e.g. in XDR-TB). However, it is debated whether capreomycin should not be the first-choice second-line injectable drug in MDR-TB, as it seems that resistance develops in the sequence of capreomycin, then kanamycin and finally amikacin, related to the probability of resistance mutations in *Mycobacterium tuberculosis*. Thus, if amikacin resistance is present, there is a high chance of resistance to other second-line injectables. Alternatively, if a strain is capreomycin resistant, susceptibility to amikacin is still likely [3]. High rates of capreomycin resistance have been shown in kanamycin/amikacin-resistant strains by molecular gene sequencing in a retrospective study of XDR-TB in the Western Cape, South Africa (33 of 57; 58%), where capreomycin had not been used for decades [4]. However, contrary to other reports, the same study also reported 6 deaths due to capreomycin in patients treated for XDR-TB, 5 with acute renal failure and 1 with severe hypokalaemia. Careful monitoring of renal function and potassium levels is essential, even in resource-limited settings, whenever capreomycin, and probably any second-line injectable agent, is used [4].

The suggestion that capreomycin should be used before kanamycin in retreatment cases with streptomycin resistance is not new. McClatchy et al. [5] suggested this sequence in 1977 because of 'variable cross-resistance' between kanamycin and capreomycin and fewer adverse effects with capreomycin compared to kanamycin. They do not, however, state which adverse effects are referred to or how they differ between the two drugs. Even earlier, Tsukamura [6] found that tuberculous bacilli, resistant to low kanamycin concentrations, were susceptible to both capreomycin and viomycin, but those resistant to high concentrations of kanamycin were usually resistant to capreomycin but susceptible to viomycin. However, bacilli resistant to capreomycin were resistant to viomycin but usually susceptible to kanamycin. These results suggested a preferential order in the administration of these drugs.

Recently, wild-type *M. tuberculosis* isolates were tested for critical concentrations of different injectable agents in Middlebrook 7H10 medium to determine their highest minimum inhibitory concentration (MIC) [7]. This study

**Table 2.** Characteristics of the described second-line drugs from the WHO anti-TB drug groups 2, 4 and 5

| Drug | Year discovered | Mechanism of action | Resistance genes | Current recommended dose | Formulation size | Main adverse effects |
|---|---|---|---|---|---|---|
| Kanamycin | 1957 | inhibition of protein synthesis | *rrs* | 15–20 mg/kg daily | 1-gram vial | ototoxicity, nephrotoxicity |
| Amikacin | 1972 | inhibition of protein synthesis | *rrs* | 15–20 mg/kg daily | 100-mg, 250-mg, 500-mg and 1-gram vials | ototoxicity, nephrotoxicity |
| Streptomycin | 1944 | inhibition of protein synthesis | *rrs, gidB, rpsL* | 15–20 mg/kg daily | 1-gram vial | ototoxicity, nephrotoxicity |
| Capreomycin | 1959 | inhibition of protein synthesis | *rrs, tlyA* | 15–20 mg/kg daily | 1-gram vial | ototoxicity, nephrotoxicity |
| Ethionamide, prothionamide | 1950s | inhibition of mycolic acid synthesis | *inhA, mabA, fabG1, ethA* | 15–20 mg/kg daily, 500–750 mg daily (adults) | 125-mg and 250-mg tablets | gastrointestinal disturbance, metallic taste, hypothyroidism |
| Cycloserine, terizidone | 1952 | inhibition of peptidoglycan cell wall synthesis | unclear but possibly involving AlrA, Ddl or PBP4 | 10–20 mg/kg daily | 250-mg capsules | neurological and psychological effects |
| Clofazimine | 1954 | unknown – possibly inhibition of mycobacterial DNA replication | unclear | 5 mg/kg daily or 100–300 mg daily (adults) | 50-mg, 100-mg tablets | skin discolouration |
| PAS | 1943 | unclear – possibly disruption of folic acid metabolism or inhibition of iron uptake | unclear but possibly involving *thyA* | 150 mg/kg granules daily | PAS sodium salt tablets (500 mg) or PAS acid granules (4-gram sachets) | gastrointestinal intolerance, hypothyroidism, hepatitis |
| Linezolid | 2000 | inhibition of protein synthesis (23S rRNA) | unclear | 600 mg daily (or 300 mg daily) | 600-mg tablets (and intravenous solution) | diarrhoea, headache, nausea, myelosuppression, neurotoxicity, lactic acidosis and pancreatitis |
| Amoxicillin/ clavulanate, imipenem, meropenem | 1980s–1990s | inhibition of cell wall synthesis | *M. tuberculosis* intrinsically resistant to β-lactams | as for bacterial infections | amoxicillin/clavulanate – various formulations; meropenem – 500-mg and 1-gram vials; imipenem – 250-mg and 500-mg vials | gastrointestinal intolerance, hypersensitivity reactions, seizures, liver and renal dysfunction |
| Thiacetazone | 1946 | inhibition of mycolic acid synthesis | EthA | 2.5 mg/kg daily or 150 mg daily (adults) | 150-mg tablets | Stevens-Johnson syndrome in HIV-infected patients, gastrointestinal intolerance, hepatitis, skin reactions |
| Clarithromycin | 1970s | inhibition of protein synthesis | *M. tuberculosis* intrinsically resistant to macrolides | 7.5 mg/kg b.i.d. or 500 mg b.i.d. (adults) | 500-mg tablets | gastrointestinal intolerance, rash, hepatitis, prolonged QT syndrome, ventricular arrhythmias |

showed that amikacin had a lower critical concentration (1 µg/ml) than kanamycin or capreomycin (both 4 µg/ml). The authors suggested that the critical concentration for testing DST for capreomycin should be 4 µg/ml rather than the current 10 µg/ml in Middlebrook 7H10 medium. The lower critical concentration found in Middlebrook 7H10 medium for amikacin was confirmed in liquid broth MGIT 960 BACTEC. The pharmacodynamic parameter of maximum concentration ($C_{max}$) above the MIC was better for amikacin compared to kanamycin (they also compared viomycin to capreomycin and found a lower critical concentration of 2 µg/ml for viomycin compared to 4 µg/ml for capreomycin, as well as a better $C_{max}$/MIC for viomycin) [7]. Jureen et al. [7] did not find complete cross-resistance between capreomycin and viomycin as was generally accepted. A previous study also showed a lower MIC and minimal bactericidal concentration for streptomycin and amikacin compared to kanamycin and capreomycin [8].

Resistance to aminoglycosides and cyclic polypeptides is associated with mutations in the 16S rRNA gene (*rrs*). In addition, mutations in the *tlyA* gene also confer resistance to the polypeptides [7]. Maus et al. [9] showed in a molecular study that resistance to kanamycin, amikacin, capreomycin and viomycin varies depending on which mutations are present. *tlyA* gene mutations, as well as C1402T and G1484T *rrs* mutations, conferred resistance to both capreomycin and viomycin, while the A1401T *rrs* mutation conferred resistance to capreomycin but not viomycin. Kanamycin and amikacin resistance was associated with *rrs* gene mutations (A1401T, G1484T), while kanamycin resistance and amikacin susceptibility could be associated with C1402T *rrs* mutations or to an unidentified mutation [9]. It is therefore unclear which second-line injectable should be initially used, as it will depend on the mutations present in strains causing MDR-TB in a specific region.

Streptomycin was the first aminoglycoside, isolated in the USA in 1944. As with other aminoglycosides, it inhibits protein synthesis in *M. tuberculosis* by binding tightly to the conserved A site of 16S rRNA in the 30S ribosomal subunit. Because of previous frequent use, >50% of MDR-TB isolates are streptomycin resistant, but fortunately there is little cross-resistance between streptomycin and other second-line injectable agents, as *rrs* gene mutations for streptomycin are different to those of other drugs. This allows streptomycin still to be used in XDR-TB cases where isolates show streptomycin phenotypic susceptibility; DST for streptomycin remains essential in all XDR-TB cases. As the DST to streptomycin is not fully reliable, it is better to use kanamycin or capreomycin in MDR-TB cases even when the DST shows susceptibility to streptomycin. DST for streptomycin should be done in XDR-TB cases where resistance to second-line injectable agents is likely; if the isolate shows susceptibility, streptomycin may still be an alternative injectable.

However, another recent study showed that polymorphisms in the *gidB* gene can confer both resistance to streptomycin and kanamycin [10]. *rpsL* gene mutations seem to confer mainly streptomycin resistance, and not resistance to either kanamycin/amikacin or capreomycin. Via et al. [10] also found almost complete cross-resistance between kanamycin and amikacin in the strains they evaluated – especially strains with the *rrs* 1401A→G mutation. Strains with this mutation were also resistant to capreomycin. In 3 strains with *tlyA* gene mutations, none were resistant to capreomycin. The complete picture of cross-resistance between the second-line aminoglycosides and the cyclic polypeptides on a molecular basis remains confused.

Kanamycin, isolated from *Streptomyces kanamyceticus* in 1957, is probably the most commonly used second-line injectable agent. It was from kanamycin that amikacin was developed in 1972. The MIC for *M. tuberculosis* (H37Rv) is 2.0 µg/ml, which is higher than for amikacin; the half-life is 2.0–2.5 h, and elimination is by glomerular filtration [11]. Adverse effects are as for other injectable agents.

Amikacin has a broad spectrum of activity and is active against *M. tuberculosis,* but has little early bactericidal activity. Initial studies proposed complete cross-resistance between kanamycin and amikacin, and incomplete cross-resistance with capreomycin [12]. It was concluded that amikacin had no advantage over kanamycin, and because the latter was less expensive, it was the preferred aminoglycoside. Further reports showed that amikacin had the best in vivo efficacy against *M. tuberculosis* in animal models compared to kanamycin and capreomycin. The MIC for H37Rv *M. tuberculosis* was 0.5–1.0 µg/ml. Despite amikacin having the best in vivo activity, it is not widely used in adults with MDR-TB, as kanamycin is less expensive. It is often used in children however, as ampoules are available in smaller milligram sizes, and it is believed to be a less painful intramuscular injection. The elimination of amikacin and the other injectable agents is primarily renal.

Adverse effects are mainly ototoxicity (hearing loss more common than vestibular effects) and nephrotoxicity. Other observed effects are neurotoxicity (muscle paralysis and apnoea), rashes, fever, headache, tremor, nausea, anaemia and hypotension [11].

Capreomycin, a cyclic polypeptide antibiotic, was isolated from *Streptomyces capreolus* in 1959. It is active against various species of mycobacteria, including *M. tuberculosis.*

One advantage is that it has potent activity against persistent non-replicating forms of *M. tuberculosis* [11, 13]. The precise mechanism of action is unclear, although it interacts with the ribosome and inhibits protein synthesis. The drug has similar adverse effects to the aminoglycosides and varying degrees of cross-resistance with streptomycin, kanamycin and amikacin.

The MIC for drug-susceptible strains is approximately 2 μg/ml. Capreomycin is administered intravenously or intramuscularly (no absorption orally). A median $C_{max}$ of 32 μg/ml (20–47 μg/ml) is achieved after a 1-gram dose in adults (15–20 mg/kg) [11]. Time to maximum concentration ($t_{max}$) is approximately 2 h after intramuscular injection and 1.5–2 h after completion of intravenous infusion over 1 h. Because an infusion is usually over 1 h, $C_{max}$ after an intramuscular dose is higher than with intravenous infusion at the same milligram per kilogram dose. Capreomycin penetrates the cerebrospinal fluid (CSF) only in the presence of inflammation as with the aminoglycosides. It is excreted in the urine where 52% is found unchanged within 12 h.

Ototoxicity (auditory and/or vestibular) and nephrotoxicity (raised blood urea nitrogen and renal toxicity) is common and requires close monitoring; toxicity may require that capreomycin be discontinued or the dose reduced. Other possible adverse effects are severe hypokalaemia, hypersensitivity reactions such as rash, pain and excessive bleeding at injection sites and thrombocytopenia [11].

Ototoxicity is common with all second-line injectable agents and is reported to occur in 6–18% of adults under long-term treatment [14]. Duggal and Sarkar [14] demonstrated that 18.75% of 64 patients developed high-frequency hearing loss, and 6.25% also developed speech frequency hearing loss. All hearing loss was permanent and in some cases developed up to 1 year after discontinuation of the culprit drug; there was no difference in the development of hearing loss between kanamycin, amikacin and capreomycin (only 4 patients received capreomycin however). Reports of hearing loss with the injectable agents vary widely – from as low as 0% to as high as 55%. Peloquin et al. [15] found no difference in the development of ototoxicity or nephrotoxicity between daily versus thrice weekly treatment with aminoglycosides, although the total dose did increase the risk for ototoxicity. In another study, ototoxicity was not associated with treatment duration or total aminoglycoside dose, but nephrotoxicity was associated with both [16]. The presence of certain mitochondrial DNA mutations has been associated with aminoglycoside-induced deafness – at least 6 such mutations have been identified and there are probably many more; identification of these mutations before treatment initiation may help identify patients needing regular hearing testing [17]. Protective measures, including anti-oxidant therapy such as aspirin, have been shown to prevent gentamicin-induced hearing loss, but studies are needed to confirm their benefit in long-term MDR-TB treatment [18].

Nephrotoxicity is caused by reabsorption of small amounts of drug by the proximal tubules and deposition in the renal cortex. An animal model showed that amikacin had less affinity for the proximal tubules – and may therefore be less nephrotoxic [19]. Nephrotoxicity, unlike ototoxicity, is reversible.

Which second-line injectable should then be used? Amikacin has the lowest MIC and may be the most effective second-line injectable drug. Limited evidence suggests that capreomycin has fewer adverse effects than either kanamycin or amikacin. The full pattern of cross-resistance between these drugs is not clear. The choice of a second-line drug in a region/country will often depend on availability and cost, but monitoring adverse effects, such as hypokalaemia and renal toxicity and short shelf life (24 months for capreomycin) should also be considered.

### Ethionamide and Prothionamide (Thioamides)

Following the discovery of the pyridine-containing isoniazid, numerous derivatives were tested, and thio-isonicotinamide was found by several groups to have activity against *M. tuberculosis;* ethionamide was introduced by Liberman, Rist and Grumbach. Thioamides are active against *M. tuberculosis* and, to a lesser extent, other mycobacteria. Like isoniazid, the mechanism of action is inhibition of mycolic acid synthesis [20].

The thioamides ethionamide and prothionamide are important orally-administered group 4 bacteriostatic second-line drugs. The thioamides have a narrow margin between efficacy and toxicity limiting their usefulness. Further, there is important coresistance (independent gene mutations responsible for activation of prodrugs) and cross-resistance (mutation in shared target) between the thioam ides and isoniazid.

Both ethionamide/prothionamide and isoniazid are prodrugs that need activation by mycobacterial enzymes: ethionamide by EthA, a FAD-containing Bayer-Villiger mono-oxygenase that catalyses 2 steps towards activating ethionamide, and isoniazid by the catalase-peroxidase KatG. These enzymes are regulated by *ethA/ethR* and *katG* genes, respectively, and no cross-resistance between these drugs is found with these gene mutations, although coresistance may occur if mutations are present in both genes. However, following activation, these drugs both target the enoyl-acyl carrier protein reductase (InhA) component of fatty acid synthase II regulated by the *inhA* promoter region, and inhibit mycolic acid synthesis. Mutations in the *inhA* promoter region cause target associated cross-resistance with low-level isoniazid resistance and high-level ethionamide resistance [21, 22]. With the development of new polymerase-chain-reaction-based diagnostic tools such as line probe assays, it is possible to distinguish between *katG* gene mutations and *inhA* promoter region mutations. This may assist the astute clinician decide whether only low-level isoniazid resistance is present (implying that high-dose isoniazid – a group 5 drug – may be of value) while complete ethionamide resistance is likely (an *inhA* promoter region mutation), or whether the bacilli are susceptible to ethionamide, while isoniazid is unlikely to be effective even at high doses (a *katG* mutation). This is specifically helpful as DST for ethionamide critical concentrations is notoriously unreliable, although it seems that the broth-based MGIT 960 BACTEC method is more robust.

The MIC of ethionamide in broth is 0.25–0.5 μg/ml [23]. In adults, intestinal absorption of ethionamide is almost complete; food and antacids appear to have little effect [24]. Protein binding is 30% [25], and ethionamide is distributed with ease throughout the body. Peak plasma concentrations of between 1.9 and 2.5 μg/ml occur approximately 2 h after dosing following a standard oral dose of 500 mg [24, 26, 27]. With a dose of 10 mg/kg in adults, a serum level of 5.5 μg/ml is achieved [26]. Significant intra- and interindividual variation in serum concentrations occurs [28]. For clinical purposes, the recommended serum levels for susceptible strains of *M. tuberculosis* are 2.5 μg/ml [29]. After a dose of 250 mg, serum concentrations range from 0.9 to 1.1 μg/ml and are similar between adult patients with and without AIDS [30]. Ethionamide concentrations close to serum concentrations are reached in CSF [31]. Only a very small proportion of the drug is excreted unchanged, and the first step of hepatic thioamide metabolization is transformation to sulphoxide metabolites by mono-oxygenases [32]. The sulphoxide metabolite shows in vitro activity against *M. tuberculosis* comparable to the parent drug [33].

The critical concentration for ethionamide DST in the non-radiometric BACTEC MGIT 960 system in a multicentre study was 5.0 μg/ml and for prothionamide 2.5 μg/ml; they compared it to the 'gold standard' of the BACTEC 460 critical concentration for resistance of 2.5 μg/ml for ethionamide and 1.25 μg/ml for prothionamide. Both methods showed good interlaboratory reliability, although ethionamide and prothionamide DSTs are often referred to as having poor repeatability [34].

Both ethionamide and prothionamide cause severe gastrointestinal disturbance, especially in the first weeks after introduction. Prothionamide was developed hoping it would have fewer adverse effects; although some early studies reported it better tolerated, this was not confirmed in a double-blind study where the use of either ethionamide or prothionamide was the only difference in regimens [35]. These gastrointestinal effects can be reduced by initially splitting the dose into 2 or 3 daily divided doses and/or by introducing it at a lower dose and increasing the daily amount in a stepwise fashion (drug-ramping) over 1–2 weeks to a single daily dose. Metallic taste, nausea, abdominal pain and anorexia may last much longer than initial vomiting, in some patients leading to weight loss [11]. The thioamides are also hepatotoxic and should be stopped immediately, together with other hepatotoxic drugs if possible drug-related hepatitis develops. As with other hepatotoxic anti-TB agents, patients can be rechallenged after the liver enzymes have returned to normal levels usually without further hepatic disturbance in the majority of cases. A less known adverse effect is hypothyroidism, often difficult to distinguish from other causes of disturbed thyroid function in association with chronic disease (sick euthyroid syndrome). Thyroid function tests before starting these agents may assist in distinguishing drug adverse effects from other causes. Supplementation of thyroxine may be indicated during thioamide treatment; the effect is mostly reversible once these agents are stopped [36, 37]. Thioamides have several other possible adverse effects including peripheral neuropathy (preventable with pyridoxine), blurred vision, headaches and, together with excess alcohol intake, psychotic reactions [11]. Hypoglycaemia has been reported, and blood glucose should be tested in any patient receiving either drug who presents with decreased consciousness. Gynaecomastia may develop, which is reversible on stopping the thioamide.

The current recommended dose of the thioamides in adults is 15–20 mg/kg daily, but according to the above, 10–15 mg/kg could be sufficient.

### Para-Aminosalicylic acid

Para-aminosalicylic acid (PAS) was discovered by Jorge Lehman in 1943 after work on sodium benzoate and sodium salicylate by Bernheim showing in vitro activity against tubercle bacilli. It was first used in March 1944 to treat a discharging tuberculous abscess in a child at Gothenburg Children's Hospital and given orally to a young woman with pulmonary TB in October 1946 [38]. PAS was used extensively in first-line regimens for more than 25 years and effectively protected companion drugs from resistance.

There are 2 main forms of PAS: free acid PAS and sodium salt PAS. The free acid PAS is currently available in enteric coated slow-release granules and the sodium salt PAS in both granules and compressed tablets. Old studies found similar serum concentrations with free acid or sodium PAS, but late peaks with slow-release granules [39]. Duncan et al. [39] also showed fewer gastrointestinal adverse effects with the sodium salt PAS. Before 2000, sodium salt PAS was most commonly used in the majority of countries. However, in the last 10 years, with the substantial global demand for PAS to treat MDR/XDR-TB, free acid PAS was reintroduced, especially as enteric-coated PAS granules. Aminosalicylic acid has gradually replaced aminosalicylic sodium. Nonetheless, many countries use the sodium formulation, because of proven efficacy [3]. More pharmacokinetic and pharmacodynamic data are needed to confirm the belief that sodium PAS needs a dose 30% higher than free acid PAS and to determine which has fewer gastrointestinal adverse effects. The current recommended dosage for the sodium tablet form in adults is 8–12 g in 2–3 doses (200–300 mg/kg daily), while the granules are given at a lower dose of 8 g daily (4 g twice daily; 150 mg/kg daily). A major advantage of sodium PAS is that it does not need refrigeration and cold chain maintenance [3].

Despite PAS being the first effective anti-TB drug used, its mechanism of action is still not clear. Mutations in the thymidylate synthase gene, *thyA*, have been found in PAS-resistant *M. tuberculosis* strains – implying that PAS may inhibit synthesis of thymidylate. It is also suggested that it interferes with the organism's acquisition of iron [11]. Early reports showed that emergence of resistance to PAS was uncommon with resistance arising only after 22–26 weeks, when PAS was used as a single agent [40, 41].

PAS is bacteriostatic and the MIC for PAS against drug-susceptible *M. tuberculosis* strains is generally below 1 μg/ml in 7H11 agar. The drug has no postantibiotic effect, and therefore it is assumed that time above MIC is more important than $C_{max}$. Pharmacokinetic studies have shown that 4 g PAS granules twice daily maintains PAS levels almost constantly above the MIC [42].

Free acid PAS is orally administered with poor water solubility. Absorption is 60–65%, but CSF distribution is very low (10–15%). It is commonly advised that PAS should be taken with acidic fluid (e.g. orange juice) to improve absorption [11, 43]. However, Peloquin et al. [43] found better absorption when administered with food (i.e. a high-fat meal, which may increase solubility in the gastrointestinal tract), as compared to 3 other states: fasting, with orange juice or with antacid. Although the time to $C_{max}$ was longer (6–8 h compared to 4–6 h) in PAS with food compared to the 3 other states, $C_{max}$ was improved by 50% and area under the concentration curve by 70%, with time above MIC also considerably extended [43]. PAS is 50–60% protein bound and the free drug has a short serum half-life of between 0.75 and 1 h. $C_{max}$ varies widely depending on the method of administration and dose, with reported $C_{max}$ after a 4-gram single dose of 9–35 μg/ml (median 20 μg/ml) [11]. According to Peloquin et al. [43], co-administration of other second-line drugs had a minimal effect on PAS pharmacokinetics.

Elimination of PAS is either as unchanged drug or as N-acetyl-PAS mainly in urine. PAS is acetylated in the liver and intestines to N-acetyl-PAS, and the latter is an inactive, but hepatotoxic, metabolite [44]. Despite PAS being eliminated mainly by the kidneys, some suggest that renal failure is not an absolute contraindication to the use of PAS twice daily [44]. Others, however, recommend avoiding PAS in such situations [45]. Most PAS retrieved from the urine is acetylated (about 10–15 times more than the parent drug) [43]; it is possible that patients with different acetylation genotypes may eliminate PAS at different rates. No studies have evaluated this.

Low efficacy and adverse effects led to PAS becoming a second-line drug, as with many older drugs. Gastrointestinal intolerance, most frequently nausea, diarrhoea and anorexia, is common. Diarrhoea usually subsides after 1–2 weeks. Hypothyroidism and development of goitre, mainly with treatment for longer than 6 months, was documented in 1954 and was thought to be because of interference with iodine uptake by the thyroid [46]. Hepatitis occurs in up to 0.5% of patients, and other rare adverse effects include hypersensitivity reactions (contraindicated in aspirin-allergic patients), malabsorption syndrome, anaemia (because of vitamin $B_{12}$ malabsorption) and thrombocytopenia [45]. PAS may cause hypoglycaemia in diabetics. Congenital abnormalities have been described in babies exposed in the first trimester of pregnancy, and it is best avoided in early pregnancy [45].

Because of its unpleasant adverse effects, some investigators have developed large porous particles to deliver PAS by inhalation. In rats, these aerosol particles achieved remarkably good serum concentrations and high concentrations in lung tissue and lung lining fluids [47]. As for other second-line drugs, such as the injectable agents, this is an area for future investigation.

## Cycloserine and Terizidone

Cycloserine (D-4-amino-3-isoxazolidone), originally called orientomycin, was isolated in 1952 from a *Streptomyces* strain, designated strain K-300 by Kurosawa. Cycloserine can be isolated from *Streptomyces orchidaceus*, *S. garyphalus* or *S. lavendulae* [20]. Cycloserine is active against *M. tuberculosis* and several species of Gram-positive bacteria. It is a structural analogue of the amino acid D-alanine. Terizidone is a double molecule of D-cycloserine attached by 1 molecule of terephthalic dialdehyde [48]. Both drugs are manufactured only in 250-mg units (capsules). The recommended dose is 15–20 mg/kg daily in single or twice daily doses; the maximum dose is 1 g daily.

Cycloserine inhibits *M. tuberculosis* cell wall synthesis and maintenance by inhibiting the enzymes racemase and D-alanine:D-alanine ligase, both of which are essential in the synthesis of peptidoglycan and therefore the cell wall. The precise mutation for cycloserine drug resistance is unknown [11]. DST for cycloserine is difficult, and the correlation between resistant phenotype and clinical response is poor.

The MIC for cycloserine in Löwenstein-Jensen medium is approximately 10 μg/ml [49]. The pharmacodynamic parameter for optimal treatment with cycloserine, whether time above MIC or the $C_{max}$:MIC ratio, is not clear [49].

Cycloserine and terizidone are highly water soluble. Absorption after oral administration is excellent (70–100%), and it distributes to all body compartments (has a similar volume of distribution to that of total body water) reaching good concentrations in CSF.

Limited pharmacokinetic data are available for these drugs. A study in healthy volunteers found cycloserine to be best absorbed fasting, while a high-fat meal considerably delayed $t_{max}$ and decreased $C_{max}$; although $t_{max}$ was also slightly delayed by antacids or orange juice, this was not significant [49]. The median $C_{max}$ was 14.8 μg/ml (range 12.1–30.6 μg/ml) after a single dose of 500 mg cycloserine under fasting conditions, with a median $t_{max}$ of 0.75 h (range 0.25–3.00 h) – these values were similar with orange juice or antacids. The half-life of cycloserine is 8–10 h [11, 49]. From these data it seems that time above the MIC could best be achieved by not giving cycloserine with a high-fat meal and by administering it twice daily [49]. However, once daily administration is advantageous for directly observed therapy and twice daily dosing is difficult to achieve in children because the capsules are only available in 250-mg units. In another study, comparing the pharmacokinetics of cycloserine and terizidone, the $t_{max}$ was between 2 and 3 h and although the $C_{max}$ was not specifically presented, it was reported that serum terizidone concentrations were generally higher than cycloserine concentrations, although not significantly so. They reported faster elimination of drug by younger adults compared to older adults, and the half-life of both drugs was between 15 and 33 h, with that of terizidone generally longer than that of cycloserine [48]. Excretion is mainly renal, and different studies found between 26 and 92% of cycloserine in the urine after 24 h [11, 49].

Adverse effects are reported to be significantly less with terizidone compared to cycloserine, but the evidence is limited [48, 50, 51]. The nervous system is most commonly affected and many adverse effects may be prevented by co-administration of high-dose pyridoxine (150–300 mg/day). In some cases, they could be managed by lowering and/or dividing the daily dose. Neuropsychiatric adverse effects feature as drowsiness, headache, dizziness, personality changes, convulsions, tremors, paraesthesia, anxiety, slurred speech (dysarthria), depression (some with suicidal tendencies) and coma [11, 52]. Cycloserine should be used with care in alcoholics (increased risk of convulsions) and patients with mental illness or previous convulsions [11]. Some experts recommend psychiatric evaluation before use of these drugs. Neurotoxicity was recently confirmed by magnetic resonance imaging in a woman presenting with hypersomnolence and asterixis [52]. Congestive cardiac failure has been associated with cycloserine treatment in some early reports [53], and Stevens-Johnson syndrome has been described in an HIV-infected patient [54].

In light of the discussion above, consideration should be given to a proper comparative trial between terizidone and cycloserine in standard regimens.

## Clofazimine

Renewed interest in clofazimine as an effective second-line anti-TB drug was stimulated by a recent report from Bangladesh describing the successful management of MDR-TB with a 9- to 12-month regimen of first- and second-line drugs, including the fourth-generation fluoroquinolone gatifloxacin, and clofazimine replacing prothionamide in the continuation phase. Adverse effects, failure rate and default rate were lower in the treatment group where clofazimine replaced prothionamide in the continuation phase; no specific adverse effects were ascribed to clofazimine [55].

Clofazimine, a riminophenazine antibiotic first synthesized as an anti-TB drug in 1954, has never been properly evaluated as a second-line anti-TB drug, but has been used extensively for treatment of *Mycobacterium leprae* since 1969.

Although initially thought ineffective against *M. tuberculosis*, in vitro studies have shown drug-susceptible and drug-resistant strains to be susceptible to clofazimine with MICs of ≤1 μg/ml [56, 57]. A study from Ethiopia showed that all 35 MDR strains tested at 2 μg/ml by the BACTEC 460 method were susceptible to clofazimine [58]. The MIC in vitro against the reference H37Rv strain is 0.1 μg/ml. Some investigators have shown higher MICs for strains resistant to pyrazinamide and rifampicin, but this was not a consistent finding; MICs are usually ≤0.5 μg/ml for drug-susceptible and isoniazid-resistant strains, while rifampicin- and pyrazinamide-resistant strains (including MDR strains) may have a higher MIC of up to 6.25 μg/ml [11]. In vivo studies found clofazimine active in *M. tuberculosis*-infected mice when given at 20 mg/kg body weight; it prevented mortality and caused significant reduction in colony-forming units in lungs and spleen, but did not completely eradicate the organism from the spleen [56].

The mode of action of clofazimine is unknown. Clofazimine is fat soluble and administered orally as 50- and 100-mg tablets. Oral absorption is 45–62%; a high-fat meal improves absorption and bioavailability [59]. The current WHO-recommended dosage is approximately 5 mg/kg body weight (200–300 mg/day in adults), but evidence for this recommendation is not consistent. In the study from Bangladesh where high success rates (89%) were achieved with 9 months of treatment, clofazimine was used at 100 mg/day [55]. Liposome-encapsulated clofazimine may allow higher dosages to be given [60]. The drug tends to deposit in fatty tissue and cells of the reticulo-endothelial system. It concentrates in macrophages and is therefore specifically active against intracellular organisms; however, serum levels are often very low. $C_{max}$ varies between 0.145 and 2.0 μg/ml with dosages ranging from 100 to 300 mg/day [11, 59]. Because of its high macrophage concentration, the activity against *M. tuberculosis* may mainly be intracellular, with low serum concentrations giving a false impression of below-MIC values [56]. After prolonged use, clofazimine has an exceptionally long half-life of 65–70 days. Some, however, report a biphasic excretion with a half-life of between 8 h and 10 days [59]. The metabolism of clofazimine is mainly hepatic. It is not clear whether metabolites are active against *M. tuberculosis*. In addition to its antimycobacterial effect, clofazimine has an anti-inflammatory action. A recent study found excellent efficacy of clofazimine against rapidly growing mycobacteria in vitro with MICs ≤1 μg/ml; this study also noted that amikacin reduced the MIC of clofazimine against several of the mycobacteria – something that may well be worth studying in *M. tuberculosis* [61].

The frequency of drug resistance development to clofazimine seems to be low; laboratory and clinical mutants have been difficult to generate [11, 56]. Importantly, early studies showed that clofazimine, even at sub-MIC levels, prevented the development of isoniazid resistance in *M. tuberculosis* strains [62].

Gastrointestinal adverse effects such as abdominal pain, diarrhoea, nausea, vomiting and gastrointestinal intolerance are frequent (up to 50% of patients). Skin pigmentation from pink to reddish black occurs in 75–100% of patients within a few weeks of treatment, even in those dark-skinned. Reducing the usual dose of 200–300 mg to 100 mg may prevent this effect. Although reversible, it can last for months to years after treatment completion. Other adverse effects are dry skin, rash and pruritus. Discolouration of all body secretions occurs as well as eye pigmentation and irritation. Central nervous system adverse effects include headache, dizziness, drowsiness, fatigue and taste disorder. Depression has been reported due to severe skin discolouration [11]. Clofazimine crosses the placenta and may cause skin discolouration in infants.

## β-Lactam Antibiotics in Combination with Clavulanate

*Amoxicillin/Clavulanate (Amoxicillin/Clavulanic Acid, Co-Amoxiclav), Imipenem/Clavulanate and Meropenem/Clavulanate*

The combination of amoxicillin and clavulanic acid (clavulanate) is well known in the management of β-lactamase-producing bacterial infections. Both amoxicillin and clavulanate are rapidly absorbed after oral administration and have similar pharmacokinetic properties. Both have a $t_{max}$ of 1.0–2.0 h (that of amoxicillin is dose dependent), have half-lives of approximately 1–1.5 h and the same elimination mechanism. Serum levels of clavulanate, if administered in combination with amoxicillin, have been shown to be highly variable at the same dose among different patients, but this does not seem to affect its efficacy in treating bacterial infections [63].

β-Lactam antibiotics are not regarded as useful drugs against TB. Resistance is thought to be mediated by a class of β-lactamase enzymes that hydrolyse penicillins and cephalosporins. Resistance can be overcome by either inhibiting the β-lactamase or by use of an antibiotic that is not a substrate for the enzyme such as imipenem or meropenem. β-Lactamase can be inhibited with a combination of a β-lactam and a β-lactamase inhibitor, such as amoxicillin/

clavulanate, which is active against *M. tuberculosis* in vitro [3].

Some β-lactam antibiotics, such as amoxicillin and the carbapenems (imipenem and meropenem), are active against *M. tuberculosis* in vitro. Cynamon and Palmer [64] first showed that amoxicillin/clavulanate is bactericidal in vitro against *M. tuberculosis.* In 1991 Nadler et al. [65] reported 2 cases of MDR-TB with *M. tuberculosis* strains susceptible in vitro to amoxicillin/clavulanate successfully treated with the addition of amoxicillin/clavulanate to the MDR-TB regimen. Chambers et al. [66] showed that *M. tuberculosis* has several penicillin-binding proteins and that resistance could be reversed by β-lactamase inhibitors such as clavulanate. MICs for imipenem were the best (≤4 μg/ml) and, although the MIC for amoxicillin was 16 μg/ml, this was reduced to ≤2 μg/ml by the addition of clavulanate. Penetration of the *M. tuberculosis* cell wall is slow, but because of its slow replication rate (18–24 h) this does not seem to cause resistance to these drugs [66]. Others have confirmed these findings; especially that chromosomal β-lactamase is the main resistance determinant for amoxicillin (and the carbapenems). MICs in this study were much higher for amoxicillin and amoxicillin/clavulanate than in the study of Chambers et al. [66], but clavulanate, although it has no antimycobacterial activity of its own, drastically lowered the MIC for amoxicillin [67]. Another in vitro study showed that MICs for amoxicillin/clavulanate against *M. tuberculosis* can be reduced even further to <0.5 μg/ml (easily achievable even in tissue) by the synergistic effect of ethambutol at subinhibitory concentrations [68]. If this is correct, and similar effects can be expected in vivo, it may be important to add ethambutol to any MDR-TB regimen containing amoxicillin/clavulanate even in the presence of ethambutol resistance.

Early bactericidal activity, or activity from day 0–2, for amoxicillin/clavulanate was evaluated in patients in 2 studies: one showed no effect, while the other showed a relatively good early bactericidal activity [69]. This could possibly be explained by a different frequency and dose of amoxicillin in the 2 studies or by a difference in the *M. tuberculosis* strains among the different groups of patients. Recently, Gupta et al. [70] showed that a mutation in the $ldt_{Mt2}$ gene could render *M. tuberculosis* more susceptible to amoxicillin/clavulanate. They also found that this drug combination had its effect on TB infection in mice at a much later stage (chronic phase of the disease) which could also explain the lack of early bactericidal activity in the first 2 days of treatment.

The current dose recommendation of amoxicillin/clavulanate in adults is not well defined [3]. It is usually given in 2 or 3 divided doses per day, but the dose of amoxicillin varies considerably compared to clavulanate in the available preparations. Extended-release tablets have also been marketed. The optimal dose, combination and frequency of administration for treatment of drug-resistant TB needs further investigation. Until then, a dose of 1 g amoxicillin/62.5 mg clavulanate twice daily seems reasonable.

As explained above, the carbapenems offer another approach to overcome the β-lactam resistance of *M. tuberculosis.* They are poor substrates for class A and class C β-lactamases, and 2 carbapenems, meropenem and imipenem, are active in vitro against *M. tuberculosis.* Efficacy has been shown in some reports of patients with MDR-TB treated with imipenem and meropenem with clavulanic acid [2].

In a recent in vitro study, Hugonnet et al. [71] showed that meropenem is the best β-lactam to use in combination with clavulanate. In this study it showed low MICs (≤1 μg/ml) for both drug-susceptible and drug-resistant *M. tuberculosis* strains when compared to amoxicillin, imipenem and other β-lactams that had variable MICs. In vitro studies also showed meropenem/clavulanate to be active against 'persistent' *M. tuberculosis* strains, implying that it could be a good sterilizing drug in the treatment of TB [71].

In contrast to amoxicillin/clavulanate which is well absorbed orally, the carbapenems are only administered intravenously. Meropenem has the advantage of good CSF penetration, which makes it a useful drug for central nervous system TB.

Adverse effects for all the above drugs are mainly gastrointestinal and hypersensitivity reactions. Seizures, increased liver enzymes and elevations in serum creatinine and blood urea may occur with the carbapenems.

Despite these encouraging reports, limited clinical experience, unknown long-term toxicity, high costs and the need to treat intravenously restrict carbapenem use to severe cases only [2].

## Linezolid

Linezolid, the first oxazolidinone antibiotic approved for clinical use against mainly aerobic Gram-positive organisms, has good activity against drug-susceptible and drug-resistant *M. tuberculosis* strains in vitro and in animal studies. Several case series of off-label use in MDR and XDR-TB have confirmed its anti-TB efficacy, but optimal dosage and duration of therapy have not been established [72–75]. Severe, sometimes irreversible adverse effects, its current exorbitant cost and lack of studies confirming efficacy are likely the main reasons for it not being used more often.

Linezolid has a unique mechanism of action, inhibiting protein synthesis at an early stage of translation. Binding to the 23S rRNA, it inhibits early-phase translation and prevents proper binding of formylmethionine tRNA; because of this unique mechanism, cross-resistance with any existing anti-TB agent is unlikely [11]. *M. tuberculosis* strains resistant to linezolid have been found, but mutations conferring resistance have not been identified [11, 76].

The MICs for linezolid vary between studies, but the majority of strains tested, both pan-susceptible and MDR/XDR, have MICs ≤1 μg/ml. Several strains have MICs of <0.5 μg/ml, while the mutant prevention concentration has been estimated at 1.2 μg/ml [11, 77]. Linezolid is either administered orally or intravenously: absorption/bioavailability after oral administration is 100% and the volume of distribution is high [72]. Plasma protein binding is 31% [11]. It has excellent tissue and CSF penetration and could therefore be a useful drug in the management of MDR/XDR-TB meningitis, which generally has a poor prognosis. $C_{max}$ in adults after a single dose of 600 mg administered either intravenously or orally is the same at 12.7–12.9 μg/ml, and the half-life is similar at 4–4.5 h. In another study, $C_{max}$ after a 300-mg daily dose was 11.6 ± 4.4 μg/ml in 10 patients, 7 days after starting linezolid. Concentration above the MIC was maintained for 24 h in a number of patients with $C_{min}$ at 24 h of 2.1 ± 1.3 μg/ml [74], and $t_{max}$ was 1–2 h. From a study in healthy volunteers it seems as if there is limited drug accumulation if given at 600 mg twice daily: on day 1 $C_{max}$ was 14.5 ± 4.6 μg/ml with $t_{max}$ <1 h; $C_{max}$ on day 7 was significantly higher at 24.0 ± 6.9 μg/ml [78]. Linezolid is almost fully excreted in urine, either as linezolid (30%) or as inactive metabolites (70%); a small amount is excreted in the faeces (<10%) [11].

Adverse effects have frequently been reported, especially with long-term use; the most common are diarrhoea, headache and nausea. More important severe adverse effects are reversible myelosuppression (anaemia, leucopenia, thrombocytopenia and pancytopenia), neurotoxicity (peripheral neuropathy – sometimes irreversible – and optic neuritis – mostly reversible), lactic acidosis and pancreatitis [11]. These effects were common at the previously recommended adult dose of 600 mg twice daily, but the myelosuppression and, to a lesser extent, the neurotoxicity are greatly reduced at the lower doses of 600 mg daily (either single or divided dose) and 300 mg daily, while still retaining efficacy against *M. tuberculosis* [72–74, 79, 80].

The current dose recommendation for linezolid, for those that can afford it, is 600 mg/day. Strict monitoring for adverse effects is essential and patients should be advised to immediately report any unusual gum bleeding. Studies are needed to assess the efficacy of low-dose linezolid in MDR/XDR-TB [2].

## Clarithromycin

Clarithromycin, a macrolide antibiotic, has proven efficacy against non-tuberculous mycobacteria, especially *M. avium,* as well as *M. leprae*. However, although according to MICs clarithromycin is currently the preferred macrolide against *M. tuberculosis*, its activity is uncertain, as in vitro extracellular MICs range from 4 to ≥16 μg/ml. Initial reports of in vitro and in vivo animal experimental studies gave conflicting results. Some studies showed low but confirmed activity, more intracellular than extracellular and with efficacy comparable to thiacetazone in a mouse model [81], while others in similar studies showed that clarithromycin was inactive against *M. tuberculosis* [82]. Mycobacteria are said to be intrinsically resistant to macrolides as a characteristic of the *ermB* gene. This resistance gene can be induced by clarithromycin and similar agents [83].

Despite this, studies have found clarithromycin to have a synergistic effect on first-line anti-TB drugs such as isoniazid, rifampicin, ethambutol and pyrazinamide with enhanced intracellular effectiveness against *M. tuberculosis* [84, 85]. In addition, ethambutol exerted a synergistic effect on clarithromycin, increasing its effectiveness despite MICs >4 μg/ml in all strains tested [86]. This could be due to ethambutol inhibiting cell wall integrity allowing clarithromycin to attach to its ribosomal target even in the presence of ethambutol resistance.

Clarithromycin inhibits protein synthesis by binding to the 50S ribosomal subunit. An early study showed that the MIC against different *M. tuberculosis* strains varied from 1.3 to 10 μg/ml [11, 87]. The $C_{max}$ after a 200-mg dose in healthy adults is low at 0.6 ± 0.43 μg/ml, and the half-life is 2.33 h [11]. The drug is well absorbed after oral administration and is acid stable. The peak concentration at higher doses in the serum is approximately 2.16 ± 0.5 μg/ml, while the peak concentration in the lung is 13.5 μg/g, with even higher intracellular concentrations in lung tissue [88].

Adverse effects include gastrointestinal disturbances, rash, hepatotoxicity, prolonged QT syndrome and ventricular arrhythmias. In animal models (monkeys, rats, mice) it causes foetal abnormalities; therefore its use in pregnancy is currently contraindicated [11].

DST for clarithromycin of 69 *M. tuberculosis* strains from Rwanda in a liquid broth BACTEC 460 radiometric system found only 1 strain resistant to clarithromycin at a concentration of 4 μg/ml [89]. Where clarithromycin is not frequently used for other bacterial infections, it could play a more prominent role in MDR-TB treatment, especially if combined with drugs with a possible synergistic action.

Although there are no studies to confirm it, the current recommended dose is 500 mg twice daily [3].

## Thiacetazone

Thiacetazone (4-acetylaminobenzaldehyde thiosemicarbazone, thioacetazone, para-acetylaminobenzaldehyde thiosemicarbazone) was developed in Germany in 1946 by Domagk et al. [90] after investigations of sulphonamides had revealed that thiazoles and thiodiazole derivatives had antimycobacterial activity. Good clinical activity against TB was found, but it fell into disuse because of toxicity at higher doses given at the time, in addition to the discovery of the excellent antituberculous activity of isoniazid. However, when a cheap effective drug was sought to accompany isoniazid to prevent resistance in regimens used in low-income countries, thiacetazone was reintroduced early in the 1960s [91]. After a number of pilot studies to determine the optimal dose of both drugs, a controlled clinical trial demonstrated that the combination of isoniazid and thiacetazone was as effective as the standard combination of isoniazid and PAS in producing sputum conversion and preventing isoniazid resistance [92]. Streptomycin in the initial 8-week phase improved these results, with significantly less isoniazid resistance developing in the streptomycin group and a considerably higher rate of bacteriologically negative sputa at 6 and 12 months [93, 94]. This regimen was used for many years in resource-limited countries [95].

Thiacetazone fell into almost complete disuse and was withdrawn in many countries, because of the severe adverse effect of Stevens-Johnson syndrome and even death following its use in HIV-infected patients. It is still contraindicated for use in those HIV-infected [3, 96]. However, it is reasonable to question whether thiacetazone should not have a more prominent role in the management of HIV-uninfected MDR/XDR-TB patients, as the armamentarium of available drugs is limited. One argument against its use is cross-resistance between thiacetazone and other agents such as ethionamide. Mutations in the *ethA* gene confer activation-associated cross-resistance between ethionamide and thiacetazone [33]. Cross-resistance between ethionamide and thiacetazone varies from 29 to 79%; other mechanisms of resistance or inactivation of thiacetazone have recently been described.

The mechanism of action is inhibition of cell wall synthesis, possibly by the inhibition of mycolic acid cyclopropanation [97]. Thiacetazone is a weak bacteriostatic agent with poor sterilizing activity. It is administered orally and is well absorbed, but little is known about its bioavailability. The MIC for thiacetazone against *M. tuberculosis* seems to be between 0.4 and 1.0 μg/ml for wild-type strains [98, 99]. The $C_{max}$ was on average 1.8 μg/ml after a daily dose of 150 mg [100], and 2.9 μg/ml after a dose of 4 mg/kg [101], while $t_{max}$ was 4–5 h [99, 101]. The half-life was 11 h [101]. Peloquin et al. [102] found the $C_{max}$ to be a mean of 1.59 ± 0.47 μg/ml, $t_{max}$ 3.30 ± 1.18 h and serum half-life 15–16 h after a daily dose of 150 mg in healthy volunteers. It is partially excreted unchanged in the urine, but the major form of excretion is unknown.

The observed in vitro susceptibility of *M. tuberculosis* varies considerably depending on the technique of DST and the strain origin. In a comparison of *M. tuberculosis* strains, those from India were less susceptible to thiacetazone than UK strains; this geographic variation was later confirmed. The susceptibility of strains may vary even within the same country. The correlation between in vitro and in vivo results is often very poor [20].

Recently, François et al. [103] showed that human flavin-containing mono-oxygenase 2.1, expressed predominantly in the lung, catalyses oxygenation of thiacetazone. The metabolites generated, the sulphenic acid, sulphinic acid and carbodi-imide derivatives, are the same as those produced by EthA and are inactive against *M. tuberculosis*. Because of a genetic polymorphism, Europeans and Asians lack flavin-containing mono-oxygenase 2.1, but in sub-Saharan Africa a substantial proportion of individuals express it. This may have the implication that thiacetazone may not be as effective in MDR/XDR-TB treatment in sub-Saharan Africa as in other regions.

Adverse effects with thiacetazone were common and severe at the higher doses previously used. Although adverse effects with a reduced dose of 150 mg daily were still common (21%), they were relatively mild before the advent of HIV. The current recommended dose of thiacetazone is 2.5 mg/kg body weight as a single daily dose. It may cause nausea, vomiting and anorexia, skin reactions (possibly immune-related), hepatotoxicity, haemolytic anaemia and agranulocytosis. The last was a rare, but occasionally fatal, adverse effect [104]. Skin reactions, presenting early and with increased severity, especially the often fatal Stevens-Johnson syndrome and toxic epidermal necrolysis, occurred significantly more frequently in HIV-infected as compared to HIV-uninfected patients [96, 100, 105].

The WHO does not recommend the reserve drugs of group 5 for routine use in drug-resistant TB treatment because their contribution to the efficacy of multidrug regimens is unclear. While thiacetazone is a drug with known efficacy against TB [95], it is placed in group 5 because its role in drug-resistant TB treatment is not well established. However, although it was removed from several countries because of the severe and sometimes fatal adverse effects in HIV-infected patients, thiacetazone is still a useful drug in HIV-uninfected patients, especially to protect companion drugs with better efficacy from the emergence of drug resistance.

## References


1 World Health Organization: Multidrug and Extensively Drug-Resistant TB (M/XDR-TB): 2010 Global Report on Surveillance and Response. WHO/HTM/TB/2010.3. Geneva, WHO, 2010.

2 World Health Organization: Guidelines for the Programmatic Management of Drug-Resistant Tuberculosis – Emergency Update. WHO/HTM/TB/2008.402. Geneva, WHO, 2008.

3 Caminero JA, Sotgiu G, Zumla A, Migliori GB: Best drug treatment for multidrug-resistant and extensively drug-resistant tuberculosis. Lancet Infect Dis 2010;10:621–629.

4 Dheda K, Shean K, Zumla A, Badri M, Streicher EM, Page-Shipp L, Willcox P, John MA, Reubenson G, Govindasamy D, Wong M, Padanilam X, Dziwiecki A, van Helden PD, Siwendu S, Jarand J, Menezes CN, Burns A, Victor T, Warren R, Grobusch MP, van der Walt M, Kvasnovsky C: Early treatment outcomes and HIV status of patients with extensively drug-resistant tuberculosis in South Africa: a retrospective cohort study. Lancet 2010;375:1798–1807.

5 McClatchy JK, Kanes W, Davidson PT, Moulding TS: Cross-resistance in *M. tuberculosis* to kanamycin, capreomycin and viomycin. Tubercle 1977;58:29–34.

6 Tsukamura M: Cross-resistance relationships between capreomycin, kanamycin, and viomycin resistances in tubercle bacilli from patients. Am Rev Respir Dis 1969;99:780–782.

7 Jureen P, Angeby K, Sturegard E, Chryssanthou E, Giske CG, Werngren J, Nordvall M, Johansson A, Kahlmeter G, Hoffner S, Schon T: Wild-type MIC distributions for aminoglycoside and cyclic polypeptide antibiotics used for treatment of *Mycobacterium tuberculosis* infections. J Clin Microbiol 2010;48:1853–1858.

8 Heifets L, Lindholm-Levy P: Comparison of bactericidal activities of streptomycin, amikacin, kanamycin, and capreomycin against *Mycobacterium avium* and *M. tuberculosis*. Antimicrob Agents Chemother 1989;33:1298–1301.

9 Maus CE, Plikaytis BB, Shinnick TM: Molecular analysis of cross-resistance to capreomycin, kanamycin, amikacin, and viomycin in *Mycobacterium tuberculosis*. Antimicrob Agents Chemother 2005;49:3192–3197.

10 Via LE, Cho SN, Hwang S, Bang H, Park SK, Kang HS, Jeon D, Min SY, Oh T, Kim Y, Kim YM, Rajan V, Wong SY, Shamputa IC, Carroll M, Goldfeder L, Lee SA, Holland SM, Eum S, Lee H, Barry CE 3rd: Polymorphisms associated with resistance and cross-resistance to aminoglycosides and capreomycin in *Mycobacterium tuberculosis* isolates from South Korean patients with drug-resistant tuberculosis. J Clin Microbiol 2010;48:402–411.

11 Handbook of anti-tuberculosis agents. Tuberculosis (Edinb) 2008;88:1–169.

12 Allen BW, Mitchison DA, Chan YC, Yew WW, Allan WG, Girling DJ: Amikacin in the treatment of pulmonary tuberculosis. Tubercle 1983;64:111–118.

13 Heifets L, Simon J, Pham V: Capreomycin is active against non-replicating *M. tuberculosis*. Ann Clin Microbiol Antimicrob 2005;4:6.

14 Duggal P, Sarkar M: Audiologic monitoring of multi-drug resistant tuberculosis patients on aminoglycoside treatment with long term follow-up. BMC Ear Nose Throat Disord 2007;7:5.

15 Peloquin CA, Berning SE, Nitta AT, Simone PM, Goble M, Huitt GA, Iseman MD, Cook JL, Curran-Everett D: Aminoglycoside toxicity: daily versus thrice-weekly dosing for treatment of mycobacterial diseases. Clin Infect Dis 2004;38:1538–1544.

16 De Jager P, van Altena R: Hearing loss and nephrotoxicity in long-term aminoglycoside treatment in patients with tuberculosis. Int J Tuberc Lung Dis 2002;6:622–627.

17 Bardien S, de Jong G, Schaaf HS, Harris T, Fagan J, Petersen L: Aminoglycoside-induced hearing loss: South Africans at risk. S Afr Med J 2009;99:440–441.

18 Sha SH, Qiu JH, Schacht J: Aspirin to prevent gentamicin-induced hearing loss. N Engl J Med 2006;354:1856–1857.

19 Luft FC, Bloch R, Sloan RS, Yum MN, Costello R, Maxwell DR: Comparative nephrotoxicity of aminoglycoside antibiotics in rats. J Infect Dis 1978;138:541–545.

20 Rieder HL: Interventions for Tuberculosis Control and Elimination. Paris, International Union against Tuberculosis and Lung Disease, 2002.

21 Banerjee A, Dubnau E, Quemard A, Balasubramanian V, Um KS, Wilson T, Collins D, de Lisle G, Jacobs WR Jr: *inhA*, a gene encoding a target for isoniazid and ethionamide in *Mycobacterium tuberculosis*. Science 1994;263:227–230.

22 Schaaf HS, Victor TC, Venter A, Brittle W, Jordaan AM, Hesseling AC, Marais BJ, van Helden PD, Donald PR: Ethionamide cross- and co-resistance in children with isoniazid-resistant tuberculosis. Int J Tuberc Lung Dis 2009;13:1355–1359.

23 Rastogi N, Labrousse V, Goh KS: In vitro activities of fourteen antimicrobial agents against drug susceptible and resistant clinical isolates of *Mycobacterium tuberculosis* and comparative intracellular activities against the virulent H37Rv strain in human macrophages. Curr Microbiol 1996;33:167–175.

24 Auclair B, Nix DE, Adam RD, James GT, Peloquin CA: Pharmacokinetics of ethionamide administered under fasting conditions or with orange juice, food, or antacids. Antimicrob Agents Chemother 2001;45:810–814.

25 Dover LG, Corsino PE, Daniels IR, Cocklin SL, Tatituri V, Besra GS, Futterer K: Crystal structure of the TetR/CamR family repressor *Mycobacterium tuberculosis* EthR implicated in ethionamide resistance. J Mol Biol 2004;340:1095–1105.

26 Eule H: Ethionamide concentration in the blood and urine of healthy persons and lung patients (in German). Beitr Klin Erforsch Tuberk Lungenkr 1965;132:339–342.

27 Zhu M, Namdar R, Stambaugh JJ, Starke JR, Bulpitt AE, Berning SE, Peloquin CA: Population pharmacokinetics of ethionamide in patients with tuberculosis. Tuberculosis (Edinb) 2002;82:91–96.

28 Mattila MJ, Koskinen R, Takki S: Absorption of ethionamide and prothionamide in vitro and in vivo. Ann Med Intern Fenn 1968;57:75–79.

29 Heifets L: Qualitative and quantitative drug-susceptibility tests in mycobacteriology. Am Rev Respir Dis 1988;137:1217–1222.

30 Conte JE Jr, Golden JA, McQuitty M, Kipps J, Lin ET, Zurlinden E: Effects of AIDS and gender on steady-state plasma and intrapulmonary ethionamide concentrations. Antimicrob Agents Chemother 2000;44:1337–1341.

31 Hughes IE, Smith H: Ethionamide: its passage into the cerebrospinal fluid in man. Lancet 1962;1:616–617.
32 Henderson MC, Siddens LK, Morre JT, Krueger SK, Williams DE: Metabolism of the anti-tuberculosis drug ethionamide by mouse and human FMO1, FMO2 and FMO3 and mouse and human lung microsomes. Toxicol Appl Pharmacol 2008;233:420–427.
33 De Barber AE, Mdluli K, Bosman M, Bekker LG, Barry CE 3rd: Ethionamide activation and sensitivity in multidrug-resistant *Mycobacterium tuberculosis*. Proc Natl Acad Sci USA 2000;97:9677–9682.
34 Rusch-Gerdes S, Pfyffer GE, Casal M, Chadwick M, Siddiqi S: Multicenter laboratory validation of the BACTEC MGIT 960 technique for testing susceptibilities of *Mycobacterium tuberculosis* to classical second-line drugs and newer antimicrobials. J Clin Microbiol 2006;44:688–692.
35 A comparison of the toxicity of prothionamide and ethionamide: a report from the research committee of the British Tuberculosis Association. Tubercle 1968;49:125–135.
36 McDonnell ME, Braverman LE, Bernardo J: Hypothyroidism due to ethionamide. N Engl J Med 2005;352:2757–2759.
37 Hallbauer UM, Schaaf HS: Ethionamide induced hypothyroidism in children. S Afr J Epidemiol Infect, in press.
38 Schaaf HS, Donald PR: The epidemiology and management of drug-resistant tuberculosis in childhood; in Spiegelburg DD (ed): New Topics in Tuberculosis Research. New York, Nova Science Publishers, 2007, pp 71–102.
39 Duncan DK, Carr DT, Pfuetze KH, Power MH: Serum concentrations of para-aminosalicylic acid (PAS) produced by various forms of PAS. Dis Chest 1951;19:138–148.
40 Carstensen B: Para-aminosalicylic acid (PAS) in pulmonary and extrapulmonary tuberculosis. Am Rev Tuberc 1950;61:613–620.
41 Karlson AG, Pfuetze KH, Carr T, Feldman WH, Hinshaw HC: The effect of combined therapy with streptomycin, para-aminosalicylic acid and promin on the emergence of streptomycin-resistant strains of tubercle bacilli; a preliminary report. Mayo Clin Proc 1949;24:85–88.
42 Peloquin CA, Berning SE, Huitt GA, Childs JM, Singleton MD, James GT: Once-daily and twice-daily dosing of *p*-aminosalicylic acid granules. Am J Respir Crit Care Med 1999;159:932–934.
43 Peloquin CA, Zhu M, Adam RD, Singleton MD, Nix DE: Pharmacokinetics of para-aminosalicylic acid granules under four dosing conditions. Ann Pharmacother 2001;35:1332–1338.
44 Peloquin CA: Pharmacological issues in the treatment of tuberculosis. Ann NY Acad Sci 2001;953:157–164.
45 McIlleron H. Tuberculosis drug information; in Schaaf HS, Zumla A (eds): Tuberculosis: A Comprehensive Clinical Reference. London, Saunders Elsevier, 2009, pp 958–971.
46 Balint JA, Fraser R, Hanno MG: Radio-iodine measurements of thyroid function during and after PAS treatment of tuberculosis. Br Med J 1954;i:1234–1237.
47 Tsapis N, Bennett D, O'Driscoll K, Shea K, Lipp MM, Fu K, Clarke RW, Deaver D, Yamins D, Wright J, Peloquin CA, Weitz DA, Edwards DA: Direct lung delivery of para-aminosalicylic acid by aerosol particles. Tuberculosis (Edinb) 2003;83:379–385.
48 Zitkova L, Tousek J: Pharmacokinetics of cycloserine and terizidone: a comparative study. Chemotherapy 1974;20:18–28.
49 Zhu M, Nix DE, Adam RD, Childs JM, Peloquin CA: Pharmacokinetics of cycloserine under fasting conditions and with high-fat meal, orange juice, and antacids. Pharmacotherapy 2001;21:891–897.
50 Galletti F: Tolerability of terizidone. Minerva Med 1991;82:477–481.
51 Weyer K: Annexure 2: DOTS-Plus for multidrug resistant tuberculosis patients in South Africa. Systematic evaluation of a standardised treatment regimen applied under tuberculosis control programme conditions. 2004. http://wwwsa-healthinfoorg/tb/annexures1-4pdf (accessed October 30, 2010).
52 Kwon HM, Kim HK, Cho J, Hong YH, Nam H: Cycloserine-induced encephalopathy: evidence on brain MRI. Eur J Neurol 2008;15:e60–e61.
53 Walker WC, Murdoch JM: Cycloserine in the treatment of pulmonary tuberculosis: a report on toxicity. Tubercle 1957;38:297–302.
54 Akula SK, Aruna AS, Johnson JE, Anderson DS: Cycloserine-induced Stevens-Johnson syndrome in an AIDS patient with multidrug-resistant tuberculosis. Int J Tuberc Lung Dis 1997;1:187–190.
55 Van Deun A, Maug AK, Salim MA, Das PK, Sarker MR, Daru P, Rieder HL: Short, highly effective, and inexpensive standardized treatment of multidrug-resistant tuberculosis. Am J Respir Crit Care Med 2010;182:684–692.
56 Reddy VM, Nadadhur G, Daneluzzi D, O'Sullivan JF, Gangadharam PR: Antituberculosis activities of clofazimine and its new analogs B4154 and B4157. Antimicrob Agents Chemother 1996;40:633–636.
57 Van Ingen J, Simons S, de Zwaan R, van der Laan T, Kamst-van Agterveld M, Boeree MJ, van Soolingen D: Comparative study on genotypic and phenotypic second-line drug resistance testing of *Mycobacterium tuberculosis* complex isolates. J Clin Microbiol 2010;48:2749–2753.
58 Abate G, Miorner H, Ahmed O, Hoffner SE: Drug resistance in *Mycobacterium tuberculosis* strains isolated from re-treatment cases of pulmonary tuberculosis in Ethiopia: susceptibility to first-line and alternative drugs. Int J Tuberc Lung Dis 1998;2:580–584.
59 Nix DE, Adam RD, Auclair B, Krueger TS, Godo PG, Peloquin CA: Pharmacokinetics and relative bioavailability of clofazimine in relation to food, orange juice and antacid. Tuberculosis (Edinb) 2004;84:365–373.
60 Adams LB, Sinha I, Franzblau SG, Krahenbuhl JL, Mehta RT: Effective treatment of acute and chronic murine tuberculosis with liposome-encapsulated clofazimine. Antimicrob Agents Chemother 1999;43:1638–1643.
61 Shen GH, Wu BD, Hu ST, Lin CF, Wu KM, Chen JH: High efficacy of clofazimine and its synergistic effect with amikacin against rapidly growing mycobacteria. Int J Antimicrob Agents 2010;35:400–404.
62 Barry VC, Conalty ML: The antimycobacterial activity of B 663. Lepr Rev 1965;36:3–7.
63 Vree TB, Dammers E, Exler PS: Identical pattern of highly variable absorption of clavulanic acid from four different oral formulations of co-amoxiclav in healthy subjects. J Antimicrob Chemother 2003;51:373–378.
64 Cynamon MH, Palmer GS: In vitro activity of amoxicillin in combination with clavulanic acid against *Mycobacterium tuberculosis*. Antimicrob Agents Chemother 1983;24:429–431.
65 Nadler JP, Berger J, Nord JA, Cofsky R, Saxena M: Amoxicillin-clavulanic acid for treating drug-resistant *Mycobacterium tuberculosis*. Chest 1991;99:1025–1026.
66 Chambers HF, Moreau D, Yajko D, Miick C, Wagner C, Hackbarth C, Kocagoz S, Rosenberg E, Hadley WK, Nikaido H: Can penicillins and other beta-lactam antibiotics be used to treat tuberculosis? Antimicrob Agents Chemother 1995;39:2620–2624.
67 Segura C, Salvado M, Collado I, Chaves J, Coira A: Contribution of beta-lactamases to beta-lactam susceptibilities of susceptible and multidrug-resistant *Mycobacterium tuberculosis* clinical isolates. Antimicrob Agents Chemother 1998;42:1524–1526.
68 Abate G, Miorner H: Susceptibility of multidrug-resistant strains of *Mycobacterium tuberculosis* to amoxycillin in combination with clavulanic acid and ethambutol. J Antimicrob Chemother 1998;42:735–740.
69 Donald PR, Diacon AH: The early bactericidal activity of anti-tuberculosis drugs: a literature review. Tuberculosis (Edinb) 2008;88(suppl 1):S75–S83.
70 Gupta R, Lavollay M, Mainardi JL, Arthur M, Bishai WR, Lamichhane G: The *Mycobacterium tuberculosis* protein LdtMt2 is a nonclassical transpeptidase required for virulence and resistance to amoxicillin. Nat Med 2010;16:466–469.
71 Hugonnet JE, Tremblay LW, Boshoff HI, Barry CE 3rd, Blanchard JS: Meropenem-clavulanate is effective against extensively drug-resistant *Mycobacterium tuberculosis*. Science 2009;323:1215–1218.
72 Condos R, Hadgiangelis N, Leibert E, Jacquette G, Harkin T, Rom WN: Case series report of a linezolid-containing regimen for extensively drug-resistant tuberculosis. Chest 2008;134:187–192.
73 Fortun J, Martin-Davila P, Navas E, Perez-Elias MJ, Cobo J, Tato M, de la Pedrosa EG, Gomez-Mampaso E, Moreno S: Linezolid for the treatment of multidrug-resistant tuberculosis. J Antimicrob Chemother 2005;56:180–185.

74 Koh WJ, Kwon OJ, Gwak H, Chung JW, Cho SN, Kim WS, Shim TS: Daily 300 mg dose of linezolid for the treatment of intractable multidrug-resistant and extensively drug-resistant tuberculosis. J Antimicrob Chemother 2009;64:388–391.
75 Yew WW, Leung CC: How should we treat 'difficult' multidrug-resistant tuberculosis? Chest 2009;135:587–588.
76 Richter E, Rusch-Gerdes S, Hillemann D: First linezolid-resistant clinical isolates of *Mycobacterium tuberculosis*. Antimicrob Agents Chemother 2007;51:1534–1536.
77 Rodriguez JC, Cebrian L, Lopez M, Ruiz M, Jimenez I, Royo G: Mutant prevention concentration: comparison of fluoroquinolones and linezolid with *Mycobacterium tuberculosis*. J Antimicrob Chemother 2004;53:441–444.
78 Burkhardt O, Borner K, von der Hoh N, Koppe P, Pletz MW, Nord CE, Lode H: Single- and multiple-dose pharmacokinetics of linezolid and co-amoxiclav in healthy human volunteers. J Antimicrob Chemother 2002;50:707–712.
79 Park IN, Hong SB, Oh YM, Kim MN, Lim CM, Lee SD, Koh Y, Kim WS, Kim DS, Kim WD, Shim TS: Efficacy and tolerability of daily-half dose linezolid in patients with intractable multidrug-resistant tuberculosis. J Antimicrob Chemother 2006;58:701–704.
80 Nam HS, Koh WJ, Kwon OJ, Cho SN, Shim TS: Daily half-dose linezolid for the treatment of intractable multidrug-resistant tuberculosis. Int J Antimicrob Agents 2009;33:92–93.
81 Luna-Herrera J, Reddy VM, Daneluzzi D, Gangadharam PR: Antituberculosis activity of clarithromycin. Antimicrob Agents Chemother 1995;39:2692–2695.
82 Truffot-Pernot C, Lounis N, Grosset JH, Ji B: Clarithromycin is inactive against *Mycobacterium tuberculosis*. Antimicrob Agents Chemother 1995;39:2827–2828.
83 Andini N, Nash KA: Intrinsic macrolide resistance of the *Mycobacterium tuberculosis* complex is inducible. Antimicrob Agents Chemother 2006;50:2560–2562.
84 Cavalieri SJ, Biehle JR, Sanders WE Jr: Synergistic activities of clarithromycin and antituberculous drugs against multidrug-resistant *Mycobacterium tuberculosis*. Antimicrob Agents Chemother 1995;39:1542–1545.
85 Mor N, Esfandiari A: Synergistic activities of clarithromycin and pyrazinamide against *Mycobacterium tuberculosis* in human macrophages. Antimicrob Agents Chemother 1997;41:2035–2036.
86 Bosne-David S, Barros V, Verde SC, Portugal C, David HL: Intrinsic resistance of *Mycobacterium tuberculosis* to clarithromycin is effectively reversed by subinhibitory concentrations of cell wall inhibitors. J Antimicrob Chemother 2000;46:391–395.
87 Gorzynski EA, Gutman SI, Allen W: Comparative antimycobacterial activities of difloxacin, temafloxacin, enoxacin, pefloxacin, reference fluoroquinolones, and a new macrolide, clarithromycin. Antimicrob Agents Chemother 1989;33:591–592.
88 Stoffels K, Traore H, Vanderbist F, Fauville-Dufaux M: The effect of combined tobramycin-clarithromycin on *Mycobacterium tuberculosis* isolates. Int J Tuberc Lung Dis 2009;13:1041–1044.
89 Umubyeyi A, Rigouts L, Shamputa IC, Dediste A, Struelens M, Portaels F: Low levels of second-line drug resistance among multidrug-resistant *Mycobacterium tuberculosis* isolates from Rwanda. Int J Infect Dis 2008;12:152–156.
90 Domagk G, Behnisch R, Mietzsch F, Schmidt H: On a new class of compounds effective in vitro against tubercle bacilli. Naturwissenschaften 1946;33:315.
91 Leowski J: Thioacetazone – a review. Indian J Chest Dis Allied Sci 1982;24:184–189.
92 East African Hospitals and British Medical Research Council: Comparative trial of isoniazid in combination with thiacetazone or a substituted diphenylthiourea (SU1906) or PAS in the treatment of acute pulmonary tuberculosis in East Africans. Tubercle 1960;41:399–423.
93 East African Hospitals and British Medical Research Council: Isoniazid with thiacetazone (thioacetazone) in the treatment of pulmonary tuberculosis in East Africa – third investigation: the effect of an initial streptomycin supplement. Tubercle 1966;47:1–32.
94 East African Hospitals and British Medical Research Council: Isoniazid with thiacetazone (thioacetazone) in the treatment of pulmonary tuberculosis in East Africa – fifth investigation: a co-operative study in East African hospitals, clinics and laboratories with the collaboration of the East African and British Medical Research Councils. Tubercle 1970;51:123–151.
95 Van Deun A, Aung KJ, Hamid Salim MA, Ali MA, Naha MS, Das PK, Hossain MA, Declercq E: Extension of the intensive phase reduces unfavourable outcomes with the 8-month thioacetazone regimen. Int J Tuberc Lung Dis 2006;10:1255–1261.
96 Nunn P, Kibuga D, Gathua S, Brindle R, Imalingat A, Wasunna K, Lucas S, Gilks C, Omwega M, Were J, McAdam K: Cutaneous hypersensitivity reactions due to thiacetazone in HIV-1 seropositive patients treated for tuberculosis. Lancet 1991;337:627–630.
97 Alahari A, Trivelli X, Guerardel Y, Dover LG, Besra GS, Sacchettini JC, Reynolds RC, Coxon GD, Kremer L: Thiacetazone, an antitubercular drug that inhibits cyclopropanation of cell wall mycolic acids in mycobacteria. PLoS One 2007;2:e1343.
98 Cavanagh P, McPherson K: The thiacetazone sensitivity of *Mycobacterium tuberculosis*. J Med Microbiol 1969;2:237–242.
99 Ellard GA, Dickinson JM, Gammon PT, Mitchison DA: Serum concentrations and antituberculosis activity of thiacetazone. Tubercle 1974;55:41–54.
100 Nunn P, Porter J, Winstanley P: Thiacetazone – avoid like poison or use with care? Trans R Soc Trop Med Hyg 1993;87:578–582.
101 Sen PK, Chatterjef R: Anti-TB drug regimens: an approach through pharmacotherapeutic basis. Ind J Tub 1981;28:191–199.
102 Peloquin CA, Nitta AT, Berning SE, Iseman MD, James GT: Pharmacokinetic evaluation of thiacetazone. Pharmacotherapy 1996;16:735–741.
103 Francois AA, Nishida CR, de Montellano PR, Phillips IR, Shephard EA: Human flavin-containing monooxygenase 2.1 catalyzes oxygenation of the antitubercular drugs thiacetazone and ethionamide. Drug Metab Dispos 2009;37:178–186.
104 Gupta SK, Bedi RS, Maini VK: Agranulocytosis due to thiacetazone. Ind J Tub 1983;30:146–148.
105 Chintu C, Luo C, Bhat G, Raviglione M, Dupont H, Zumla A: Cutaneous hypersensitivity reactions due to thiacetazone in the treatment of tuberculosis in Zambian children infected with HIV-I. Arch Dis Child 1993;68:665–668.



Prof. H.S. Schaaf
Department of Paediatrics and Child Health
Stellenbosch University, PO Box 19063
Tygerberg 7505 (South Africa)
Tel. +27 21 9389 112, E-Mail hss@sun.ac.za

Chapter 11

Donald PR, van Helden PD (eds): Antituberculosis Chemotherapy.
Prog Respir Res. Basel, Karger, 2011, vol 40, pp 96–104

# Acquisition, Transmission and Amplification of Drug-Resistant Tuberculosis

Borna Müller[a] · Robin M. Warren[a] · Monique Williams[a] · Erik C. Böttger[b] · Nicolaas C. Gey van Pittius[a] · Thomas C. Victor[a]

[a]DST/NRF Centre of Excellence for Biomedical TB Research/MRC Centre for Molecular and Cellular Biology, Division of Molecular Biology and Human Genetics, Faculty of Health Science, Stellenbosch University, Tygerberg, South Africa; [b]Institut für Medizinische Mikrobiologie, Nationales Zentrum für Mykobakterien, Universität Zürich, Zürich, Schweiz

**Abstract**

Multidrug-resistant tuberculosis (MDR-TB) is a man-made problem that constitutes a serious threat to TB management and consumes a considerable amount of resources allocated to TB control. Drug-resistant TB only emerges as a result of exposure to anti-TB drugs, and acquisition of resistance in a patient is classically attributed to non-compliance, inappropriate treatment or poor drug quality, while primary resistance results from transmission of drug-resistant strains of *Mycobacterium tuberculosis*. Herein, we discuss dogmas associated with acquired and primary drug resistance, their origins and how most of these assumptions are changing in the light of recent discoveries. Based on empirical data, we suggest that current control programmes have contributed considerably to the rise of MDR-TB throughout the world and that curbing the MDR-TB epidemic in certain settings may only be possible by the very early detection of drug-resistant strains. The emergence of extensively drug-resistant TB and totally drug-resistant TB in several settings illustrates how continuous use of obviously ineffective control measures creates an ever deadlier disease. Failure to address these issues will threaten the effectiveness of any new drugs and regimens that may be introduced.

Copyright © 2011 S. Karger AG, Basel

Bacteria are constantly exposed to substances with the potential to disrupt crucial metabolic processes. They therefore possess intrinsic resistance or tolerance-conferring mechanisms to minimize the detrimental effect of toxic molecules, including antibiotics [1]. The cell envelope surrounding a bacterium is the first line of defence against such agents and is designed to reduce their penetration [1]. A mechanism that acts synergistically with reduced cell permeability is efflux, an energy-dependent process which involves pumping molecules out of the cell against a concentration gradient [1–3]. Efflux is also utilized by bacteria to extrude toxic substances generated within the cell, either by metabolic processes or owing to the incidental activity of enzymes. In addition, certain enzymes in bacteria are able to modify toxic molecules into non-toxic derivatives, effectively reducing their concentration [1].

As opposed to intrinsic drug resistance and tolerance, resistance in bacteria may evolve by natural selection. Such newly developed resistance may be defined pragmatically as a significant decrease in susceptibility in a given bacterium to a given drug when compared to susceptible strains that have never been exposed to this drug. In the laboratory the critical concentration of a particular drug is used to group strains as susceptible or resistant [4], although this concentration has no relation to the concentration which is present in the infected patient [5]. The development of antibiotic resistance in *Mycobacterium tuberculosis* occurs by a process of spontaneous chromosomal mutations [5, 6]. The detection of these mutations forms the foundation on which many drug resistance genotyping tests are based [7, 8]. Simple mutations include base substitutions (incorrect nucleotide base is incorporated) or frameshifts (insertion or deletion of a nucleotide base), and occur because of the intrinsic error rate of the enzyme catalysing DNA replication and the spontaneous or chemical modification of nucleotide bases. While in most cases these mutations are deleterious to the organism, they may confer a selective advantage in the presence of certain antibiotics enabling the mutant clones to out-compete the wild-type clones.

Therefore, when spontaneous mutants of *M. tuberculosis* in a patient are exposed to a given agent, those harbouring resistance-conferring mutations become the predominant populations (fig. 1) [6, 9]. The known drug resistance mutations in *M. tuberculosis* are localized mainly in the targets of the antibiotics, in the enzymes which activate or deactivate these drugs or the promoter regions upstream of genes [6, 9, 10]. There is a fraction of clinical and in vitro resistant mutants which does not possess these classical mutations, suggesting that other unknown mechanisms may also confer resistance. This is supported by differences observed in the level of resistance to a particular drug (expressed as the minimum inhibitory concentration) of strains harbouring the same mutation [3]. It can be hypothesized that other unknown resistance-conferring mutations act by increasing the efficiency of any of the intrinsic resistance mechanisms discussed above.

From a clinical perspective, drug-resistant tuberculosis (TB) may emerge in a patient through two distinct mechanisms. It may be acquired by a previously drug-sensitive strain of *M. tuberculosis* in a given patient due to e.g. inadequate treatment, poor drug quality or patient non-adherence. Alternatively, drug resistance may be defined as primary resistance if a given patient is infected by an already resistant strain (fig. 1) [11]. Drug resistance initially emerges by the acquisition of resistance, and patients developing drug-resistant TB may then spread resistant strains to other susceptible individuals in their communities. Transmitted drug-resistant strains can then acquire additional resistance to other anti-TB drugs in a process referred to as drug resistance amplification (fig. 2) [11].

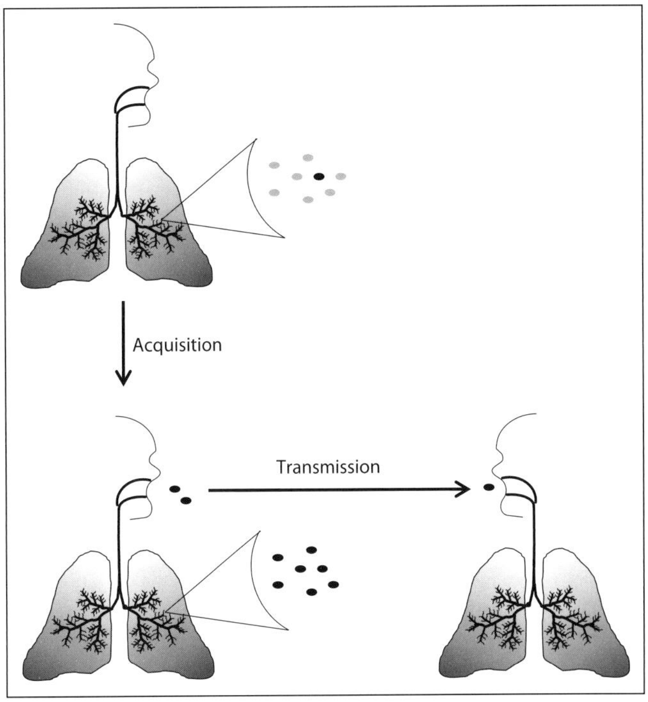


**Fig. 1.** Acquisition and transmission of drug-resistant TB. The selection of spontaneously occurring drug-resistant bacteria (black dots) in a population of predominantly drug-sensitive bacteria (grey dots) leads to 'acquired resistance' in a TB patient. This occurs as a result of patient non-compliance, wrong treatment or poor drug quality. Transmission of drug-resistant strains to contacts leads to primary drug-resistant TB.

## Can Combination Therapy Prevent the Acquisition of Drug Resistance?

The World Health Organization (WHO) guidelines for the therapy of new TB patients recommend a standard regimen (formerly called 'category I' regimen) including isoniazid, rifampicin, pyrazinamide and ethambutol during the first 2 months of chemotherapy (intensive phase) followed by medication with isoniazid and rifampicin for a period of 4 months (continuation phase) [15]. For smear-positive pulmonary TB patients, after the completion of the intensive phase therapy, sputum smear microscopy should be performed. In the absence of sputum conversion (if acid-fast bacilli are still detected in the sputum), patients may be put on continuation phase therapy but sputum microscopy should be repeated at the end of treatment month 3. In the case of a repeated detection of acid-fast bacilli, sputum culture and drug susceptibility testing should be performed [15]. Rapid molecular-based drug susceptibility tests may provide results within 1–2 days [7, 8]. However, many high-burden countries lack the laboratory capacity to conduct molecular drug sensitivity testing, or lengthy culture-based methods, requiring weeks or months to produce results, are the only tests available [8]. Moreover, in general, developing countries lack sufficiently equipped laboratories, qualified technical personnel and laboratories with well-implemented information management, sample logistics and workflow automation. In settings where rapid molecular-based drug susceptibility testing is routinely performed, the drug regimen should be guided by the test results. If only culture-based testing can be performed, patients may receive an empirical second-line regimen until drug susceptibility results are available and the regimen is adjusted appropriately. In settings where drug susceptibility testing is not routine, the empirical second-line regimens will continue throughout treatment.

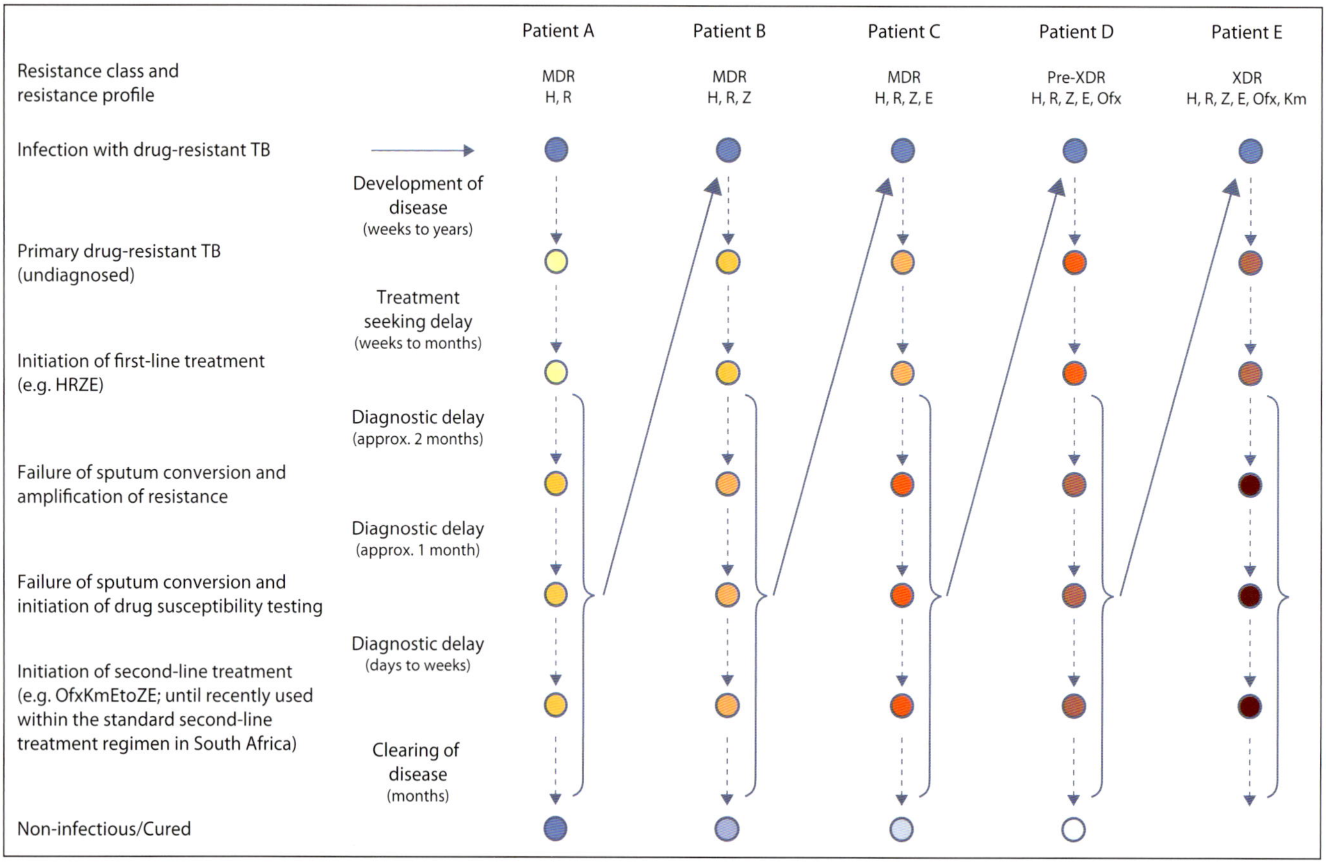


**Fig. 2.** A scenario for the amplification and spread of drug resistance and the emergence of extensively drug-resistant (XDR) TB. The scenario is based on the previous standard second-line treatment regimen in South Africa [12]. Emergence of extensively drug-resistant TB can occur through a stepwise amplification of resistance in transmitting multidrug-resistant (MDR) strains [13]. The course of disease (dashed arrows) for primary multidrug-resistant TB patients (circles) is illustrated. Solid arrows indicate the transmission of drug-resistant strains during the period of diagnostic delay to patient contacts. The light yellow to dark red filled circles indicate increasingly resistant active TB disease in infectious patients. The fading blue circles indicate the decreasing effectiveness of a second-line treatment regimen [14]. Diagnostic delay in combination with the use of empirical regimens thus contributes to both, amplification of resistance and spread of drug-resistant TB. Treatment seeking delay similarly contributes to the transmission of resistance, however, without amplification of resistance. H = Isoniazid; R = rifampicin; Z = pyrazinamide; E = ethambutol; Ofx = ofloxacin; Km = kanamycin; Eto = ethionamide.

Combination therapy for TB treatment was introduced in 1949 as a result of early observations of the emergence of antibiotic resistance and treatment failure in initial trials of streptomycin monotherapy for TB treatment [16–18]. Combination therapy initially included two drugs (streptomycin and para-aminosalicylic acid) and was found to lower the failure rate significantly [17, 18]. In theory, the simultaneous application of multiple effective drugs makes emergence of drug resistance highly improbable. The frequency of spontaneously evolving mutations in *M. tuberculosis* conferring resistance to isoniazid and rifampicin was estimated from in vitro experiments at $2.56 \times 10^{-8}$ and $3.32 \times 10^{-9}$ mutations per bacterium per cell division, respectively [19, 20]. The formula $p = 1 - (1 - r)^n$ can be used to calculate the probability of a bacterium to spontaneously acquire resistance to one or a combination of drugs with p being the probability of drug resistance emerging, r being the mutation rate and n being the number of bacilli in a lesion [19]. Assuming a number of $10^8$ bacteria per lesion and a combined mutation rate of $10^{-16}$ for the acquisition of resistance to both isoniazid and rifampicin, this probability would be virtually zero ($10^{-6}$%) [19]. Based on these theoretical considerations, the WHO-recommended TB treatment regimen should be efficient in preventing the acquisition of drug resistance in TB, and this assumption forms the basis of present-day treatment regimens.

The dogma that combination therapy can prevent the emergence of resistance could be challenged by the frequent occurrence and observed outbreaks of drug-resistant TB in many parts of the world [14, 21–30]. The WHO and International Union against Tuberculosis and Lung Disease Global Surveillance Project for Anti-Tuberculosis Drug Resistance recently revealed proportions of resistance to at least 1 drug ranging from 0 to 56% and from 0 to 86% for new TB cases and previously treated cases, respectively [31]. The respective percentages for multidrug-resistant TB (MDR-TB) ranged from 0 to 19% and from 0 to 60%. The projected numbers worldwide were estimated at 285,718 and 203,230 MDR-TB cases among new and previously treated TB patients for the year 2006, respectively, corresponding to 3.1 and 19.3% of all new and previously treated patients or 4.8% of the total number of estimated incident TB cases [31]. The amplification of resistance in MDR-TB constitutes a particular threat to TB control, and extensively drug-resistant TB (XDR-TB), defined by MDR-TB with additional resistance to any fluoroquinolone and any of the injectable drugs amikacin, kanamycin and capreomycin used in second-line therapy, has been reported worldwide [11, 21, 31].

The acquisition of drug resistance under combination therapy is commonly attributed to patient non-compliance, poor drug quality or drug supply or incorrect treatment. However, in many settings the drug-resistant TB epidemic is often due to the absence of effective control programmes or an effect of the spread of resistance that emerged before effective control was implemented [32]. Therefore, the widespread occurrence of drug-resistant TB does not, as such, contradict the dogma that currently applied standard treatment regimens effectively prevent the acquisition of drug resistance. Nevertheless, acquisition of resistance in compliant patients treated under standardized combination therapy has been observed and may be a particular problem in individuals co-infected with HIV [13, 23, 33, 34]. Antiretroviral therapy may interfere with the pharmacokinetic properties of anti-TB drugs facilitating the emergence of drug resistance. Although some mechanisms of drug-drug interactions have been described, more studies in this respect are urgently needed [23, 33]. Malabsorption of anti-TB drugs is an additional independent factor facilitating the acquisition of drug resistance [23, 33]. In HIV-positive patients, active TB is often paucibacillary, leading to the mycobacteria being more difficult to detect in sputum and disease being more difficult to diagnose. Therefore, preventive isoniazid therapy, although helpful to reduce the chances of reactivation of latent TB in HIV co-infected individuals and to prevent TB transmission, is associated with the risk of subjecting patients with undetected active TB to monotherapy, which may quickly lead to emergence of isoniazid resistance [23, 35]. These observations may be of particular importance in areas with a high prevalence of HIV infection and where TB and drug-resistant TB are highly prevalent [21, 23]. Moreover, this demonstrates that the prevention of drug resistance acquisition through current treatment regimens is not absolute.

## The Dogma that Tuberculosis Control Programmes Prevent Transmission of *M. tuberculosis* Strains

The occurrence of primary resistance and therefore transmission of drug-resistant strains of *M. tuberculosis* has been associated with chronically flawed dogmas. The most important may be the assumption that drug-resistant TB is primarily acquired and rarely transmitted. This assumption is based on studies in the 1950s which argued that a defective catalytic activity, owing to drug resistance mutations in the *katG* gene, reduced the virulence of isoniazid-resistant strains leading to attenuation and reduced fitness of *M. tuberculosis* drug-resistant strains [36, 37]. Consequently, it was believed that drug-resistant strains would not pose a threat to TB control given their presumed low rate of transmission [5, 38]. The assumption of drug-resistant TB being primarily acquired was also suggested by the observation of a significantly higher frequency of drug-resistant TB in retreatment cases than in new TB cases [15, 31]. Thus, according to the concept of spontaneous mutation, patients who had received prior treatment were more likely to develop drug resistance during a second treatment period by selection of resistant mutants that had emerged during previous treatment. Accordingly, retreatment cases became the focus of surveillance aimed at identifying factors driving the drug resistance epidemic and developing policies to respond to these factors.

The dogma of a decreased fitness of drug-resistant TB strains was challenged in more recent studies demonstrating that certain drug resistance mutations were propagated efficiently through transmission and only conferred a low fitness cost [5, 38–42]. In *M. tuberculosis*, a selection appears to exist in vivo for low-cost resistance mutations as demonstrated by the inverse correlation between the frequency of certain resistance mutations in clinical strains and the fitness cost of these mutations as determined by in vitro fitness assays [39, 42]. Alternatively, the genetic background of a strain may be sufficient to overcome the fitness cost of the mutation conferring resistance [38]. Also, restoration of fitness has been explained by the concurrent accumulation of compensatory mutations which ameliorate the fitness cost associated with the resistance-conferring mutation [5, 43]. However, the likelihood of a costly resistance mutation to emerge in conjunction with an additional compensatory mutation is lower than the probability of the appearance of a single low-cost resistance mutation. Therefore, the observation of costly resistance mutations in clinical isolates may reflect epidemiological bottlenecks, e.g. resulting from a limited inoculum size during transmission [43].

Outbreaks of drug-resistant TB have been widely reported [14, 23–30]. Among the earliest and best characterized outbreaks were multiple nosocomial clusters of MDR-TB in patients co-infected with mostly HIV in New York City, in the early 1990s [28–30]. A majority of these clusters were caused by a single *M. tuberculosis* strain named 'W'; this strain was also shown to have been responsible for MDR-TB outbreaks in the New York State prison system [28–30]. In 2006, a nosocomial outbreak of XDR-TB was reported in a rural area of KwaZulu-Natal Province, South Africa [14]. The outbreak was characterized by an extreme mortality rate, 52 of 53 patients with XDR-TB died within the study period with a median survival of 16 days from the time of diagnosis. All XDR-TB patients who were tested were HIV positive [14]. Various examples of institutional outbreaks, mostly involving patients co-infected with HIV, have also been described in other settings and further supported the idea that drug-resistant strains are readily transmitted [13, 23, 44]. However, many early reports also suggested that outbreaks may predominantly occur in institutional or congregate settings such as hospitals, prisons and mines, and the association with HIV initiated the theory that drug-resistant TB was only able to spread in vulnerable populations. Nevertheless, transmission of drug-resistant TB was also demonstrated in community settings with a low HIV prevalence, suggesting that drug-resistant strains were not only transmissible in immunosuppressed individuals but in fact can be as transmissible as drug-sensitive strains [24–26]. Van Rie et al. described a cluster of *M. tuberculosis* causing MDR-TB in non-institutionalized, HIV-negative patients in Cape Town, South Africa [26]. A recent report from the Western Cape Province in South Africa showed that a different drug-resistant strain, Beijing R220, accounted for 27% of the MDR-TB cases in this setting in 2006. The authors suggest that this strain has evolved unique properties that allow both acquisition and transmission of drug resistance [25, 27].

In the light of these findings, it may be questioned whether current control programmes can effectively prevent transmission of drug-resistant TB. Considering the recommended diagnostic algorithm for the detection of drug-resistant cases denoted above, it can take more than 3 months to detect and effectively treat patients infected with primary MDR strains [8, 15]. It is likely that these patients remain infectious throughout the whole first-line treatment period and thereby further fuel the drug resistance epidemic by transmission to contacts. This situation is exacerbated considerably by generally lower cure rates and high rates of treatment default in MDR-TB patients (fig. 2). For 2008, the WHO estimated 13,000 new MDR-TB patients in South Africa but only 8,200 were diagnosed by the National Laboratory Health Services [unpubl. data; 31]. If these numbers are correct, the case detection rate for MDR-TB was only 63% and considerably lower than the estimated case detection rate for all TB cases, i.e. 78% of smear-positive cases within the directly observed treatment short-course (DOTS) programme in 2007 [45]. All these factors may contribute to MDR-TB transmission and are likely to be important in many parts of the world.

## How Tuberculosis Control Programmes Promoted the Amplification of Resistance

Inefficient TB control programmes can play a major role in the escalation of drug resistance by promoting additional acquisition of resistance. The main reason for drug resistance amplification under combination therapy, and if treatment adherence is ensured, is diagnostic delay for the detection of primary resistant cases in combination with the use of standardized treatment regimens [11, 21]. This is exemplified by a recent study amongst miners in South Africa with a well-implemented TB control programme and excellent treatment adherence rates [13]. As explained before, infection with MDR strains may remain undetected for at least 3 months if WHO treatment guidelines are followed [15]; consequently, affected patients are treated with only 2 effective drugs (pyrazinamide and ethambutol). While isoniazid and rifampicin are effective in preventing the emergence of resistance to companion drugs, pyrazinamide and ethambutol are much less effective in preventing further resistance amplification. Therefore, if infecting MDR bacteria survive the 2-month intensive phase, they are likely to have acquired resistance to at least one additional drug (fig. 2). Again, these patients remain infectious thereby amplifying the drug resistance epidemic through transmission to contacts as effective treatment may only occur when MDR-TB is diagnosed. If pyrazinamide and ethambutol are blindly used in second-line regimens, as until recently in South Africa

[12], efficiently transmitted MDR strains may rapidly lead to further amplification of resistance to second-line anti-TB drugs [12] (fig. 2).

An additional problem, especially for MDR-TB treatment, arises from mutations conferring resistance to more than one anti-TB drug, e.g. mutations in the promoter region of the *fabG1(mabA)-inhA* operon are known to decrease isoniazid susceptibility, a first-line drug, and to confer resistance to ethionamide which is often used in second-line regimens. A recent study showed how strains with this mutation are overrepresented in XDR-TB, in 2 provinces in South Africa [46]. One explanation for this could be that strains evolving with an *inhA* promoter mutation when exposed to isoniazid during first-line treatment will be exposed to a treatment regimen with one less effective drug if ethionamide resistance remains undetected during second-line treatment. This increases the chance to acquire additional resistance to other second-line drugs [46]. Cross-resistance or simultaneous resistance to more than one drug has also been shown to occur in vitro through efflux-pump-derived mechanisms [2, 47]. The induction of efflux through one drug could lead to efflux of other drugs either by the same pump or by different pumps that become co-activated as a result of the presence of antibiotics [2]. However, our knowledge about cross-resistance in drug-resistant TB or more generally how resistance or exposure to one drug influences resistance to other drugs is sadly lacking. Understanding such interactions is crucial for the design of effective treatment regimens.

## Who Is to Blame?

From an epidemiological and public health perspective, it is important to quantify the contribution of acquired resistance and primary resistance to the overall burden of drug-resistant TB. This proportion is critical to guide interventions and control programmes. More specifically, a high percentage of acquired resistance suggests that available resources to prevent drug-resistant TB should mostly be employed to assist patient compliance, the correct administration of drugs and to ensure good drug quality. However, if drug resistance is primarily transmitted, a rising prevalence in drug-resistant TB can be attributed to an ineffective control programme. The proportion of acquired and primary drug resistance in TB is directly calculated from the percentage of retreatment and new TB cases among all drug-resistant cases, respectively. This is based on the assumption that all drug-resistant TB episodes classified as retreatment cases represent cases of acquired resistance while all drug-resistant cases classified as new TB cases should represent primary resistant cases. Recurrent TB episodes from reinfections with primary drug-resistant strains after cure from a previous drug-sensitive TB infection would be classified as retreatment cases and accordingly wrongly categorized as cases of acquired resistance. Reports of such occurrences in high-incidence settings suggest that primary drug resistance could be considerably underestimated [48].

Although the concept of new cases and retreatment cases is simple, an additional potentially more important problem may be the incorrect classification of patients, especially in high-incidence, resource-limited settings. Patients may not correctly disclose any previous treatment, e.g. to avoid treatment with an injectable drug (i.e. streptomycin in the retreatment or category II regimen and kanamycin, amikacin or capreomycin in the second-line treatment regimen) [15]. Patients may change health clinics during an ongoing treatment, e.g. if not satisfied with the health care services or treatment they received [49]. They may then be incorrectly classified as retreatment cases even if no treatment default occurred. Patient mistrust towards health care professionals could be exacerbated in cases where people were infected with an MDR strain and no clinical improvement is experienced during treatment for several months (fig. 2). Little is known about the importance of such factors in distorting drug resistance statistics although their influence seems probable. Importantly, in high-incidence settings with highly standardized treatment and control programmes, single episodes of primary MDR-TB cases may be frequently misclassified as two distinct episodes. This may happen when patients are reregistered and reclassified as retreatment cases if their sputum smear or culture is positive at month 5 or later during treatment [15]. Also, first-line treatment may be able to lower the bacterial load of MDR strains sufficiently for infected patients to be diagnosed sputum negative and cured at the end of treatment. In these cases, relapse may quickly occur after completion of therapy; such a patient will be classified as a retreatment case. Mixed infections involving drug-resistant and drug-sensitive strains have been shown to cause changing drug resistance patterns [50], and relapse due to the drug-resistant strain may quickly occur after cure from infection by the drug-sensitive strain. These scenarios suggest that the classification of primary and acquired resistance may be flawed in several ways.

There is mounting evidence that at present MDR-TB in South Africa is primarily a result of the transmission of MDR strains of *M. tuberculosis* [24–27]. WHO estimates modeled on 2002 data suggested that 59% of all MDR-TB cases in South Africa were primary MDR cases [45]. According to our experience, this number is likely to be an underestimate (e.g. due to the above-mentioned factors) or has increased considerably, more recently. The importance of transmission to the occurrence of drug-resistant TB is probably underestimated in many high-incidence and poorly investigated areas [51, 52], and our inability to accurately quantify the contribution of transmission and acquisition to drug-resistant TB and particularly MDR-TB is deeply disturbing. This suggests that failure of national control programmes to limit transmission of drug-resistant TB is, in many settings, the main driver of the drug-resistant TB epidemic which is to a lesser extent caused by patient non-compliance. Emergence of XDR-TB may mostly occur in patients initially infected with primary MDR strains that acquired additional resistance to second-line drugs. These cases therefore illustrate the failure of TB control programmes to prevent the transmission and amplification of MDR-TB [11, 21, 32]. Moreover, the emergence of XDR-TB in many places worldwide suggests that mistakes made in the past that caused the MDR-TB pandemic are being repeated.

## Curbing the Multidrug-Resistant Tuberculosis Pandemic

Comprehensive analyses of the factors leading to the current drug-resistant TB pandemic and recommendations for control are provided by several recent review articles [11, 21, 23, 32]. Basic requirements to control drug-resistant TB and TB in general still need to be implemented and improved in many high-incidence areas and underinvestigated regions (notably sub-Saharan Africa). These requirements are encompassed by the DOTS strategy and consist of (1) political commitment with increased and sustained financing, (2) case detection by quality-assured bacteriology, (3) standardized treatment with supervision and patient support, (4) an effective drug supply and management system and (5) a monitoring and evaluation system and impact measurement [45].

Countries with a high prevalence of drug-resistant and MDR-TB may be differentiated based on the existence or absence of functional TB control programmes applying the DOTS strategy [13]. Since DOTS includes approaches aiming to ensure proper treatment for patients, anti-TB drug supply and quality and patient adherence, it targets all key factors involved in the acquisition of drug resistance and can be considered effective in preventing it. Therefore, DOTS implementation is a cornerstone for the prevention of TB drug resistance and a prerequisite in every setting with high levels of drug-resistant TB [13]. However, as pointed out above, its effectiveness to prevent drug resistance acquisition is not absolute and can be compromised by factors such as malabsorption and drug-drug interactions, especially in HIV-positive individuals. This could be of particular importance in areas with a high prevalence of HIV co-infection in TB patients.

In settings with high levels of drug resistance, despite effective implementation of DOTS, drug resistance is likely to have emerged before the implementation of effective control measures [13]. In these areas, an ongoing drug resistance epidemic could be a result of transmission of drug-resistant TB as suggested by multiple studies [24, 26, 27, 41, 51, 53]. As indicated before, national TB control programmes even if in accordance with DOTS may not be effective in preventing the transmission of drug resistance as patients infected with primary MDR strains are only detected several months after TB diagnosis. Therefore, it seems imperative to considerably accelerate the detection of drug-resistant cases in order to curb or prevent the transmission of resistance.

It must be acknowledged that WHO treatment guidelines suggest that drug sensitivity testing should ideally be performed at the start of any TB treatment [15]. Considering that access to drug sensitivity testing cannot be easily provided to everyone in many resource-limited high-incidence settings, risk groups were defined that may prioritize early drug sensitivity testing [15]. Specifically, all new patients in countries where the level of MDR-TB in new patients is higher than 3% should be tested for susceptibility to isoniazid and rifampicin [15]. However, as indicated previously, the accuracy of these classifications may be doubted, e.g. in South Africa, where the contribution of transmission to drug-resistant TB is large and drug sensitivity testing at the onset of treatment would be advisable, the level of MDR-TB in new patients was reported to be only 1.8% [31]. Irrespective of this, the proposed threshold value is rather arbitrary. The decision should rather be based on an assessment of the contribution of transmission to all drug-resistant TB cases rather than the total number of TB cases (including drug-sensitive TB).

New technologies such as molecular probe assays that allow early detection of drug resistance are readily available and their implementation for early drug sensitivity testing will be essential to fight the transmission and amplification of drug-resistant TB [7, 8, 46, 54]. Along with reliable information about resistance to anti-TB drugs, molecular probe assays can provide information on resistance-conferring mutations, which may allow the use of adapted TB regimens, e.g. *inhA* promoter mutations confer low-level resistance to isoniazid as well as resistance to ethionamide while mutations in the *katG* gene confer high-level resistance to isoniazid only [6, 9]. This means that patients infected with strains exhibiting *inhA* promoter mutations should not be treated with ethionamide but might respond to high doses of isoniazid if no other high-level resistance-conferring mutations are present [46, 54]. Importantly, molecular drug resistance typing techniques should rather assist than replace culture-based phenotypic drug susceptibility testing. Otherwise, this will inevitably lead to the selection and spread of resistant strains with properties that remain undetected by the molecular identification methods currently in use [46].

In conclusion, drug-resistant TB is a man-made problem with incorrect treatment, poor drug quality and non-compliance of patients and control programmes at the root of the emergence of resistance and ineffective disease control (i.e. failure to prevent transmission of drug resistance) having contributed to a large extent to the amplification of resistance and spread of the MDR-TB pandemic. Cases of untreatable totally drug-resistant TB have been reported and reflect the continuous use of obviously ineffective control measures that do not address the ultimate causes of drug resistance transmission and amplification. The adaptation of the strategies to eradicate MDR-TB as well as prevent amplification of resistance in MDR-TB is urgent as we are rapidly running out of treatment options. Finally, failure to apply the basic tenets of the DOTS strategy will always lead us down the same road and annul all efforts to develop new anti-TB drugs and regimens. Evolution is unforgiving; allowing drug-resistant mutants a selective advantage by not implementing supervised therapy and relying on our present inefficiencies will rapidly make TB deadlier than ever.

## References


1 Nguyen L, Pieters J: Mycobacterial subversion of chemotherapeutic reagents and host defense tactics: challenges in tuberculosis drug development. Annu Rev Pharmacol Toxicol 2009; 49:427–453.

2 Srivastava S, Musuka S, Sherman C, Meek C, Leff R, Gumbo T: Efflux-pump-derived multiple drug resistance to ethambutol monotherapy in *Mycobacterium tuberculosis* and the pharmacokinetics and pharmacodynamics of ethambutol. J Infect Dis 2010;201:1225–1231.

3 Louw GE, Warren RM, Gey van Pittius NC, McEvoy CR, van Helden PD, Victor TC: A balancing act: efflux/influx in mycobacterial drug resistance. Antimicrob Agents Chemother 2009;53: 3181–3189.

4 World Health Organization: Guidelines for Surveillance of Drug Resistance in Tuberculosis. Geneva, WHO, 2009.

5 Bottger EC, Springer B: Tuberculosis: drug resistance, fitness, and strategies for global control. Eur J Pediatr 2008;167:141–148.

6 Johnson R, Streicher EM, Louw GE, Warren RM, van Helden PD, Victor TC: Drug resistance in *Mycobacterium tuberculosis*. Curr Issues Mol Biol 2006;8:97–111.

7 Barnard M, Allbert H, Coetzee G, O'Brien R, Bosiman ME: Rapid molecular screening for multidrug-resistant tuberculosis in a high-volume public health laboratory in South Africa. Am J Respir Crit Care Med 2008;177:787–792.

8 Van Deun A, Martin A, Palomino JC: Diagnosis of drug-resistant tuberculosis: reliability and rapidity of detection. Int J Tuberc Lung Dis 2010;14:131–140.

9 Zhang Y, Yew WW: Mechanisms of drug resistance in *Mycobacterium tuberculosis*. Int J Tuberc Lung Dis 2009;13:1320–1330.

10 Sandgren A, Strong M, Muthukrishnan P, Weiner BK, Church GM, Murray MB: Tuberculosis drug resistance mutation database. PLoS Med 2009;6:e2.

11 Jassal M, Bishai WR: Extensively drug-resistant tuberculosis. Lancet Infect Dis 2009;9:19–30.

12 Hoek KG, Schaaf HS, Gey van Pittius NC, van Helden PD, Warren RM: Resistance to pyrazinamide and ethambutol compromises MDR/XDR-TB treatment. S Afr Med J 2009;99:785–787.

13 Calver AD, Falmer AA, Murray M, Strauss OJ, Streicher EM, Hanekom M, Liversage T, Masibi M, van Helden PD, Warren RM, Victor TC: Emergence of increased resistance and extensively drug-resistant tuberculosis despite treatment adherence, South Africa. Emerg Infect Dis 2010;16:264–271.

14 Gandhi NR, Moll A, Sturm AW, Pawinski R, Govender T, Lalloo U, Zeller K, Andrews J, Friedland G: Extensively drug-resistant tuberculosis as a cause of death in patients co-infected with tuberculosis and HIV in a rural area of South Africa. Lancet 2006;368:1575–1580.

15 World Health Organization: Treatment of Tuberculosis – Guidelines. Geneva, WHO, 2009.

16 Medical Research Council: Streptomycin treatment of pulmonary tuberculosis. Br Med J 1948;ii:769–782.

17 Dunner E, Brown WB, Wallace J. The effect of streptomycin with para-aminosalicylic acid on the emergence of resistant strains of tubercle bacilli. Dis Chest 1949;16:661–666.

18 Medical Research Council: Treatment of pulmonary tuberculosis with streptomycin and para-amino-salicylic acid. Br Med J 1950;ii:1073–1085.

19 Gillespie SH: Evolution of drug resistance in *Mycobacterium tuberculosis:* clinical and molecular perspective. Antimicrob Agents Chemother 2002;46:267–274.

20 David HL: Probability distribution of drug-resistant mutants in unselected populations of *Mycobacterium tuberculosis*. Appl Microbiol 1970;20:810–814.

21 Donald PR, van Helden PD: The global burden of tuberculosis – combating drug resistance in difficult times. N Engl J Med 2009;360:2393–2395.

22 Dye C, Espinal MA, Watt CJ, Mbiaga C, Williams BG: Worldwide incidence of multidrug-resistant tuberculosis. J Infect Dis 2002;185:1197–1202.

23 Wells CD, Cegielski JP, Nelson LJ, Laserson KF, Holtz TH, Finlay A, Castro KG, Weyer K: HIV infection and multidrug-resistant tuberculosis: the perfect storm. J Infect Dis 2007;196(suppl 1):S86–S107.

24 Victor TC, Streicher EM, Kewley C, Jordaan AM, van der Spuy GD, Bosman M, Louw H, Murray M, Young D, van Helden PD, Warren RM: Spread of an emerging *Mycobacterium tuberculosis* drug-resistant strain in the Western Cape of South Africa. Int J Tuberc Lung Dis 2007;11:195–201.

25 Johnson R, Warren R, Strauss OJ, Jordaan AM, Falmer AA, Beyers N, Schaaf HS, Murray M, Cloete K, van Helden PD, Victor TC: An outbreak of drug-resistant tuberculosis caused by a Beijing strain in the Western Cape, South Africa. Int J Tuberc Lung Dis 2006;10:1412–1414.

26 Van Rie A, Warren RM, Beyers N, Gie RP, Classen CN, Richardson M, Sampson SL, Victor TC, van Helden PD: Transmission of a multidrug-resistant *Mycobacterium tuberculosis* strain resembling 'strain W' among noninstitutionalized, human immunodeficiency virus-seronegative patients. J Infect Dis 1999;180:1608–1615.

27 Johnson R, Warren RM, van der Spuy GD, Gey van Pittius NC, Theron D, Streicher EM, Bosman M, Coetzee GJ, van Helden PD, Victor TC: Drug-resistant tuberculosis epidemic in the Western Cape driven by a virulent Beijing genotype strain. Int J Tuberc Lung Dis 2010;14:119–121.
28 Alland D, Kalkut GE, Moss AR, McAdam RA, Hahn JA, Bosworth W, Drucker E, Bloom BR: Transmission of tuberculosis in New York City – an analysis by DNA fingerprinting and conventional epidemiologic methods. N Engl J Med 1994;330:1710–1716.
29 Frieden TR, Sterling T, Pablos-Mendez A, Kilburn JO, Cauthen GM, Dooley SW: The emergence of drug-resistant tuberculosis in New York City. N Engl J Med 1993;328:521–526.
30 Valway SE, Greifinger RB, Papania M, Kilburn JO, Woodley C, Di Ferdinando GT, Dooley SW: Multidrug-resistant tuberculosis in the New York State prison system, 1990–1991. J Infect Dis 1994;170:151–156.
31 The World Health Organization/International Union against Tuberculosis and Lung Disease (WHO/UNION) Global Project on Anti-Tuberculosis Drug Resistance Surveillance: Anti-Tuberculosis Drug Resistance in the World. Geneva, WHO, 2008.
32 Caminero JA: Multidrug-resistant tuberculosis: epidemiology, risk factors and case finding. Int J Tuberc Lung Dis 2010;14:382–390.
33 March F, Garriga X, Rodriguez P, Moreno C, Garrigo M, Coll P, Prats G: Acquired drug resistance in *Mycobacterium tuberculosis* isolates recovered from compliant patients with human immunodeficiency virus-associated tuberculosis. Clin Infect Dis 1997;25:1044–1047.
34 Han LL, Sloutsky A, Canales R, Naroditskaya V, Shin SS, Seung KJ, Timperi R, Becerra MC: Acquisition of drug resistance in multidrug-resistant *Mycobacterium tuberculosis* during directly observed empiric retreatment with standardized regimens. Int J Tuberc Lung Dis 2005;9:818–821.
35 Cohen T, Lipsitch M, Walensky RP, Murray M: Beneficial and perverse effects of isoniazid preventive therapy for latent tuberculosis infection in HIV-tuberculosis coinfected populations. Proc Natl Acad Sci USA 2006;103:7042–7047.
36 Middlebrook G: Isoniazid-resistance and catalase activity of tubercle bacilli: a preliminary report. Am Rev Tuberc 1954;69:471–472.
37 Middlebrook G, Cohn ML: Some observations on the pathogenicity of isoniazid-resistant variants of tubercle bacilli. Science 1953;118:297–299.
38 Borrell S, Gagneux S: Infectiousness, reproductive fitness and evolution of drug-resistant *Mycobacterium tuberculosis*. Int J Tuberc Lung Dis 2009;13:1456–1466.
39 Gagneux S, Long CD, Small PM, Van T, Schoolnik GK, Bohannan BJ: The competitive cost of antibiotic resistance in *Mycobacterium tuberculosis*. Science 2006;312:1944–1946.
40 Gagneux S, Burgos MV, Deriemer K, Enciso A, Munoz S, Hopewell PC, Small PM, Pym AS: Impact of bacterial genetics on the transmission of isoniazid-resistant *Mycobacterium tuberculosis*. PLoS Pathog 2006;2:603–610.
41 Cohen T, Murray M: Modeling epidemics of multidrug-resistant *M. tuberculosis* of heterogeneous fitness. Nat Med 2004;10:1117–1121.
42 Pym AS, Saint-Joanis B, Cole ST: Effect of *katG* mutations on the virulence of *Mycobacterium tuberculosis* and the implication for transmission in humans. Infect Immun 2002;70:4955–4960.
43 Shcherbakov D, Akbergenov R, Matt T, Sander P, Andersson DI, Bottger EC: Directed mutagenesis of *Mycobacterium smegmatis* 16S rRNA to reconstruct the in-vivo evolution of aminoglycoside resistance in *Mycobacterium tuberculosis*. Mol Microbiol 2010, E-pub ahead of print.
44 Portugal I, Covas MJ, Brum L, Viveiros M, Ferrinho P, Moniz-Pereira J, David H: Outbreak of multiple drug-resistant tuberculosis in Lisbon: detection by restriction fragment length polymorphism analysis. Int J Tuberc Lung Dis 1999;3:207–213.
45 World Health Organization: Global Tuberculosis Control 2009 – Epidemiology, Strategy, Financing. Geneva, WHO, 2009.
46 Müller B, Streicher EM, Hoek KG, Tait M, Trollip A, Bosman ME, Coetzee GJ, Chabula-Nxiweni EM, Hoosain E, Gey van Pittius NC, Victor TC, van Helden PD, Warren RM: *inhA* promoter mutations: a gateway to extensively drug-resistant tuberculosis in South Africa? Int J Tuberc Lung Dis 2011;15:344–351.
47 Colangeli R, Helb D, Sridharan S, Sun J, Varma-Basil M, Hazbon MH, Harbacheuski R, Megjugorac NJ, Jacobs WR Jr, Holzenburg A, Sacchettini JC, Alland D: The *Mycobacterium tuberculosis iniA* gene is essential for activity of an efflux pump that confers drug tolerance to both isoniazid and ethambutol. Mol Microbiol 2005;55:1829–1840.
48 Van Rie A, Warren R, Richardson M, Victor TC, Gie RP, Enarson DA, Beyers N, van Helden PD: Exogenous reinfection as a cause of recurrent tuberculosis after curative treatment. N Engl J Med 1999;341:1174–1179.
49 Holtz TH, Lancaster J, Laserson KF, Wells CD, Thorpe L, Weyer K: Risk factors associated with default from multidrug-resistant tuberculosis treatment, South Africa, 1999–2001. Int J Tuberc Lung Dis 2006;10:649–655.
50 Van Rie A, Victor TC, Richardson M, Johnson R, van der Spuy GD, Murray EJ, Beyers N, Gey van Pittius NC, van Helden PD, Warren RM: Reinfection and mixed infection cause changing *Mycobacterium tuberculosis* drug-resistance patterns. Am J Respir Crit Care Med 2005;172:636–642.
51 Luciani F, Sisson SA, Jiang H, Francis AR, Tanaka MM: The epidemiological fitness cost of drug resistance in *Mycobacterium tuberculosis*. Proc Natl Acad Sci USA 2009;106:14711–14715.
52 Ben AY, Nemser B, Singh A, Sankin A, Schluger N: Underreported threat of multidrug-resistant tuberculosis in Africa. Emerg Infect Dis 2008;14:1345–1352.
53 Strauss OJ, Warren RM, Jordaan A, Streicher EM, Hanekom M, Falmer AA, Albert H, Trollip A, Hoosain E, van Helden PD, Victor TC: Spread of a low-fitness drug-resistant *Mycobacterium tuberculosis* strain in a setting of high human immunodeficiency virus prevalence. J Clin Microbiol 2008;46:1514–1516.
54 Warren RM, Streicher EM, van Pittius NC, Marais BJ, van der Spuy GD, Victor TC, Sirgel F, Donald PR, van Helden PD: The clinical relevance of mycobacterial pharmacogenetics. Tuberculosis (Edinb) 2009;89:199–202.

Borna Müller, PhD
DST/NRF Centre of Excellence for Biomedical Tuberculosis Research/MRC Centre for Molecular and Cellular Biology
Division of Molecular Biology and Human Genetics, Faculty of Health Sciences, Stellenbosch University
Francie van Zyl Avenue, Tygerberg 7505 (South Africa)
Tel. +27 21 938 9482, E-Mail bmuller@sun.ac.za

Chapter 12
Donald PR, van Helden PD (eds): Antituberculosis Chemotherapy.
Prog Respir Res. Basel, Karger, 2011, vol 40, pp 105–115

# The Treatment of Tuberculosis in Children

Andrea T. Cruz · Jeffrey R. Starke
Department of Pediatrics, Baylor College of Medicine, Houston, Tex., USA

**Abstract**
The treatment of childhood tuberculosis (TB) is influenced by a number of factors specific to the host and pathogen. Children often have lower bacterial loads and a higher incidence of extrapulmonary disease than adults, meaning that many of the diagnostic parameters used to ensure clinical response to treatment in adults are not applicable to children. On the other hand, regimens that are successful in treating adults with pulmonary TB should be successful in children; establishing the pharmacokinetic parameters of drugs, drug safety and minimum required treatment are the major issues for children. The rationale behind empirical medication selection, regimens used for commonly encountered clinical scenarios and special situations will be reviewed. The latter include treatment of the child co-infected with HIV and TB, extrapulmonary TB, treatment of children with drug-resistant TB and management of medication adherence and intolerance issues. Finally, we review future directions for the treatment of TB, including shorter treatment regimens and new agents.

Copyright © 2011 S. Karger AG, Basel

It is estimated that 5% of tuberculosis (TB) cases in low-prevalence nations and up to 40% in high-prevalence countries occur in children [1]. Childhood TB differs from TB in adults in several ways. First, children often have short incubation periods between exposure and disease onset, meaning that the diagnosis of TB in a child is a marker of recent TB transmission in the community. Second, childhood TB is often paucibacillary in nature; the relatively smaller organism burden compared with adults with cavitary disease means that the risk of selection for spontaneous mutations conferring antituberculous drug resistance should be lower. Third, childhood TB is more often extrapulmonary in nature, even in immunocompetent children, when compared with adults [2]; this may affect duration of therapy, empirical drug selection and the decision to utilize corticosteroids. Fourth, children generally tolerate TB medications better than adults, changing the risk-benefit relationship for offering TB chemoprophylaxis. Finally, the fact that it is uncommon for children to be contagious with TB, including that they are less likely to have sputum smears positive for acid-fast bacilli, unfortunately has led to a reduced emphasis on the diagnosis and subsequent treatment of childhood TB in some public health programmes. However, doing so ignores the individual and population burdens of childhood TB, as effective therapy can decrease morbidity and mortality for the child and prevent cases of reactivation in adolescence and adulthood.

Children can be classified as being exposed to or infected with TB, or having TB disease. TB *exposure* is a category of most relevance in low-prevalence nations, where resources allow for active surveillance following identification of a person with suspected contagious TB (a source case). Children with TB exposure are asymptomatic young (<4 years old) children with normal chest radiographs, negative initial tuberculin skin tests or γ-interferon release assays, and normal physical examination in contact with a source case; here, insufficient time has elapsed to determine if the child is infected. Children with latent TB *infection* (LTBI) have a positive tuberculin skin test or γ-interferon release assay in the absence of clinical or radiographic findings. Children with *disease* are symptomatic or have radiographic or physical examination findings caused by *Mycobacterium tuberculosis*.

## Microbiological Basis for Treatment

The basis of treatment for TB is unique among infectious diseases because it is based upon the estimated microbial burden. This estimated microbial burden is a marker of the potential for drug resistance. For example, the frequency of spontaneous mutations conferring resistance is estimated to be 1 in $10^8$ for isoniazid (INH) and streptomycin, 1 in $10^{10}$ for rifampicin (RIF) and 1 in $10^7$ for ethambutol (EMB) [3]. The greater the number of organisms, the higher the probability of having subpopulations in which spontaneous point mutations have conferred resistance to anti-TB medications. The microbial burden is estimated by physical examination and radiographic findings. For TB exposure and infection, the microbial burden can be considered to be small enough that the mathematical chances of having naturally occurring resistant organisms is low, and children can be treated with monotherapy. In contrast, persons with TB disease have a higher organism burden (a cavity is estimated to harbour $10^9$–$10^{12}$ organisms), and the risk of resistant organisms is no longer negligible; consequently, multidrug therapy is required. Selection for resistant organisms and disease recurrence or relapse has been documented for all drugs used as monotherapy to treat TB disease in adult patients.

The slow replication cycle of *M. tuberculosis* also impacts treatment, requiring longer treatment courses and affecting the structure of TB disease treatment regimens. TB bacilli are killed during replication, and replication is most common during the exponential growth phase. Thus, more drugs are used during the initial 2-month intensive phase than are used during the remaining months of therapy (the consolidative phase).

When considering the selection of antituberculous agents, it is important to consider how TB differs in children and adults. Children often have lower bacterial burdens, lessening the likelihood of spontaneous mutations conferring resistance. For children with primary TB, this means that theoretically, the regimens could use fewer drugs for a shorter period of time; however, there are few controlled studies that have evaluated this. However, an adolescent with TB disease, or a child with cavitary TB of any age should be treated similarly to adults. Also, children often have primary progressive TB, as opposed to reactivation disease. This has epidemiological importance, as a new diagnosis in a child often reflects recent community transmission, and often a specific source case with TB may be identified, particularly in regions with low TB prevalence. This knowledge facilitates empirical antibiotic selection for the paediatric patient.

## Current Treatment Regimens

*TB Exposure and Infection*

Young or immunocompromised children with TB exposure, given the risk of rapid disease progression, can be started on monotherapy for prophylaxis until the definitive tuberculin skin test is performed, usually 8–10 weeks after the exposure has ended. Children with LTBI can be treated with a number of regimens (table 1) to decrease their 5–40% (depending on age) overall likelihood of developing TB disease [4, 5]. The most efficacy data are available for INH-based regimens, but more recently, shorter-course multidrug regimens have been described for LTBI. The theoretical advantages of shorter therapeutic courses are enhanced patient adherence, decreased health care costs and increased efficacy in children with INH monoresistance [6]. However, shorter-course regimens are not recommended in national and international guidelines. Children with TB exposure and infection historically have only been identified and treated in low-prevalence nations. However, studies of HIV-infected children (most of whom were not under antiretroviral therapy) in countries with high TB disease prevalence showed decreased mortality in children receiving INH and co-trimoxazole when compared with placebo [7]. This demonstrates the efficacy of relatively low-cost INH prophylaxis, once TB disease has been excluded, in at-risk HIV-infected children in high-prevalence settings [8].

For children with TB exposure or infection, therapy can be administered daily via the family or intermittently via directly observed therapy (DOT), where a dispassionate third party supervises medication administration. DOT is preferred for high-risk children or in circumstances when adherence for taking medications is suspected or anticipated to be low, but may not be feasible in resource-poor settings. One study in HIV-infected children showed 95% adherence using self-supervised therapy with INH prophylaxis in children receiving either daily or thrice weekly therapy [9]. However, adherence to therapy outside of study parameters has typically been poor [10].

Management of children with TB exposure and infection whose source cases have drug-resistant TB is more challenging. If 1–2 drugs can be found to which the source case isolate is susceptible and the child is tolerant, children with TB infection can be treated for 9–12 months. For children with TB exposure whose source case has extensively drug-resistant TB, sequential skin testing and close follow-up may be a more viable option. However, in countries whose TB incidence is high, children may be exposed to more than one source case, and identification of particular isolates may

**Table 1.** Regimens for the treatment of children with TB exposure and infection

| Category | Agent | Duration of therapy, months | Other |
|---|---|---|---|
| Exposure, <4 years old | INH | 2–3 | Repeat TST 8–10 weeks after contact with source case is broken physically or microbiologically; if positive, see section on infection |
| Exposure, ≥4 years old | None | n.a. | |
| Infection | INH | 6–9 | Medications may be administered daily by family or intermittently via directly observed therapy |
| | RIF | 6 | |
| | INH + RIF | 3 | |
| | RIF | 4 | |
| Disease | See table 2 | ≥6 months[1] | Medications should be administered via directly observed therapy if at all possible |

The agent used may need to be modified based upon source case susceptibilities. TST = Tuberculin skin test; n.a. = not assessed. Adapted from American Academy of Pediatrics [4] and Spyridis et al. [5].
[1] Duration of therapy may be influenced by disease site and severity, immunological status of the child and the isolate's drug susceptibilities.

not be possible. There are no trials on the effectiveness of drugs in preventing TB in people exposed to or infected with multidrug-resistant (MDR) TB.

*TB Disease in Children – General Considerations*
The decision of which medications to initiate depends upon several factors: minimizing drug toxicities and interactions; manner in which medications are administered (suspension, tablet) and by whom (self/family administered versus DOT); location of disease (meningeal or non-meningeal), and concern for drug-resistant isolates, based upon knowledge of local epidemiology.

In the mid-20th century, children with isolated pulmonary disease were often treated for over 1 year. Fortunately, the last 30 years have witnessed an expanded body of data on the efficacy of shorter-course treatments, and 6-month courses of therapy are now routinely utilized for most HIV-uninfected children with non-meningeal forms of TB disease. The regimens for the most commonly encountered clinical scenarios in children with TB disease are summarized in table 2 [4, 11]. The first- and second-line anti-TB agents are listed in table 3 [12, 13]. An in-depth discussion of these drugs is outside the scope of this article, but is explored in great detail in many of the accompanying articles in this volume. Briefly, the backbone of TB regimens in children is INH, RIF, pyrazinamide (PZA) and EMB; these form the basis for empirical therapy unless drug resistance in a source case is recognized before the initiation of therapy. INH and RIF are the bactericidal agents and are utilized in both the intensification and continuation phases of therapy. PZA is used during the first 2 months of therapy to enable shorter treatment durations (for drug-susceptible isolates). In recent years with increased rates of drug-resistant TB isolates, EMB was added to the initial intensification phase. EMB can be stopped if drug susceptibility testing demonstrates a susceptible isolate. EMB had been underutilized in the past because of concerns for ocular toxicity that could not be easily assessed in the preverbal child. However, children achieve lower serum levels than adults when given the same milligram per kilogram dose, potentially explaining the rarity of EMB side effects in paediatrics, and why the paediatric dose has been increased to 20 mg/kg daily [16].

First-line and second-line medications are generally better tolerated by children than adults with fewer adverse reactions. Consequently, routine laboratory monitoring is not needed in the otherwise healthy child receiving first-line TB medications. However, as there are fewer data on adverse effects of second-line medications in children, particularly infants and toddlers, laboratory monitoring should be considered (table 4). Fluoroquinolones have proven efficacy in TB but have been used infrequently in children, as there have been concerns about the theoretical risk of arthropathy, based on juvenile animal models. However, as the fluoroquinolones have been used with increasing frequency for a variety of infections in childhood, the incidence of bone and joint abnormalities has been extremely low. While there are good pharmacokinetic data for ciprofloxacin in children, there are sparse data for levofloxacin and no published data

**Table 2.** Regimens for the treatment of children with TB disease

| TB patient | Intensive regimen | Consolidation regimen | Notes |
|---|---|---|---|
| Uncomplicated pulmonary TB or non-meningeal extrapulmonary TB | 2 HRZE | 4 HR | If source case is known to have a pan-susceptible isolate, the intensification regimen does not require E<br>In HIV-uninfected children with isolated intrathoracic lymphadenopathy, 6 months of HR have been used |
| Severe disease, considerable disease at the conclusion of 6 months or concern for drug resistance | 2 HRZE | ≥4 HRE | If the isolate is pan-susceptible, E may be stopped |
| TB meningitis | 2 HRZ(Eth or I) | 7–10 HR | Adjunctive corticosteroids should be initiated with TB therapy |
| HIV-infected, uncomplicated pulmonary TB | 2 HRZE | 7 HR | Risk of relapse is higher in HIV-infected persons treated for 6 months versus 9 months [8] |
| HIV-infected, extrapulmonary TB | 2 HRZE | 10 HR | Concomitant administration of R with PI or NNRTI is not recommended |
| Isolated H resistance | 2 RZE | 4–7 RZE | F may be added for children with extensive disease |
| Isolated R resistance | 2 HZEF | 10–16 HEF | An injectable agent may be added to the intensification regimen of children with extensive disease |
| H + R resistance | ≥6 EZFI | ≥10 EZF | Children with extensive disease should receive at least 18 months of therapy; the optimal duration of therapy with I is not established |
| MDR-TB with additional resistance | 3–5 drugs to which the isolate is susceptible | | The optimal duration of therapy and efficacy of different regimens have not been established |

E = EMB; Eth = ethionamide; F = fluoroquinolone; H = INH; I = injectable agent (amikacin, capreomycin, kanamycin); NNRTI = non-nucleoside reverse-transcriptase inhibitor; PI = protease inhibitor; R = RIF; Z = pyrazinamide. During the intensive phase, therapy is administered daily for the first 2 weeks, then changed to intermittent therapy, often biweekly or thrice weekly; in neonates and young infants, consideration should be given to continuing daily therapy for a longer period of time, as the incremental increase in medication volume between daily and intermittent therapy can induce emesis. During the consolidation phase, therapy may be administered biweekly or thrice weekly. For patients on alternative regimens (e.g. fluoroquinolones), there is insufficient data to recommend intermittent dosing. Adapted from American Academy of Pediatrics [4] and Swaminathan et al. [11].

for moxifloxacin in children. The putative risk of the use of a fluoroquinolone in a child with TB needs to be balanced against the benefit of a generally well-tolerated, bactericidal medication with central nervous system penetrance and activity against many drug-resistant isolates.

For cases of drug-susceptible TB in a child, medications are usually given daily for the first 2–4 weeks of therapy, then may be changed to biweekly or thrice weekly dosing. While American organizations support biweekly therapy via DOT, international recommendations are to administer medications 3 times a week via DOT to minimize the impact of missed doses. As the pill count (and medication volume, for suspensions) increases considerably when a child transitions from daily to intermittent therapy, there are situations when a child might benefit from continued daily therapy. This includes neonates and young infants, in whom the

**Table 3.** Drugs used for the treatment of TB in children

| Agent | Daily dose | | Biweekly dose | | Thrice weekly dose | | Weekly dose | | CNS penetrance % | Available formulations |
|---|---|---|---|---|---|---|---|---|---|---|
| | mg/kg/ day | max. dose mg | mg/kg/ day | max. dose mg | mg/kg/ day | max. dose mg | mg/kg/ day | max. dose mg | | |
| INH | 10–15 | 300 | 20–30 | 900 | 10–15 | 900 | – | – | 100 | tablet (100, 300 mg) |
| RIF | 10–20 | 600 | | 600 | 10 | 600 | – | – | 10–20 | capsule (150 mg) |
| Rifabutin | 5 | 300 | 5 | 300 | 5 | 300 | – | – | 10–20 | capsule (150 mg) |
| Rifapentine | – | – | – | – | – | – | 10 | 600 | unknown | tablet (150 mg) |
| Pyrazinamide | 30–40 | 2,000 | 50 | 4,000 | 30–40 | 3,000 | – | – | 100 | tablet (500 mg) |
| EMB | 15–25 | 1,600–2,500 | 50 | 4,000 | 25–35 | 2,400 | – | – | minimal | tablet (100, 400 mg) |
| Amikacin | 15–30 | 1,000 | 15–30 | 1,000 | – | – | – | – | low | i.v., i.m. (aqueous solution) |
| Capreomycin | 15–30 | 1,000 | 15–30 | 1,000 | – | – | – | – | minimal | i.m. (aqueous solution) |
| Cycloserine | 10–15 | 1,000 | – | – | – | – | – | – | 100 | tablet (250 mg) |
| Ethionamide | 15–20 | 1,000 | – | – | – | – | – | – | 100 | tablet (250 mg) |
| Kanamycin | 15–30 | 1,000 | | | – | – | – | – | low | i.v., i.m. (aqueous solution) |
| Levofloxacin | 7.5–10 | 1,000 | – | – | – | – | – | – | 16–20 | i.v. (aqueous solution), tablet (250, 500, 750 mg) |
| Linezolid | 10 b.i.d. | 600 b.i.d. | – | – | – | – | – | – | 70–98 | tablet (600 mg), i.v. (aqueous solution), suspension (20 mg/ml) |
| Para-aminosalicylic acid | 150–300 | 10,000 | – | – | – | – | – | – | 10–50 | granules (4 g/packet), tablet (500 mg) |
| Streptomycin | 20–40 | 1,000 | 20 | 1,000 | – | – | – | – | minimal | i.v., i.m. (aqueous solution) |

For rifabutin, appropriate dosing for children is unknown; rifapentine is not approved for use in children. – = no data on intermittent dosing; i.v. = intravenous; i.m. = intramuscular. Adapted from Centers for Disease Control and Prevention [12], World Health Organization [13], Schaaf et al. [14] and Anger et al. [15].

increased volume of required medications might result in emesis or refusal. Another group for whom daily therapy is preferable is children being treated for drug-resistant TB; for most second-line medications, data on the efficacy of intermittent dosing are not available.

Other considerations relate to medication formulations. Although specific paediatric drug formulations are often lacking, all first-line TB drugs are available in formulations that can be administered to young children. However, INH suspension in some countries (such as the USA) is sorbitol based and causes an osmotic diarrhoea in many children when the required volume exceeds 5 ml. Consequently, we only utilize INH suspension in young babies who are exclusively formula-fed or breastfed. Once a young baby is taking

**Table 4.** Possible side effects and drug interactions with anti-TB medications in children

| Agent | Toxicities | Drug interactions | Laboratory monitoring parameters | Modified dosing for hepatic or renal impairment | Pregnancy category and considerations |
|---|---|---|---|---|---|
| INH[1] | Hepatitis, peripheral neuropathy | + | n.n. | c.b.u. | C; pregnant women and exclusively breastfed infants receiving INH should be given pyridoxine (vitamin $B_6$) |
| RIF | Hepatitis | ++ | n.n. | c.b.u. | C; administer vitamin K at birth to mothers receiving rifamycins |
| Rifabutin | Hepatitis | ++ | n.n. | c.b.u. | B; administer vitamin K at birth to mothers receiving rifamycins |
| Rifapentine | Hepatitis | ++ | n.n. | c.b.u. | C; administer vitamin K at birth to mothers receiving rifamycins |
| PZA | Gout, rash | – | n.n. | Renal | C; routine use in first trimester not recommended by CDC/ATS |
| EMB | Optic neuritis, colour blindness | – | n.n. | Renal | C |
| Amikacin | Ototoxicity, nephrotoxicity | – | Baseline/ monthly creatinine and hearing screens | Renal | D; routine use in pregnancy not recommended by CDC/ATS |
| Capreomycin | Nephrotoxicity, ototoxicity | – | Baseline/ monthly creatinine, potassium and hearing screens | Renal | C; routine use in pregnancy not recommended by CDC/ATS |
| Cycloserine | CNS stimulation (seizures, psychosis, depression), rash, paraesthesia | – | Monthly neuropsychiatric evaluation | Renal | C; use in pregnancy recommended by CDC/ATS only when no alternative exists; mothers should not breastfeed while taking cycloserine |
| Ethionamide[1] | Hepatitis, peripheral neuropathy, optic neuritis, gastrointestional distress, hypothyroidism | – | Baseline hepatic transaminases and thyroid function tests | c.b.u.; renal | C; excreted in breast milk; consider laboratory monitoring in breastfed infants of mothers receiving ethionamide |
| Kanamycin | Ototoxicity, nephrotoxicity | – | Baseline/ monthly creatinine and hearing screens | Renal | D; routine use in pregnancy not recommended by CDC/ATS |

**Table 4.** Continued

| Agent | Toxicities | Drug interactions | Laboratory monitoring parameters | Modified dosing for hepatic or renal impairment | Pregnancy category and considerations |
|---|---|---|---|---|---|
| Levofloxacin[2] | Arthropathy, CNS stimulation, prolongation of QTc, gastrointestinal distress | + | Consider uric acid if given with PZA | Renal | C; excreted in breast milk; consider cessation of breastfeeding while mothers are taking fluoroquinolones |
| Linezolid | Lactic acidosis, myelosuppression, optic neuritis, pancreatitis, peripheral neuropathy | + | Complete blood count, lactate monthly; vision testing, amylase as indicated | Renal | C; lactation information unavailable |
| Para-aminosalicylic acid | Gastrointestinal distress, hepatitis, hypothyroidism, hypersensitivity reactions | + | Baseline hepatic transaminases and thyroid function tests; check monthly if used >3 months | Renal | C |

– = Minimal interactions; + = few interactions; ++ = multiple interactions; n.n. = routine baseline laboratory evaluation not necessary unless the child has known hepatic dysfunction or is receiving other (non-antituberculous) potentially hepatotoxic medications; c.b.u. = can be used, with more frequent monitoring, in patients with underlying hepatic dysfunction; ATS = American Thoracic Society; CDC = Centers for Disease Control and Prevention; CNS = central nervous system. Rifapentine is not approved for use in children. Pregnancy categories: B = no controlled studies in pregnant women, but studies in non-human animals demonstrate no teratogenicity; C = studies in animals either demonstrate teratogenic effects, or no studies are available in pregnant human or non-human animals; D = there is evidence of human fetal risk. Adapted from Centers from Disease Control and Prevention [12] and World Health Organization [13].

[1] Concomitant administration of pyridoxine (vitamin $B_6$) can decrease neurological side effects.

[2] Other fluoroquinolones not included as ciprofloxacin is no longer a recommended antituberculous agent and there are few data for use of gatifloxacin and moxifloxacin in children.

any pureed foods, we transition to INH tablets that are crushed and mixed with food. RIF suspension has a standard pharmacopoeia formulation, but the shelf life is short and it must be refrigerated. Fixed-dose combinations are available internationally for many first-line TB medications. They are attractive because of the ease of administration, the increased adherence due to the decreasing pill burden, the decreased risk of medication errors and the decreased risk of selection of resistant isolates by inadvertent monotherapy. However, the weight based dosing used in young children precludes the use of some fixed-dose combination formulations.

Supplementation with pyridoxine (vitamin $B_6$) is routinely added to children receiving INH who are exclusively breastfed infants, have intestinal malabsorption, are HIV infected, postpubertal or pregnant. While vitamin $B_6$ prevents peripheral neuropathy associated with INH and ethionamide, it does not prevent hepatotoxicity.

## Specific Scenarios

### *Treatment of TB Disease in the HIV-Infected Child*

Treating TB disease in the child co-infected with HIV poses a number of challenges [17]. First, HIV-infected persons often have more adverse events caused by TB medications than HIV-uninfected persons. Second, the rifamycins interact with several classes of antiretroviral (ARV) medications. Third, there is the issue of when to begin TB therapy in relation to ARV drugs to avoid immune reconstitution inflammatory syndrome (IRIS). Fourth, standard 6-month courses of TB therapy have been associated with treatment failure or relapse in HIV-infected persons.

HIV-infected children with TB disease have an increased risk of medication side effects than HIV-uninfected children with TB [18]. In part, this is because first-line TB medications and ARV agents share many side effects: neuropathy, gastrointestinal distress, dermatitis and hepatitis [19]. In one South African study, almost 10% of children undergoing treatment for both TB and HIV had adverse medication effects, of which approximately 40% were attributed to TB agents [18]. One common and occasionally life-threatening complication seen primarily in HIV-infected children is IRIS. There are 2 types of IRIS: paradoxical IRIS, where children have a paradoxical worsening of TB symptoms and often radiographic findings after initiation of therapy, and unmasking IRIS, where an HIV-infected child with undiagnosed TB disease begins to receive ARV drugs then develops TB symptoms. Although IRIS has been associated with other opportunistic infections, it has been most commonly described in persons co-infected with TB, with some series noting up to 16–38% incidence of IRIS within 2–4 months of ARV initiation [20]. Adults with CD4+ cell counts <50/μl, disseminated TB, greater reduction in viral load after starting ARV therapy and a shorter time period between initiation of TB medications and ARV drugs are at the highest risk [19, 21]. One study in HIV-infected South African infants showed IRIS rates of 21%, a third of which were due to TB [22]. Non-steroidal anti-inflammatory drugs have been used for moderate IRIS cases, and corticosteroids have been used for severe IRIS.

RIF decreases the serum concentrations of all protease inhibitors except for ritonavir by 75–89% and decreases non-nucleoside reverse-transcriptase inhibitors (NNRTIs) by 25–96%, requiring an NNRTI dose increase for all except nevirapine (though nevirapine concentrations can be reduced up to 55%). In contrast, the use of rifabutin in children receiving protease inhibitors can lead to 190–435% increases in rifabutin levels, requiring thrice weekly rifabutin dosing. For NNRTIs, delavirdine should be avoided, and efavirenz requires dose reduction; rifabutin dosing does not need to be altered [19]. Nucleoside reverse-transcriptase inhibitor concentrations are not significantly affected by rifamycin administration. Time to sputum conversion and risk of relapse were not significantly different in HIV-infected patients who received RIF versus rifabutin-containing regimens. While rifabutin is the rifamycin offering the least interaction with ARV agents, widespread use is limited by cost considerations. Rifapentine is not recommended for use in HIV-infected patients because of the risk of relapse with rifamycin-resistant organisms during therapy; rifapentine is not currently recommended for use in children either. Despite the potential drug interactions with rifamycins, it is not recommended that rifamycins be excluded from TB treatment regimens, as exclusion of these bactericidal and sterilizing drugs will likely prolong duration of therapy and may result in poorer outcomes.

Many children receive the diagnosis of HIV after presenting with TB. The optimal timing of starting a child on TB and HIV medications is unclear. When treatment for both co-infections was started simultaneously, adverse effects were noted frequently, the pill burden posed a challenge for young children, and IRIS rates increased. Consequently, therapy for HIV was often delayed until after TB therapy had been completed, leading to increased mortality from other opportunistic infections. One randomized trial in HIV-infected (CD4+ <500/μl), acid-fast bacillus smear-positive adults showed that starting ARV therapies within 4 weeks of initiation of TB therapy led to reduced mortality and similar rates of adverse events when compared with the group started on ARV treatments after completing TB therapy. While patients started on ARV treatments sooner had higher rates of IRIS (12 vs. 4%), no deaths or changes in medication regimens were attributable to IRIS [23]. In the absence of equivalent paediatric data, earlier initiation of ARV therapy in children co-infected with TB should be considered.

A recent meta-analysis showed that rates of TB relapse and failure in adults were higher when rifamycins were given for only 6 months versus ≥9 months and when therapy was given intermittently during the intensification phase [24]. The recommendation is that HIV-infected children receive at least 9 months of therapy for TB [4]. Intermittent therapy during the continuation phase of TB therapy is not recommended for patients with CD4+ cell counts <100/μl [12].

*Extrapulmonary Disease*

Most forms of extrapulmonary TB are amenable to 6-month courses of therapy. However, meningeal, miliary, skeletal or disseminated forms of TB should be treated for 9–12 months. The empirical selection of anti-TB agents is the same for extrapulmonary disease as for pulmonary TB, with the exception of TB meningitis. As EMB crosses the blood-brain barrier poorly, use of ethionamide is beneficial in children with TB meningitis; however, emesis is commonly seen with ethionamide, and it is necessary to assure that children can tolerate all medicines orally prior to discharge. An alternative for children with TB meningitis is to empirically add an injectable agent, changing to ethionamide when the child is ready to be discharged from the hospital.

*Role of Corticosteroids*

Corticosteroids should never be administered to children with TB without concomitant administration of antituberculous agents. The benefit of corticosteroid use has been best described for children with TB meningitis, where use of steroids decreases morbidity and mortality. However, other children with TB in whom the host inflammatory response is thought to be causing tissue damage might benefit from corticosteroids. These include children with massive intrathoracic lymphadenopathy causing airway compression, tuberculous pericarditis and miliary disease. There are few data on the efficacy of steroids in HIV-infected persons with TB meningitis [25]. The route of administration should be guided by the patient's clinical course. A common regimen is prednisone 1–2 mg/kg/day for 4–8 weeks, followed by a slow taper. There is no evidence of the superiority of any one steroid formulation for TB.

*Drug Resistance*

In the relative absence of data specific to paediatric cases, the principles of treating children with drug-resistant TB are the same as in adults. Daily therapy with at least 3 agents to which the isolate has known susceptibility is recommended. In adults, one problem is that in vitro susceptibilities do not correlate with clinical response as well for second-line drugs as for first-line medications. In children, this problem is exacerbated because there are fewer published data on pharmacokinetics and drug dosing for second-line drugs as compared with first-line drugs [14]. While children have fewer side effects from second-line drugs than adults, this may be due, in part, to more rapid drug metabolism and lower serum levels [26], potentially compromising efficacy. Also, many recommendations on duration of therapy in adults are based on sputum smear conversion, a marker of little relevance for most cases of childhood TB. As children generally have paucibacillary disease, the need to continue medications for 18–24 months for children with minimal (and radiographically resolved) pulmonary disease is unclear.

The decision of what medications to begin once susceptibilities are available should be guided by maximizing the number of bactericidal drugs and minimizing adverse events. Fluoroquinolones in combination with other anti-TB agents and surgical debulking of pulmonary disease have been used with success in adults. More recently, linezolid has been used in adults with drug-resistant disease [15]; while its utility is limited by high rates of myelosuppression, a risk of lactic acidosis that may be higher in HIV-infected patients and cost considerations, at least 1 paediatric case report describes long-term use without side effects [27]. However, there are no trials showing superiority of one regimen over another for drug-resistant TB.

*Medication Intolerance, Treatment Interruptions and Medication Adherence*

Children generally tolerate TB medications better than adults. However, a child will occasionally have adverse events. In these circumstances, the risk of exacerbating symptoms must be balanced with the understanding that there are a finite number of medications with paediatric formulations, and a move from a first-line to a second-line medication is suboptimal. The most common side effects seen in children are gastrointestinal distress, hepatitis and rash. If gastrointestinal symptoms occur, medications should be held until transaminases are checked; if elevated, screening for other forms of hepatitis should be done. If there is evidence of hepatitis, all hepatically metabolized TB drugs should be stopped and a liver-sparing regimen begun (e.g. EMB, a fluoroquinolone, an injectable agent, and a second-line oral medication). When transaminases return to <2 times the upper limit of normal, standard TB medications can be resumed, one per week. Generally, RIF is restarted first, followed by INH and PZA. In children with severe rashes with mucosal involvement or angio-oedema, the order of restarting medications is the same but can be done every 2–3 days. However, most rashes caused by TB medications are mild, respond well to antihistamines and do not require regimen modification.

Treatment interruptions are managed depending on the stage of therapy, the number of doses missed, and the initial presentation of the child. Interruptions over 14 days during the intensive phase should prompt re-initiation of all therapy. Interruptions over 3 months in the continuation phase should also prompt restarting all medications. Shorter interruptions during continuation therapy are managed based upon the number of doses missed, and often these doses are added to the end of therapy. For children who were sputum smear negative initially, have a normal chest radiograph after starting therapy and have received up to 80% of doses, continuation of therapy may not be beneficial. In contrast, children who were initially sputum smear positive should receive 100% of doses [12]. These guidelines, with their emphasis on sputum smears, were developed for adults and have questionable applicability to young children, who often have paucibacillary disease. Nonetheless, the importance of medication adherence in preventing secondary resistance cannot be overstated.

Medication adherence has historically been poor for persons receiving unsupervised therapy for TB disease, and a recent study of Indian adults with newly diagnosed, smear-positive pulmonary TB showed a 6% default rate even among patients treated via DOT short course [28]. Recently published comparable data are not available for children with TB disease, but many of the risk factors for default in adults (social stressors, poor relationship between patient and caregiver) could be applied to the child's caregivers. DOT is the preferred method of administering medications to a child with TB disease. In the USA, this role is fulfilled by local health departments. In resource-poor settings, this role may be fulfilled by a village elder or other respected person in the community.

### Following the Child Receiving Antituberculosis Chemotherapy

Children on multidrug therapy for TB disease should be seen monthly to assess adherence, response to therapy and monitor for adverse effects. Baseline and serial evaluation of liver transaminases in the asymptomatic child without pre-existing liver disease and not taking other hepatotoxic drugs (such as anticonvulsant drugs) receiving INH monotherapy or first-line TB medications is not recommended, as hepatotoxicity is very uncommon in children. However, if the child develops any symptoms compatible with hepatitis, the threshold for checking hepatic transaminases should be low. Generally, chest radiography is performed prior to initiation of therapy, after 1–2 months of medications, and (if the second chest radiograph is abnormal) at the end of therapy to establish a new radiographic baseline for the child. Approximately 60% of children have abnormal radiographs at the conclusion of anti-TB chemotherapy. While children are not treated until radiographic normalcy, in a child with significant cavitary lesions after 6 months of therapy, consideration should be given to continuing therapy for 9 months.

### Future Directions

One future direction for treatment of TB is to expand the armamentarium of drugs that can be used for MDR-TB and extensively drug-resistant TB. The use of fluoroquinolones has improved outcomes of patients with MDR-TB, but few other medications have become licensed. Consequently, many older TB drugs, such as para-aminosalicylic acid, have been resurrected. Additionally, existing antibiotics have been tested for antimycobacterial activity; however, the pharmacokinetics, efficacy and, in some cases, safety of these drugs have not been well established for children of various ages. In this fashion, linezolid, macrolides, amoxicillin-clavulanate and other drugs have been utilized, with varying degrees of success, in patients with MDR-TB and extensively drug-resistant TB. While there are several new drugs in the pipeline, data for utilization in children generally lag far behind similar adult data. This does not preclude paediatricians using these medications in children, but does mean that the medications may not be used to maximal impact until details of pharmacokinetics in children are established. The issues surrounding drug development and children are described in another paper in this volume.

The last quarter century has seen a decline in treatment duration for children with TB disease. The next step is to study if treatment duration for children with LTBI can be shortened. Adherence with therapy for LTBI has historically been poor, with fewer than half of adults in industrialized nations and <20% of children in the developing world completing therapy [10], though children receiving INH in the context of a study had higher adherence [9]. Adherence is often inversely correlated with duration of therapy and adverse effects from medications. There are several international studies [5] on the use of shorter courses of INH and RIF for LTBI therapy. One recent modelling study showed that 4 months of RIF monotherapy was more cost-effective than 9 months of INH [29], while another study demonstrated that LTBI patients receiving 4 months of RIF had lower rates of side effects and higher adherence than persons receiving 9 months of INH [30]. As a third of the global population is estimated to have LTBI and serve as reservoirs for future disease cases, finding short courses of well-tolerated, cost-effective medications to treat LTBI is imperative.

## References


1 Swaminathan S, Rekha B: Pediatric tuberculosis: global overview and challenges. Clin Infect Dis 2010;50:S184–S194.
2 Peto HM, Pratt RH, Harrington TA, LoBue PA, Armstrong LR: Epidemiology of extrapulmonary tuberculosis in the United States, 1993–2006. Clin Infect Dis 2009;49:1350–1357.
3 David HL: Probability distribution of drug-resistant mutants in unselected populations of *Mycobacterium tuberculosis*. Appl Microbiol 1970;20:810–814.
4 American Academy of Pediatrics: Tuberculosis; in Pickering LJ, Baker CJ (eds): Red Book Report of the Committee on Infectious Disease, ed 28. Chicago, American Academy of Pediatrics, 2009.
5 Spyridis NP, Sypridis PG, Gelesme A, Sypsa V, Valianatou M, Metsou F, Gourgiotis D, Tsolia MN: The effectiveness of a 9-month regimen of isoniazid alone versus 3- and 4-month regimens of isoniazid plus rifampin for treatment of latent tuberculosis infection in children: results of an 11-year randomized study. Clin Infect Dis 2007;45:715–722.
6 Finnell SM, Christenson JC, Downs SM: Latent tuberculosis infection in children: a call for revised treatment guidelines. Pediatrics 2009;123:816–822.
7 Gray DM, Young T, Cotton M, Zar H: Impact of tuberculosis preventive therapy on tuberculosis and mortality in HIV-infected children. Cochrane Database Syst Rev 2009;1:CD006418.
8 Marais BJ, Ayles H, Graham SM, Godfrey-Faussett P: Screening and preventive therapy for tuberculosis. Clin Chest Med. 2009;30:827–846.
9 Le Roux SM, Cotton MF, Golub JE, le Roux DM, Workman L, Zar HJ: Adherence to isoniazid prophylaxis among HIV-infected children: a randomized controlled trial comparing two dosing schedules. BMC Med 2009;7:67.
10 Horsburgh CR, Goldberg S, Bethel J, Chen S, Colson PW, Hirsch-Moverman Y, Hughes S, Shrestha-Kuwahara R, Sterling TR, Wall K, Weinfurter P, Tuberculosis Epidemiologic Studies Consortium: Latent TB infection treatment acceptance and completion in the United States and Canada. Chest 2010;137:401–409.
11 Swaminathan S, Narendran G, Venkatesan P, Iliayas S, Santhanakrishnan R, Menon PA, Padmapriyadarsini C, Ramachandran R, Chinnaiyan P, Suhadev M, Sakthivel R, Narayanan PR: Efficacy of a 6-month versus 9-month intermittent treatment regimen in HIV-infected patients with tuberculosis. Am J Respir Crit Care Med 2010;181:743–751.
12 Centers for Disease Control and Prevention (CDC), American Thoracic Society, and Infectious Disease Society of America: Treatment of tuberculosis. MMWR Recomm Rep 2003;52:RR-11.
13 World Health Organization: Treatment of Tuberculosis: Guidelines. 2009. http://www.who.int/tb/publications/tb_treatmentguidelines/en/index.html (accessed May 29, 2010).
14 Schaaf HS, Moll AP, Dheda K: Multidrug- and extensively drug-resistant tuberculosis in Africa and South America: epidemiology, diagnosis, and management in adults and children. Clin Chest Med 2009;30:667–683.
15 Anger HA, Dworkin F, Sharma S, Munsiff SS, Nilsen DM, Ahuja SD: Linezolid for treatment of multidrug-resistant and extensively drug-resistant tuberculosis, New York City, 2000–2006. J Antimicrob Chemother 2010;65:775–783.
16 Donald PR, Maher D, Maritz JS, Qazi S: Ethambutol dosage for the treatment of children: literature review and recommendations. Int J Tuberc Lung Dis 2006;10:1318–1330.
17 Marais BJ, Graham SM, Cotton MF, Beyers N: Diagnostic and management challenges for childhood tuberculosis in the era of HIV. J Infect Dis 2007;196:S76–S85.
18 Walters E, Cotton MF, Rabie H, Schaaf HS, Walters LO, Marais BJ: Clinical presentation and outcome of tuberculosis in human immunodeficiency virus infected children on anti-retroviral therapy. BMC Pediatr 2008;8:1.
19 McIlleron H, Meinties G, Burman WJ, Maartens G: Complications of antiretroviral therapy in patients with tuberculosis: drug interactions, toxicity, and immune reconstitution inflammatory syndrome. J Infect Dis 2007;196:S63–S75.
20 Orikiiriza J, Bakeera-Kitaka S, Musiime V, Mworozi EA, Mugyenyi P, Boulware DR: The clinical pattern, prevalence, and factors associated with immune reconstitution inflammatory syndrome in Ugandan children. AIDS 2010;24:2009–2017.
21 Müller M, Wandel S, Colebunders R, Attia S, Furrer H, Eggers M, leDEA Southern and Central Africa: Immune reconstitution inflammatory syndrome in patients starting antiretroviral therapy for HIV infection: a systematic review and meta-analysis. Lancet Infect Dis 2010;10:251–261.
22 Smith K, Kuhn L, Coovadia A, Meyers T, Hu CC, Reitz C, Barry G, Strehlau R, Sherman G, Abrams EJ: Immune reconstitution inflammatory syndrome among HIV-infected South African infants initiating antiretroviral therapy. AIDS 2009;23:1097–1107.
23 Abdool-Karim SS, Naidoo K, Grobler A, Padayatchi N, Baxter C, Gray A, Gengiah T, Nair G, Bamber S, Singh A, Khan M, Pienaar J, El-Sadr W, Friedland G, Abdool-Karim Q: Timing of initiation of antiretroviral drugs during tuberculosis therapy. N Engl J Med 2010;362:697–706.
24 Khan FA, Minion J, Pai M, Royce S, Burman W, Harries AD, Menzies D: Treatment of active tuberculosis in HIV-coinfected patients: a systematic review and meta-analysis. Clin Infect Dis 2010;50:1288–1299.
25 Prasad K, Singh MB: Corticosteroids for managing tuberculous meningitis. Cochrane Database Syst Rev 2006;1:CD002244.
26 Donald PR, Schaaf HS: Old and new drugs for the treatment of tuberculosis in children. Paediatr Resp Rev 2007;8:134–141.
27 Schaaf HS, Willemse M, Donald PR: Long-term linezolid treatment in a young child with extensively drug-resistant tuberculosis. Pediatr Infect Dis J 2009;28:748–750.
28 Vijay S, Kumar P, Chauhan LS, Vollepore BH, Kizhakkethil UP, Rao SG: Risk factors associated with default among new smear positive TB patients treated under DOTS in India. PLoS One 2010;5:e10043.
29 Holland DP, Sanders GD, Hamilton CD, Stout JE: Costs and cost-effectiveness of four treatment regimens for latent tuberculosis infection. Am J Respir Crit Care Med 2009;179:1055–1060.
30 Menzies D, Long R, Trajman A, Dion M-J, Yang J, Al Jahdali H, Memish Z, Khan K, Gardam M, Hoeppner V, Benedetti A, Schwartzman K: Adverse events with 4 months of rifampin therapy or 9 months of isoniazid therapy for latent tuberculosis infection. Ann Intern Med 2008;149:689–697.



Andrea T. Cruz, MD, MPH
Texas Children's Hospital, MC 3-2371
1102 Bates Street, Suite 1850
Houston, TX 77030 (USA)
Tel. +1 832 824 5584, E-Mail acruz@bcm.edu

# The Future

Donald PR, van Helden PD (eds): Antituberculosis Chemotherapy.
Prog Respir Res. Basel, Karger, 2011, vol 40, pp 118–127

# Issues and Challenges in the Development of Novel Tuberculosis Drug Regimens

Ngozi Erondu · Ann Ginsberg

Global Alliance for TB Drug Development, New York, N.Y., USA

**Abstract**

Due to the limitations of current tuberculosis (TB) treatment, there is an urgent need for the development of novel TB drug regimens to address the persistent and worsening global TB epidemic. The main goals for developing new regimens are: shortening and simplifying the treatment of active, drug-sensitive and drug-resistant TB; effectively treating TB in patients co-infected with HIV with drugs that do not adversely interact with antiretroviral agents, and shortening the treatment of latent TB infection. Key challenges for novel regimen development include the need for multiple safe, efficacious drugs with novel mechanisms of action, and the long duration and high cost of TB clinical trials. There are now 9 drugs in various stages of clinical development, belonging to 6 different chemical classes with distinct mechanisms of action. This represents the most active pipeline for TB drug development in history. The status of the clinical development of these drugs – AZD5847, PNU-100480, rifapentine, PA-824, delamanid, TMC207, SQ109, moxifloxacin and gatifloxacin – will be reviewed in this chapter. To significantly reduce the long development timelines, a new paradigm, which considers the whole multidrug combination rather than the individual drug as the unit of clinical development and target for registration, has been proposed and will also be discussed.

Copyright © 2011 S. Karger AG, Basel

Limitations and inadequacies of the current tuberculosis (TB) treatment regimens contribute significantly to the global burden of TB, the emergence and spread of multidrug-resistant (MDR) and extensively drug-resistant TB, and the difficulty of controlling this disease and reaching the Millennium Development Goals and Stop TB Partnership global targets for reducing disease burden. Current TB treatment regimens are described in detail elsewhere in this volume. However, some key features include the following: (1) adequate treatment of drug-sensitive TB requires the use of a 4-drug combination (1-letter abbreviations will be used for combinations as follows: H = isoniazid, R = rifampicin, Z = pyrazinamide and E = ethambutol) for 6–9 months; (2) the rifamycins, a key component of first-line TB treatment, have significant interactions with the cytochrome (CYP) P450 system; specifically, they cause the induction of enzymes/transporters that are involved in the metabolism of several drugs including some antiretroviral agents, which makes the treatment of TB patients co-infected with HIV challenging, especially in resource-limited settings; (3) the long duration of therapy and the side effects of the current drugs lead to non-compliance, a major contributor to the emergence and spread of drug-resistant TB, treatment of which often lasts for 2 or more years and requires more expensive drugs (including injectables) with limited or uncertain efficacy and worse safety profiles; (4) treatment of latent TB, key to controlling the epidemic especially in regions of the world with high HIV infection rates, currently requires lengthy treatment (up to 9 months) with isoniazid although shorter regimens [e.g. 3 months of weekly rifapentine (P) + isoniazid] are being evaluated (see below; NCT00023452).

Given the limitations and challenges described above, the need for the development of new treatment regimens of both active and latent TB cannot be overemphasized. The ultimate goals are to develop a regimen for active TB that can shorten and simplify the treatment of both drug-sensitive (DS) and MDR-TB in both HIV-infected and uninfected individuals, and an ultrashort, simple, safe regimen

**Table 1.** Drugs in clinical development

| Drug | Class | Phase of clinical development | Sponsor(s) |
|---|---|---|---|
| AZD5847 | oxazolidinone | I | Astra Zeneca |
| PNU-100480 | oxazolidinone | I | Pfizer |
| Rifapentine | rifamycin | II | sanofi-aventis, TB Trials Consortium |
| PA-824 | nitro-imidazole | II | TB Alliance |
| Delamanid | nitro-imidazole | II | Otsuka |
| TMC207 | diarylquinoline | II | Tibotec, TB Alliance |
| SQ109 | ethylene diamine | II | Sequella, NIH |
| Moxifloxacin | fluoroquinolone | III | TB Alliance, UCL, Bayer |
| Gatifloxacin | fluoroquinolone | III | OFLOTUB consortium |

to eradicate latent TB infection. The optimal or ideal target profile of drugs in such novel regimen(s) includes:

- novel mechanism of action with equal efficacy against both DS- and MDR-TB;
- no cross-resistance with current drugs, minimizing the likelihood of pre-existing resistance;
- no significant cytochrome P450-mediated drug-drug interactions, thereby allowing safe and effective co-administration with antiretroviral agents;
- good pharmacokinetic profile in both adult and paediatric populations reflected by being able to be administered orally, once daily or less frequently, and suitability for development in a fixed dose combination;
- excellent safety and tolerability profile;
- low cost of goods, making the regimen affordable in resource-limited regions of the world where TB is highly prevalent.

## Drugs in Clinical Development

As shown in table 1, there are at least 9 drugs currently in various stages of clinical development. Compared to currently approved anti-TB medications, all these drugs with the exception of rifapentine have novel mechanisms of action and are active against both DS- and MDR-TB.

*Phase I*

There are 2 drugs in this phase of development, both poised to enter phase II in the near future. AZD5847 and PNU-100480 both belong to the oxazolidinone class of antimicrobial agents and are being developed by Astra Zeneca and Pfizer, respectively. The mycobactericidal activity of these drugs results from inhibition of protein synthesis. The prototype for this class, linezolid, although used off label for the treatment of MDR-TB, is hampered by a side effect profile that includes haematological and neurological toxicity.

PNU-100480 (PNU) is derived from linezolid but is more potent and appears to have a better safety profile. In the mouse model of TB infection [1], it has been shown that PNU is more bactericidal than linezolid and causes a 2-log reduction in lung CFU counts when added to standard therapy (HRZ) or a 2-drug regimen such as moxifloxacin (M) and pyrazinamide. Interestingly, PNU + MZ was more active than HRZ. In another mouse study, PNU had better sterilizing activity than linezolid, and when combined with HRZ, shortened the duration of treatment required for cure [2]. These data support the potential of a PNU-containing regimen to result in treatment shortening for both DS- and MDR-TB. A number of studies with PNU in healthy volunteers have been completed, including single- and multiple-dose studies as well as assessment of food effect and bactericidal activity using the whole-blood assay. Available data indicate that PNU was well tolerated in single doses up to 1,500 mg and multiple doses up to 600 mg b.i.d. for 28 days. Its mycobactericidal activity determined with the whole-blood assay was superior to that of linezolid, and for both drugs, the maximum activity occurred at $\geq 2$ times the minimum inhibitory concentration [3]. Simulations using PNU as monotherapy indicate that optimal efficacy would require a total daily dose of 800–1,200 mg [4]. The next planned study is a phase II extended early bactericidal activity (eEBA) study in patients with pulmonary TB.

The other oxazolidinone in early development is AZD5847. A single-dose phase I study in healthy volunteers, which included the assessment of food effects, has been completed while a 14-day multiple ascending dose study to assess the safety, tolerability and pharmacokinetics of an oral suspension is ongoing (NCT01116258). No data have been publicly released.

*Phase II*

The 5 drugs in this phase are: rifapentine, a rifamycin with a long half-life being evaluated for use with currently available drugs by sanofi-aventis in collaboration with the TB Trials Consortium of the US Centers for Disease Control; PA-824 and delamanid, 2 nitro-imidazoles being developed by the TB Alliance and Otsuka, respectively; TMC207, a diarylquinoline being jointly developed by Tibotec (for MDR-TB) and the TB Alliance (for DS-TB), and SQ109, an ethylene diamine being developed by Sequella Inc., in collaboration with the National Institutes of Health.

Rifapentine was approved for the treatment of TB in the USA in 1998 but based on data from patients and the mouse model of TB infection, the currently approved dosing recommendation (600 mg twice weekly) may not be optimal. It appears that substantially superior efficacy may be achieved by administering higher doses of the drug, potentially enabling a significant reduction in treatment duration [5]. In addition, multidrug regimens containing rifapentine, e.g. PMZ and TMC207 + PZ, have been shown to be highly effective in mice infected with *Mycobacterium tuberculosis* [6, 7]. There are several ongoing clinical studies with rifapentine including: a 14-day study evaluating the pharmacokinetics, safety and tolerability of escalating doses (up to 20 mg/kg) in healthy volunteers (NCT01162486); an 8-week study comparing the efficacy, safety and tolerability of daily rifapentine (approx. 10 mg/kg/dose) to that of daily rifampicin (approx. 10 mg/kg/dose) when added to HZE in patients with pulmonary TB (NCT00694629); an 8-week study comparing the efficacy, safety and tolerability of the experimental regimen HPMZ to the standard therapy (HRZE) in patients with pulmonary TB (NCT00728507); a non-inferiority study (Rifaquin) comparing 2 experimental regimens containing high-dose rifapentine (15 mg/kg body weight, 2 months of daily EMRZ followed by 2 months of MP given twice weekly; 20 mg/kg body weight, 2 months of daily EMRZ followed by 4 months of MP given once weekly) to the standard regimen (2 months of daily HRZE followed by 4 months of daily HR) in the treatment of pulmonary TB, and a study comparing the efficacy, safety and tolerability of a 3-month course of weekly rifapentine and isoniazid (3HP) to a 9-month course of daily isoniazid (9H) in preventing TB among high-risk tuberculin skin test reactors, including children and HIV-infected persons, who require treatment for latent TB infection (NCT00023452). Preliminary results presented at the International Union against Tuberculosis and Lung Disease (IUATLD) meeting in November 2010 from the latent TB infection study (TB Trials Consortium Study 26) indicate that 3 months of weekly HP was non-inferior to 9 months of daily isoniazid and the completion rate was significantly higher in the 3HP group compared to the 9H group (81.9 vs. 69.5%). However, the use of rifapentine will be limited to DS-TB due to its cross-resistance with rifampicin, and its use in TB patients co-infected with HIV will be complicated by cytochrome P450-mediated drug-drug interactions with antiretroviral agents.

PA-824 is a nitro-imidazo-oxazine with anti-TB activity and a unique mechanism of action which has not yet been fully defined. It has been demonstrated to inhibit mycobacterial protein and lipid synthesis, and to inhibit the oxidation of hydroxymycolate to ketomycolate, thereby interfering with mycobacterial cell wall biosynthesis. In addition, activation of PA-824 results in the generation of highly reactive species such as nitric oxide, and this has been postulated as a possible mechanism for its activity against non-replicating *M. tuberculosis* [8]. PA-824 demonstrated in vitro activity against both DS- and MDR-TB, and in vivo activity in a mouse model of TB. In mice infected with *M. tuberculosis*, the combination of PA-824 and pyrazinamide displayed mycobactericidal activity that was equivalent to that of the first-line regimen (HRZ), while the combination of PA-824, moxifloxacin and pyrazinamide cured mice more rapidly than the first-line regimen [9, 10]. Thus, these novel regimens, which contain neither isoniazid nor rifampicin, may have the potential to (1) shorten the duration of TB chemotherapy and (2) treat both DS- and MDR-TB. Several phase I and phase II studies have been completed with PA-824, and these include: single- and multiple-dose, dose escalation studies; 2 food effect studies; a midazolam drug-drug interaction study in healthy volunteers, and 2 eEBA studies in patients with newly diagnosed, smear-positive, drug-sensitive pulmonary TB [11–13]. In these studies, PA-824 was well tolerated at doses up to 1,200 mg daily for 14 days; its pharmacokinetics was consistent with once daily dosing or less; there was a less than 2-fold food effect with a high-fat, high-calorie meal at the anticipated clinical dose of ≤200 mg/day, and PA-824 was not a significant inhibitor/inducer of CYP3A4. The efficacy data from the first eEBA study indicated that all doses studied of PA-824 (200, 600, 1,000 and 1,200 mg) produced an equivalent decrease in sputum CFU counts over the 14-day treatment period [14]. However, in the second eEBA study, with a similar design to the first except for the use of lower doses of PA-824 (50,

100, 150 and 200 mg/day), preliminary results indicated a dose response. All doses of PA-824 used in this study produced a measurable decrease in sputum CFU counts over the 14-day treatment period with the 100-, 150- and 200-mg doses of PA-824 having similar efficacy, greater than that of the 50-mg dose. Given the data from preclinical studies evaluating regimens consisting of PA-824 and pyrazinamide or PA-824, pyrazinamide and moxifloxacin, a 14-day eEBA study has recently been initiated by the TB Alliance to determine whether these combinations are as bactericidal in man as has been demonstrated in the mouse model of TB (NCT01215851).

Delamanid, a nitro-imidazo-oxazole, is the second member of the nitro-imidazole class in clinical development. Mycobactericidal activity has been demonstrated in vitro, and in vivo in the mouse model as well as in humans [14]. Two EBA studies have been conducted, and an 8-week study evaluating the efficacy, safety and tolerability of the drug + optimized second-line regimen (O2R) in MDR-TB patients has recently been completed but the results have not yet been publicly released at the time of writing this review. There is also an ongoing open-label, dose escalation study to assess safety, tolerability, pharmacokinetics and efficacy in MDR-TB patients (NCT01131351).

TMC207 is a diarylquinoline investigational anti-TB compound that specifically targets the F0 subunit of mycobacterial adenosine triphosphate synthase, thereby inhibiting the proton pump of the enzyme. Due to this drug's unique and novel mechanism of action, it exhibits no cross-resistance with current anti-TB drugs. In vitro, TMC207 potently inhibits both DS and MDR *M. tuberculosis* isolates, and is also bactericidal against non-replicating bacilli. In the murine model of TB, TMC207 was as active as the standard regimen (HRZ), while addition of TMC207 to this drug regimen resulted in accelerated mycobactericidal activity [15]. It appears to have a synergistic interaction with pyrazinamide: 100% of mice were culture negative after 8 weeks of treatment with TMC207 and pyrazinamide compared to 0% of mice treated with HRZ [16]. Collectively, these findings in the mouse model have led to the suggestion that a regimen that includes TMC207 and pyrazinamide could be effective in the treatment of both DS- and MDR-TB and shorten treatment duration. Several phase I studies have been conducted evaluating TMC207; available data indicate it was generally well tolerated up to single doses of 700 mg and multiple doses up to 400 mg daily for 15 days. It has a long terminal half-life and is extensively metabolized by CYP3A4, with the result that its plasma concentration decreased and increased in the presence of CYP3A4 inducers and inhibitors, respectively. This is likely to make its use in HIV-TB co-infected patients on antiretroviral agents quite challenging. TMC207 has also been studied in 1 phase II dose-ranging 7-day EBA trial in patients with DS-TB [17]. The results from this study showed clinically relevant bactericidal activity only at the highest TMC207 dose (400 mg) tested with a delay in onset of response (activity detected from day 4 onwards). No clinically relevant changes were seen with the lower doses of TMC207 (25 and 100 mg) during the 7 days of treatment. The reason for this delayed onset of activity (400 mg) or lack of bactericidal activity (at lower doses) is not yet clear but may be partly due to suboptimal plasma concentrations initially or throughout the 7-day duration of treatment and may also reflect the time needed to deplete mycobacterial adenosine triphosphate stores. Based on mouse data, the average target plasma concentration of TMC207 for efficacy in humans is approximately 600 ng/ml. Thus, in a 14-day dose-ranging EBA study recently conducted by the TB Alliance in patients with DS-TB, different dosing regimens were studied to obtain average plasma concentrations ranging from 500 to 2,000 ng/ml throughout most of the dosing period. Results from this study are pending. To determine whether TMC207-containing combinations are as bactericidal in man as has been demonstrated in the mouse model of TB, the TB Alliance recently initiated an eEBA study of TMC207 + pyrazinamide and TMC207 + PA-824 in patients with newly diagnosed, smear-positive, drug-sensitive pulmonary TB (NCT01215851).

Tibotec is also conducting a 2-stage phase IIb study in patients with MDR-TB [18], treated with 400 mg of TMC207 daily for 2 weeks followed by 200 mg 3 times a week for an additional 6 weeks (stage 1) or with 400 mg daily for 2 weeks followed by 200 mg 3 times a week for an additional 22 weeks (stage 2). In stage 1, involving a total of 47 patients randomized to either TMC207 + O2R or to placebo + O2R, the addition of TMC207 resulted in a faster sputum conversion rate versus placebo (hazard ratio of 11.8 with 95% confidence interval of 2.3–61.3; $p = 0.003$). In addition, the proportion of patients with conversion of sputum culture at the end of the 8-week treatment was 48 versus 9% (TMC207 vs. placebo). There were no significant differences in the occurrence of adverse events in the 2 treatment groups with the exception of nausea, which was more frequent in the TMC207 group. Preliminary results from stage 2 (involving a total of 161 patients), presented at the IUATLD meeting in November 2010, revealed a faster sputum conversion rate with TMC207 versus placebo (hazard ratio of 2.2 with 95% confidence interval of 1.4–3.4; $p = 0.003$), and at the end of the 24-week treatment period, the proportion of patients with negative cultures was

79 versus 58% (TMC207 vs. placebo). Adverse events were evenly distributed between the treatment groups. Enrolment of a 6-month open-label study in MDR-TB patients using TMC207 + O2R has recently been completed.

SQ109, an ethylene diamine being developed by Sequella Inc., was originally selected from a compound library generated using the ethylene diamine pharmacophore of ethambutol. However, it appears to be substantially distinct from ethambutol and is active against both drug-sensitive and drug-resistant *M. tuberculosis* including ethambutol-resistant strains [19]. Its mechanism of action has not been precisely elucidated but it is believed to involve the inhibition of mycobacterial cell wall synthesis [20]. In vitro studies have shown that its mycobactericidal activity is synergistic with isoniazid, rifampicin and TMC207 but no additivity or synergy was seen with ethambutol or pyrazinamide [21, 22]. Interestingly, the synergy with rifampicin was also seen in rifampicin-resistant strains, where it lowered the minimum inhibitory concentration of rifampicin. Single- and multiple-dose studies in healthy subjects have been completed and SQ109 appears to be generally well tolerated up to 300 mg as a single dose and up to 150 mg daily for 14 days. The half-life has been estimated at 61 h, with steady state attained by 7 days. A phase II eEBA study in patients with newly diagnosed, uncomplicated, smear-positive pulmonary TB has been initiated (NCT01218217).

*Phase III*

The 2 drugs in this phase of development, gatifloxacin (G) and moxifloxacin, belong to the fluoroquinolone class of antimicrobial agents, which act by targeting DNA gyrase. These drugs have been shown to have significant mycobactericidal activity, and a number of them have been and are still being used off label for the treatment of MDR-TB. The newer 8-methoxy fluoroquinolones represented by gatifloxacin and moxifloxacin have demonstrated more potent in vitro and in vivo activity against *M. tuberculosis* compared to the older fluoroquinolones such as ciprofloxacin, levofloxacin and ofloxacin [23]. In the mouse model, moxifloxacin-containing regimens have demonstrated the potential to reduce the duration of treatment for drug-sensitive TB from 6 to 4 months [24]. Additional results suggesting potential for superior efficacy have come from phase II studies in patients with drug-sensitive TB in which gatifloxacin was substituted for ethambutol, or moxifloxacin was substituted for either ethambutol or isoniazid [25–28]. In all these clinical studies, the safety and tolerability profiles of these 2 fluoroquinolones have been acceptable. However, some concern remains regarding the dysglycemic effects of gatifloxacin especially in the elderly and the QT-prolonging effects of moxifloxacin especially in patients at risk of developing torsades de pointes due to family/medical history, concurrent illness or concomitant medications.

Moxifloxacin is being developed by the TB Alliance and Bayer Healthcare in collaboration with the University College London and the British Medical Research Council. The ongoing phase III, pivotal registration study (REMox TB) is a randomized, double-blind trial consisting of 3 arms: standard, 6-month therapy (2HRZE/4HR), substitution of moxifloxacin for isoniazid (2EMRZ/2MR) and substitution of moxifloxacin for ethambutol (2HRZM/2HRM). The objective is to evaluate the potential of each of the moxifloxacin-containing regimens to shorten treatment of DS-TB to 4 months.

Gatifloxacin is being evaluated by the OFLOTUB consortium in a randomized, double-blind, phase III study comparing the standard, 6-month therapy (2HRZE/4HR) to a regimen in which gatifloxacin replaces ethambutol (2HRZG/2HRG). The objective of this study is to evaluate the potential of the gatifloxacin-containing regimen to shorten DS-TB treatment from 6 to 4 months. A total of 1,836 patients were enrolled, and analysis of 1-year post-treatment data is ongoing. The completed trial will include results from 2 years of posttreatment follow-up.

*Approaches to Novel TB Regimen Development*

The multidrug nature of TB treatment regimens is a key driver of the strategy underpinning clinical development programmes of new TB therapies. TB treatment must consist of multiple drugs given in combination in order to prevent drug-resistant strains from being selected and to maximize efficacy. This creates a challenge, because in TB, as in all other therapeutic areas, the regulatory 'unit of development' has traditionally been a single drug. Having 9 drugs currently in clinical development is making it feasible for the first time since the early days of antibiotic discovery to evaluate completely novel regimens for TB.

The current development programme for a moxifloxacin-based, treatment-shortening regimen for DS-TB provides an example of the more traditional approach in developing new multidrug combination regimens in TB, having been initiated in approximately 2005 when other new TB drugs were not yet available. In this approach, 1 new drug is substituted into the current standard of care (SOC) regimen for 1 of the current drugs, and the target of registration is technically the single new drug. Figure 1 depicts a simplified sketch of this approach. The new drug is evaluated first in the acute and then relapse mouse model for

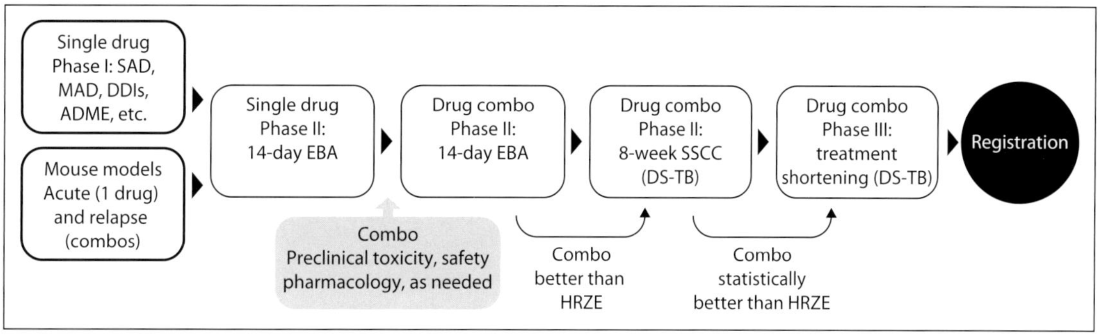


**Fig. 1.** Novel TB drug: schematic of the proposed clinical development path for DS-TB. SAD = single ascending dose; MAD = multiple ascending dose; DDI = drug-drug interaction; ADME = absorption, distribution, metabolism and excretion; combo = combination therapy; SSCC = serial sputum colony counting; see text for detailed explanation.

efficacy. If it appears promising, full preclinical and phase I human safety, tolerability and pharmacokinetic evaluation of the drug is undertaken. If successful, it is then advanced into a phase II eEBA trial to evaluate its bactericidal activity against *M. tuberculosis* in patients with sputum culture-positive TB. This trial is also used to perform dose ranging and to evaluate safety, tolerability and pharmacokinetics. In parallel with phase I testing of the individual new drug, potential substitution regimens are evaluated in a relapse mouse model and if one demonstrates adequate potential for treatment-shortening, and the individual, new drug has met preset preclinical and phase I evaluation criteria, the new drug substituted into the standard multidrug combination regimen is advanced into a 14-day eEBA study. If in the eEBA study, the new drug combination shows potential to be superior to first-line SOC treatment (HRZE) in efficacy (qualitatively; not powered for statistical significance) and continues to demonstrate good safety and tolerability, the combination is advanced into an 8-week phase II safety and efficacy trial with a primary end point based on reduction in colony counts over time in sputum – for example, serial sputum colony counting (SSCC) – rather than the binary 8-week sputum culture conversion rate which has traditionally been used as a primary end point in phase II TB drug trials. This approach provides greater sensitivity in evaluation of efficacy and enables smaller sample sizes than a binary end point (approx. 50 per arm rather than 200 or more). In this trial, the regimen must demonstrate statistically significant and clinically meaningful superiority to HRZE in order to be advanced into a pivotal, phase III registration trial. The phase III trial would be designed to demonstrate treatment shortening (e.g. to 2, 3 or 4 months) with non-inferiority with respect to microbiologically proven failure plus relapse rates relative to the current (i.e. 6-month), first-line SOC.

Figure 2 depicts the current drug development approach to registering a drug as a novel agent for MDR-TB treatment (e.g. being followed presently for TMC207 and delamanid). In this scheme, a single, novel TB drug with a new mechanism of action and no cross-resistance to current first-line TB drugs is developed for an MDR-TB treatment indication in combination with current MDR-TB drugs. The novel drug is evaluated as described above in the mouse models through phase II EBA testing. If it appears to have potential to shorten time to sputum conversion to negative, it is advanced into an 8-week phase II safety and efficacy trial, added on to an O2R or potentially in place of one of the less efficacious, more toxic, second-line drugs, such as cycloserine, ethionamide or para-aminosalicylate sodium. TMC207 and delamanid development programmes have taken the approach of adding the new drug onto a current second-line regimen rather than substituting for one of the current drugs – rendering the pill burden of the new regimen even greater than that of the current second-line regimens. The phase IIb trial in this paradigm would typically have a primary end point based on SSCC. In this trial, the experimental regimen (new drug added to or substituted into a current O2R) must demonstrate statistically significant and clinically meaningful superiority to the O2R in order to be advanced into a pivotal, registration trial. The new drug must meet predetermined criteria at each stage in order to advance. The pivotal trial is designed primarily to demonstrate superiority of the experimental regimen (novel drug added to or substituted into the O2R) relative to the O2R with respect to 6-month sputum culture conversion rates. Meeting the efficacy and safety end points

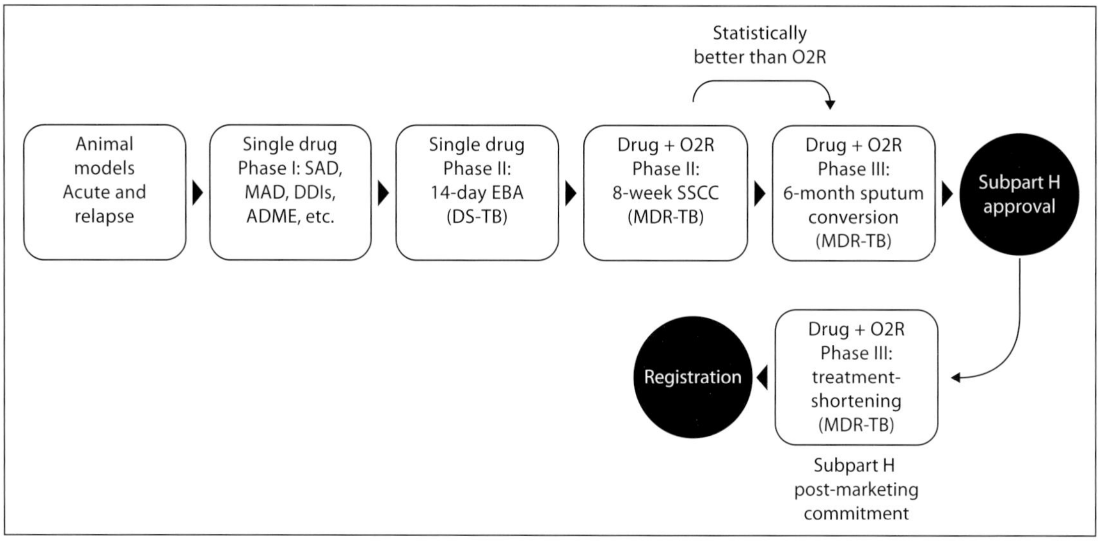


**Fig. 2.** Novel TB drug: schematic of the proposed clinical development path for MDR-TB. See figure 1 for abbreviations and text for detailed explanation.

could lead to successful subpart H accelerated registration in the USA. Accelerated registration should be followed by a phase III programme to evaluate the ability of the novel regimen to improve efficacy and/or shorten MDR-TB treatment relative to the O2R with respect to a stable, microbiological cure end point rather than a 6-month sputum culture conversion rate end point.

To speed the rate of progress in developing improved TB regimens for DS- and MDR-TB, the paradigm for development programmes is now shifting from considering a single new drug as the unit of development and target of registration to defining the whole multidrug combination as the development and registration unit. There are 2 major, underlying factors helping to drive this shift. First, to markedly improve TB treatment, it is likely that entirely new multidrug combinations will be needed – both to shorten and simplify therapy for DS-TB and MDR-TB, and to improve efficacy, safety and tolerability of MDR- and extensively drug-resistant TB therapies. The current drugs have largely not been optimized in terms of their pharmacokinetic properties, safety, tolerability and/or efficacy profiles and therefore all or most will need to be replaced. Second, it is not ethical to test a single drug in TB patients for longer than 14 days, both due to the risk of selecting drug-resistant strains and due to creating an unacceptably long delay in providing the current SOC without an anticipated adequate benefit from the single, new drug. As a result, trying to fulfil the urgent medical need for improved TB treatments would not only take several decades if approached 1 drug at a time, but in many ways is not feasible. Therefore, the TB Alliance and other stakeholders have started pursuing a strategy for the development of improved TB treatments that considers the multidrug regimen to be the unit of development and target of registration.

Figure 3 schematically depicts a possible approach to the development of a novel combination regimen containing more than 1 new chemical entity and composed of drugs without cross-resistance to either isoniazid or rifampicin – that is, a novel regimen that would be appropriate for the treatment of most TB cases, whether considered DS or MDR with respect to current first-line therapy. First, promising 3-drug combinations, with potential to improve both DS- and MDR-TB treatment, are identified by testing in both acute infection and relapse animal models [11, 29]. In parallel with this non-clinical triaging of potential drug combinations, each individual drug is evaluated in a full, investigational new drug-enabling preclinical efficacy, toxicity, absorption/distribution/metabolism/excretion and safety pharmacology programme, and then a robust phase I set of studies to identify the maximally tolerated dose, pharmacokinetic profile and key drug-drug interactions in healthy volunteers. Promising individual drugs are then evaluated for their bactericidal activity in phase II eEBA trials for up to 14 days, to evaluate their safety, tolerability, bactericidal activity and pharmacokinetic profiles in

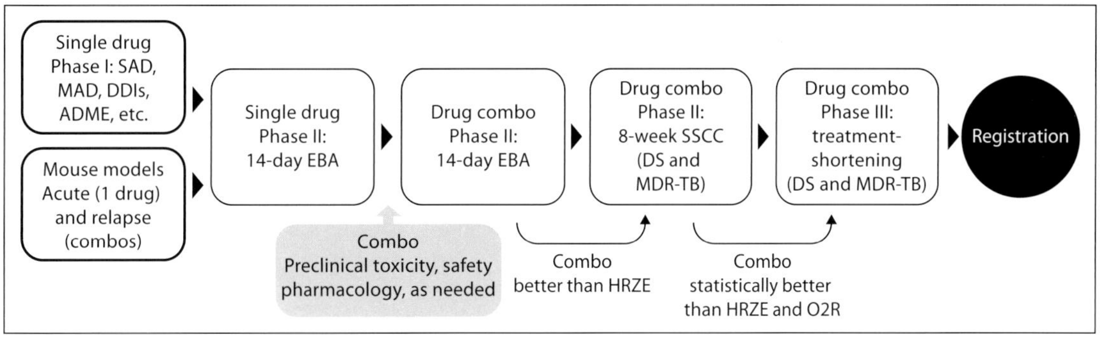


**Fig. 3.** Novel multidrug combinations: schematic of the proposed clinical development path for DS- and MDR-TB. See figure 1 for abbreviations and text for detailed explanation.

pulmonary TB patients. These studies can also be used for dose finding – i.e. to help choose 1 or 2 doses to use in late-stage clinical development.

Next, promising 2- or 3-drug combinations (based on the previous preclinical and clinical results) are evaluated, also in eEBA trials. If appropriate, non-clinical toxicology and safety pharmacology studies of the proposed combination are also conducted. The eEBA studies are not typically powered for statistical comparisons amongst treatment arms, but if a drug combination qualitatively looks as or more efficacious than first-line SOC treatment (HRZE), that combination would be proposed for further development as a regimen potentially appropriate for use in treating both DS- and MDR-TB patients (relative to current first-line treatment). If this candidate combination consists of only a 2-drug combination, and it looks qualitatively as efficacious or more so than HRZE (and demonstrates an appropriate safety and tolerability profile), it would be further evaluated in eEBA trials as a key 'building block' for 3- or 4-drug final combinations. If the promising candidate combination consists of at least 3 drugs, it could be moved next into a trial (or 2 parallel trials) consisting of an 8-week treatment period – compared to HRZE for patients sensitive to first-line SOC treatment and compared to an O2R or even, potentially, historical controls, for MDR-TB patients. These trials could make use of SSCC as a primary efficacy end point. The results of this trial(s) would have to demonstrate superiority to the SOC regimens for the novel combination to be moved into phase III development for DS- and/or MDR-TB treatment. Optimized phase III trial designs for evaluating a novel regimen simultaneously for DS- and MDR-TB are currently under development by the TB Alliance and other stakeholders.

A more automated measure than the labour-intensive SSCC for evaluating drug efficacy in phase II and III trials is currently being evaluated by the TB Alliance in collaboration with Professors Andreas Diacon, Peter Donald and Stefan Maritz in Cape Town, South Africa, as a potential alternate end point: time to positivity in the MGIT liquid culture system. The ability to use this more automated end point would substantially simplify the laboratory support of late-stage TB drug trials.

In 2010, the Bill and Melinda Gates Foundation, the TB Alliance and the Critical Path Institute launched a new initiative, the Critical Path to TB Regimens, to help enable the paradigm shift from registration of single, new TB drugs to development and registration of novel multidrug regimens. This initiative engages drug sponsors, regulators, scientists, clinical researchers, funders and other stakeholders to work together on multiple aspects of regimen development and approval. The range of activities includes building the needed clinical trial capacity, advancing relevant regulatory science (e.g. biomarker qualification, clinical end point definition), facilitating cooperative development programmes by multiple drug sponsors and helping to secure funding. As of this writing, at least 12 sponsors have signed on, the US Food and Drug Administration has expressed support, and other, global regulators are becoming engaged.

## Conclusion

After many decades of relative neglect, substantial efforts are again being made to develop improved TB treatments. To protect successfully developed novel TB drugs against the development of drug resistance, multiple safeguards must be implemented. The new regimens should be manufactured and administered whenever possible as fixed dose combinations and single drugs should be available only under tight regulation and medical supervision. A second, crucial component of introducing novel TB treatment regimens should be developing and implementing rapid, affordable, point of care drug sensitivity tests for both current first-line drugs and for each drug in the proposed novel treatment combination. Coordinated testing, introduction and utilization of a novel regimen with the appropriate drug sensitivity testing will be crucial to ensuring both appropriate patient care and prevention of the rapid development of drug resistance to the next generation of TB drugs.

## References


1 Williams KN, Stover CK, Zhu T, Tasneen R, Tyagi S, Grosset JH, Nuermberger E: Promising antituberculosis activity of the oxazolidinone PNU-100480 relative to that of linezolid in a murine model. Antimicrob Agents Chemother 2009;53:1314–1319.

2 Williams KN, Brickner SJ, Stover CK, Zhu T, Ogden A, Tasneed R, Tyagi S, Grosset JH, Nuermberger EL: Addition of PNU-100480 to first-line drugs shortens the time needed to cure murine tuberculosis. Am J Respir Crit Care Med 2009;180:371–376.

3 Wallis RS, Jakubiec WM, Kumar V, Silvia AN, Paige D, Dimitrova D, Li X, Ladutko L, Campbell S, Friedland G, Mitton-Fry M, Miller PF: Pharmacokinetics and whole-blood bactericidal activity against *Mycobacterium tuberculosis* of single doses of PNU-100480 in healthy volunteers. J Infect Dis 2010;202:745–751.

4 Kumar V, Liu J, Wallis RS, Jakubiec W, Silvia AM, Zhu T, Paige D, Nucci G: Population PK-PD modeling of phase 1 data of PNU-100480 to guide doses for phase 2a study. 3rd Int Workshop Clin Pharmacol TB Drugs, Boston, September 2010.

5 Burman WJ: Rip Van Winkle wakes up: development of tuberculosis treatment in the 21st century. Clin Infect Dis 2010;50:S165–S172.

6 Rosenthal IM, Zheng M, Almeida D, Grosset JH, Nuermberger EL: Isoniazid or moxifloxacin in rifapentine-based regimens for experimental tuberculosis? Am J Respir Crit Care Med 2008;178:989–993.

7 Veziris N, Ibrahim M, Lounis N, Chauffour A, Truffot-Pernot C, Andries K, Jarlier V: A once-weekly R207919-containing regimen exceeds activity of the standard daily regimen in murine tuberculosis. Am J Respir Crit Care Med 2008;179:75–79.

8 Singh R, Manjunatha U, Boshoff HIM, Ha YH, Niyomrattanakit P, Ledwidge R, Dowd CS, Lee IY, Kim P, Zhang L, Kang S, Keller TH, Jiricek J, Barry CE 3rd: PA-824 kills nonreplicating *Mycobacterium tuberculosis* by intracellular NO release. Science 2008;322:1392–1395.

9 Tasneen R, Tyagi S, Williams K, Grosset J, Nuermberger E: Enhanced bactericidal activity of rifampin and/or pyrazinamide when combined with PA-824 in a murine model of tuberculosis. Antimicrob Agents Chemother 2008:52:3664–3668.

10 Nuermberger E, Tyagi S, Tasneed R, Williams KN, Almeida D, Rosenthal I, Grosset JH: Powerful bactericidal and sterilizing activity of a regimen containing PA-824, moxifloxacin, and pyrazinamide in a murine model of tuberculosis. Antimicrob Agents Chemother 2008;52:1522–1524.

11 Ginsberg AM, Laurenzi MW, Rouse DJ, Whitney KD, Spigelman MK: Safety, tolerability, and pharmacokinetics of PA-824 in healthy subjects. Antimicrob Agents Chemother 2009;53:3720–3725.

12 Ginsberg AM, Laurenzi MW, Rouse DJ, Whitney KD, Spigelman MK: Assessment of the effects of the nitroimidazo-oxazine PA-824 on renal function in healthy subjects. Antimicrob Agents Chemother 2009;53:3726–3733.

13 Diacon AH, Dawson R, Hanekom M, Narunsky K, Maritz SJ, Venter A, Donald PR, van Niekerk C, Whitney K, Rouse DJ, Laurenzi MW, Ginsberg AM, Spigelman MK: Early bactericidal activity and pharmacokinetics of PA-824 in smear-positive tuberculosis patients. Antimicrob Agents Chemother 2010;54:3402–3407.

14 Matsumoto M, Hashizume H, Tomishige T, Kawasaki M, Tsubouchi H, Sasaki H, Shimokawa Y, Komatsu M: OPC-67683, a nitro-dihydro-imidazooxazole derivative with promising action against tuberculosis in vitro and in mice. PLoS Med 2006;3:2131–2144.

15 Andries K, Verhasselt P, Guillmont J, Göhlmann HWH, Neefs J-M, Winkler H, van Gestel J, Timmerman P, Zhu M, Lee E, Williams P, de Chaffoy D, Huitric E, Hoffner S, Cambau E, Truffot-Pernot C, Lounis N, Jarlier V: A diarylquinoline drug active on the ATP synthase of *Mycobacterium tuberculosis*. Science 2005;307:223–227.

16 Ibrahim M, Andries K, Lounis N, Chauffour A, Truffot-Pernot C, Jarlier V, Verizis N: Synergistic activity of R207910 combined with pyrazinamide against murine tuberculosis. Antimicrob Agents Chemother 2007;51:1011–1015.

17 Rustomjee R, Diacon AH, Allen J, Venter A, Reddy C, Patientia RF, Mthiyane TCP, De Marez T, van Heeswijk R, Kerstens R, Koul A, de Beule K, Donald PR, McNeeley DF: Early bactericidal activity and pharmacokinetics of the diarylquinoline TMC207 in treatment of pulmonary tuberculosis. Antimicrob Agents Chemother 2008;52:2831–2835.

18 Diacon AH, Pym A, Grobusch M, Patientia R, Rustomjee R, Page-Shipp L, Pistorius C, Krause R, Bogoshi M, Churchyard G, Venter A, Allen J, Palomino JC, de Marez T, van Heeswijk RPG, Lounis N, Meyvisch P, Verbeeck J, Parys W, de Beule K, Andries K, McNeeley D: The diarylquinoline TMC207 for multidrug-resistant tuberculosis. N Engl J Med 2009;360:2397–2405.

19 Protopova M, Hanrahan C, Nikonenko B, Samala R, Chen P, Gearhart J, Einck L, Nacy CA: Identification of a new antitubercular drug candidate, SQ109, from a combinatorial library of 1,2-ethylenediamines. J Antimicrob Chemother 2005;56:968–974.

20 Nikonenko BV, Protopova M, Samala R, Einck L, Nacy CA: Drug therapy of experimental tuberculosis (TB): improved outcome by combining SQ109, a new diamine antibiotic, with existing TB drugs. Antimicrob Agents Chemother 2007;51:1563–1565.

21 Chen P, Gearhart J, Protopova M, Einck L, Nacy CA: Synergistic interactions of SQ109, a new ethylene diamine, with front-line antitubercular drugs in vitro. J Antimicrob Chemother 2006;58:332–337.

22 Reddy VM, Einck L, Andries K, Nacy CA: In vitro interactions between new antitubercular drug candidates SQ109 and TMC207. Antimicrob Agents Chemother 2010;54:2840–2846.

23 Rodriguez JC, Ruiz M, Climent A, Royo G: In vitro activity of four fluoroquinolones against *Mycobacterium tuberculosis*. Int J Antimicrob Agents 2001;17:229–231.

24 Nuermberger EL, Yoshimatsu T, Tyagi S, O'Brien RJ, Vernon AN, Chaisson RE, et al: Moxifloxacin-containing regimen greatly reduces time to culture conversion in murine tuberculosis. Am J Respir Crit Care Med 2003;169:421–426.
25 Burman W, Goldberg S, Johnson JL, et al: Moxifloxacin versus ethambutol in the first 2 months of treatment for pulmonary tuberculosis. Am J Respir Crit Care Med 2006;174:331–338.
26 Rustomjee R, Lienhardt C, Kanyok T, Davies GT, Levin J, Mthiyane T, Reddy C, Sturm AW, Sirgel FA, Allen J, Coleman DJ, Fourie B, Mitchison DA, Gatifloxacin for TB (OFLOTUB) Study Team. A phase II study of the sterilizing activities of ofloxacin, gatifloxacin and moxifloxacin in pulmonary tuberculosis. Int J Tuberc Lung Dis 2008;12:128–138.
27 Conde MB, Efron A, Loredo C, Muzy de Souza GR, Graça NP, Cezar MC, Ram M, Chaudhary MA, Bishai WR, Kritski AL, Chaisson RE: Moxifloxacin versus ethambutol in the initial treatment of tuberculosis: a double-blind, randomized, controlled phase II trial. Lancet 2009;373:1183–1189.
28 Dorman SE, Johnson JL, Goldberg S, Muzanye G, Padayatchi N, Bozeman L, Heilig CM, Bernardo J, Choudhri S, Grosset JH, Guy E, Guyadeen P, Corazon Leus M, Maltas G, Menzies D, Nuermberger EL, Villarino M, Vernon A, Chaisson RE, Tuberculosis Trials Consortium: Substitution of moxifloxacin for isoniazid during intensive phase treatment of pulmonary tuberculosis. Am J Respir Crit Care Med 2009;180:273–280.
29 Nuermberger E: Using animal models to develop new treatments for tuberculosis. Semin Respir Crit Care Med 2008;29:542–551.

Ngozi Erondu
Global Alliance for TB Drug Development
40 Wall Street, 24th Floor
New York, NY 10005 (USA)
E-Mail ngerondu@aol.com

Donald PR, van Helden PD (eds): Antituberculosis Chemotherapy.
Prog Respir Res. Basel, Karger, 2011, vol 40, pp 128–144

# Drug Resistance in *Mycobacterium tuberculosis*: Molecular Mechanisms and Laboratory Susceptibility Testing

Erik C. Böttger

Institut für Medizinische Mikrobiologie, Nationales Zentrum für Mykobakterien, Universität Zürich, Zürich, Schweiz

**Abstract**

Evidence is accumulating that drug resistance in *Mycobacterium tuberculosis* is by no means a homogeneous biological entity. This perception implies limitations of current procedures for in vitro drug susceptibility testing, based on unique but often poorly understood techniques in diagnostic mycobacteriology. The aim of this paper is to briefly review the molecular mechanisms of mycobacterial drug resistance, to critically reflect the principles involved in drug susceptibility testing of *M. tuberculosis* in the diagnostic laboratory and to discuss possible implications for therapy.

Copyright © 2011 S. Karger AG, Basel

Die Philosophen haben die Welt nur verschieden interpretiert, es kommt darauf an, sie zu verändern.

*Karl Marx, Thesen über Feuerbach (1845)*

The treatment of tuberculosis (TB) faces 3 problems: (1) interruption of further transmission, (2) curing of the acute disease and (3) preventing relapse. Anti-TB drugs were first introduced for TB therapy in the 1940s [1, 2]. However, despite a positive initial clinical response, single-drug therapy resulted in the rapid emergence of drug-resistant strains [3]. By combining the 2 anti-TB drugs available at that time – streptomycin (STM) and para-aminosalicylic acid – the emergence of resistance was reduced to approximately 10% [4]. When isoniazid (INH) was introduced in the early 1950s, and combined with STM and para-aminosalicylic acid, this combination effectively prevented the emergence of resistance but required 18 months of treatment to ensure cure of the disease [5]. Subsequently, pyrazinamide (PZA) [6], rifampicin (RIF) [7] and ethambutol (EMB) [8] were introduced (for an overview of anti-TB agents and drug targets, see table 1). Extensive studies were carried out by the British Medical Research Council to define the optimal drug combination and the minimal duration of therapy [9, 10; for a review, see 11, 12]. The outcome consisted of a therapeutic regimen comprised of an initial 2-month treatment with INH, RIF and PZA, followed by a 4-month treatment with INH and RIF. Combination therapy is necessary for the successful treatment of disease and to avoid the emergence of resistance, while a minimum 6-month treatment is required to prevent relapse [13]. This protocol, further developed and now termed standard therapy short course, is still in use today and is recommended with slight modifications (including the addition of EMB or STM) by the International Union against Tuberculosis and Lung Disease, the World Health Organization and the American Thoracic Society. While drug-resistant TB was reported in the past before the emergence of HIV, the increased susceptibility of HIV patients to disease following infection with *Mycobacterium tuberculosis* has contributed greatly to the current situation.

## Genetic Aspects of Drug Resistance

In contrast to other bacterial pathogens, plasmid-mediated mechanisms of resistance are absent in *M. tuberculosis*, but acquired drug resistance is exclusively due to chromosomal alterations such as mutations or deletions. These chromosomal alterations affect either the drug target itself or bacterial enzymes activating/modifying the drug. Drug resistance in *M. tuberculosis* occurs when resistant mutants

**Table 1.** Anti-TB drugs: mechanisms of action and cellular targets

| Drug | Cellular function inhibited | Target |
|---|---|---|
| First-line drugs | | |
| INH | Mycolic acid synthesis | Enoyl reductase |
| RIF | RNA synthesis | RNA polymerase |
| EMB | Arabinogalactan synthesis | Arabinosyl transferase |
| PZA | Unclear | Unclear |
| Second-line drugs | | |
| Quinolones | DNA supercoiling | DNA gyrase |
| Ethionamide | Mycolic acid synthesis | Enoyl reductase |
| STM | Protein synthesis | 30S ribosomal subunit |
| KAN, AMK | Protein synthesis | 30S ribosomal subunit |
| Capreomycin | Protein synthesis | 30S/50S ribosomal subunit |

that are present naturally in the mycobacterial population are selected out by inadequate or interrupted treatment. Mutants resistant to a single drug occur approximately in every $10^{-6}$ to $10^{-8}$ cells [14]. In theory, the effective presence of a mutant which is resistant to 2 drugs would require a population of $10^{12}$–$10^{16}$ mycobacterial cells. This mathematical concept provides the basis for the successful use of combination drug therapy to prevent the emergence of resistance.

During the past 15 years, significant knowledge has been gained concerning the molecular mechanisms of mycobacterial drug resistance [for a review, see 15–17; see also http://www.tbdreamdb.com]. These studies have unequivocally established that the chromosomal loci responsible for the resistance to various drugs are not linked. Thus, clinical poly- or multidrug resistance in *M. tuberculosis* is not due to a single genetic locus, such as upregulation of an efflux pump or induction of a transcriptional regulator, but rather due to an accumulation of multiple different mutations.

In general, there is a clear correlation between the genetic mechanism and the resistance phenotype. Thus, mutations in *rpsL* (STM), *rpoB* (RIF) or 16S ribosomal RNA (KAN, AMK; 2-deoxystreptamine aminoglycosides) are associated with high-level drug resistance, and mutations in *gldB* (STM), *eis* (kanamycin, KAN), and *inhA* (INH) confer a low-level resistance phenotype. Resistance-conferring chromosomal alterations in a drug target gene, as observed in clinical isolates, are highly restricted. Presumably this reflects the in vivo selection for resistance mutations which maintain gene function, readily explaining the predominance of certain resistance mutations, e.g. RpsL 42 Lys→Arg (STM), KatG 315 serine → threonine (INH), 16S rRNA 1408A→G (KAN, amikacin, AMK). In contrast, resistance-conferring chromosomal alterations in genes involved in prodrug conversion, for example *pncA* and *ethA*, often display a wide diversity, indicating that there is little functional constraint as a loss of gene function phenotype is apparently well tolerated [for a review, see 18, 19].

Intuitively, a strain's background – that is, nucleic acid sequence polymorphisms and unknown genetic alterations – would be expected to affect the phenotype of a chromosomal resistance determinant. It is perhaps surprising that the resistance level associated with a defined resistance mutation is a rather stable characteristic. Significant levels of phenotypic heterogeneity for a given resistance mutation have been observed only rarely, for example the *katG* S315T alteration and INH resistance (see below). In addition, resistance to a single drug may involve multiple genetic alterations locating to different genes, as well as multiple genetic alterations within a single gene. Presumably, this accumulation of various resistance mutations, all associated with resistance to a single drug, will either affect (increase) phenotypic resistance [20] or ameliorate the fitness cost associated with a defined resistance mutation [21, 22].

## Principles of Drug Susceptibility Testing in the Laboratory

During the 1950s, the establishment of laboratory methods for *M. tuberculosis* drug susceptibility testing was a tremendous challenge. At that time, when diagnostic procedures for drug susceptibility testing of bacteria were largely unexplored, sensitivity and resistance in *M. tuberculosis* were defined as follows: 'sensitive' strains are those that have never been exposed

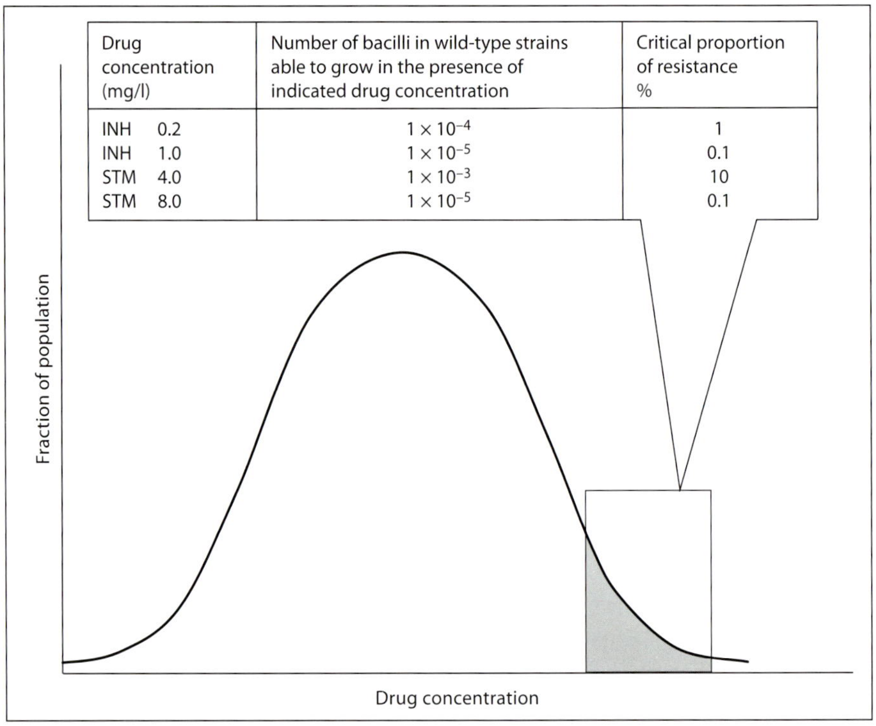


**Fig. 1.** Critical concentration and proportion testing: drug susceptibility of a wild-type bacterial population follows a gaussian distribution.

to anti-TB drugs ('wild' strains); 'resistant' strains are those that differ from sensitive strains in their capacity to grow in the presence of higher concentrations of the drug [23]. Fortuitously, it was found that drug-susceptible strains of *M. tuberculosis* that have not been exposed to anti-TB drugs (wild-type strains) do not exhibit much variation in minimum inhibitory concentrations (MICs) to those drugs. Depending on which laboratory method was used for susceptibility testing, significant differences were found in the drug concentrations which discriminate most efficiently between susceptible wild-type strains and probably resistant strains. For example, with proportion testing of STM a maximum discrimination was achieved with a resistance proportion of 1% on 4 mg/l dihydro-STM, while with the absolute-concentration method maximum discrimination was at 16 μg/ml [23].

Current procedures for drug susceptibility testing of mycobacteria are characterized by 2 peculiarities: (1) the 'critical concentration' and (2) the 'critical proportion' [24]. The drug concentration which categorizes a clinical *M. tuberculosis* isolate as either susceptible or resistant is defined as the concentration that inhibits the growth of wild-type strains, without appreciably affecting the growth of strains with alterations in drug susceptibility – this concentration is termed the 'critical concentration'. Proportion testing in mycobacteriology is based on the observation that '. . . all strains of tuberculosis contain some bacilli that are resistant to antibacillary drugs – in resistant strains the *proportion* of such bacilli is considerably higher than in sensitive strains' [25]. The drug susceptibility of a bacterial wild-type population follows a gaussian distribution. Thus, depending on the drug concentration, a small fraction of the population will show phenotypic resistance (fig. 1). This observation forms the basis for combining proportion testing and 'critical concentration' (table 2).

Standardization of the 'critical concentration' has not been without controversy. For example, the recommended concentrations for EMB underwent adjustments over time [26, 27], not the least because of low interlaboratory reproducibility of EMB susceptibility testing [28]. Most likely, this is due to the very small differences between the concentration used for in vitro drug susceptibility testing and the natural drug susceptibility of wild-type isolates of *M. tuberculosis* (table 3). Thus, minute changes in drug susceptibility will have a major impact on interpretation of in vitro test results, with only a narrow range between the MICs of susceptible isolates and resistant isolates.

Among mycobacteriologists a misperception of 'critical proportion' and clinical resistance frequently prevails. While the critical proportion of cells (subpopulation) able to grow in the presence of the critical concentration is mostly defined as equal or greater than 1% of the population (1 in 100) [24], the frequency of mutational resistance is much lower, approximately $10^{-7}$ (i.e. 0.00001%, or 1 in ten million).

**Table 2.** Critical concentration and critical proportion

| Antimicrobial agent | Critical concentration used for testing, mg/l | Critical proportion, % |
|---|---|---|
| INH | 0.1 | 1 |
| RIF | 1.0 | 1 |
| EMB | 5.0 | 1 |
| PZA | 100 | 10 |

The critical proportion of drug-resistant mutants is defined as proportion of bacilli resistant to the anti-TB drug in vitro, above which a clinical response is unlikely.

**Table 3.** Mycobacterial drug susceptibility testing: the critical concentration (mg/l)

| Antimicrobial agent | MIC of susceptible *M. tuberculosis* | Concentration in serum | Concentration used for testing | |
|---|---|---|---|---|
| | | | low | high |
| INH | 0.05–0.2 | 5–10 | 0.1 | 0.4 |
| RIF | 0.5 | 10 | 1 | – |
| PZA | 20 | 40–50 | 100 | – |
| EMB | 1–5 | 2–5 | 5 | 7.5 |
| Ofloxacin | 0.25–0.5 | 2–10 | 2 | – |
| Ethionamide | 0.5–2.5 | 2–20 | 2.5 | – |
| STM | 0.5–1.0 | 25–50 | 2 | 6 |
| AMK | 0.5–1.0 | 20–40 | 1 | – |
| Capreomycin | 2–5 | 10–30 | 5 | – |

It is, however, the mutational resistance which is responsible for treatment failure and for the emergence of resistance following inappropriate drug regimens. The critical proportion of resistance is a technical term and should not be confused with mutational resistance. In combination with the critical concentration, the critical proportion is a laboratory term used in in vitro drug susceptibility testing to define the epidemiological cut-off.

## Isoniazid

Isonicotinic acid hydrazide (INH) is a highly specific antimycobacterial agent, being exquisitely potent against the *M. tuberculosis* complex. INH is a prodrug which needs to be converted into its active form by the bacterial enzyme KatG, a catalase-peroxidase [29]. Biochemical and genetic studies suggest that activated INH targets InhA [30], an enoyl-acyl carrier protein reductase, which takes part in fatty acid biosynthesis. INH resistance is genetically heterogeneous and may involve mutations in *inhA* and/or *katG* [31–34]. While mutational alterations in *inhA* mainly affect the gene's promoter resulting in InhA overexpression and are associated with low-level resistance to INH, mutations in *katG* confer moderate- to high-level drug resistance (fig. 2). The clinically most prevalent moderate- to high-level resistance mutation is the serine → threonine exchange at amino acid position 315 of KatG; this single genetic alteration accounts for more than 60–80% of INH resistance due to *katG* mutations [35, 36]. Of note, the KatG S315T replacement is associated with a surprisingly heterogeneous phenotype of resistance [37, 38] – all clinical strains with this mutation are able to grow in the presence of at least 1 mg/l INH; however, the exact MIC values may range from 2 to >10 mg/l INH (fig. 3).

More recently, it has been suggested that the strain genetic background may impact on the type of INH resistance mutation associated with a particular isolate, explaining why different phylogenetic lineages of *M. tuberculosis* may be associated with different resistance mutations [39]. However, several words of caution are necessary here. (1)

| Genes involved in resistance | Role in resistance | Phenotypic resistance | Frequency in clinical strains[1] |
|---|---|---|---|
| *katG* | prodrug conversion | moderate- to high-level (>1 mg/l) | 70–80% |
| *inhA* | drug target | low-level (<1 mg/l) | 20–30% |

**a** [1]Frequency based on clinical strains categorized as resistant as per critical concentration testing.

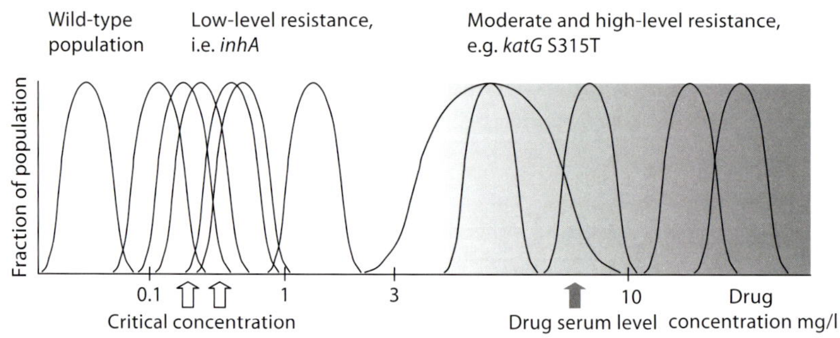


**b**

**Fig. 2.** INH resistance: molecular mechanisms and phenotypic drug susceptibility. **a** Molecular mechanisms and phenotypic resistance level. **b** Schematized changes in drug susceptibility – exemplary gaussian distributions of a population's drug susceptibility.

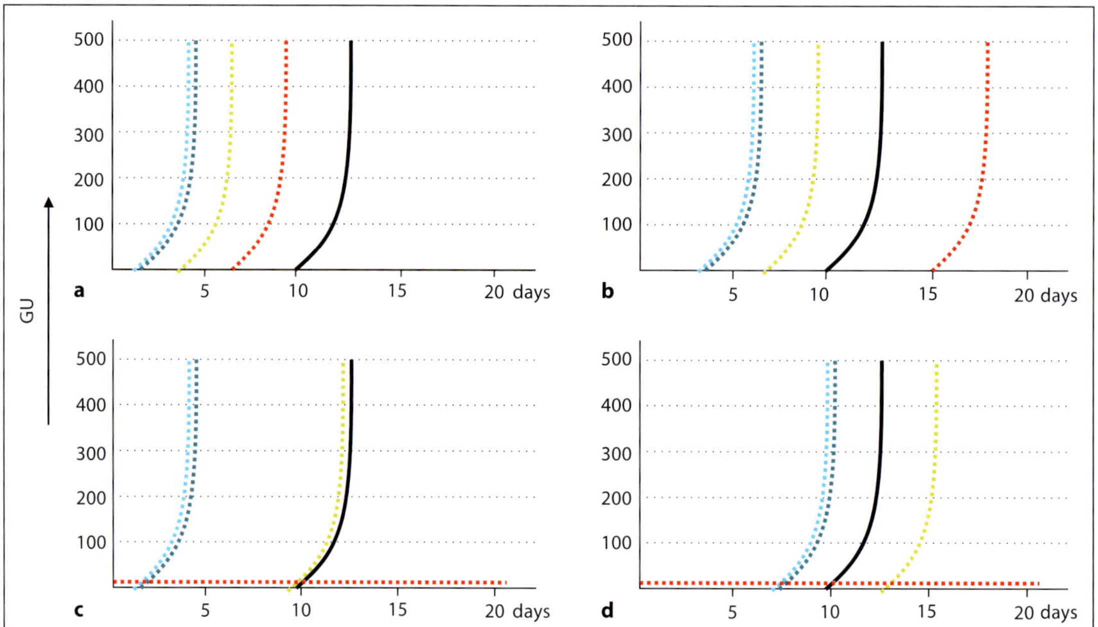


**Fig. 3.** Phenotypic heterogeneity in INH-resistant clinical isolates with the *katG* S315 mutation. Drug susceptibility was determined using MGIT 960 instrumentation equipped with the EpiCenter TBeXiST software. As per proportion testing, the bacterial inoculum for the drug-free growth control is 1% of the inoculum used for the drug-containing vial. The drug-containing vial is incubated an additional 7 days following positivity of the drug-free growth control to facilitate quantitation of resistance, both at a drug concentration and at a population level. The term 'intermediate' indicates that a drug concentration significantly inhibits bacterial growth, although not completely. For example, as indicated in **d**, 3.0 mg/l INH inhibits the growth of more than 99.9% of the population of isolate 176291. Drug concentrations are represented by colours as follows: blue = 0.1 mg/l; green = 1.0 mg/l; yellow = 3.0 mg/l; red = 10.0 mg/l; black = drug-free growth control; GU = growth units. The figure is taken from Springer et al. [38], with permission of the publisher. **a** Isolate 177836: resistant at 0.1, 1.0, 3.0 and 10.0 mg/l. **b** Isolate 186137: resistant at 0.1, 1.0 and 3.0 mg/l and intermediate at 10.0 mg/l. **c** Isolate 186069: resistant at 0.1, 1.0 and 3.0 mg/l and susceptible at 10.0 mg/l. **d** Isolate 176291: resistant at 0.1 and 1.0 mg/l, intermediate at 3.0 mg/l and susceptible at 10.0 mg/l.

**Table 4.** Are different phylogenetic lineages associated with different resistance mutations?

| Study | INH-resistant isolates | Mutation katG | Mutation inhA | No mutation | Laboratory drug susceptibility testing |
|---|---|---|---|---|---|
| New York State, USA [29] | 92 (100) | 51 (55) | 20 (22) | 21 (23) | proportion method 0.1 mg/l |
| | 35 (100) | 2 (6) | 18 (52) | 15 (42) | proportion method <0.4 mg/l |
| | 57 (100) | 49 (86) | 2 (4) | 6 (10) | proportion method >0.4 mg/l |
| Various geographical regions, Russian Federation [37] | 319 (100) | 287 (89) | 3 (1) | 29 (10) | absolute concentration method 1.0 mg/l |

Data are expressed as numbers, with percentages in parentheses.

In vitro laboratory generation of INH-resistant mutants by selection for spontaneous resistance cannot be used to faithfully reconstruct clinical resistance, as the resistant mutants selected in vitro do not reflect the in vivo mechanism of INH resistance [40]. In addition, the unique strain-specific phenotypic heterogeneity for a given INH resistance mutation (see above) points to methodological problems in choosing the appropriate drug concentration for in vitro selection. (2) Strain-specific differences in resistance-associated mutations may reflect geographic-specific differences in the way drug susceptibility testing is performed in the diagnostic laboratory rather than differences in strain genetic background. For example, in one study from New York 20% of INH resistance was associated with mutations in *inhA*, while this was less than 1% in a study from the Russian Federation [34, 41]. However, this difference does not necessarily reflect an impact of a strain genetic background, but more likely differences in drug susceptibly testing (table 4). Thus, in Europe and in North America the established procedure is proportion testing using INH at a concentration of 0.1 mg/l. However, in Russia the established procedure is absolute concentration testing using INH at a concentration of 1.0 mg/l. Limiting the New York study to strains with INH resistance >0.4 mg/l changes the results significantly. Now, the data between the two studies become virtually identical with the vast majority of INH resistance (>85%) due to mutations in *katG*. Mutations in *inhA* are not associated with INH resistance in Russia, presumably not because of differences in strain genetic background, but more likely because of the procedures used in the diagnostic laboratory to define resistance.

## Rifampicin

RIF is not specific for mycobacteria but affects many bacteria by interacting with the RNA polymerase β-subunit and preventing transcription. Clinical RIF resistance is mostly high-level resistance and associated with distinct mutations in *rpoB* [42, 43] (fig. 4). Resistance mutations cluster in a region comprising amino acids 500–540 in RpoB. While there is some heterogeneity in the type of replacement and the position of the amino acid affected, e.g. positions 531 and 526, the 531 serine → leucine replacement is the most prevalent alteration, accounting for more than 50% of clinical RIF resistance.

## Ethambutol

EMB is thought to act on the mycobacterial cell wall, with arabinan synthesis as the primary site of action [44, 45]. As discussed above, drug susceptibility testing for EMB is particularly problematic [27]. Several reasons may account for this, e.g. the bacteriostatic nature of EMB and the reduced activity of the drug in culture medium. Most important, however, is the small difference between the drug concentration used for in vitro drug susceptibility testing and the natural drug susceptibility of wild-type isolates of *M. tuberculosis* (table 3). Thus, minute changes in drug susceptibility will have a major impact on the interpretation of the in vitro test result, with only a narrow range between MICs of susceptible and MICs of resistant isolates of *M. tuberculosis*. Acquired EMB resistance is associated with mutations

| Genes involved in resistance | Role in resistance | Phenotypic resistance | Frequency in clinical strains[1] |
|---|---|---|---|
| *rpoB* | drug target | mostly high-level (>20 mg/l) | > 95% |

**a** [1]Frequency based on clinical strains categorized as resistant as per critical concentration testing.

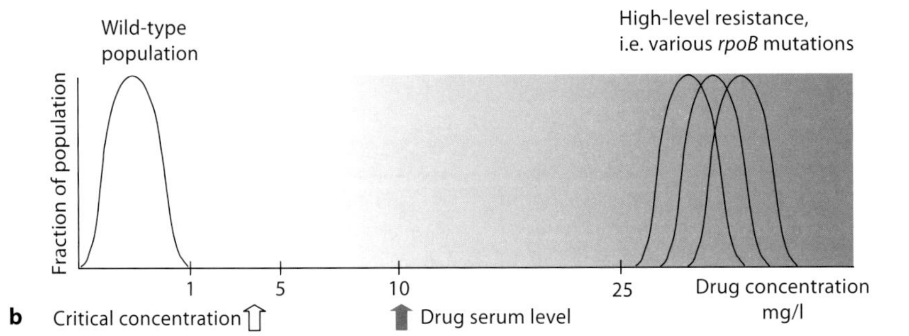


**Fig. 4.** RIF resistance: molecular mechanisms and phenotypic drug susceptibility. **a** Molecular mechanisms and phenotypic resistance levels. **b** Schematized changes in drug susceptibility – exemplary gaussian distributions of a population's drug susceptibility.

| Genes involved in resistance | Role in resistance | Phenotypic resistance | Frequency in clinical strains[1] |
|---|---|---|---|
| *embB* | drug target | low- to moderate-level (<25 mg/l) | >80% |

**a** [1]Frequency based on clinical strains categorized as resistant as per critical concentration testing.

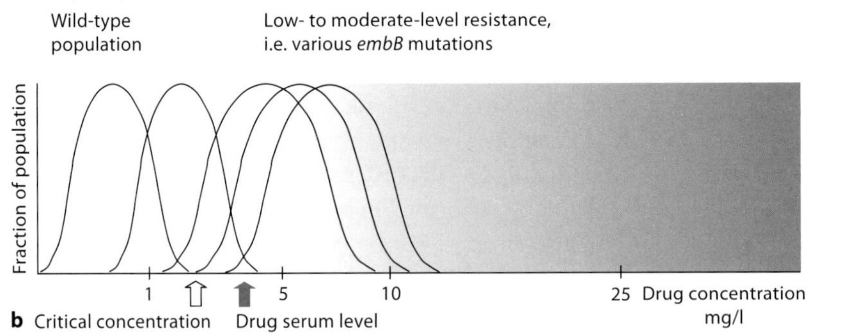


**Fig. 5.** EMB resistance: molecular mechanisms and phenotypic drug susceptibility. **a** Molecular mechanisms and phenotypic resistance levels. **b** Schematized changes in drug susceptibility – exemplary gaussian distributions of a population's drug susceptibility.

in *embB*, in particular codon 306 [46–49]. However, these mutations confer only a small increase in MIC (2- to 4-fold; fig. 5). The clinical implications of laboratory-assessed phenotypic resistance are unclear at present, as is the finding of an *embB* mutation.

## Pyrazinamide

PZA is a nicotinamide analogue, which is converted into its active form by the bacterial pyrazinamidase PncA. While the drug target is still unclear, clinical resistance is mostly associated with various mutations, including non-sense mutations, in *pncA* [50–54]. The testing of PZA is problematic. PZA is a unique and unconventional antibiotic that is not active in vitro under normal culture conditions [55]. A paradox limiting analysis of PZA resistance is that the critical concentration used for in vitro testing largely exceeds the drug concentrations present in vivo (table 3). While the conditions established for PZA testing in vitro are highly artificial, they allow for recognition of resistance – in particular in combination with a determination of pyrazinamidase activity. The quantitative analysis of resistance levels, for example low-level versus high-level resistance, is not possible with the procedures currently in place. However, as PZA is ineffective against *Mycobacterium bovis*, which is naturally *pncA*–, it has to be assumed that *pncA* negativity confers high-level drug resistance – at least in clinical terms.

| Genes involved in resistance | Role in resistance | Phenotypic resistance | Frequency in clinical strains[1] |
|---|---|---|---|
| *gyrA* | drug target | moderate-level (>1 <10 mg/l) | >80% |

**a** [1]Frequency based on clinical strains categorized as resistant as per critical concentration testing.

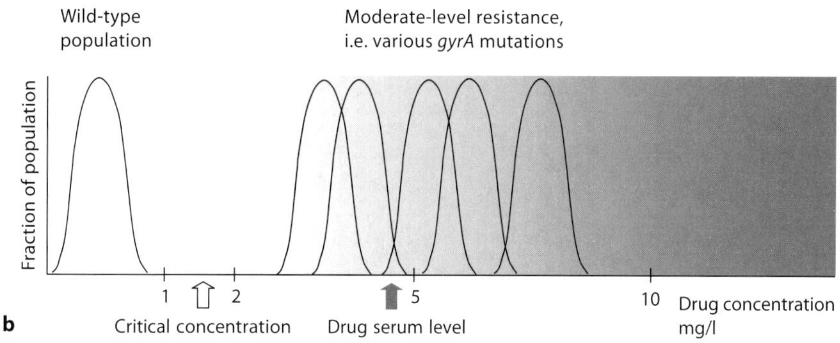


**Fig. 6.** Fluoroquinolone resistance: molecular mechanisms and phenotypic drug susceptibility. **a** Molecular mechanisms and phenotypic resistance levels. **b** Schematized changes in drug susceptibility – exemplary gaussian distributions of a population's drug susceptibility.

## Fluoroquinolones

Fluoroquinolones target bacterial topo-isomerase and are broad-spectrum antibacterial agents. Mutations in DNA gyrase, a type II DNA topo-isomerase, confer quinolone resistance in *M. tuberculosis*. DNA gyrase is made up of 2 A and 2 B subunits encoded by *gyrA* and *gyrB*. Fluoroquinolone resistance in *M. tuberculosis* is mostly associated with mutations in the quinolone resistance-determining region of *gyrA*, in particular involving codons 90 and 94 [56–59]. Corresponding mutations confer a 5- to 10-fold increase in MIC [57, 58, our unpubl. observations] (fig. 6). Given the drug concentrations present in vivo (table 3) and that *M. tuberculosis* is intrinsically not particularly susceptible to quinolones [60], these mutations are presumably sufficient to confer clinical resistance to ofloxacin. However, circumstantial evidence has been provided that, owing to more favourable MICs associated with the corresponding mutations, the later-generation fluoroquinolones, such as moxifloxacin, may still improve treatment outcome [60b, 60c]. While double mutations are quite rare, e.g. Ala 90 → Val plus Ala 94 → Asn [59], mixed resistant populations within an individual patient are observed [unpubl. observations]. Most likely, this finding indicates emerging acquired resistance reflecting the stochasticity of resistance mutations, with individual resistance mutations being largely functionally equivalent with respect to both resistance level conferred and fitness cost associated [for similar phenomena in macrolide-resistant *Mycobacterium avium*, see 61].

There is a word of caution necessary: besides the problematic issue of the intrinsically rather low quinolone susceptibility of *M. tuberculosis* with the potential of rapid resistance development, the widespread use of quinolones for long-term treatment of TB in developing countries may lead to a build-up of resistance to these drugs in other pathogens of major significance, such as *Salmonella* or *Escherichia coli*. This is a lesson to be learnt from the past when these drugs were used for long-term treatment of patients with chronic urinary tract problems – not only did quinolone resistance in *E. coli*, which was once thought to be impossible, emerge under these circumstances, but corresponding isolates are now present in the community. The cost-benefit ratio of strategies for combating TB should be carefully weighed as focussing too much on one aspect may have undesirable consequences in others.

## Ethionamide

Ethionamide (ETH) is a structural analogue of INH used as a second-line drug. ETH is thought to inhibit mycolic acid biosynthesis in *M. tuberculosis*. ETH and INH share a common drug target, InhA [30]. Like INH, ETH is a prodrug which needs to be activated by a bacterial enzyme. However, in this case it is not KatG but EthA [62, 63]. Similar to INH, resistance-conferring mutations either affect the gene encoding the activating enzyme *ethA* or the gene encoding the putative drug target *inhA* [64]. Loss-of-function mutations in *ethA* confer resistance to ETH but not to INH, mutations in *inhA* (overexpression) confer significant ETH resistance and low-level resistance to INH. The *ethA* and *inhA* mutational alterations typically confer

| Genes involved in resistance | Role in resistance | Phenotypic resistance | Frequency in clinical strains[1] |
|---|---|---|---|
| *inhA* | drug target | low- to moderate-level | approx. 30–50% |
| *ethA* | prodrug conversion | moderate- to high-level | approx. 30–50% |

**a** [1]Frequency based on clinical strains categorized as resistant as per critical concentration testing.

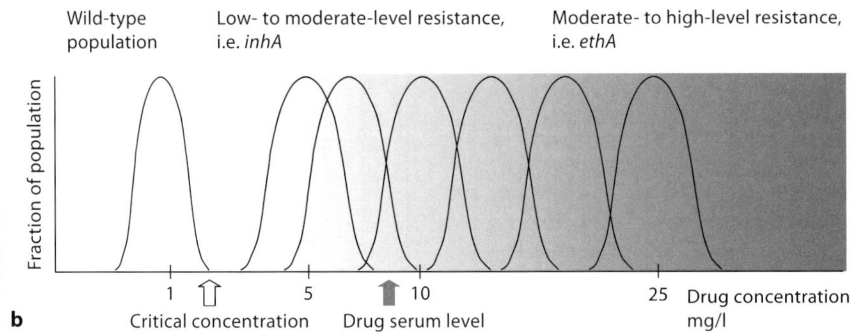


**b**

**Fig. 7.** ETH resistance: molecular mechanisms and phenotypic drug susceptibility. **a** Molecular mechanisms and phenotypic resistance levels. **b** Schematized changes in drug susceptibility – exemplary gaussian distributions of a population's drug susceptibility.

moderate (and presumably high) levels of drug resistance (fig. 7). However, a high-level resistance phenotype is difficult to assess, as ETH is barely soluble at concentrations higher than 20 mg/l.

## Streptomycin, Amikacin, Kanamycin and Capreomycin

Protein synthesis is one of the most complex of the basic cell-biological processes. The ribosome is the target for many broad-spectrum antibacterial agents with many of these having potent antimycobacterial activity, e.g. STM, AMK and KAN. In general, these compounds bind to the nucleic acid part of the ribosome, i.e. the rRNAs, and interfere with key steps in translation, such as decoding or translocation. Sensitivity to drugs that act by inhibiting protein synthesis is frequently dominant over antibiotic resistance. Most eubacteria carry several rRNA operons in their genome; correspondingly, mutations in rRNA are rarely associated with drug resistance [65]. It was in the early 90s that mutations in rRNA were first observed to confer drug resistance in clinical pathogens, i.e. *M. tuberculosis* [20, 66, 67], *M. avium*, *M. intracellulare* [61, 68], *M. chelonae* and *M. abscessus* [69]. This is largely due to the fact that these organisms carry a single set of rRNA genes in their chromosome [70, 71]. Under these circumstances normally recessive mutations can exert a dominant phenotype, allowing clinical resistance to be conferred by mutations in genes coding for rRNA.

### Streptomycin

STM, discovered by Albert Sachs and Selman Waksman in 1944 [1], was the first antibiotic active against the aetiological agent of TB, *M. tuberculosis*, and was used in control programmes for many years. However, as a result of the availability of other drugs, in particular INH, RIF and PZA, STM usage declined in industrialized countries. Nevertheless, STM is still a first-line drug in the treatment of TB in certain geographic regions.

STM is an aminocyclitol glycoside antibiotic which interferes with prokaryotic protein synthesis. At the phenotypic level STM resistance is heterogeneous and involves low-level, moderate-level and high-level drug resistance – distinct phenotypic resistance levels are associated with distinct chromosomal mutations [20, 66, 72–76] (fig. 8). Clinically, the most prevalent resistance mutation is the Lys→Arg alteration at amino acid position 42 of RpsL – this mutation alone accounts for 80–90% of clinically relevant resistance (for the discussion of laboratory vs. clinical resistance see below).

### Amikacin, Kanamycin and Capreomycin

AMK and KAN are classical aminoglycosides with broad-spectrum antibacterial activity. These aminoglycosides target the ribosome by binding to the decoding A site of the small ribosomal subunit and they affect protein synthesis by inducing codon misreading and by inhibiting translocation of the

| Genes involved in resistance | Role in resistance | Phenotypic resistance | Frequency in clinical strains[1] |
|---|---|---|---|
| *rpsL* | drug target | high-level (>20 mg/l) | >70% |
| *rrs* | drug target | moderate-level (>5 <20 mg/l) | <10% |
| *gldB* | drug target | low-level (>2 <10 mg/l) | approx. 20% |

**a** [1]Frequency based on clinical strains categorized as resistant as per critical concentration testing.

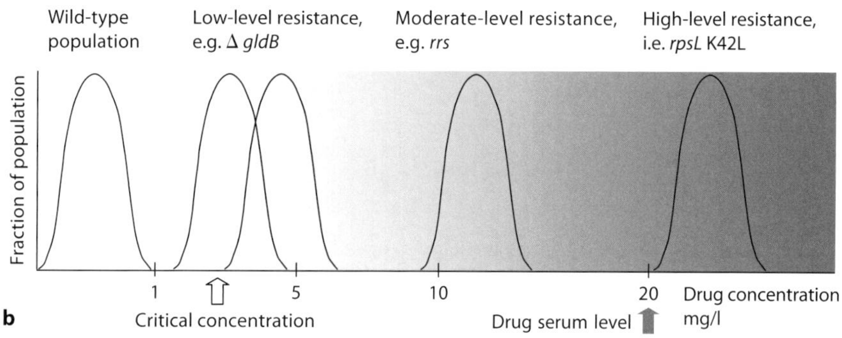


**b**

**Fig. 8.** STM resistance: molecular mechanisms and phenotypic drug susceptibility. **a** Molecular mechanisms and phenotypic resistance levels. **b** Schematized changes in drug susceptibility – exemplary gaussian distributions of a population's drug susceptibility.

transfer-messenger RNA complex. Resistance to these compounds is heterogeneous and involves low-level, moderate-level and high-level drug resistance. Distinct phenotypic resistance levels are associated with different chromosomal mutations [22, 67, 77–80] (fig. 9). With the exception of low-level KAN resistance due to *eis* overexpression [81, 82], these 2 compounds in general show cross-resistance. Clinically, the adenine → guanine replacement at 16S rRNA position 1408 is the most prevalent resistance mutation, accounting for more than 95% of clinically relevant resistance [22].

Capreomycin (CAP), a cyclic peptide antibiotic, is particularly active against mycobacteria [83]. CAP like the structurally similar compound viomycin inhibits bacterial growth by blocking ribosomal protein synthesis [84]. CAP/viomycin bind at the interface between helix 44 of the small ribosomal subunit and helix 69 of the large ribosomal subunit [85, 86]. The drug binding site of these compounds in part overlaps that of AMK and KAN involving residues 1491, 1492 and 1493 of the 16S rRNA. The same mutational alterations in 16S rRNA H44 involved in resistance to AMK/KAN may also confer resistance to CAP. Thus, there is a certain degree of cross-resistance [79, 80, 87–89]. 16S rRNA A1408G mediates high-level resistance to AMK/KAN, but low-level resistance to CAP; conversely, mutations C1409U and G1491U confer moderate levels of resistance to AMK/KAN and high levels of resistance to CAP [22; unpubl. observations]. In addition, and unique to CAP, various loss-of-function mutations in rRNA methylase TlyA confer low-level CAP resistance [90].

## Diagnostic Drug Susceptibility Testing

The 'gold standard' in bacteriology for drug susceptibility testing is MIC testing. This procedure is defined by 2 elements: (1) the drug concentration – a series dilution is used to titrate the minimal amount of the drug needed to inhibit bacterial growth in vitro; (2) the inoculum – the inoculum and the test conditions are chosen such that a single resistant cell in the population tested (1 in $10^5$ bacteria) is sufficient to give a resistant test result.

In contrast, in the diagnostic mycobacteriology laboratory, proportion testing and mostly a single drug concentration – the 'critical concentration' – are used to study drug susceptibility and to categorize a clinical isolate of *M. tuberculosis* as susceptible or resistant [24]. Note that the procedure in place defines only 2 possible test outcomes: susceptible or resistant. The 'critical concentration' in part bears little relationship to the drug concentrations which are present in vivo in the patient (table 3). For example, the in vivo concentrations for STM are 10- to 20-fold higher compared to the 'critical concentration'. When we studied the mechanisms of STM resistance in *M. tuberculosis* in the early 1990s [72], we made the following observations (fig. 9): (1) there is a strict correlation between the molecular mechanism of resistance and the phenotypic resistance level conferred; thus, mutations in *rpsL* mediate high-level drug resistance and those in rRNA confer moderate levels of resistance; (2) a significant part of drug-resistant clinical strains exhibits a low-level

| Genes involved in resistance | Role in resistance | Phenotypic resistance | Frequency in clinical strains[1] |
|---|---|---|---|
| *rrs* A1408G | drug target | high-level (>20 mg/l) | >70% |
| *rrs* C1409U | drug target | low- to moderate-level (>5 <20 mg/l) | <5% |
| *rrs* G1491U | drug target | moderate- to high-level (>5 mg/l) | < 5% |
| *eis*[2] | drug | low-level (>1 <10 mg/l) | approx. 20% |

[1]Frequency based on clinical strains categorized as resistant as per critical concentration testing
[2]Note that *eis* only modifies KAN, but not AMK [82]; the molecular mechanisms involved in low-level AMK resistance still need to be identified.

**a**

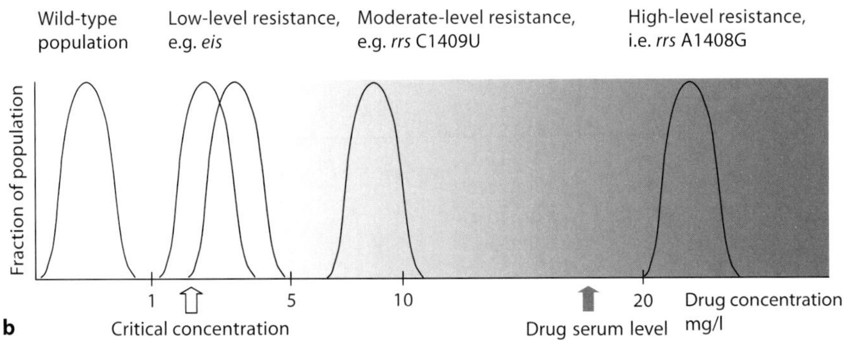


**b**

**Fig. 9.** AMK/KAN resistance: molecular mechanisms and phenotypic drug susceptibility. **a** Molecular mechanisms and phenotypic resistance levels. **b** Schematized changes in drug susceptibility – exemplary gaussian distributions of a population's drug susceptibility.

resistance phenotype. Here, no mutational target alteration in either *rpsL* or *rrs* is present. These observations were the first to unequivocally demonstrate that low-level resistance in clinical isolates of *M. tuberculosis* is a genetic entity on its own, distinct from moderate- or high-level drug resistance. Similar low-level resistance phenotypes, each associated with a unique genetic alteration, have been identified e.g. for INH and KAN.

Different levels of phenotypic resistance are in general not taken into account when using critical concentrations for mycobacterial in vitro drug susceptibility testing. Regardless of whether high-level, moderate-level or low-level drug resistance is present, and as a result of the procedure used, any corresponding isolate is categorized uniformly as resistant in the diagnostic laboratory. However, the biological implications of low-level versus high-level drug resistance are different for a number of reasons. (1) In vivo drug concentrations need to be taken into account, i.e. the resistance phenotype determined in vitro should be related to the drug concentrations which can be achieved in vivo. In bacteriology, this is commonly addressed by the definition of clinical break points. (2) From experience in the treatment of endocarditis, the problem of low-level resistance is well known. Streptococci naturally exhibit a low-level resistance phenotype to aminoglycosides. This is due to impermeability of their cell wall; the drug target itself – the ribosome – is susceptible. In the presence of drugs which target cell wall synthesis, such as β-lactams, aminoglycosides become bactericidal. The current perception is that β-lactams interfere with the integrity of the cell wall allowing aminoglycosides to penetrate and to reach their target.

While it is feasible to define the MIC distributions based on laboratory data, caution is necessary when attempting to define the clinical break point on the basis of pharmacokinetic (PK) and pharmacodynamic (PD) calculations and Monte Carlo simulations. The clinical break point is the quantitative MIC corresponding to clinical resistance, i.e. treatment failure/poor outcome. Laboratory MIC data and PK modelling can be used to calculate PK/PD characteristics and to provide measures of drug bioavailability, such as area under the curve over MIC, the maximum concentration over MIC and the time above MIC. However, while these PK/PD characteristics allow to tentatively suggest break points, they cannot be directly linked to clinical outcome. In addition, significant differences in calculated PK/PD properties may exist for different clinically effective TB drugs [91, 92]. An issue to be considered is that TB chemotherapy is a combination therapy involving compounds, which in part act in additive/synergistic fashion including agents targeting cell wall synthesis. If, for example, the antibacterial effects of a 2-drug regimen are additive, the MIC values decrease by half as compared with the MIC of each drug alone. If the antibacterial effect is synergistic, the MIC would be one fourth of each drug alone. In as much as PK/PD considerations are relevant, a logical consequence is that compounds with favourable PK/PD characteristics, i.e. high in vivo drug concentrations compared to the MIC, should be more active than compounds with a small difference. Along these lines of thought, the aminoglycosides STM and AMK/KAN should be equivalent, but – most likely – superior to CAP (table 3).

## Clinical Implications of Drug Resistance

The definition of drug resistance in mycobacteriology dates back to 1962: 'Resistance is defined as a decrease in sensitivity of sufficient degree to be reasonably certain that the strain concerned is different from a sample of wild strains of human type that have never come into contact with the drug. . . This definition is based on the laboratory response; strains that are resistant in this sense do not *necessarily* fail to respond' [23]. Thus, rather than based on clinical outcome, this definition is epidemiological and corresponds to what is defined as epidemiological cut-off. As early as 1969 the prognostic significance of in vitro determined drug resistance was found to be limited. 'There is evidence that the presence of resistance to a single drug has little or no effect on the outcome of treatment with the three drugs isoniazid, streptomycin, and para-amino salicylic acid. Furthermore, even in the presence of primary resistance to 2 first-line drugs, a bacteriological response is not infrequently obtained with the 3-drug regimen' [25].

For INH, a significant fraction of clinical TB isolates categorized as resistant in the diagnostic laboratory exhibits only a low-level resistant phenotype [93]. While the use of INH for the treatment of INH-resistant TB has been discussed controversially [94–96], several studies have demonstrated a benefit of adding INH to treatment regimens of INH-resistant TB [97–99]. A successful treatment outcome despite a resistant phenotype – as determined by routine drug susceptibility testing – most likely reflects limitations of the procedures used to determine drug susceptibility, and indicates that low-level drug resistance may not correspond to clinical resistance [93, 100]. The National Committee for Clinical Laboratory Standards subcommittee has incorporated parts of these considerations in its guidelines. 'In the case of isoniazid, if an isolate is resistant to the critical concentration of 0.1 μg/ml but susceptible to the higher concentration of 0.4 μg/ml, the following comment should be given – the test results indicate low-level resistance to isoniazid: some evidence suggests that patients infected with corresponding strains may benefit from continuing therapy with isoniazid' [101].

Limitations in mycobacterial drug susceptibility testing were noted already in the early 1960s when the principles of the current procedures were established. 'We consider that the best type of sensitivity test is a fully quantitative determination in which the organisms' capability of growth on medium containing a wide range of drug concentrations is known. This type of test would provide full information on the degree of resistance. However, since such a test requires large amounts of medium and is time-consuming, it cannot be recommended as a routine procedure' [24]. As discussed above, the evidence is overwhelming that the term 'resistance' in *M. tuberculosis* is by no means a simple dichotomy, but quite heterogeneous and composed of low-level, moderate-level and high-level drug resistance. This presumably has important biological implications. It is conceivable that low-level drug resistance in part does not correspond to clinical resistance; conversely, in the presence of a high-level resistant phenotype the drug is presumably of little, if any, clinical benefit. While low-level resistance may not correspond to clinical resistance, the failure to appropriately recognize high-level drug resistance may result in the build-up of further resistance. The clinical implications of moderate levels of resistance are less clear and need to be addressed in future studies. However, the conclusion is inescapable: changes in our means of drug susceptibility testing are required to address these issues.

## Quantitative Drug Susceptibility Testing

With the global rise in multidrug-resistant strains, there is an increasing need to determine susceptibility to first- and second-line anti-TB agents precisely. Treatment of patients with drug-resistant TB should be based on reliable and quantitative measures of susceptibility testing, a cornerstone for preventing further amplification of resistance and for optimally exploiting available compounds. Detailed knowledge of quantitative drug resistance may guide empirical treatment of drug-resistant TB, e.g. addressing whether and when to add second-line drugs. A fundamental drawback to this strategy is that even in the developed countries only a limited panel of anti-TB drug concentrations is tested, leaving the exact resistance levels of clinical *M. tuberculosis* isolates vestigial.

In principle, automated systems for cultural propagation of mycobacteria have the potential to meet the challenge of

**Table 5.** Suggested recommendations for quantitative drug susceptibility testing based on TBeXiST-equipped MGIT 960

| |
|---|
| INH<br>• 0.1 mg/l is used for screening<br>• 1.0 mg/l is used to separate low (0.1 R, 1.0 S) from moderate (1.0 R, 10.0 S) resistance<br>• 10.0 mg/l is used to recognize high-level drug resistance<br>• test results R at 1.0 mg/l and S at 10.0 mg/l need further clinical data for interpretation<br>• 1.0 mg/l presumably is the most important concentration to test<br>• mutations in *inhA* typically lead to low-level resistance (0.1 R, 1.0 S)<br>• mutations in *katG* result in R at 1.0 mg/l and show varying test results at 3.0 mg/l and 10.0 mg/l |
| RIF<br>• 1.0 mg/l is used for screening<br>• 10.0 mg/l is used to recognize high-level drug resistance<br>• most, if not all, mutations in *rpoB* are associated with R >50.0 mg/l (high-level drug resistance) |
| EMB<br>• 5.0 mg/l is used for screening<br>• 25.0 mg/l is used to recognize high-level drug resistance<br>• strains with mutations in *embB* are mostly, if not always, susceptible or intermediate at 25.0 mg/l |
| STM<br>• 1.0 mg/l is used for screening<br>• 4.0 mg/l is used to separate low (1.0 R, 4.0 S) from moderate (1.0 R, 4.0 R, 20.0 S) resistance<br>• 20.0 mg/l is used to recognize high-level drug resistance<br>• mutations in *rspL* are associated with high-level resistance (>20.0 mg/l)<br>• good correlation between genotype and phenotype |
| AMK<br>• 1.0 mg/l is used for screening<br>• 4.0 mg/l is used to separate low (1.0 R, 4.0 S) from moderate (1.0 R, 4.0 R, 20.0 S) resistance<br>• 20.0 mg/l is used to recognize high-level drug resistance<br>• mutation at *rrs* position 1408 (A→G) results in high-level resistance (>20.0 mg/l)<br>• good correlation between genotype and phenotype |
| ETH<br>• 2.5 mg/l is used for screening<br>• additional testing at 12.5 mg/l<br>• mutations in *inhA* (C15T) may show phenotypic variability: unanimously R at 2.5 mg/l and 5.0 mg/l; I or R at 12.5 mg/l<br>• mutations in *ethA* are mostly R at 12.5 mg/l |
| Ofloxacin<br>• 0.5 mg/l is used for screening<br>• additional testing at 2.0 and 10.0 mg/l<br>• mutations in *gyrA* are R at 0.5 and 2.0 mg/l and mostly S at 10.0 mg/l |

R = Resistant; S = susceptible; I = intermediate.

precise determinations of drug resistance levels with reasonable labour input. Since 2004 we have implemented measures of quantitative drug susceptibility testing [37]. More recently, we have adopted a fully automated platform for this purpose by combining the liquid MGIT 960 culture instrumentation with a software developed by the manufacturer according to our specifications, i.e. the EpiCenter TBeXiST module [38]. In this instrumentation, a fluorescence-based oxygen sensor is used for growth detection. The general principle of proportion testing is maintained, i.e. the inoculum for the drug-free growth control is 1% of the inoculum used for the drug-containing vial. To categorize a test result the terms 'resistant', 'susceptible' and 'intermediate' are used [38]. The term 'intermediate' has been defined to categorize a test result where a given drug concentration significantly inhibits bacterial growth, although not completely. An example is given in figure 3. Conditions proposed for semiquantitative testing and suggested criteria for interpretation are summarized in table 5. The procedure developed provides a fully automated walk-away system for semiquantitative drug susceptibility testing of *M. tuberculosis* equipped with an expert system for interpretation which can readily be implemented in any specialized laboratory. In principle, the procedure developed also offers the possibility to identify mixed populations ('heteroresistance'), e.g. a mixture of wild-type and resistant mutants [102]. Corresponding attempts are facilitated by the use of various inocula for the drug-free control, as this allows to define the fraction of resistant mutants more precisely. Note that the terms 'intermediate' and 'heteroresistance' define 2 entirely different issues and must not be confused: intermediate drug susceptibility refers to reduced drug susceptibility of the population, i.e. the population is homogeneous; heteroresistance refers to a mixture of susceptible wild-type and resistant mutant populations, i.e. the population is heterogeneous, as may be observed when resistance is acquired under therapy or in case of mixed infections. When using the proportion method (i.e. the inoculum for the drug-free growth control is 1% of that used for the drug-containing vial) any heteroresistance >1% (resistant mutant vs. susceptible wild type) may be detected.

The emergence and rise of drug-resistant TB urgently requires means to make optimal use of available drugs. The consequences of erratic drug susceptibility testing are particularly severe in terms of treatment options for apparent multidrug-resistant or extensively drug-resistant TB. Following 40 years of proportion-based testing at critical concentrations, and in view of the techniques available today, it is time to adapt mycobacterial drug susceptibility testing to standard bacteriology procedures. Whilst critical concentration testing is appropriate for screening, it should be complemented by measures of quantitative drug susceptibility in case of resistant test results, in particular for those drugs where heterogeneity in phenotypic resistance is frequently present (low-, moderate-, high-level resistance), such as INH, STM and AMK/KAN. The widespread implementation of standardized protocols for quantitative drug susceptibility testing of both first-line and second-line drugs will be the most important prerequisite to correlate data from quantitative resistance testing with clinical outcome and to address the biological relevance of low and moderate drug resistance. Hopefully, this will allow the assembly of available compounds into effective regimens to fully exploit their potential in the treatment of what is currently perceived as drug-resistant TB. Given the limited number of drugs available for the management of extensively drug-resistant TB, it is essential to take advantage of those that could possibly be used in a multidrug regimen to treat a significant proportion of corresponding cases.

## Acknowledgements

I apologize to all those colleagues whose work could not be cited due to space limitations. I am indebted to my coworkers and collaborators, with whom I had the privilege to share ideas and views. I thank Susanna Salas for help with the manuscript. I hasten to give credit to Georges Canetti. His ideas, as brilliantly summarized in the J. Burns Amberson lecture [103], are among the most thoughtful and incisive intellectual contributions to the field, which have largely influenced my perceptions and ways of thinking. In contrast to currently advocated mechanistic studies which are rather simplistic and greatly overestimated in today's world of science, Canetti's thoughts exemplify what is at the heart of any scientific endeavour – careful observation combined with intellectual reflection to precisely define what the problem is about. Studies conducted in my laboratory have been supported by the German Research Council, the Bundesministerium für Forschung und Technologie (Germany), the European Commission, the Swiss National Research Foundation, the Bundesamt für Gesundheit (Switzerland), the University of Zurich, the Niedersächsischer Verein zur Bekämpfung der Tuberkulose (Germany), and the UBS Optimus Foundation (Switzerland).

## References

1 Schatz A, Bugie E, Waksman SA: Substance exhibiting activity against Gram-positive and Gram-negative bacteria. Proc Soc Exp Biol Med 1944;55:66–69.
2 Lehman J: Para-aminosalicylic acid in the treatment of tuberculosis. Lancet 1946;250:15–16.
3 Pyle MM: Relative numbers of resistant tubercule bacilli in sputa of patients before and during treatment with streptomycin. Proc Mayo Clin 1947;22:465–473.
4 Medical Research Council: Treatment of pulmonary tuberculosis with streptomycin and para-amino salicylic acid. Br Med J 1950;ii:1073–1085.
5 Medical Research Council: Various combinations of isoniazid with streptomycin or with PAS in the treatment of pulmonary tuberculosis. Br Med J 1955;i:435–445.
6 Yeager R, Monroe WE, Dessaus FI: Pyrazinamide (aldinamide) in the treatment of pulmonary tuberculosis. Am Rev Tuberc 1952;65:523–546.
7 Maggi NC, Pasqualucci CR, Ballota R, Sensi P: Rifampicin: a new orally active rifamycin. Chemotherapia 1966;11:285–292.
8 Thomas JP, Baughn CO, Wilkinson RG, Shephard RG: A new synthetic compound with antituberculous activity in mice: ethambutol (dextro-2,2'-(ethylenediimino)-di-L-butanol). Am Rev Respir Dis 1961;83:891–893.
9 British Medical Research Council: Controlled clinical trial of short-course (6 months) regimens of chemotherapy for treatment of pulmonary tuberculosis. Lancet 1972;i:1072–1085.
10 British Thoracic Association: A controlled trial of six month chemotherapy in pulmonary tuberculosis: second report results during the 24 months after the end of chemotherapy. Am Rev Respir Dis 1982;126:460–462.

11 Mitchison DA: Mechanisms of the action of drugs in short-course chemotherapy. Bull Int Union Tuberc 1985;60:36–40.
12 Fox W, Ellard GA, Mitchison DA: Studies on the treatment of tuberculosis undertaken by the British Medical Research Council tuberculosis units, 1946–1986, with relevant subsequent publications. Int J Tuberc Lung Dis 1999;10(suppl 2):S231–S279.
13 Connolly LE, Edelstein PH, Ramakrishnan L: Why is long-term therapy required to cure tuberculosis? PLoS Med 2007;4:e120.
14 David HL: Probability distribution of drug-resistant mutants in unselected populations of *Mycobacterium tuberculosis*. Appl Microbiol 1970;20:810–814.
15 Ramaswamy S, Musser JM: Molecular genetic basis of antimicrobial agent resistance in *Mycobacterium tuberculosis*: 1998 update. Tuberc Lung Dis 1998;79:3–29.
16 Wade MM, Zhang Y: Mechanisms of drug resistance in *Mycobacterium tuberculosis*. Front Biosci 2004;9:975–994.
17 Pym AS, Cole ST: Mechanisms of drug resistance in *Mycobacterium tuberculosis;* in Wax RG, Lewis K, Salyers AA, Taber H (eds): Bacterial Resistance to Antimicrobials, ed 2. Boca Raton, CRC Press-Taylor & Francis Group, 2008, pp 313–342.
18 Böttger EC: Mechanisms of mycobacterial drug resistance: implications for treatment and prevention strategies. Chemotherapy 2006;15:23–28.
19 Böttger EC, Springer B: Tuberculosis: drug resistance, fitness and strategies for global control. Eur J Pediatr 2008;167:141–148.
20 Meier A, Kirschner P, Bange FC, Vogel U, Böttger EC: Genetic alterations in streptomycin-resistant *Mycobacterium tuberculosis*: mapping of mutations conferring resistance. Antimicrob Agents Chemother 1994;38:228–233.
21 Sherman DR, Mdluli K, Hickey MJ, Arain TM, Morris SL, Barry CE, Stover CK: Compensatory *ahpC* gene expression in isoniazid-resistant *Mycobacterium tuberculosis*. Science 1996;272:1641–1643.
22 Shcherbakov D, Akbergenov R, Matt T, Sander P, Andersson DI, Böttger EC: Directed mutagenesis of *Mycobacterium smegmatis* 16S rRNA to reconstruct the in-vivo evolution of aminoglycoside resistance in *Mycobacterium tuberculosis*. Mol Microbiol 2010;77:830–840.
23 Canetti G, Froman S, Grosset J, Hauduroy P, Langerová M, Mahler HT, Meissner G, Mitchison DA, Sula L: Mycobacteria: laboratory methods for testing drug sensitivity and resistance. Bull World Health Org 1963;29:565–578.
24 Inderlied CB, Salfinger M: Antimicrobial agents and susceptibility tests: mycobacteria; in Murray PR, Baron EJ, Pfaller MA, Tenover FC, Yolken RH (eds): Manual of Clinical Microbiology. Washington, American Society for Microbiology, 1995, pp 1385–1404.
25 Canetti G, Fox W, Khomenko A, Mahler HT, Menon NK, Mitchison DA, Rist N, Smelev NA: Advances in techniques of testing mycobacterial drug sensitivity and the use of sensitivity tests in tuberculosis control programmes. Bull World Health Org 1969;41:21–43.
26 Woodley CL: Evaluation of streptomycin and ethambutol concentrations for susceptibility testing of *Mycobacterium tuberculosis* by radiometric and conventional procedures. J Clin Microbiol 1986;23:385–386.
27 Madison B, Robinson-Dunn B, George I, Gross W, Lipman H, Metchuck B, Sloctsky, A, Washabange G, Mazurek G, Riddershof J: Multicenter evaluation of ethambutol susceptibility testing of *Mycobacterium tuberculosis* by agar proportion and radiometric methods. J Clin Microbiol 2002;40:3976–3979.
28 Laszló A, Rahman M, Raviglione M, Bustreo F, WHO/IUATLD Network of Supranational Reference Laboratories: Quality assurance programme for drug susceptibility testing of *Mycobacterium tuberculosis* in the WHO/IUATLD supranational laboratory network: first round of proficiency testing. Int J Tuberc Lung Dis 1997;1:231–238.
29 Zhang Y, Heym B, Allen B, Young D, Cole S: The catalase-peroxidase gene and isoniazid resistance of *Mycobacterium tuberculosis*. Nature 1992;358:591–593.
30 Banerjee A, Dubnau E, Quemard A, Balasubramanian V, Um SK, Wilson T, Collins, D, De Lisle G, Jacobs WR Jr: *inhA*, a gene encoding a target for isoniazid and ethionamide in *Mycobacterium tuberculosis*. Science 1994;263:227–230.
31 Rouse DA, Li Z, Bai GH, Morris SL: Characterization of the *katG* and *inhA* genes of isoniazid resistant clinical isolates of *Mycobacterium tuberculosis*. Antimicrob Agents Chemother 1995;39:2472–2477.
32 Musser JM, Kapur V, Williams DL, Kreiswirth BN, van Soolingen D, van Embden, JD: Characterization of the catalase-peroxidase gene (*katG*) and *inhA* locus in isoniazid-resistant and -susceptible strains of *Mycobacterium tuberculosis* by automated DNA sequencing: restricted array of mutations associated with drug resistance. J Infect Dis 1996;173:196–202.
33 Dobner P, Rusch-Gerdes S, Bretzel G, Feldmann K, Rifai M, Loscher T, Rinder H: Usefulness of *Mycobacterium tuberculosis* genomic mutations in the genes *katG* and *inhA* for the prediction of isoniazid resistance. Int J Tuberc Lung Dis 1997;1:365–369.
34 Somoskovi A, Dormandy J, Mitsani D, Rivenburg J, Salfinger M: Use of smear-positive samples to assess the PCR-based genotype MTBDR assay for rapid, direct detection of the *Mycobacterium tuberculosis* complex as well as its resistance to isoniazid and rifampicin. J Clin Microbiol 2006;44:4459–4463.
35 Marttila HJ, Soini H, Eerola E, Vyshnevskya E, Vyshnevskaya BI, Otten TF, Vasilyef AV, Viljanen MK: A Ser315Thr substitution in KatG is predominant in genetically heterogeneous multidrug-resistant *Mycobacterium tuberculosis* isolates originating from the St Petersburg area in Russia. Antimicrob Agents Chemother 1998;42:2443–2445.
36 Van Soolingen D, Borgdorff MW, de Haas PE, Sebek MM, Veen J, Dessens M, Kremer K, van Embden JD: Molecular epidemiology of tuberculosis in the Netherlands: a nationwide study from 1993 through 1997. J Infect Dis 1999;180:726–736.
37 Springer B, Calligaris-Maibach RC, Ritter C, Böttger EC: Tuberculosis drug resistance in an area of low endemicity in 2004 to 2006: semiquantitative drug susceptibility testing and genotyping. J Clin Microbiol 2008;46:4064–4067.
38 Springer B, Lucke K, Calligaris-Maibach RC, Ritter C, Böttger EC: Quantitative drug susceptibility testing of *Mycobacterium tuberculosis* by use of MGIT 960 and EpiCenter instrumentation. J Clin Microbiol 2009;47:1773–1780.
39 Gagneux S, Burgos MV, De Riemer K, Encisco A, Muñoz S, Hopewell PC, Small PM, Pym AS: Impact of bacterial genetics on the transmission of isoniazid-resistant *Mycobacterium tuberculosis*. PLoS Pathog 2006;2:e61.
40 Bergval IL, Schuitema AR, Klatser PR, Anthony RM: Resistant mutants of *Mycobacterium tuberculosis* selected in vitro do not reflect the in vivo mechanism of isoniazid resistance. J Antimicrob Chemother 2009;64:512–523.
41 Afanas'ev MV, Ikryannikova LN, Il'ina EN, Sidorenko SV, Kuz'min AV, Larionova EE, Smirnova, TG, Chernousova LN, Kamaev EY, Skorniakov SN, Kinsht VN, Cherednichenko AG, Govorun VM: Molecular characteristics of rifampicin- and isoniazid-resistant *Mycobacterium tuberculosis* isolates from the Russian Federation. J Antimicrob Chemother 2007;59:1057–1064.
42 Telenti A, Imboden P, Marchesi F, Lowrie D, Cole ST, Colston MJ, Matter L, Schopfer K, Bodmer T: Detection of rifampicin-resistance mutations in *Mycobacterium tuberculosis*. Lancet 1993;341:647–650.
43 Huitric E, Werngren J, Juréen P, Hoffner S: Resistance levels and *rpoB* gene mutations among in vitro-selected rifampicin-resistant *Mycobacterium tuberculosis* mutants. Antimicrob Agents Chemother 2006;50:2860–2862.
44 Takayama K, Kilburn JO: Inhibition of synthesis of arabinogalactane by ethambutol in *Mycobacterium smegmatis*. Antimicrob Agents Chemother 1989;33:1493–1499.
45 Telenti A, Philipp WJ, Screevatsan S, Bernasconi C, Stockbauer KE, Wieles B, Musser JM, Jacobs WR Jr: The *emb* operon, a gene cluster of *Mycobacterium tuberculosis* involved in resistance to ethambutol. Nat Med 1997;3:567–570.

46 Johnson R, Jordaan AM, Pretorius L, Engelke E, van der Spuy G, Kewley C, Bosman M, van Helden PD, Warren R, Victor TC: Ethambutol resistance testing by mutation detection. Int J Tuberc Lung Dis 2006;10:68–73.
47 Starks AM, Gumusboga A, Plikaytis BB, Shinnick TM, Posey JE: Mutations at *embB* codon 306 are an important molecular indicator of ethambutol resistance in *Mycobacterium tuberculosis*. Antimicrob Agents Chemother 2009;53:1061–1066.
48 Safi H, Fleischmann RD, Peterson SN, Jones MB, Jarrahi B, Alland D: Allelic exchange and mutant selection demonstrate that common clinical embCAB gene mutations only modestly increase resistance to ethambutol in *Mycobacterium tuberculosis*. Antimicrob Agents Chemother 2010;54:103–108.
49 Plinke C, Cox HS, Kalon S, Doshetov D, Rusch-Gerdes S, Niemann S: Tuberculosis ethambutol resistance: concordance between phenotypic and genotypic test results. Tuberculosis 2009;89:448–452.
50 Scorpio A, Zhang Y: Mutations in *pncA*, a gene encoding pyrazinamidase/nicotinamidase, cause resistance to the antituberculous drug pyrazinamide in tubercle bacillus. Nat Med 1996;2:662–667.
51 Scorpio A, Lindholm-Levy P, Heifets L, Gilman R, Siddiqi S, Cynamon M, Zhang Y: Characterization of *pncA* mutations in pyrazinamide-resistant *Mycobacterium tuberculosis*. Antimicrob Agents Chemother 1997;41:540–543.
52 Mestdagh M, Fonteyne PA, Realini L, Rossau R, Jannes G, Mijs W, De Smet KA, Portaels F, van den Eeckhout E: Relationship between pyrazinamide resistance, loss of pyrazinamidase activity, and mutations in the *pncA* locus in multidrug-resistant clinical isolates of *Mycobacterium tuberculosis*. Antimicrob Agents Chemother 1999;43:2317–2319.
53 Lemaitre N, Sougakoff W, Truffot-Pernot C, Jarlier V: Characterization of new mutations in pyrazinamide resistant strains of *Mycobacterium tuberculosis* and identification of conserved regions important for the catalytic activity of the pyrazinamidase *pncA*. Antimicrob Agents Chemother 1999;43:1761–1763.
54 Morlock GP, Crawford JT, Butler WR, Brim SE, Sikes D, Mazurek GH, Woodley CL, Cooksey RC: Phenotypic characterization of *pncA* mutants of *Mycobacterium tuberculosis*. Antimicrob Agents Chemother 2000;44:2291–2295.
55 Zhang Y, Mitchison D: The curious characteristics of pyrazinamide: a review. Int J Tuberc Lung Dis 2003,7.6–21.
56 Takiff HE, Salazar L, Guerrero C, Philipp W, Huang WM, Kreiswirth B, Cole ST, Jacobs WR Jr, Telenti A: Cloning and nucleotide sequence of *Mycobacterium tuberculosis gyrA* and *gyrB* genes and detection of quinolone resistance mutations. Antimicrob Agents Chemother 1994;38:773–780.
57 Kam KM, Yip CW, Cheung TL, Tang HS, Leung OC, Chan MY: Stepwise decrease in moxifloxacin susceptibility amongst clinical isolates of multidrug-resistant *Mycobacterium tuberculosis*: correlation with ofloxacin susceptibility. Microb Drug Res 2006;12:7–11.
58 Chan RC, Hui M, Chan EW, Au TK, Chin ML, Yip CK, Au Yeang CK, Yeung CY, Kam KM, Yip PC, Cheng AF: Genetic and phenotypic characterization of drug-resistant *Mycobacterium tuberculosis* isolates in Hong Kong. J Antimicrob Chemother 2007;59:866–873.
59 Von Groll A, Martin A, Jureen P, Hoffner S, Vandamme P, Portaels F, Palomino JC, da Silva PA: Fluoroquinolone resistance in *Mycobacterium tuberculosis* and mutations in *gyrA* and *gyrB*. Antimicrob Agents Chemother 2009;53:4498–500.
60 Matrat S, Aubry A, Mayer C, Jarlier V, Cambau E: Mutagenesis in the 34 GyrA helix and in the toprim domain of GyrB refines the contribution of *Mycobacterium tuberculosis* DNA gyrase to intrinsic resistance to quinolones. Antimicrob Agents Chemother 2008;52:2909–2914.
60b Jacobson KR, Tierney DB, Jeon CY, Mitnick CD, Murray MB: Treatment outcomes among patients with extensively drug-resistant tuberculosis. Clin Infect Dis 2010;51:6–14.
60c Poissy J, Aubry A, Fernandez C, Lott MC, Chauffour A, Jarlier V, Farinotti R, Veziris N: Should moxifloxacin be used for the treatment of extensively drug-resistant tuberculosis? An answer from a murine model. Antimicrob Agents Chemother 2010;54:4765–4771.
61 Meier A, Heifets L, Wallace RJ Jr, Zhang Y, Brown BA, Sander P, Böttger EC: Molecular mechanisms of clarithromycin resistance in *Mycobacterium avium*: observation of multiple 23S rDNA mutations in a clonal population. J Infect Dis 1996;174:354–360.
62 De Barber AE, Mdluli K, Bosman M, Bekker, LG, Barry CE 3rd: Ethionamide activation and sensitivity in multidrug-resistant *Mycobacterium tuberculosis*. Proc Natl Acad Sci USA 2000;97:9677–9682.
63 Wang F, Langley R, Gulten G, Dover LG, Besra GS, Jacobs WR Jr, Sacchettini JC: Mechanism of thioamide drug action against tuberculosis and leprosy. J Exp Med 2007;204:73–78.
64 Morlock GP, Metchock B, Sikes D, Crawford JT, Cooksey RC: *ethA*, *inhA*, and *katG* loci of ethionamide-resistant clinical *Mycobacterium tuberculosis* isolates. Antimicrob Agents Chemother 2003;47:3799–3805.
65 Hobbie SN, Bruell C, Kalapala S, Akshay S, Schmidt S, Pfister, P, Böttger EC: A genetic model to investigate drug-target interactions at the ribosomal decoding site. Biochimie 2006;88:1033–1043.
66 Finken M, Kirschner P, Meier A, Wrede A, Böttger EC: Molecular basis of streptomycin resistance in *Mycobacterium tuberculosis*: alteration of the ribosomal protein S12 gene and point mutations within a functional 16S ribosomal RNA pseudoknot. Mol Microbiol 1993;9:1239–1246.
67 Sander P, Prammananan T, Böttger EC: Introducing mutations into a chromosomal rRNA gene using a genetically modified eubacterial host with a single rRNA operon. Mol Microbiol 1996;22:841–848.
68 Meier A, Kirschner P, Springer B, Steingrube VA, Brown BA, Wallace RJ Jr, Böttger EC: Identification of mutations in 23S rRNA gene of clarithromycin-resistant *Mycobacterium intracellulare*. Antimicrob Agents Chemother 1994;38:381–384.
69 Prammananan T, Sander P, Brown BA, Frischkorn K, Onyi GO, Zhang Y, Böttger EC, Wallace RJ Jr: A single 16S ribosomal RNA substitution is responsible for resistance to amikacin and other 2-deoxystreptamine aminoglycosides in *Mycobacterium abscessus* and *Mycobacterium chelonae*. J Infect Dis 1998;177:1573–1581.
70 Bercovier H, Kafri O, Sela S: Mycobacteria possess a surprisingly small number of ribosomal RNA genes in relation to the size of their genome. Biochem Biophys Res Commun 1986;136:1136–1141.
71 Springer B, Kidan YG, Prammananan T, Ellrott K, Böttger EC, Sander P: Mechanisms of streptomycin resistance: selection of mutations in the 16S rRNA gene conferring resistance. Antimicrob Agents Chemother 2001;45:2877–2884.
72 Meier A, Sander P, Schaper KJ, Scholz M, Böttger EC: Correlation of molecular resistance mechanism and phenotypic resistance level in streptomycin-resistant *M. tuberculosis*. Antimicrob Agents Chemother 1996;40:2452–2454.
73 Honore N, Cole ST: Streptomycin resistance in mycobacteria. Antimicrob Agents Chemother 1994;38:238–242.
74 Sreevatsan S, Pan X, Stockbauer K, Williams D, Kreiswirth B, Musser JM: Characterization of *rpsL* and *rrs* mutations in streptomycin-resistant *Mycobacterium tuberculosis* isolates from diverse geographical localities. Antimicrob Agents Chemother 1996;40:1024–1026.
75 Cooksey RC, Morlock GP, McQueen A, Glickman SE, Crawford JT: Characterization of streptomycin resistance mechanisms among *Mycobacterium tuberculosis* isolates from New York City. Antimicrob Agents Chemother 1996;40:1186–1188.
76 Okamoto S, Tamaru A, Nakajima C, Nishimura K, Tanaka Y, Tokuyama S, Suzuki Y, Ochi K: Loss of a conserved 7-methylguanosine modification in 16S rRNA confers low-level streptomycin resistance in bacteria. Mol Microbiol 2007;63:1096–1106.
77 Suzuki Y, Katsukava C, Tamaru A, Abe C, Makino M, Mizuguchi Y, Taniguchi H: Detection of kanamycin-resistant *Mycobacterium tuberculosis* by identifying mutations in the 16S rRNA gene. J Clin Micobiol 1998;36:1220–1225.
78 Alangaden GJ, Kreiswirth B, Aouad A, Khetarpal M, Igno FR, Moghazeh SL, Manavathu EK, Lerner SA: Mechanism of resistance to amikacin and kanamycin in *Mycobacterium tuberculosis*. Antimicrob Agents Chemother 1998;42:1295–1297.

79 Maus CE, Plikaytis BB, Shinnick TM: Molecular analysis of cross-resistance to capreomycin, kanamycin, amikacin, and viomycin in *Mycobacterium tuberculosis*. Antimicrob Agents Chemother 2005;49:3192–3197.
80 Jugheli L, Bzekalava N, de Rijk P, Fissette K, Portaels F, Rigouts L: High level of cross-resistance between kanamycin, amikacin, and capreomycin among *Mycobacterium tuberculosis* isolates from Georgia and a close relation with mutations in the *rrs* gene. Antimicrob Agents Chemother 2009;53:5064–5068.
81 Zaunbrecher MA, Sikes RD, Metchock B, Shinnick TM, Posey JE: Overexpression of the chromosomally encoded aminoglycoside acetyltransferase *eis* confers kanamycin resistance in *Mycobacterium tuberculosis*. Proc Natl Acad Sci USA 2009;106:20004–20009.
82 Krüüner A, Jureen P, Levina K, Ghebremichael S, Hoffner S: Discordant resistance to kanamycin and amikacin in drug-resistant *Mycobacterium tuberculosis*. Antimicrob Agents Chemother 2003;47:2971–2973.
83 Sutton WB, Gordee RS, Wick WE, Stanfield L: In-vitro and in-vivo laboratory studies on the antituberculous activity of capreomycin. Ann NY Acad Sci 1966;135:947–959.
84 Liou YF, Tanaka N: Dual actions of viomycin on the ribosomal functions. Biochem Biophys Res Commun 1976;71:477–483.
85 Johansen SK, Maus CE, Plikaytis BB, Douthwaite S: Capreomycin binds across the ribosomal subunit interface using *tlyA*-encoded 2'-O-methylations in 16S and 23S rRNAs. Mol Cell 2006;23:173–182.
86 Stanley RE, Blaha G, Grodzicki RL, Strickler MD, Steitz TA: The structures of the anti-tuberculosis antibiotics viomycin and capreomycin bound to the 70S ribosome. Nat Struct Mol Biol 2010;17:289–293.
87 Tsukamura M: Cross-resistance relationships between capreomycin, kanamycin, and viomycin resistances in tubercle bacilli from patients. Am Rev Respir Dis 1969;99:780–782.
88 McClatchy JK, Kanes W, Davidson PT, Moulding TS: Cross-resistance in *M. tuberculosis* to kanamycin, capreomycin and viomycin. Tubercle 1977;58:29–34.
89 Feuerriegel S, Cox HS, Zarkua N, Karimovich HA, Braker A, Rüsch-Gerdes S, Niemann S: Sequence analyses of just four genes to detect extensively drug-resistant *Mycobacterium tuberculosis* strains in multidrug-resistant tuberculosis patients undergoing treatment. Antimicrob Agents Chemother 2009;53:3353–3356.
90 Maus CE, Plikaytis BB, Shinnick TM: Mutation of *tlyA* confers capreomycin resistance in *Mycobacterium tuberculosis*. Antimicrob Agents Chemother 2005;49:571–577.
91 Vaddady PK, Lee RE, Meibohm B: In vitro pharmacokinetic/pharmacodynamic models in anti-infective drug development: focus on TB. Future Med Chem 2010;2:1355–1369.
92 Schön T, Juréen P, Giske CG, Chryssanthou E, Sturegård E, Werngren J, Kahlmeter G, Hoffner SE, Angeby KA: Evaluation of wild-type MIC distributions as a tool for determination of clinical breakpoints for *Mycobacterium tuberculosis*. J Antimicrob Chemother 2009;64:786–793.
93 Victor TC, Warren R, Butt JL, Jordaan AM, Felix JV, Venter A, Sirgel FA, Schaaf HS, Donald PR, Richardson M, Cynamon MH, van Helden PD: Genome and MIC stability in *Mycobacterium tuberculosis* and indications for continuation of use of isoniazid in multidrug-resistant tuberculosis. J Med Microbiol 1997;46:847–857.
94 Stewart SM, Crofton JW: The clinical significance of low degrees of drug resistance in pulmonary tuberculosis. Am Rev Respir Dis 1964;89:811–829.
95 Moulding TS: Should isoniazid be used in retreatment of tuberculosis despite acquired isoniazid resistance? Am Rev Respir Dis 1981;123:262–264.
96 Cynamon MH, Zhang Y, Harpster T, Cheng S, De Stefano MS: High-dose isoniazid therapy for isoniazid-resistant murine *Mycobacterium tuberculosis* infection. Antimicrob Agents Chemother 1999;43:2922–2924.
97 Tripathy SP, Menon NK, Mitchison DA, Narayana AS, Somasundaram PA, Stott H, Velu S: Response to treatment with isoniazid plus PAS of tuberculous patients with primary isoniazid resistance. Tubercle 1969;50:257–268.
98 Devadatta S, Bhatia AL, Andrews RH, Fox W, Mitchison DA, Radhakrishna S, Ramakrishnan CV, Selkon JB, Velu S: Response of patients infected with isoniazid-resistant tubercle bacilli to treatment with isoniazid plus PAS or isoniazid alone. Bull World Health Org 1961;25:807–829.
99 Petty TL, Mitchell RS: Successful treatment of advanced isoniazid- and streptomycin-resistant pulmonary tuberculosis with ethionamide, pyrazinamide, and isoniazid. Am Rev Respir Dis 1962;86:503–512.
100 Böttger EC: Drug resistant tuberculosis. Lancet 2001;357:1288–1289.
101 NCCLS: Susceptibility testing of mycobacteria, nocardiae, and other aerobic actinomycetes. Approved standard NCCLS document M24-A. Wayne, NCCLS, 2003.
102 Rinder H, Mieskes KT, Löscher T: Heteroresistance in *Mycobacterium tuberculosis*. Int J Tuberc Lung Dis 2001;5:339–345.
103 Canetti G: Present aspects of bacterial resistance in tuberculosis. Am Rev Respir Dis 1965;92:687–703.

Erik C. Böttger, MD, Professor of Medicine and Microbiology, Director and Chairman
Institut für Medizinische Mikrobiologie
Nationales Zentrum für Mykobakterien, Universität Zürich
Gloriastrasse 30/32, CH–8006 Zürich (Switzerland)
Tel. +41 44 634 26 60, E-Mail boettger@imm.uzh.ch

Donald PR, van Helden PD (eds): Antituberculosis Chemotherapy.
Prog Respir Res. Basel, Karger, 2011, vol 40, pp 145–152

# The Role of the Mouse Model in the Evaluation of New Antituberculosis Drugs

Eric L. Nuermberger

Center for Tuberculosis Research, Department of Medicine, Johns Hopkins University School of Medicine, and Department of International Health, Johns Hopkins Bloomberg School of Public Health, Baltimore, Md., USA

**Abstract**

For the first time in 4 decades, new agents with novel mechanisms of action have entered clinical trials designed to evaluate their potential to improve the treatment of tuberculosis. Much of the optimism surrounding these new drugs comes from promising results observed in animal models. Moreover, selection of the most promising combinations of new and existing drugs to form entirely novel regimens for future trials will also rely on information from animal studies. This review describes the historical track record of experimental animal chemotherapy models, their potential pitfalls and recent efforts to improve their utility. Although the mouse model is featured, the role of other animal models is also briefly considered.

Copyright © 2011 S. Karger AG, Basel

Tuberculosis (TB) continues to exact a terrible toll on humankind while the emergence and spread of multidrug-resistant strains of *Mycobacterium tuberculosis* threatens to undermine what is currently our strongest line of defence, combination chemotherapy. Fortunately, after a decades-long drought in which no new class of drugs was approved for use against TB, renewed discovery efforts and repurposing of existing antibacterial agents have produced a global portfolio of at least 10 potential new drugs for TB from 6 new classes which are currently under evaluation in clinical trials [1]. Another previously approved agent, rifapentine, is being re-examined to identify the optimal dose [2]. Promising developments at earlier stages of discovery and preclinical development also continue to emerge. It is hoped that new drug combinations containing 1 or more new agents will improve the treatment of drug-susceptible as well as drug-resistant forms of TB, as well as treatment of latent infection. To better understand this potential and inform clinical trial designs, drug developers often turn to animal models, most commonly the mouse. A recent review described mice as an efficient and economical model which represents the relative contributions of existing TB drugs remarkably well and outlined our typical sequential approach to evaluating new drug candidates in this species [3]. In this review, I will describe recent developments related to the role of animal models of TB chemotherapy and their utility in preclinical evaluations of promising drugs and combinations.

## The Potential for More Rapid Assessment of Drug Efficacy in Mice

Early in the discovery and development process, once bioavailability is established, the most important question is whether a compound is active or inactive in vivo. A straightforward approach is to challenge mice with a lethal dose of *M. tuberculosis* and then determine whether, and at what dose, a compound prevents the development of terminal disease. Nikonenko et al. [4] suggested a 7-day incubation period after infection, 2 weeks of treatment, and then simply monitoring body weight is sufficient to discriminate active from inactive compounds. We and others have used an incubation period of 1–3 days followed by 4 weeks of treatment, with observations of mortality and body weight as well as gross examination for lung lesions and splenomegaly at treatment completion to identify whether complete bacteriostasis or even bactericidal activity occurred. While both of these approaches may constitute relatively simple screening approaches to identify active compounds and the minimum effective doses, neither will distinguish bactericidal from bacteriostatic activity nor quantify a bactericidal effect.

Bactericidal effects are traditionally confirmed by comparing the number of colony-forming units (CFU) present in organ homogenates at some time point during treatment to the CFU count at the initiation of treatment. The activity of compounds with early bactericidal effects may be revealed with as few as 2 daily doses when treatment is started soon after high-dose infection [5], when the bacteria are actively multiplying in the pre-immune phase of infection. The attraction of such an assay is its speed, the small compound requirement and the ability to assess drug activity in the absence of adaptive host immunity. However, the dynamic range of such an assay is limited and compounds which have predominantly bacteriostatic effects (e.g. ethambutol), delayed bactericidal effects (e.g. TMC207) or poor activity against actively multiplying bacteria (e.g. pyrazinamide) may appear inactive. A longer treatment period permits a wider dynamic range, better resolves the comparative activity of various drugs and may better inform dose selection for further mouse studies [6], but assessing compound activity in the absence of host immunity still has the potential to mislead the investigator about the therapeutic potential of compounds that are not as bactericidal against actively multiplying bacteria but have important activity against slowly multiplying or non-multiplying bacteria. For example, rifampicin and pyrazinamide at human-equivalent doses (10 and 150 mg/kg, respectively) are, at best, bacteriostatic in this model [6], despite having the greatest treatment-shortening potential among existing TB drugs in mice as well as humans. Therefore, caution is advised before discounting the potential of a new agent based solely on the assessment of activity in a pre-immune or immunocompromised mouse model [7].

Although organ CFU counts are a commonly used outcome measure, they require (1) that mice be killed for the assessment at each time point, (2) substantial time and effort for necropsy, homogenization and plating in serial dilutions, and (3) 3–4 weeks for colonies to grow before counting can take place. Efforts to reduce the number of animals as well as the time and other resources needed to evaluate new compounds have focused on a variety of real-time surrogate markers. A bioluminescent reporter strain of *Mycobacterium bovis* bacille Calmette-Guérin (BCG) expressing firefly luciferase, which produces light from organ homogenates after addition of luciferin, was employed at Pathogenesis Corp. to screen a library of nitro-imidazole derivatives that ultimately produced PA-824 [8], a drug currently in phase II trials. Because the firefly luciferase reaction requires ATP, the ratio of relative light units produced to CFU may change as organisms enter the stationary phase or other non-replicating conditions or are targeted by antibacterial drug mechanisms which affect ATP levels. This may limit the ability to discriminate bacteriostatic from bactericidal effects. Bacterial luciferases, on the other hand, do not require ATP. The engineering of recombinant bacteria expressing both the bacterial luciferase and its aldehyde substrate, together with the advent of sensitive charge-coupled device cameras, has made it possible to serially evaluate drug effects in real time in live animals. However, despite significant progress [9], this has not proven feasible for *M. tuberculosis* to date.

Other real-time imaging methods also have promise for serial, non-invasive monitoring of the response to chemotherapy. For example, [$^{18}$F]-2-fluorodeoxy-D-glucose is a radiotracer for monitoring tissue inflammation using positron emission tomography. It was recently used to monitor the response to 2 combination chemotherapy regimens in different species of mice [10], although its greatest application is probably in larger animal models in which the reduction in the number of animals required for study has very significant cost implications. Still, [$^{18}$F]-2-fluorodeoxy-D-glucose positron emission tomography imaging does not image the organism in question, and the downgrading of the inflammatory response lags behind that of the bacterial burden during effective treatment. Other recently reported modalities for imaging the infecting organisms themselves have demonstrated proof of concept, but must overcome sensitivity issues before they have much utility as a means of monitoring the response to effective chemotherapy [11].

## Measuring Sterilizing Activity

Most evaluations of new compounds in vivo begin with an assessment of activity against actively multiplying bacteria. However, TB is rather unique in that the duration of treatment necessary to cure patients is ultimately determined by a regimen's ability to eradicate bacilli which persist in a viable state despite exposure to bactericidal drugs which eradicate the vast majority of the population. These antibiotic-tolerant 'persisters' cause relapse after treatment of insufficient duration or potency, and the ability of a drug or regimen to eradicate them and shorten the duration of treatment needed to prevent relapse is commonly referred to as 'sterilizing' activity. Existing TB drugs have differing degrees of sterilizing activity, and the extent of a drug's sterilizing activity does not always correlate with its activity against actively multiplying bacteria. The dramatic early bactericidal activity of isoniazid compared with the treatment-shortening potential of rifampicin is the best case in point. Since the development of drugs with improved sterilizing activity is a principal objective of TB drug development, all compounds showing even modest activity in the initial in vivo efficacy screen should, in principle, be evaluated for the ability to clear *M. tuberculosis* from the lungs of mice. However, demonstrating the absence of cultivable organisms in organ homogenates during treatment does not necessarily confirm absence of viable bacilli. If the treatment is of inadequate duration or insufficient sterilizing activity, persisters which are initially non-cultivable bacteria may regrow in the ensuing 3–6 months and give rise to a 'relapse'. Hence, prevention of relapse must be the 'gold standard' outcome measure of sterilizing activity, at least as it pertains to mouse infection. The speed with which a drug or regimen reduces the organ CFU count to zero during treatment is commonly a reliable indicator of sterilizing potential but this is not always the case. Caution is advised if this method is used to rank drugs or regimens for their treatment-shortening ability. For example, Andries et al. [12] have recently treated intravenously infected mice with a variety of combinations including rifapentine, pyrazinamide, moxifloxacin and the new diarylquinoline TMC207. In comparing the contributions of TMC207 and rifapentine to the various regimens, it was evident that inclusion of TMC207 was associated with the most rapid fall in lung CFU counts, but rifapentine had the greatest contribution in terms of the duration of treatment necessary to prevent relapse.

## More Rapid Appraisal of Potential Sterilizing Activity

While relapse remains the gold standard outcome measure for sterilizing activity, less labour- and time-intensive methods of estimating a compound's sterilizing activity are needed for earlier points in the development path. Recent efforts to develop abbreviated surrogate models capable of ranking compounds in terms of their potential sterilizing activity have promise.

Traditionally, mouse models for evaluating sterilizing activity have used several months of intensive combination chemotherapy to select for persisters prior to evaluating the new drugs in question [3]. More rapid methods should seek more efficient ways of enriching for persisters. While there is considerable debate over the location and metabolic state of the bacterial persisters in TB and the extent to which they are present at the initiation of treatment (as opposed to being induced or created in response to drug exposure), they are generally thought to be slowly multiplying or not multiplying at all. Achieving the non- or slowly replicating persistent state with a virulent *M. tuberculosis* strain in mice requires (1) production of an initial bacterial burden large enough to contain a sufficiently large subpopulation of persisters followed by a selective treatment that is long enough and/or potent enough to sufficiently enrich the remaining viable population for persisters and/or (2) elicitation of an adaptive immune response which results in growth containment. Therefore, the most straightforward and representative approach to a shorter surrogate model for sterilizing activity may be to simply intensify the selective chemotherapy regimen so that the persister subpopulation is revealed in a shorter time frame (e.g. by increasing the dose of rifampicin and/or other drugs in the pretreatment selection regimen).

One seemingly attractive option for an extremely short alternative model is to infect mice directly with a culture of non-replicating *M. tuberculosis* produced in vitro by various means (e.g. hypoxia or nutrient starvation). However, in our experience with nutrient starvation, the bacteria resume active growth within a few days in the non-immune host and, therefore, present only a small window for evaluating drug activity against non-multiplying bacteria. Woolhiser et al. [13] had similar results with the use of hypoxic cultures. Another approach is to infect mice with a mutant strain of *M. tuberculosis* with defective growth. Sala et al. [14] have recently provided intriguing preliminary data after infecting mice with the streptomycin-dependent 18b mutant of *M. tuberculosis* which multiplies (poorly) in mice supplemented with streptomycin injections but stops multiplying (slowly declines, in fact) when streptomycin is withdrawn. These investigators infected mice with the 18b strain, treated them with daily streptomycin for 3 weeks to establish the infection, then withdrew the streptomycin for 1 week before treating the mice with the test drugs for up to 8 weeks. The ranking of drugs in terms of activity in this model was consistent with evidence of their sterilizing activity in mice. Rifampicin was most active, followed by moxifloxacin and PA-824. Consistent with its limited sterilizing activity in humans, isoniazid was not active and neither was another cell-wall-acting agent, the benzthiazinone BTZ043. Therefore, this simple and rapid model of non-multiplying persistence may be able to rank drug candidates in terms of their sterilizing potential. Further validation and efforts to reduce the time needed to set up the model are warranted. However, because the mutant has defective ribosomal function, it may

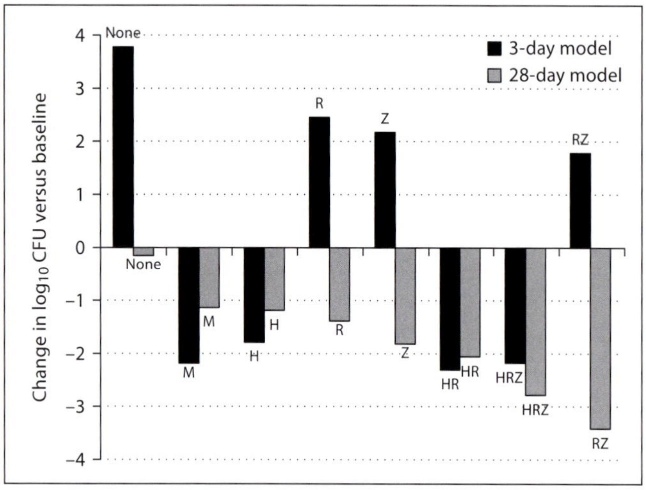


**Fig. 1.** Comparison of the activity of first-line anti-TB drugs after 4 weeks of treatment in acute (3-day incubation period) and established (28-day incubation period) infection models. M = Moxifloxacin; H = isoniazid; R = rifampicin; Z = pyrazinamide.

not be appropriate for evaluating compounds which act on the ribosome.

While we continue to seek a simple, rapid means to estimate the potential sterilizing activity of new compounds, our current approach (provided there is a sufficient amount of compound) is to evaluate compounds with promising in vitro activity and evidence of bioavailability in an acute infection model (high-dose aerosol implantation followed by 3-day incubation period prior to infection) and a more chronic infection (low-dose aerosol implantation followed by 28- to 42-day incubation). In the acute model, bacterial multiplication continues for at least 2 weeks of the treatment period in untreated control mice, and isoniazid, a drug known for its potent bactericidal activity against actively multiplying organisms, is the most active drug. Rifampicin, despite its demonstrated ability to dramatically shorten the duration of TB therapy, is largely bacteriostatic at human-equivalent doses and may actually permit some multiplication (fig. 1, black bars). Pyrazinamide also has limited inhibitory effects in this model. Similar results have been observed by others when treatment is initiated in the pre-immune phase of infection [6] and suggest that caution is warranted when trying to interpret a new compound's treatment-shortening potential when using an acute infection model or the analogous situation of immunocompromised mice [7]. In the more chronic model, there is no increase in CFU counts in untreated control mice during the treatment period, indicating that the bacterial burden has been enriched for slowly multiplying or non-multiplying bacilli. Rifampicin and pyrazinamide become more active than isoniazid (fig. 1, gray bars). Although the chronic model does not measure sterilizing activity, comparative studies of other new drugs in development indicate that rankings in this model correlate better with the sterilizing activity of drugs in mice than do rankings based on the 3-day or 14-day incubation models [unpubl. data]. Using the short and long incubation models in concert is likely to give a good representation of the compound's activity against both bacterial growth phases and better defines its potential contribution to the treatment of TB.

## Modelling the Chemotherapy of Latent Tuberculosis Infection

With the exception of non-human primates, no available animal model mimics the conditions of latent TB infection (LTBI). However, Lecoeur et al. [15] developed a mouse model that has become an accepted model for the experimental chemotherapy of LTBI after demonstrating its utility in several studies. It involves immunization of mice with *M. bovis* BCG 4–6 weeks before infection with virulent *M. tuberculosis* to limit multiplication and establish an infection of low burden and, at most, limited replication (i.e. CFU counts remain stable over time). This model garnered attention after demonstrating that 2 months of rifampicin-pyrazinamide had a sterilizing activity superior to 6 months of isoniazid [15], giving rise to clinical trials which established the efficacy of short-course rifampicin-pyrazinamide. Although this regimen is no longer recommended due to concerns of hepatotoxicity, this is no reason for questioning the ability of the mouse model to represent drug efficacy [16]. The BCG immunization model has also been used to test newer antituberculous drugs. Once weekly administration of isoniazid and rifapentine for 3 months was as effective as daily administration of isoniazid for 6 months [17], a hypothesis under study in a large ongoing clinical trial.

Use of a more immunogenic BCG mutant and a very low aerosol challenge dose with *M. tuberculosis* produces a stable paucibacillary state (<$10^4$ CFU) even more representative of LTBI. The refined model was recently validated by testing 4 clinically relevant LTBI regimens [18]. The ranking of the regimens in order of increasing activity and the duration needed to cure the infection in this model are consistent with the decreasing treatment durations recommended when these regimens are used in humans (i.e. 6–9 months of isoniazid, 4 months of rifampicin, 3 months of rifampicin-isoniazid, 2 months of rifampicin-pyrazinamide; table 1). No

**Table 1.** Results of treatment with clinically relevant LTBI regimens in the paucibacillary murine model

| Regimen | Lung CFU ± SD at initiation | Results after treatment for | | | |
|---|---|---|---|---|---|
| | | 4 weeks | | 8 weeks | |
| | | lung CFU | relapse, % | lung CFU | relapse, % |
| 1 Untreated | 3.65±0.30 | 3.71±0.56 | n.d. | 3.64±0.51 | n.d. |
| 2 INH | | 2.61±0.44 | n.d. | 1.71±0.54 | n.d. |
| 3 RIF | | 1.87±0.49 | n.d. | 0.33±0.30 | n.d. |
| 4 RIF + INH | | 1.08±0.47 | 100 | 0 | 47 |
| 5 RIF + PZA | | 0.18±0.15 | 53 | 0 | 0 |

n.d. = Not done; INH = isoniazid; RIF = rifampicin; PZA = pyrazinamide.

other model, including the commonly cited Cornell model, has been validated in this way. In the same experiment, it was observed that regimens including daily rifapentine (10 mg/kg) were as effective as rifampicin-pyrazinamide and prevented relapse after 6–8 weeks of treatment [18], suggesting that daily rifapentine regimens may make treatment of LTBI in 2 months or less possible again. Studies of new drugs in development should inform the design of regimens capable of treating LTBI in contacts of multidrug-resistant or extensively drug-resistant TB patients.

## Understanding the Pharmacodynamics of Antituberculosis Drugs

Knowledge of a drug's pharmacodynamic (PD) properties, especially (1) whether it exhibits time- or concentration-dependent killing, and (2) the drug exposure targets necessary for bactericidal effects (and the maximal effect $E_{max}$, if achievable), is crucial to optimize drug dosing. Once elucidated, the PD parameter linked to efficacy and the magnitude of that parameter which correlates with efficacy against a given infection are generally similar between host species and predictably influenced by the susceptibility of the infecting organism [19]. Therefore, results from animal studies using a suitable model should be applicable to human infections.

The most widely used experimental design for linking PD variables with antibacterial activity is the dose fractionation study wherein a range of total doses given over a set time period is divided into regimens with different dosing frequencies (e.g. daily, thrice weekly etc.) so that the independent relationship of each of the 3 main PD parameters – maximum concentration/minimum inhibitory concentration (MIC), area under the curve (AUC)/MIC and time above MIC – to activity can be determined. The PD-linked variable is identified by the strength of the correlation between parameter values and some measure of drug effect, usually CFU counts. If done properly, such a study will define the PD parameter(s) and the magnitude of the parameter(s) that correlate with efficacy in the mouse and may be used to establish target drug exposures for future clinical trials. Moreover, because the PD-linked variables are likely the same among members of a particular drug class, the information gained from one compound may be applicable to other compounds in development.

The dose fractionation methodology has recently been adapted to study the PD of anti-TB drugs in mice. For example, Jayaram et al. [20] have demonstrated that the AUC/MIC ratio correlates best with the bactericidal activity of isoniazid and that the serum AUC necessary for the $E_{max}$ of isoniazid in mice was 25 μg/ml•h. Similarly, the early bactericidal activity of isoniazid has been shown to plateau as the dose exceeds 300 mg in slow acetylators of the drug for whom the AUC is expected to be approximately 20–25 μg/ml•h, whereas doses above 600 mg may be necessary to attain $E_{max}$ in rapid acetylators for whom the AUC after the 300-mg dose is approximately 6–8 μg/ml•h [21, 22]. There is excellent concordance with in vitro results as well, as the AUC/MIC value associated with 50% of the $E_{max}$ is remarkably similar between the murine model, an in vitro hollow-fibre model and human early bactericidal activity studies [23]. Thus, results with isoniazid in mice correlate well with its effect in humans and define the exposure above which no additional therapeutic benefit is observed.

While the $E_{max}$ of isoniazid occurs at an AUC/MIC value of approximately 500 that is achievable even in humans who are rapid acetylators (albeit with a higher dose than 5 mg/kg), the $E_{max}$ for rifampicin occurs at an AUC/MIC that is more than 2 orders of magnitude higher than the values typically achieved with a 600-mg dose [22, 24]. These data would have obvious implications for experimental compounds entering phase II clinical trials today. A PD profile like that of isoniazid would provide a rationale for not testing doses which exceed the exposure necessary to achieve the $E_{max}$, while a PD profile like that of rifampicin suggests that increasing doses beyond the clinically tolerable range will continue to confer increasing activity and that the maximal dose should be determined by factors such as tolerability and toxicity. Application of such an approach during the preclinical evaluation of rifapentine would have suggested that more frequent administration and/or administration of higher doses, compared to 600 mg once weekly, should improve the sterilizing activity of the drug and shorten the duration of TB treatment, as recently demonstrated in the murine model [2]. Only now, 40 years after the introduction of rifampicin and 12 years after FDA approval of rifapentine for once weekly use, are clinical trials under way to establish the optimal dose of these critical sterilizing drugs. A higher priority should be placed on PD optimization of new drugs in development [25].

### Utility of Other Animal Models

While historical results qualify mice as reasonable surrogates for assessing the sterilizing activity of drugs and combinations [3, 16], it is well known that conventional mouse strains infected with *M. tuberculosis* do not develop caseous necrosis, the pathological hallmark of human TB. Instead, mice develop only loose aggregates of mononuclear cells without tissue necrosis. Lesions in guinea pigs, rabbits and non-human primates are more similar pathologically to humans, including central necrosis and caseation. If such lesions or an associated micro-environmental condition (e.g. hypoxia, nutrient depletion, acidic pH) are determinants of bacterial persistence in human TB, the sterilizing activity of new TB drug candidates could be misjudged in mice if the bacterial target involved in persistence or the drug's mechanism of sterilizing activity is not relevant to the pathogenesis of mouse infection. In this case, the use of other models may provide important information on sterilizing activity. On the other hand, persistence might represent probabilistic and/or stochastic bacterial events which are relatively independent of the environment since similar treatments require just as long or longer to cure a mouse as compared to a human, despite the differences in pathology [3]. Debate over whether the pathological incongruity between mice and humans limits the ability of mouse models to forecast the sterilizing activity of future drug candidates [16] has created uncertainty among sponsors seeking to develop new TB drugs and combinations. At stake is whether results in mice should be confirmed in guinea pigs or another more expensive model before a new drug or combination is advanced to clinical trials or removed from development.

Although used successfully in the past to demonstrate the anti-TB activity of a variety of agents, guinea pigs remain poorly characterized as a model of TB chemotherapy [26]. Previous guinea pig studies have used various infectious doses, routes of infection, drug doses, incubation periods prior to treatment and outcome measures, making direct comparisons between experiments difficult and comparisons with mice impossible [3]. Using similar lung bacterial densities and human-equivalent drug doses, Ahmad et al. [27] have recently compared the efficacy of the standard first-line regimen of rifampicin-isoniazid-pyrazinamide, given predominantly twice weekly, in BALB/c mice and guinea pigs after both high- and low-dose infection. Remarkably, the duration of rifampicin-isoniazid-pyrazinamide treatment needed to prevent relapse was at least 2 months shorter in guinea pigs compared to mice, suggesting that the robust host response in the guinea pigs aided, rather than inhibited, the sterilizing action of rifampicin and/or pyrazinamide. The remarkable efficacy of rifampicin-isoniazid-pyrazinamide in guinea pigs contrasts with bacterial persistence observed with isoniazid or streptomycin monotherapy [26, 28], indicating this model may reliably and quickly discriminate drugs and regimens on the basis of their sterilizing activity. However, whether the sterilizing activity of new drugs in development will be better represented in guinea pigs remains to be determined.

Rabbits have been used to demonstrate that metronidazole has anti-TB activity in necrotic lesions with sufficient hypoxia, a result that has not been observed in various mouse models lacking sufficient tissue hypoxia [29, 30] or in guinea pigs due to drug toxicity and insufficient drug exposures [31]. That metronidazole appeared to have similar activity to rifampicin in rabbits is notable [30]. However, no pharmacokinetic information was provided to compare drug exposures in rabbits relative to human doses. A recently described rabbit model of cavitary disease also has interest as a model for early bactericidal activity, evaluation of drug penetration into cavities and studies devoted to the emergence of resistance [32].

Additional comparative studies with new drugs are needed to determine whether more pathologically accurate animal models have a role in TB drug development. The principal drawback of these larger animals is the significantly higher expense. The ideal model would blend the lower cost and superior tractability of mice with more human-like pathology. Recent reports suggest that C3HeB/FeJ mice could fill this niche. After low-dose aerosol infection, these mice develop discrete, well-formed granulomas with central necrosis and predominantly extracellular bacilli [10, 33]. Additional studies are under way to determine whether these pathological differences affect the way new and existing TB drugs and regimens perform in mice.

## Conclusions

With unprecedented numbers of new drugs in clinical trials for the treatment of TB and productive ongoing new discovery efforts, we are more reliant than ever on animal models to inform drug development. From first-in-animal experiments to late preclinical studies which aim to define the most promising combinations of new and existing drugs, the mouse has been the workhorse of the last few decades. However, the availability of new agents with new mechanisms of action in clinical trials also provides an opportunity to probe limitations of this model and better understand the contribution of other animal models to TB drug development. A faster path from discovery to approval may be a fortunate by-product of current drug development efforts.

## References


1 Nuermberger EL, Spigelman MK, Yew WW: Current development and future prospects in chemotherapy of tuberculosis. Respirology 2010;15:764–778.
2 Rosenthal IM, Zhang M, Williams KN, Peloquin CA, Tyagi S, Vernon AA, Bishai WR, Chaisson RE, Grosset JH, Nuermberger EL: Daily dosing of rifapentine cures tuberculosis in three months or less in the murine model. PLoS Med 2007;4:e344.
3 Nuermberger E: Using animal models to develop new treatments for tuberculosis. Semin Respir Crit Care Med 2008;29:542–551.
4 Nikonenko BV, Samala R, Einck L, Nacy CA: Rapid, simple in vivo screen for new drugs active against *Mycobacterium tuberculosis*. Antimicrob Agents Chemother 2004;48:4550–4555.
5 Shoen CM, De Stefano MS, Sklaney MR, Monica BJ, Slee AM, Cynamon MH: Short-course treatment regimen to identify potential antituberculous agents in a murine model of tuberculosis. J Antimicrob Chemother 2004;53:641–645.
6 Rullas J, Garcia JI, Beltran M, Cardona PJ, Caceres N, Garcia-Bustos JF, Angulo-Barturen I: Fast standardized therapeutic-efficacy assay for drug discovery against tuberculosis. Antimicrob Agents Chemother 2010;54:2262–2264.
7 Lenaerts AJ, Gruppo V, Brooks JV, Orme IM: Rapid in vivo screening of experimental drugs for tuberculosis using gamma interferon gene-disrupted mice. Antimicrob Agents Chemother 2003;47:783–785.
8 Stover CK, Warrener P, Van Devanter DR, Sherman DR, Arain TM, Langhorne MH, Anderson SW, Towell JA, Yuan Y, McMurray DN, Kreiswirth BN, Barry CE, Baker WR: A small-molecule nitroimidazopyran drug candidate for the treatment of tuberculosis. Nature 2000;405:962–966.
9 Andreu N, Zelmer A, Fletcher T, Elkington PT, Ward TH, Ripoll J, Parish T, Bancroft GJ, Schaible U, Robertson BD, Wiles S: Optimisation of bioluminescent reporters for use with mycobacteria. PLoS One 2010;5:e10777.
10 Davis SL, Nuermberger EL, Um PK, Vidal C, Jedynak B, Pomper MG, Bishai WR, Jain SK: Noninvasive pulmonary [$^{18}$F]-2-fluoro-deoxy-D-glucose positron emission tomography correlates with bactericidal activity of tuberculosis drug treatment. Antimicrob Agents Chemother 2009;53:4879–4884.
11 Davis SL, Be NA, Lamichhane G, Nimmagadda S, Pomper MG, Bishai WR, Jain SK: Bacterial thymidine kinase as a non-invasive imaging reporter for *Mycobacterium tuberculosis* in live animals. PLoS One 2009;4:e6297.
12 Andries K, Gevers T, Lounis N: Bactericidal potencies of new regimens are not predictive for their sterilizing potencies in a murine model of tuberculosis. Antimicrob Agent Chemother 2010;54:4540–4544.
13 Woolhiser L, Tamayo MH, Wang B, Gruppo V, Belisle JT, Lenaerts AJ, Basaraba RJ, Orme IM: In vivo adaptation of the Wayne model of latent tuberculosis. Infect Immun 2007;75:2621–2625.
14 Sala C, Dhar N, Hartkoorn RC, Zhang M, Ha YH, Schneider P, Cole ST: Simple model for testing drugs against nonreplicating *Mycobacterium tuberculosis*. Antimicrob Agents Chemother 2010;54:4150–4158.
15 Lecoeur HF, Truffot-Pernot C, Grosset JH: Experimental short-course preventive therapy of tuberculosis with rifampin and pyrazinamide. Am Rev Respir Dis 1989;140:1189–1193.
16 Mitchison DA, Chang KC: Experimental models of tuberculosis: can we trust the mouse? Am J Respir Crit Care Med 2009;180:201–202.
17 Nuermberger E, Tyagi S, Williams KN, Rosenthal I, Bishai WR, Grosset JH: Rifapentine, moxifloxacin, or DNA vaccine improves treatment of latent tuberculosis in a mouse model. Am J Respir Crit Care Med 2005;172:1452–1456.
18 Zhang T, Zhang M, Rosenthal IM, Grosset JH, Nuermberger EL: Short-course therapy with daily rifapentine in a murine model of latent tuberculosis infection. Am J Respir Crit Care Med 2009;180:1151–1157.
19 Craig WA: Pharmacokinetic/pharmacodynamic parameters: rationale for antibacterial dosing of mice and men. Clin Infect Dis 1998;26:1–10.
20 Jayaram R, Shandil RK, Gaonkar S, Kaur P, Suresh BL, Mahesh BN, Jayashree R, Nandi V, Bharath S, Kantharaj E, Balasubramanian V: Isoniazid pharmacokinetics-pharmacodynamics in an aerosol infection model of tuberculosis. Antimicrob Agents Chemother 2004;48:2951–2957.
21 Donald PR, Sirgel FA, Botha FJ, Seifart HI, Parkin DP, Vandenplas ML, Van de Wal BW, Maritz JS, Mitchison DA: The early bactericidal activity of isoniazid related to its dose size in pulmonary tuberculosis. Am J Respir Crit Care Med 1997;156:895–900.
22 Peloquin CA, Jaresko GS, Yong CL, Keung AC, Bulpitt AE, Jelliffe RW: Population pharmacokinetic modeling of isoniazid, rifampin, and pyrazinamide. Antimicrob Agents Chemother 1997;41:2670–2679.
23 Gumbo T, Louie A, Liu W, Brown D, Ambrose PG, Bhavnani SM, Drusano GL: Isoniazid bactericidal activity and resistance emergence: integrating pharmacodynamics and pharmacogenomics to predict efficacy in different ethnic populations. Antimicrob Agents Chemother 2007;51:2329–2336.

24 Jayaram R, Gaonkar S, Kaur P, Suresh BL, Mahesh BN, Jayashree R, Nandi V, Bharat S, Shandil RK, Kantharaj E, Balasubramanian V: Pharmacokinetics-pharmacodynamics of rifampin in an aerosol infection model of tuberculosis. Antimicrob Agents Chemother 2003;47:2118–2124.
25 Ahmad Z, Peloquin CA, Singh RP, Derendorf H, Tyagi S, Ginsberg A, Grosset JH, Nuermberger EL: PA-824 exhibits time-dependent activity in a murine model of tuberculosis. Antimicrob Agents Chemother 2011;55:239–245.
26 Ahmad Z, Klinkenberg LG, Pinn ML, Fraig MM, Peloquin CA, Bishai WR, Nuermberger EL, Grosset JH, Karakousis PC: Biphasic kill curve of isoniazid reveals the presence of drug-tolerant, not drug-resistant, *Mycobacterium tuberculosis* in the guinea pig. J Infect Dis 2009;200:1136–1143.
27 Ahmad Z, Nuermberger EL, Tasneen R, Pinn ML, Williams KN, Peloquin CA, Grosset JH, Karakousis PC: Comparison of the 'Denver regimen' against acute tuberculosis in the mouse and guinea pig. J Antimicrob Chemother 2010;65:729–734.
28 Ahmad Z, Pinn ML, Nuermberger EL, Peloquin CA, Grosset JH, Karakousis PC: The potent bactericidal activity of streptomycin in the guinea pig model of tuberculosis ceases due to the presence of persisters. J Antimicrob Chemother 2010;65:2172–2175.
29 Klinkenberg LG, Sutherland LA, Bishai WR, Karakousis PC: Metronidazole lacks activity against *Mycobacterium tuberculosis* in an in vivo hypoxic granuloma model of latency. J Infect Dis 2008;198:275–283.
30 Via LE, Lin PL, Ray SM, Carrillo J, Allen SS, Eum SY, Taylor K, Klein E, Manjunatha U, Gonzales J, Lee EG, Park SK, Raleigh JA, Cho SN, McMurray DN, Flynn JL, Barry CE III: Tuberculous granulomas are hypoxic in guinea pigs, rabbits, and nonhuman primates. Infect Immun 2008;76:2333–2340.
31 Hoff DR, Caraway ML, Brooks EJ, Driver ER, Ryan GJ, Peloquin CA, Orme IM, Basaraba RJ, Lenaerts AJ: Metronidazole lacks antibacterial activity in guinea pigs infected with *Mycobacterium tuberculosis.* Antimicrob Agents Chemother 2008;52:4137–4140.
32 Nedeltchev GG, Raghunand TR, Jassal MS, Lun S, Cheng QJ, Bishai WR: Extrapulmonary dissemination of *Mycobacterium bovis* but not *Mycobacterium tuberculosis* in a bronchoscopic rabbit model of cavitary tuberculosis. Infect Immun 2009;77:598–603.
33 Pan H, Yan BS, Rojas M, Shebzukhov YV, Zhou H, Kobzik L, Higgins DE, Daly MJ, Bloom BR, Kramnik I: *Ipr1* gene mediates innate immunity to tuberculosis. Nature 2005;434:767–772.

Eric L. Nuermberger, MD
1550 Orleans Street
Baltimore, MD 21231-1002 (USA)
Tel. +1 410 502 0580, E-Mail enuermb@jhmi.edu

Chapter 16

Donald PR, van Helden PD (eds): Antituberculosis Chemotherapy.
Prog Respir Res. Basel, Karger, 2011, vol 40, pp 153–160

# Current Issues in Tuberculosis Pharmacokinetics

Eric F. Egelund · Charles A. Peloquin

University of Florida, Gainesville, Fla., USA

## Abstract

The treatment of tuberculosis (TB) has remained mostly unchanged for the last 40 years. A renewed effort by public and private agencies around the world to slow the spread of the disease has led to an increased interest in finding a superior anti-TB drug regimen. The current doses recommended for first-line treatment of TB (isoniazid, rifampicin, pyrazinamide, ethambutol) may be inadequate for certain patients. Additionally, efforts are being made to reduce the length of treatment by utilizing other medications with activity against *Mycobacterium tuberculosis*, such as the fluoroquinolones. While the pharmacokinetic (PK) profile of a drug helps to explain a drug's action in the body, equally important is the management of that drug's PK profile clinically. Herein we review current PK questions being asked by leading researchers in the field and the role that therapeutic drug management may play in the treatment of TB.

Copyright © 2011 S. Karger AG, Basel

In contrast to the treatment of many common infectious diseases, the treatment of tuberculosis (TB) involves a multidrug regimen given for at least 6 months. The combination therapy used for TB attempts to accomplish 2 things: kill as many *Mycobacterium tuberculosis* bacilli as possible and avoid the selection of drug-resistant mutations. However, the length of treatment, the potential for drug interactions and adverse drug reactions conspire against the successful and timely completion of therapy.

Comorbid conditions, especially HIV, complicate TB in several ways. First, already TB-infected patients are much more likely to develop active disease. Next, they may present with atypical signs and symptoms, delaying the diagnosis of TB and the start of effective treatment. Finally, changes in drug absorption as well as several potential drug interactions impact TB drug pharmacokinetics, adversely affecting treatment outcomes. As with TB, HIV patients require multiple medications for treatment. The high pill burdens, multidrug interactions and overlapping presentations of adverse drug reactions make treating TB and HIV simultaneously a real challenge. Patients with diabetes, cystic fibrosis or those who have experienced gastrointestinal surgery may absorb their TB drugs more slowly or less completely than healthy persons, eroding the effectiveness of treatment [1–3].

How often should a patient take isoniazid? How much rifampicin can be given? The current TB regimens were developed empirically decades ago and have undergone very little modification since their inception. Several studies indicate that higher doses of anti-TB drugs are needed and are well tolerated in specific patient populations [4–6]. A helpful tool in unravelling the complicated tangle of drug interactions, comorbid conditions and patient-specific traits is therapeutic drug monitoring, or therapeutic drug management (TDM). TDM is the process of modifying a drug's dose based on its serum concentrations and can be a great resource to the clinician if used properly. This paper focusses on recent issues in the field of TB pharmacokinetics which need to be researched if we are to improve patient care. Other issues impacting TB pharmacokinetics which will be discussed include: practical considerations of TDM, the optimization of dosing strategies and when TDM may be of most benefit to the clinician.

## Practical Considerations

Pharmacokinetics may be thought of as what the body does to the drug. Pharmacodynamics may be thought of as what the drug does to the body [7]. In the case of antimicrobials, 2 separate objects of drug action exist. First, the organism (*Mycobacterium tuberculosis* in this case) is the object of drug efficacy. The patient is the object of any drug toxicity. Both aspects of pharmacodynamics must be managed simultaneously.

A significant limitation to the assessment of efficacy is that the available markers are delayed and not specific. Further, they are reversible, so even if sputum smears or cultures convert to negative, they can revert to positive. Therefore, a change in these parameters is not indicative of a durable response.

Proper assessment of a drug's effect on the body is only as good as the data provided to the clinician. Logistical issues may hinder the process in many different ways. Collecting multiple serum samples in a clinical setting to achieve an enhanced pharmacokinetic (PK) profile is not feasible, financially or logistically, for the clinician. Therefore, we must rely on 1 or 2 blood samples to make an assessment. Many steps in the sample collection process are required to ensure integrity. The nurse must verify that the patient actually receives the medication, and, if given orally, ensure the patient does not vomit shortly after ingestion. Blood samples must be drawn at the requested time points and recorded accurately. For drug monitoring of TB agents a 2-hour time sample and a 6-hour time sample are often taken. The 2-hour time sample captures the peak of most TB drugs while the 6-hour sample aids in evaluating the rate and completeness of drug absorption. Once the nurse collects the blood samples they have to be centrifuged, the serum harvested, and then frozen. Isoniazid and ethionamide are not stable at room temperature in blood so these two medications need to be processed quickly.

## Therapeutic Drug Monitoring/Therapeutic Drug Management

TDM has successfully been used in a variety of settings, including the clinical management of TB. Not all patients will require monitoring. In many instances, however, the monitoring of serum concentrations and subsequent individualization of therapy is recommended. Reduced serum concentrations may result from malabsorption, drug-drug interactions or inadequate drug dose [8].

For a TB drug to be effective it has to reach its site of action in sufficient quantity to kill *M. tuberculosis*. The first potential barrier to efficacy is absorption. Many factors influence the absorption of TB drugs: disease state, concomitant food or antacids, transporters in the gut, etc., which may result in a time to maximum concentration later than expected, or a maximum concentration ($C_{max}$) or area under the curve (AUC) lower than expected. Thankfully, with 2 time points malabsorption or delayed absorption may be captured and the dosing increased if warranted. Diabetes and HIV are 2 of the most common comorbid conditions in which absorption is affected, and patients with either condition are candidates for TDM.

## Ethambutol

A study of ethambutol by Zhu et al. [9] suggests that not all TB patients are receiving adequate doses of the drug. The empirical normal serum concentration range for daily dosing of ethambutol is 2–6 µg/ml, based on proven achievable concentrations, rather than pharmacodynamic (PD) relationships established from dose-ranging studies. In the cited study, maximum concentrations below the modest goal of 2 µg/ml were common in adults given standard doses on a milligram per kilogram basis (<25 mg/kg). More alarming, maximum concentrations of less than 1 µg/ml were common in children. A review of ethambutol dosage in children by Donald et al. [5] also found low concentrations to be common. These authors conclude that doses in the range of 15–25 mg/kg given daily may be used in children of all ages.

For HIV patients in the Zhu study, the $C_{max}$ values were on average 20% lower than their HIV-negative counterparts. With a maximum inhibitory concentration (MIC) for *M. tuberculosis* around 1–2 µg/ml, concern arises that the free drug concentrations at 15 mg/kg are too low to be effective.

Ethambutol is included in the regimen as a 'safety check' in case of yet-to-be-determined isoniazid resistance. Parsons et al. [10] showed that isoniazid-resistant strains, with a mutation at *katG* Ser315, are associated with increased ethambutol resistance. Additionally, the *ini*A gene, which encodes an efflux pump, is associated with resistance to both drugs [11]. Studies indicate that the transporter is induced by isoniazid, which may then act as a substrate for both or induce a pathway which leads to multiple efflux pumps, one or more of which would act on ethambutol [12]. Thus, a domino-type scenario may occur where isoniazid resistance leads to ethambutol resistance which leads to rifampicin resistance, though this has yet to be proven clinically.

Higher doses of ethambutol (and possibly isoniazid) may render the point moot. The concern with higher ethambutol doses is increasing the risk of ocular toxicity. As doses increase, a greater percentage of patients may experience optic neuritis. In studies of ethambutol from the 1960s, for patients given daily doses of 50, 25 and 12.5 mg/kg, the incidence of optic neuritis was 15, 3 and 1–<2%, respectively [13, 14]. In the study undertaken by Zhu et al. [9], simulations suggested that daily doses of 25 mg/kg would be the preferred regimen for most patients, especially in special populations such as HIV patients or patients with suspected rifampicin- or isoniazid-resistant isolates.

## Isoniazid

Isoniazid has been a mainstay of TB therapy for nearly 5 decades. For much of that time the standard dose has been 300 mg. As isoniazid did not undergo rigorous randomized trials, and the standard dose was established before the advent of modern pharmacogenetics, the question has been raised if this is the most appropriate dose for all patient populations. Additionally, increasing the dose of isoniazid has been suggested to overcome the 'low-level' resistance of some isolates. In short, 300 mg may not be the optimal dose for all TB patients.

During the first 2 days of therapy, isoniazid has a high kill rate against *M. tuberculosis*. Following this period of time its activity begins to decline. During this second phase, resistance to isoniazid begins to occur. *M. tuberculosis* develops resistance to isoniazid more easily than to other TB medications. The proportion of resistance among new cases worldwide is believed to be around 10.3–27.7% among previously treated cases [15]. 'Low-level' resistance to isoniazid spans the range of 0.1–0.2 μg/ml. Isoniazid may still be useful despite this resistance. The drug remains effective at rapid killing of non-resistant *M. tuberculosis*, resulting in a reduced number of bacilli. A rapid reduction in mycobacterial counts allows other drugs such as rifampicin and pyrazinamide to be more effective.

A review by Mitchison and Nunn [16] of 12 studies supports this view. The study shows that initial isoniazid resistance has little impact on sterilizing activity in 6-month multidrug regimens containing rifampicin and/or pyrazinamide [16]. A murine study by Cynamon et al. [17] revealed similar results. They demonstrated that isoniazid in combination with other anti-TB drugs may be useful in patients with MICs of 0.2–0.5 μg/ml. However, they noted no difference in cell counts between mice treated with lower doses of isoniazid (25 mg/kg) as compared to those treated with higher doses (100 mg/kg), leading the authors to conclude 'that doses of isoniazid greater than 300 mg/day are unlikely to be more effective for treatment of human pulmonary tuberculosis than is the standard dose' but when used in combination with other anti-TB drugs to be beneficial in patients with isoniazid MICs ≤5 μg/ml [17]. Clearly, this question warrants further clinical study. While empirically including higher doses of isoniazid (such as 600 mg daily or 900 mg 3 times weekly) in cases where it might be of benefit is relatively easy and inexpensive, we need unequivocal data to show that this is both effective and safe. The risk of liver and nervous system toxicities is warranted only if the drug actually reduces the mycobacterial burden.

## Pyrazinamide

The current recommended daily dose of pyrazinamide is 15–30 mg/kg in TB-infected adults with a maximum dose of 2 g; despite the fact that the British Medical Research Council studies established pyrazinamide's use as a first-line treatment using 35 mg/kg [18, 19]. Recent PK-PD studies suggest that higher doses will be more efficacious in the treatment of TB than those used currently. Utilizing a hollow-fibre model, Gumbo et al. [20] demonstrated that AUC/MIC best correlated with pyrazinamide's sterilizing effect. Subsequent Monte Carlo simulations showed that doses greater than the standard 2 g/day were necessary to produce the AUC/MIC ratio associated with the pyrazinamide $EC_{90}$ (concentration which leads to 90% maximum killing) [20].

A weight-based dosing method appears to provide the best approach to treatment. For example, in a recent population PK model of 227 South African TB patients, the volume of distribution and clearance both increased with weight (4.33 litres and 0.545 l/h, respectively, with each 10-kg increase in weight) [21]. While current guidelines provide recommendations for 3 distinct groups of patients based on weight (40–55, 56–75, 76–90 kg), no recommendations for patients over 90 kg – an ever increasing population – exist. Also, the guidelines do not provide a strict milligram per kilogram dosing schedule [18].

How would an increase in dose affect the incidence of adverse events? Of primary concern with high-dose pyrazinamide is the risk of hepatotoxicity. Initial concerns rose from 2 studies undertaken in 1954 in which doses ranging from 40 up to 70 mg/kg resulted in elevated rates of toxicity [22, 23]. However, a recent meta-analysis combined with population PK-PD modelling suggests no more risk of hepatotoxic side effects with high-dose than low-dose pyrazinamide [6]. Arthralgia was the most common side effect experienced, with a 16% frequency in studies using pyrazinamide as monotherapy and 2.5% in combination therapy. Thankfully, arthralgia is not the treatment-ending adverse event that hepatotoxicity can be and is generally well tolerated with the use of non-steroidal anti-inflammatory drugs. As with isoniazid above, a comparative clinical trial is needed to prove that the commonly used lower doses (20–25 mg/kg daily) of pyrazinamide are actually equally effective as higher doses (such as 35 mg/kg) and actually reduce toxicity. If the lower doses fail to reduce toxicity while concurrently slowing the sterilization process, the higher doses should be used.

### Rifampicin

Rifampicin given at 600 mg/day has been one of the cornerstones of therapy since the drug was approved by the FDA in 1971. The 600-mg dose is currently the recommended maximum dose despite the lack of studies regarding optimal dosing. Rifampicin has long been known to have a dose response regarding efficacy [24, 25]. Rifampicin's peak occurs approximately 2 h after dosing and has a serum concentration range of 8–24 μg/ml for a 600-mg dose. For rifampicin the MIC of *M. tuberculosis* lies in the 0.15–0.5 μg/ml range, thus one would expect adequate eradication of *M. tuberculosis* at this dose [26, 27]. More recent studies are contributing to a better understanding of rifampicin's activity. First, in vitro and mouse model studies have shown that the AUC/MIC is highly correlated with rifampicin's bactericidal activity. Second, modelling of broncho-alveolar lavage data suggests that the distribution of rifampicin within compartments inside the lungs may be an important consideration [28].

A recent PK-PD analysis utilizing a hollow-fibre model looked at an overall rifampicin dose of 4,200 mg divided into 3 scheduling formats: 600 mg daily for 7 days, 2,100 mg twice weekly and a one-time dose of 4,200 mg. In all 3 treatment groups, reduction of microbial growth was comparable, suggesting that the AUC/MIC is associated with rifampicin bactericidal activity. However, when looking at the resistant subpopulation, $C_{max}$/MIC was the parameter which best explained suppression. Similarly, the postantibiotic effect was best explained by the $C_{max}$/MIC. The authors argue that rifampicin is concentration dependent and doses higher than 600 mg would optimize rifampicin's ability to kill *M. tuberculosis*, with the caveat that patients are able to tolerate the increased doses, a position we too have long advocated [4, 29]. A murine model by Jayaram et al. [30] points to AUC/MIC as the PK-PD parameter most associated with rifampicin's bactericidal activity. Using an aerosol infection model, the researchers noted a greater correlation with AUC/MIC with reduction in bacterial load than either $C_{max}$/MIC or time/MIC [30]. This result was confirmed by Rosenthal et al. [31] and Zhang et al. [32].

Several human studies have used doses beyond 600 mg, with doses of 750, 900 and 1,200 mg having all been tested [33–36]. Of major concern with higher doses is the potential for increased adverse events, specifically the 'flu-like' syndrome experienced by some patients. The flu-like syndrome occurs primarily with patients receiving once or twice weekly rifampicin [37]. Additionally, while rifampicin's maximum recommended dose is 600 mg for TB disease, higher doses are utilized in other disease states: 900 mg has been used for treating leprosy, brucellosis and staphylococcal infections while 1,200 mg has been used in 1 patient with *Legionella*, several patients with leishmaniasis and is the maximum recommended dose for meningococcal prophylaxis [38–40]. Very few adverse events have been seen at these elevated doses thus far.

A limited number of trials exist comparing 600 mg rifampicin with greater than 600 mg [33, 35]. In a comparison of 450, 600 and 750 mg of rifampicin (all with 300 mg isoniazid), no difference in the rate of relapse or sputum conversion was seen in the 600- and 750-mg groups, but the 450-mg group had a significantly higher rate of relapse and lower rate of sputum conversion [35]. Kreis et al. [33], using ultrashort 3-month regimens with 1,200 mg of rifampicin (+ isoniazid and streptomycin), had a nearly 100% sputum conversion, though 16% of patients did experience a relapse after 1 year. Had a longer duration of treatment been employed, very high durable cures may have been achieved. Based on the accumulated data a case can be made that the 600-mg dose needs to be further evaluated as the 'optimal' dose to be used in the treatment of *M. tuberculosis* [29, 36].

### Rifapentine

Similar arguments for increased doses may be made for rifapentine. Rifapentine, with its long half-life, has been used in once weekly maintenance regimens to facilitate directly observed therapy. Unfortunately, intermittent therapy is more likely to lead to rifamycin resistance, especially in patients with HIV. In a comparison of once weekly rifapentine and isoniazid to that of twice weekly rifampicin and isoniazid in HIV-negative patients, a higher rate of relapse existed in the rifapentine arm [41].

One solution is to increase the dose of rifapentine. A study of 35 TB patients by Weiner et al. [42] looked at 600-, 900- and 1,200-mg doses. The AUC significantly increased as dose increased without an apparent increase in serious side effects. As the authors of this study point out, rifapentine is highly protein bound (98–99%), and higher doses may be required to reach effective concentrations.

A second solution is to combine rifapentine with another long-acting drug. A murine model utilizing once weekly moxifloxacin with 15 mg/kg rifapentine suggests that this regimen is more efficacious than twice weekly isoniazid and rifapentine [43]. Using 2 drugs with similar half-lives decreases the risk of 1 drug dipping below the MIC which would facilitate resistance. Finally, the current US Public Health Service (USPHS) TB Study 29 evaluates daily rifapentine (600 mg) as a means to improve durable cures.

## Human Immunodeficiency Virus and Rifamycins

Once a person has contracted HIV he/she becomes very susceptible to infection by *M. tuberculosis*. Researchers theorize that this susceptibility is due to the inability of alveolar macrophages to undergo cell death when infected by *M. tuberculosis*. This apoptosis of alveolar macrophages helps to eliminate *M. tuberculosis* infection by making the mycobacteria available to more competent macrophages under the influence of CD4+ T cells. HIV prevents this elimination from occurring, possibly through the involvement of tumor necrosis factor α). Further, HIV makes it more likely for latently infected patients to go on to active disease. In sum, HIV and TB make for a deadly combination.

The rifamycins induce hepatic and intestinal cytochrome (CYP) 3A4, and since a large number of medications are CYP3A4 substrates, rifamycin use leads to reduced concentrations of many drugs, and thus, reduced efficacy. Rifabutin induces CYP enzymes approximately 40% as much as rifampicin [44]. For this reason, rifabutin is recommended for HIV/TB patients to reduce the severity of drug interactions. Rifabutin itself is a CYP3A4 substrate, creating conditions for 2-way interactions with other drugs that induce or inhibit CYP3A4. If concentrations are not monitored and doses properly adjusted, resistance to rifabutin may arise [45].

Rifamycin resistance has become an increasing concern in HIV patients. Protease inhibitors conflict with rifamycin's metabolic properties and vice versa, leading to unknown serum concentrations of each. In addition, low CD4+ T cell counts and intermittent rifamycin therapy are considered risk factors for resistance [45]. The PK substudy of USPHS TB Study 23 by Weiner et al. [46] exemplifies the problem. In the study, patients were treated with rifabutin and isoniazid twice weekly. Out of the 102 patients participating in the PK portion of the study, 8 developed rifamycin resistance. Seven of the 8 were found to have low rifabutin serum concentrations ($AUC_{0-24}$)[46]. Also, the HIV-positive arm of USPHS TB Study 22 was discontinued prematurely due to rifamycin resistance in patients receiving isoniazid and rifapentine once weekly [41]. Thus, in HIV patients receiving intermittent therapy, TDM is recommended to aid in the prevention of treatment failure.

## The Fluoroquinolones

The current era of TB treatment which had emerged in the 1960s as a regimen of isoniazid, para-aminosalicylic acid and streptomycin gave way to the new rifamycins and eventually to the 4-drug regimen used today. A new era may be on the horizon as researchers look for ways to reduce the duration of therapy. The fluoroquinolones (FQs), currently used as second-line therapy, may usher in this new epoch. FQs are being studied for a role as first-line agents in the ongoing effort to shorten the length of treatment [47, 48]. Which quinolone – including levofloxacin – and what dose result in maximum efficacy has yet to be determined [49, 50].

The FQs are bactericidal and as a class have good in vitro and in vivo activity toward *M. tuberculosis*, especially moxifloxacin and gatifloxacin. Their efficacy, combined with a limited armamentarium for TB, makes them an appealing drug class to clinicians. Unfortunately we may not be maximizing their potential [47, 51].

When paired with rifampicin, moxifloxacin appears to have a synergistic effect at suppressing *M. tuberculosis* resistance, but it may come at the expense of a modest reduction in bactericidal effect [52, 53]. A hollow-fibre model by Drusano et al. [54] comparing a rifampicin and moxifloxacin 5 times weekly regimen with a daily regimen showed an increased chance of resistance in the 5-day regimen due to the discordant half-lives.

Rifapentine, with its longer half-life, may prove superior to rifampicin. As previously mentioned, a murine model combining moxifloxacin and rifapentine dosed once weekly was shown to be more efficacious than twice weekly isoniazid and rifapentine, though whether moxifloxacin should be added to a rifamycin and isoniazid, or used as a replacement for isoniazid, is unknown. Isoniazid, like rifampicin, has a much shorter half-life than moxifloxacin. Finally, daily rifapentine, perhaps with moxifloxacin, could provide nearly continuous suppression of mycobacteria. Since the timing of susceptibility to antibiotic action during the 'persister state' is poorly understood, perhaps this continuous suppression is advantageous [55].

Guidelines recommend moxifloxacin and gatifloxacin be given as 400 mg daily [56]. Data are lacking at doses above this. A hollow-fibre model combined with Monte Carlo simulations by Gumbo et al. [57] points to an 800 mg/day dose suppressing resistance in 93% of patients compared to approximately 60% with 400 mg daily. The question is, of course, if an 800-mg dose can be tolerated. Unlike the rifamycins, the FQs may be limited in dose escalation by side effects, primarily gastrointestinal, QTc prolongation, and events related to the central nervous system. In certain populations the FQs are undesirable. The FQs are contraindicated in pregnant women. In theory, FQs may have an increased risk of arthropathy in children, but limited clinical data support this. Human trials are under way to determine the appropriate dosing regimen, what TB drugs they are most compatible with and what patient population should be targeted [49, 50, 58].

## Conclusions

While most medication classes target receptors or other proteins in the human body, anti-infective agents must deal with an additional organism. The major concern with inadequate dosing or malabsorption, especially with anti-infective drugs, is the development of resistance. The World Health Organization estimates that as many as 440,000 people worldwide are infected with multidrug-resistant TB [59]. More refined dosing regimens are needed, perhaps using higher doses, using more frequent doses or using new combinations with faster killing and better suppression of resistance guided by TDM when appropriate.

## References


1 Heysell SK, Moore JL, Keller SJ, Houpt ER: Therapeutic drug monitoring for slow response to tuberculosis treatment in a state control program, Virginia, USA. Emerg Infect Dis 2010;16:1546–1553.

2 Peloquin CA: Using therapeutic drug monitoring to dose the antimycobacterial drugs. Clin Chest Med 1997;18:79–87.

3 Gilljam M, Berning SE, Peloquin CA, Strandvik B, Larsson LO: Therapeutic drug monitoring in patients with cystic fibrosis and mycobacterial disease. Eur Respir J 1999;14:347–351.

4 Gumbo T, Louie A, Deziel MR, Liu W, Parsons LM, Salfinger M, Drusano GL: Concentration-dependent *Mycobacterium tuberculosis* killing and prevention of resistance by rifampin. Antimicrob Agents Chemother 2007;51:3781–3788.

5 Donald PR, Maher D, Maritz JS, Qazi S: Ethambutol dosage for the treatment of children: literature review and recommendations. Int J Tuberc Lung Dis 2006;10:1318–1330.

6 Pasipanodya JG, Gumbo T: Clinical and toxicodynamic evidence that high-dose pyrazinamide is not more hepatotoxic than the low doses currently used. Antimicrob Agents Chemother 2010;54:2847–2854.

7 Holford N, Sheiner LB: Kinetics of pharmacologic response. Pharmacol Ther 1982;16:143–166.

8 Peloquin CA: Therapeutic drug monitoring in the treatment of tuberculosis. Drugs 2002;62:2169–2183.

9 Zhu M, Burman WJ, Starke JR, Stambaugh JJ, Steiner P, Bulpitt AE, Ashkin D, Auclair B, Berning SE, Jelliffe RW, Jaresko GS, Peloquin CA: Pharmacokinetics of ethambutol in children and adults with tuberculosis. Int J Tuberc Lung Dis 2004;8:1360–1367.

10 Parsons LM, Salfinger M, Clobridge A, Dormandy J, Mirabello L, Polletta VL, Sanic A, Sinyavskiy O, Larsen SC, Driscoll J, Zickas G, Taber HW: Phenotypic and molecular characterization of *Mycobacterium tuberculosis* isolates resistant to both isoniazid and ethambutol. Antimicrob Agents Chemother 2005;49:2218–2225.

11 Colangeli R, Helb D, Sridharan S, Sun J, Varma-Basil M, Hazbon MH, Harbacheuski R, Megjugorac NJ, Jacobs WR Jr, Holzenburg A, Sacchettini JC, Alland D: The *Mycobacterium tuberculosis iniA* gene is essential for activity of an efflux pump that confers drug tolerance to both isoniazid and ethambutol. Mol Microbiol 2005;55:1829–1840.

12 Srivastava S, Musuka S, Sherman C, Meek C, Leff R, Gumbo T: Efflux-pump-derived multiple drug resistance to ethambutol monotherapy in *Mycobacterium tuberculosis* and the pharmacokinetics and pharmacodynamics of ethambutol. J Infect Dis 2010;201:1225–1231.

13 Griffith DE, Brown-Elliott BA, Shepherd S, McLarty J, Griffith L, Wallace RJ Jr: Ethambutol ocular toxicity in treatment regimens for *Mycobacterium avium* complex lung disease. Am J Respir Crit Care Med 2005;172:250–253.

14 Leibold JE: The ocular toxicity of ethambutol and its relation to dose. Ann NY Acad Sci 1966;135:904–909.

15 World Health Organization: Anti-Tuberculosis Drug Resistance in the World, Report No 4. Geneva, WHO, 2008.

16 Mitchison DA, Nunn AJ: Influence of initial drug resistance on the response to short-course chemotherapy of pulmonary tuberculosis. Am Rev Respir Dis 1986;133:423–430.

17 Cynamon MH, Zhang Y, Harpster T, Cheng S, De Stefano MS: High-dose isoniazid therapy for isoniazid-resistant murine *Mycobacterium tuberculosis* infection. Antimicrob Agents Chemother 1999;43:2922–2924.

18 Bass JB Jr, Farer LS, Hopewell PC, O'Brien R, Jacobs RF, Ruben F, Snider DE Jr, Thornton G: Treatment of tuberculosis and tuberculosis infection in adults and children. American Thoracic Society and the Centers for Disease Control and Prevention. Am J Respir Crit Care Med 1994;149:1359–1374.

19 Investigation EABMRCP: A controlled comparison of four regimens of streptomycin plus pyrazinamide in the treatment of pulmonary tuberculosis. Tubercle 1964;50:81–112.
20 Gumbo T, Dona CS, Meek C, Leff R: Pharmacokinetics-pharmacodynamics of pyrazinamide in a novel in vitro model of tuberculosis for sterilizing effect: a paradigm for faster assessment of new antituberculosis drugs. Antimicrob Agents Chemother 2009;53:3197–3204.
21 Wilkins JJ, Langdon G, McIlleron H, Pillai GC, Smith PJ, Simonsson US: Variability in the population pharmacokinetics of pyrazinamide in South African tuberculosis patients. Eur J Clin Pharmacol 2006;62:727–735.
22 Campagna M, Calix A, Hauser G: Observations on the combined use of pyrazinamide (Aldinamide) and isoniazid in the treatment of pulmonary tuberculosis: a clinical study. Am Rev Tuberc 1954;69:334–350.
23 McDermott W, Ormond L, Muschenheim C, Deuschle K, McCune RM Jr, Tompsett R: Pyrazinamide-isoniazid in tuberculosis. Am Rev Tuberc 1954;69:319–333.
24 Pallanza R, Furesz S, Timbal MT, Carniti G: In vitro bacteriological studies on rifamycin B diethylamide (rifamide). Arzneimittelforschung 1965;15:800–802.
25 Verbist L: Rifampicin activity 'in vitro' and in established tuberculosis in mice. Acta Tuberc Pneumol Belg 1969;60:397–412.
26 Burman WJ, Gallicano K, Peloquin C: Comparative pharmacokinetics and pharmacodynamics of the rifamycin antibacterials. Clin Pharmacokinet 2001;40:327–341.
27 Lee CN, Heifets LB: Determination of minimal inhibitory concentrations of antituberculosis drugs by radiometric and conventional methods. Am Rev Respir Dis 1987;136:349–352.
28 Ziglam HM, Baldwin DR, Daniels I, Andrew JM, Finch RG: Rifampicin concentrations in bronchial mucosa, epithelial lining fluid, alveolar macrophages and serum following a single 600 mg oral dose in patients undergoing fibre-optic bronchoscopy. J Antimicrob Chemother 2002;50:1011–1015.
29 Peloquin C: What is the 'right' dose of rifampin? Int J Tuberc Lung Dis 2003;7:3–5.
30 Jayaram R, Gaonkar S, Kaur P, Suresh BL, Mahesh BN, Jayashree R, Nandi V, Bharat S, Shandil RK, Kantharaj E, Balasubramanian V: Pharmacokinetics-pharmacodynamics of rifampin in an aerosol infection model of tuberculosis. Antimicrob Agents Chemother 2003;47:2118–2124.
31 Rosenthal IM, Williams K, Tyagi S, Peloquin CA, Vernon AA, Bishai WR, Grosset JH, Nuermberger EL: Potent twice-weekly rifapentine-containing regimens in murine tuberculosis. Am J Respir Crit Care Med 2006;174:94–101.
32 Zhang T, Zhang M, Rosenthal IM, Grosset JH, Nuermberger EL: Short-course therapy with daily rifapentine in a murine model of latent tuberculosis infection. Am J Respir Crit Care Med 2009;180:1151–1157.
33 Kreis B, Pretet S, Birenbaum J, Guibout P, Hazeman JJ, Orin E, Perdrizet S, Weil J: Two three-month treatment regimens for pulmonary tuberculosis. Bull Int Union Tuberc 1976;51:71–75.
34 Constans P, Saint-Paul M, Morin Y, Bonnaud G, Bariety M: Rifampicin: initial study of plasma levels during prolonged treatment of pulmonary tuberculosis patients. Rev Tuberc Pneumol (Paris) 1968;32:991–1006.
35 Long MW, Snider DE Jr, Farer LS: US Public Health Service Cooperative trial of three rifampin-isoniazid regimens in treatment of pulmonary tuberculosis. Am Rev Respir Dis 1979;119:879–894.
36 Mitnick CD, McGee B, Peloquin CA: Tuberculosis pharmacotherapy: strategies to optimize patient care. Expert Opin Pharmacother 2009;10:381–401.
37 Martinez E, Collazos J, Mayo J: Hypersensitivity reactions to rifampin: pathogenetic mechanisms, clinical manifestations, management strategies, and review of the anaphylactic-like reactions. Medicine (Baltimore) 1999;78:361–369.
38 Dhar S, Kaur I, Sharma VK, Kumar B: 'Flu' syndrome due to rifampin: experience with four cases. Int J Lepr Other Mycobact Dis 1995;63:92–94.
39 Drancourt M, Stein A, Argenson JN, Zannier A, Curvale G, Raoult D: Oral rifampin plus ofloxacin for treatment of *Staphylococcus*-infected orthopedic implants. Antimicrob Agents Chemother 1993;37:1214–1218.
40 Clinical Pharmacology Online. Gold Standard Inc, 2010.
41 Benator D, Bhattacharya M, Bozeman L, Burman W, Cantazaro A, Chaisson R, Gordin F, Horsburgh CR, Horton J, Khan A, Lahart C, Metchock B, Pachucki C, Stanton L, Vernon A, Villarino ME, Wang YC, Weiner M, Weis S: Rifapentine and isoniazid once a week versus rifampicin and isoniazid twice a week for treatment of drug-susceptible pulmonary tuberculosis in HIV-negative patients: a randomised clinical trial. Lancet 2002;360:528–534.
42 Weiner M, Bock N, Peloquin CA, Burman WJ, Khan A, Vernon A, Zhao Z, Weis S, Sterling TR, Hayden K, Goldberg S: Pharmacokinetics of rifapentine at 600, 900, and 1,200 mg during once-weekly tuberculosis therapy. Am J Respir Crit Care Med 2004;169:1191–1197.
43 Rosenthal IM, Williams K, Tyagi S, Vernon AA, Peloquin CA, Bishai WR, Grosset JH, Nuermberger EL: Weekly moxifloxacin and rifapentine is more active than the Denver regimen in murine tuberculosis. Am J Respir Crit Care Med 2005;172:1457–1462.
44 Burman WJ, Gallicano K, Peloquin C: Therapeutic implications of drug interactions in the treatment of human immunodeficiency virus-related tuberculosis. Clin Infect Dis 1999;28:419–429.
45 Boulanger C, Hollender E, Farrell K, Stambaugh JJ, Maasen D, Ashkin D, Symes S, Espinoza LA, Rivero RO, Graham JJ, Peloquin CA: Pharmacokinetic evaluation of rifabutin in combination with lopinavir-ritonavir in patients with HIV infection and active tuberculosis. Clin Infect Dis 2009;49:1305–1311.
46 Weiner M, Benator D, Burman W, Peloquin CA, Khan A, Vernon A, Jones B, Silva-Trigo C, Zhao Z, Hodge T: Association between acquired rifamycin resistance and the pharmacokinetics of rifabutin and isoniazid among patients with HIV and tuberculosis. Clin Infect Dis 2005;40:1481–1491.
47 Burman WJ, Goldberg S, Johnson JL, Muzanye G, Engle M, Mosher AW, Choudhri S, Daley CL, Munsiff SS, Zhao Z, Vernon A, Chaisson RE: Moxifloxacin versus ethambutol in the first 2 months of treatment for pulmonary tuberculosis. Am J Respir Crit Care Med 2006;174:331–338.
48 Dorman SE, Johnson JL, Goldberg S, Muzanye G, Padayatchi N, Bozeman L, Heilig CM, Bernardo J, Choudhri S, Grosset JH, Guy E, Guyadeen P, Leus MC, Maltas G, Menzies D, Nuermberger EL, Villarino M, Vernon A, Chaisson RE: Substitution of moxifloxacin for isoniazid during intensive phase treatment of pulmonary tuberculosis. Am J Respir Crit Care Med 2009;180:273–280.
49 Peloquin CA, Hadad DJ, Molino LP, Palaci M, Boom WH, Dietze R, Johnson JL: Population pharmacokinetics of levofloxacin, gatifloxacin, and moxifloxacin in adults with pulmonary tuberculosis. Antimicrob Agents Chemother 2008;52:852–857.
50 Johnson JL, Hadad DJ, Boom WH, Daley CL, Peloquin CA, Eisenach KD, Jankus DD, Debanne SM, Charlebois ED, Maciel E, Palaci M, Dietze R: Early and extended early bactericidal activity of levofloxacin, gatifloxacin and moxifloxacin in pulmonary tuberculosis. Int J Tuberc Lung Dis 2006;10:605–612.
51 Dooley K, Flexner C, Hackman J, Peloquin CA, Nuermberger E, Chaisson RE, Dorman SE: Repeated administration of high-dose intermittent rifapentine reduces rifapentine and moxifloxacin plasma concentrations. Antimicrob Agents Chemother 2008;52:4037–4042.
52 Drusano GL, Sgambati N, Eichas A, Brown DL, Kulawy R, Louie A: The combination of rifampin plus moxifloxacin is synergistic for suppression of resistance but antagonistic for cell kill of *Mycobacterium tuberculosis* as determined in a hollow-fiber infection model. MBio 2010;1:e00139.
53 Weiner M, Burman W, Luo CC, Peloquin CA, Engle M, Goldberg S, Agarwal V, Vernon A: Effects of rifampin and multidrug resistance gene polymorphism on concentrations of moxifloxacin. Antimicrob Agents Chemother 2007;51:2861–2866.
54 Drusano GLNS, Eichas A, Kulawy R, Brown D, Louie A: Effect of administering moxifloxacin (MOX) plus rifampin (RIF) against *M. tuberculosis (Mtb)* 7/7 vs. 5/7 days. ICAAC, Boston, 2010.

55 Rosenthal IM, Zhang M, Williams KN, Peloquin CA, Tyagi S, Vernon AA, Bishai WR, Chaisson RE, Grosset JH, Nuermberger EL: Daily dosing of rifapentine cures tuberculosis in three months or less in the murine model. PLoS Med 2007;4:e344.
56 Neff M: ATS, CDC, and IDSA update recommendations on the treatment of tuberculosis. Am Fam Physician 2003;68:1854, 1857–1858, 1861–1852.
57 Gumbo T, Louie A, Deziel MR, Parsons LM, Salfinger M, Drusano GL: Selection of a moxifloxacin dose that suppresses drug resistance in *Mycobacterium tuberculosis,* by use of an in vitro pharmacodynamic infection model and mathematical modeling. J Infect Dis 2004;190:1642–1651.
58 Rustomjee R, Lienhardt C, Kanyok T, Davies GR, Levin J, Mthiyane T, Reddy C, Sturm AW, Sirgel FA, Allen J, Coleman DJ, Fourie B, Mitchison DA: A phase II study of the sterilising activities of ofloxacin, gatifloxacin and moxifloxacin in pulmonary tuberculosis. Int J Tuberc Lung Dis 2008;12:128–138.
59 World Health Organization: Multidrug and Extensively Drug-Resistant Tuberculosis: 2010 Global Report on Surveillance and Response. Geneva,WHO, 2010.

Eric F. Egelund
University of Florida
1600 SW Archer Road, Room P4-33
PO Box 100486, Gainesville, FL 32610-0486 (USA)
Tel. +1 352 273 6266, E-Mail eegelund@ufl.edu

Chapter 17

Donald PR, van Helden PD (eds): Antituberculosis Chemotherapy.
Prog Respir Res. Basel, Karger, 2011, vol 40, pp 161–175

# Pharmacological Considerations of Antitubercular Agents in Children

Jennifer L. Goldman[a] · Gregory L. Kearns[b–d] · Susan M. Abdel-Rahman[c,d]

[a]Divisions of Infectious Diseases, [b]Department of Medical Research and [c]Division of Clinical Pharmacology and Medical Toxicology, Children's Mercy Hospitals and Clinics, and [d]Department of Pediatrics, University of Missouri at Kansas City School of Medicine, Kansas City, Mo., USA

**Abstract**

This review is intended to provide a comprehensive summary of the existing paediatric clinical pharmacology data on the drugs and drug classes that are used for, or proposed for use in, the treatment of tuberculosis. It discusses antitubercular drug disposition in the context of developmental physiology (where known) and highlights the aspects of paediatric drug disposition that remain unknown for the various antitubercular agents. Finally, it introduces common problems that can arise in the conduct of paediatric pharmacokinetic studies and highlights considerations for the design of future paediatric studies on the antitubercular agents.

Copyright © 2011 S. Karger AG, Basel

In the developing world, tuberculosis (TB) remains one of the most vexing health care challenges across the age spectrum, particularly in children under 5 years where it is a major cause of childhood mortality in areas where TB is endemic [1]. As recently reviewed, the estimated annual risk of TB infection in children is 2.5% with nearly 8–20% of those who acquire the disease succumbing to it [2]. The challenge of paediatric TB is further compounded by continued evolution of drug-resistant mycobacteria, HIV co-infection, extrapulmonary disease and a paucity of new drugs and/or formulations suitable for the treatment of children, particularly the very young.

In an attempt to better address the challenges associated with paediatric TB treatment, the World Health Organization (WHO) recently revised the recommended dosages of the main first-line anti-TB drugs [3]. This re-evaluation and the resultant recommendations reflected a process including a systematic review of available data (e.g. published dosing recommendations, safety/efficacy data) by a group of experts comprising paediatricians, paediatric infectious disease specialists and clinical pharmacologists. Considerations for final dose selection included known developmental differences in physiological processes capable of altering drug disposition [4], and available pharmacokinetic and pharmacodynamic data of first-line antitubercular agents available from the very limited number of published paediatric reports. The purpose of this review is to provide a comprehensive summary of existing paediatric pharmacokinetic data on antitubercular agents, and to review recent research and pharmacological considerations necessary to optimize the TB treatment of infants and children.

## Isoniazid

Isoniazid (INH) remains a mainstay in antitubercular drug regimens, yet its dose-exposure relationship demonstrates remarkably wide interindividual variability when compared with other antitubercular agents. This may be explained, in part, by factors that influence the bioavailability and metabolism of INH as discussed below.

INH appears to be absorbed relatively quickly following peroral drug administration with time to maximal concentration ($t_{max}$) reached within 1–3 h irrespective of age [5–8]. Whether the extent of absorption is influenced by age is more difficult to assess given the methodological limitations of existing studies (e.g. limited sampling schemes, widely variant drug formulations). Nonetheless, studies suggest that children under the age of 13 years achieve maximum plasma

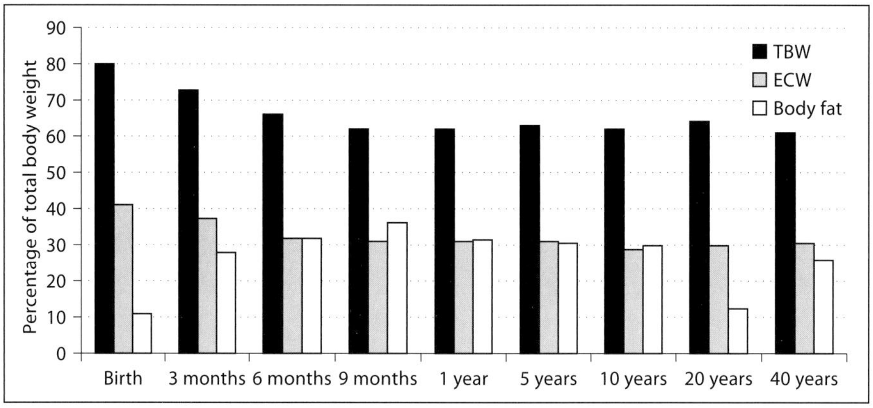


**Fig. 1.** Age-dependent changes in body composition. TBW = Total body water; ECW = extracellular water.

concentration ($C_{max}$) and area-under-the-curve (AUC) values that are 50–80% of those observed in adults after comparable weight-based (i.e. milligram per kilogram) doses [5, 6, 9]. Whether this represents a decrease in the extent of absorption alone or in combination with an increase in either the apparent volume of distribution and/or total body clearance is uncertain; however, compelling data suggest that manipulation of adult INH dosage forms for administration to children (e.g. crushing tablets into food, administering parenteral formulations orally) can markedly reduce total body INH exposure [10].

INH is well distributed throughout the body, including the central nervous system (CNS). Though maximal cerebrospinal fluid (CSF) concentrations are lower than those in plasma, CSF concentrations in young children with TB meningitis obtained 2–4 h following dosing are comparable to those in plasma [11]. The apparent distribution volume of INH approximates the total body water space. Thus, plasma concentrations in infants and young children are expected to be lower than in older children and adults following comparable weight-based doses consequent to age-associated increases in both extracellular and intracellular fluid stores (fig. 1) [4].

Interindividual differences in biotransformation represent another factor which contributes substantially to variability in INH disposition. INH undergoes acetylation by the polymorphically expressed enzyme arylamine N-acetyltransferase 2 (NAT2) present in the liver and small intestines [12]. Three metabolism phenotypes are generally recognized: homozygous fast acetylators, heterozygous fast acetylators and slow acetylators. These phenotypic differences in metabolism markedly influence INH plasma clearance and, thereby, the dose-exposure relationship for the drug [13]. Superimposed on genetic constitution of NAT2 is the developmental maturation profile of the enzyme. Although there are no well-designed, longitudinal assessments available, cross-sectional data suggest that functional NAT2 activity is acquired slowly during the first 16 months of life. Concordance between NAT2 phenotype and genotype appears to be reached by approximately 6 months of age; however, metabolic capacity may not fully mature before 4 years of age [12, 14]. The clinical relevance of this regarding INH systemic exposure profiles is difficult to discern given other factors (e.g. bioavailability, NAT2 genotype) which contribute to the variability in dose-concentration relationships.

As with most anti-infective agents, the pharmacodynamics of INH are highly dependent upon achievable drug concentrations in plasma and at the infection site. When paediatric exposure data are considered in the context of desirable pharmacokinetic targets (e.g. a 2-hour plasma concentration of 3–5 μg/ml and an associated AUC of 10.52 μg/h•ml), a substantial fraction of children will achieve the desired $C_{max}$ target at doses of 5 mg/kg but the youngest age groups will likely not achieve the desired AUC goal [15, 16]. By contrast, doses of 6–12 mg/kg attain both $C_{max}$ and AUC goals in the majority of children under the age of 12 years regardless of acetylation status [17]. Combined with other antitubercular agents, INH doses of 10 mg/kg produce $C_{max}$ and AUC values within the range of 4.4–8.2 μg/ml and 34.1–57.5 μg/h•ml, respectively in children, suggesting that current recommended doses achieve, and may even exceed, putative pharmacokinetic targets in children with TB [6].

While the clinical utility of pharmacogenetic assessment has not yet been ascribed to anti-infective drugs, INH represents an example whereby a priori knowledge of the NAT2 genotype, and by extension its phenotypic correlate, could in theory be used to refine dose selection. However, given the considerable technical resources required for this testing, it is likely that the value of pharmacogenetic assessment will largely go unrealized because of limited resources in many developing countries. The challenge that remains for clinicians is to identify an appropriate dose of INH for children that will not compromise efficacy in fast acetylators in whom bioavailability may be impaired by extemporaneous compounding, while limiting toxicity due to adequate absorption profiles or delayed drug clearance conferred by a slow acetylator phenotype. This task is simplified somewhat by the fact that children, historically, do not appear to experience adverse drug reactions (ADRs) to INH at the same rate as adults [18]. However, it is uncertain whether this finding reflects age-associated differences in ADR susceptibility or is simply a consequence of lower exposure in children. At recommended INH doses, the currently accepted pharmacokinetic targets associated with the desirable effect are likely to be attained in the vast majority of children. An important caveat associated with this recommendation is children with extrapulmonary infection (e.g. brain and bone) where the drug effect is more dependent upon tissue penetration.

## Rifamycins

*Rifampicin*

While rifampicin (RIF) has long been utilized in children as an effective component for the treatment of infections caused by *Mycobacterium tuberculosis* [19], well-described pharmacokinetic and/or pharmacodynamic data in children are limited. The interpretation of existing paediatric pharmacokinetic studies is made even more challenging by the pronounced formulation effects observed for RIF. Under selected conditions, extemporaneous compounding of adult dosage forms can restrict the amount of drug delivered to the paediatric patient. This appears most pronounced when capsule contents are dispersed in syrup and dispensed in plastic bottles [20]. Unfortunately, many paediatric pharmacokinetic reports do not describe, in detail, the nature and extent of manipulations to the oral dosage formulation prior to administration making it difficult to compare dose-exposure relationships between studies. Not surprisingly, reports of RIF's absolute bioavailability appear to be highly variable ranging from 22 to 121% in children [21]. There are some data which suggest that the rate and extent of absorption are delayed in premature neonates and young infants as compared with older children and adults ($t_{max}$: 8 vs. 2–4 h; $C_{max}$: 2.8–6.1 vs. 6.5–9.5 μg/ml) [6, 22–25]. Bioavailability of RIF appears to be further compromised by food but this too appears to have a formulation-specific component. Plasma concentrations and total body RIF exposure in children receiving a sucrose suspension mixed with apple sauce (8.9 μg/ml, AUC = 38.0 μg/h•ml) were significantly lower than those observed in children receiving the suspension alone (10.7 μg/ml, AUC = 56 μg/h•ml) or RIF powder mixed in apple sauce (11.5 μg/ml, AUC = 57 μg/h•ml) [26]. Consequently, distinguishing age-dependent effects from formulation effects and food-formulation interactions is often impossible.

Though few paediatric studies have used sensitive, chromatography-based analytical assays to describe RIF pharmacokinetics in children, existing studies suggest no appreciable difference in total body clearance, elimination rate constant or metabolite formation following intravenous administration among children aged 3–12 years. In contrast, the apparent volume of distribution observed in patients less than 4 years of age ranged from 0.37 to 1.0 l/kg as compared to 0.19–0.54 l/kg in older children suggesting a slightly higher volume of distribution in younger patients. Collectively, however, the mean volume of distribution following intravenous RIF appears similar in children when compared to adults [27]. Although RIF is widely distributed into most body fluids and tissues, its CSF penetration is variable with concentrations in the CSF ranging between 0.12 and 3.0 μg/ml at 1.3–2.3 h following an intravenous dose in children undergoing ventriculoperitoneal shunt placement [28, 29].

As with INH, differences in biotransformation contribute to the variability observed with RIF pharmacokinetics in paediatric patients. RIF undergoes desacetylation and hydrolysis within the liver. Both metabolites, desacetyl-RIF and formyl-RIF, are active against *M. tuberculosis*, though less than the parent drug. Although the specific mechanism of RIF metabolism is not well defined (making the ontogenic profile unclear), the AUC ratio of 25-O-desacetyl-RIF:RIF is variable in children following intravenous administration without an appreciable correlation between age and metabolite formation [27]. The majority of RIF is eliminated in faeces via the biliary system, thus developmental differences in renal function should not significantly impact RIF clearance [23, 27].

The proposed pharmacodynamic surrogate for RIF when treating *M. tuberculosis* is a serum concentration of ≥8 μg/ml 2 h following dose administration [30]. Among the published paediatric studies, few children appear to have achieved this therapeutic target concentration at doses of 10 mg/kg [22–25]. Pharmacokinetic simulations suggest that doses of 15 mg/kg or greater are required to assure that the majority of children attain a 2-hour concentration in excess of 8 μg/ml [31]. Prospective studies investigating higher doses of RIF are needed to confirm the adequacy of the proposed doses.

*Rifapentine*

Rifapentine is a rifamycin derivative with an exceptionally long plasma elimination half-life which would theoretically permit less frequent dosing. Although the safety and efficacy of rifapentine have not been established in the treatment of paediatric TB, 2 studies provide valuable data on the pharmacokinetics of rifapentine in children and adolescents. In children 2–12 years of age, a positive correlation between age and AUC was observed with a complementary inverse relation between age and clearance following an oral dose of 8.5 mg/kg. Younger children appear to achieve less than half the drug exposure and nearly twice the clearance as compared to older children. In children averaging 4 years of age, an AUC of 117.8 mg/h•l and total plasma clearance of 0.086 l/h/kg was observed compared to an AUC of 290.9 mg/h•l and plasma clearance of 0.047 l/h/kg in children nearly 10 years of age [32]. In contrast, adolescents ranging from 12 to 15 years of age appear to have similar pharmacokinetic parameters as adults with a mean observed $C_{max}$, AUC and clearance of 12.94 μg/ml, 330 μg/h•l and 0.030 l/h/kg, respectively, following a 600-mg oral dose [33].

These age-dependent changes in rifapentine plasma clearance suggest that younger children require a significantly higher weight-adjusted dose as compared to older children and adolescents. Although rifapentine biotransformation does appear to be increased in younger children, this does not account for all age-associated pharmacokinetic differences [33]. Crushing the tablet formulation appears to impact the pharmacokinetics by shortening the $t_{max}$ (2.5 vs. 3.7 h following ingestion of an intact tablet) while plasma $C_{max}$ values appeared similar regardless of formulation [32].

*Rifabutin*

Rifabutin is a semisynthetic rifamycin and is currently indicated for the prevention of *Mycobacterium avium* complex disease in HIV-infected adults although data suggest efficacy of rifabutin in combination TB therapy [34]. Safety and efficacy of rifabutin have not been established in children, and, at present, there are no paediatric pharmacokinetic studies.

Adult studies demonstrate that the bioavailability of rifabutin is variable with reduced absorption in patients with HIV [35]. With unpredictable bioavailability observed in adults, evaluation of both the rate and extent of rifabutin absorption in children would be warranted to establish a paediatric dose. Product-specific data indicate that the capsule formulation demonstrates relative bioavailability of 85% when compared to oral solution [36]. Assuming that the oral solution is well tolerated, children receiving the liquid formulation would be expected to have slightly higher (i.e. faster) rates of absorption.

Rifabutin is highly lipophilic, leading to intracellular tissue uptake and a prolonged terminal elimination half-life. Rifabutin undergoes extensive biotransformation resulting in numerous metabolites, at least one of which demonstrates antimicrobial activity [37]. Cytochrome 3A4 has been implicated in rifabutin metabolism although the most quantitatively relevant metabolic pathway is unclear. Consequently the impact of development on rifabutin disposition cannot be predicted apart from the fractional contribution of intestinal and hepatic cytochrome 3A4 (detailed below for TMC207).

## Pyrazinamide

Despite the fact that pyrazinamide (PZA) is a frequently used first-line agent in combination chemotherapy regimens to treat children with TB, only limited paediatric pharmacokinetic data are available. PZA is almost completely absorbed from the gastrointestinal tract following peroral administration although absorption appears delayed in children as compared to adults ($t_{max}$: 2–4 vs. 1–2 h, respectively) [38, 39]. This delay does not appear to be accounted for by comorbid diseases (e.g. HIV) so whether it is a function of age or extemporaneous formulation is unclear. Irrespective of the delay in absorption, children achieve $C_{max}$ values comparable to those of adults when PZA is administered at comparable weight-based doses (e.g. $C_{max}$ approx. 40 μg/ml at 25 mg/kg) [40, 41]. Moreover plasma concentration versus time profiles do not appear to differ substantially within paediatric populations whether under the age of 6 years, 6–10 years or 10–14 years [39].

PZA demonstrates only a modest degree of protein binding (i.e. 10–20%) and, thus, is widely distributed to most fluid compartments and tissues with penetration into the CSF in children approaching concentrations observed in plasma [42, 43]. The apparent PZA volume of distribution ranges from 0.57 to 0.84 l/kg suggesting distribution in a space comparable to total body water. Consequently, lower plasma concentrations would be expected in young children, and this is consistent with limited pharmacokinetic data demonstrating lower $C_{max}$ values in children aged less than 4 years [44].

PZA is extensively metabolized undergoing hydrolysis by a microsomal deaminase to the active metabolite pyrazinoic acid. Pyrazinoic acid is further hydroxylated to 5-hydroxypyrazinoic acid by xanthine oxidase [41]. The effect of development on the biotransformation of PZA is not known but existing pharmacokinetic data suggest that the rate of PZA elimination in children is comparable to or faster than that observed in adults [40, 45–47].

In contrast to INH and RIF, the pharmacodynamic targets for PZA are not as well defined and are complicated by the pH-dependent killing of this drug. However, current recommendations suggest that 2-hour post-dose plasma concentrations of 20 μg/ml serve as a suitable pharmacokinetic surrogate for a desirable drug effect [30]. When plasma PZA concentrations were simulated across the range of currently recommended doses using paediatric pharmacokinetic parameter estimates, predicted $C_{max}$ values ranged from 31.3 to 77.5 μg/ml, and, in every instance, infants and children were predicted to attain the proposed pharmacokinetic efficacy surrogate [31]. Simulated plasma concentration versus time profiles also suggested that infants and children spend between 32 and 91% of a 24-hour dosing interval above the susceptibility limit for *M. tuberculosis* at currently recommended doses [31]. Although the clinical relevance of this observation is unclear, evaluation of parameters such as time above minimum inhibitory concentration (MIC) and related pharmacodynamic targets that integrate pharmacokinetics and susceptibility data (e.g. AUC/MIC) may tell us whether PZA doses used in children are adequate or in excess of what is needed such that doses can be reduced to mitigate toxicity. Finally, the potential for dose-dependent PZA toxicity should be considered in paediatric patients who experience plasma concentrations far in excess of those required to ensure efficacy [48].

## Ethambutol

Ethambutol (EMB) displays good bioavailability following oral administration in adults; however, plasma $C_{max}$ values in children are nearly half of those observed in adults at comparable weight-based doses [49]. Despite a longer $t_{max}$ in children, the reduction in bioavailability does not appear to be solely accounted for by delays in the rate of absorption as compared to adults [25, 50, 51]. The bioavailability of EMB also decreases with concurrent antacid administration [51], suggesting that EMB absorption may be further impaired in the newborn infant with relative achlorhydria.

EMB has a low degree of binding to circulating plasma proteins (10–40%) and a large apparent volume of distribution in adults (≥6 l/kg) [49, 51, 52]. EMB undergoes only minimal biotransformation to dicarboxylic acid and aldehyde metabolites [28, 53]. Both findings suggest that developmental differences in body composition and drug-metabolizing enzyme activity may contribute only minimally to interindividual variability in EMB pharmacokinetics between children. By contrast, a substantial fraction of EMB clearance occurs in the kidney by glomerular filtration and active tubular secretion [54]. Consequently, dynamic maturation of renal function which occurs in the first 6 months of life would be expected to significantly impact EMB pharmacokinetics in young infants (fig. 2) [55].

Limited data on EMB pharmacokinetics in children suggest faster plasma clearance and reduced oral bioavailability as compared to adults. Thus, children under 10 years of age do frequently not achieve exposure profiles that portend therapeutic efficacy as extrapolated from adult studies (e.g. 2-hour post-dose plasma concentration in excess of 2 μg/ml) [50, 56]. At doses of 15 mg/kg/day, average $C_{max}$ values in children 2–14 years range from 0.9 to 1.2 μg/ml. Similarly, doses of 33 mg/kg thrice weekly in children fail to attain the desired pharmacokinetic surrogate [44, 56]. However, doses of 25 mg/kg/day resulted in average $C_{max}$ values ranging from 2.6 to 3.5 μg/ml, thereby demonstrating that higher weight-adjusted doses of EMB are necessary in the paediatric population [50].

## Aminoglycosides

As a class, parenterally administered aminoglycosides offer the most predictable developmental pharmacokinetic profile among antitubercular agents. The aminoglycosides distribute widely in the body (with the exception of the CNS) and have an apparent volume of distribution corresponding to the extracellular fluid space [28, 57, 58]. Consequently, their apparent volume of distribution inversely correlates with age as expected based upon developmental changes in body water spaces (fig. 1) [59–67]. Further, aminoglycosides are cleared primarily by passive renal filtration with the majority of drug accounted for in urine within 24 h following administration of a single dose [68, 69]. As the age-dependent acquisition of renal function is well characterized (fig. 2), aminoglycoside clearance can be reliably predicted

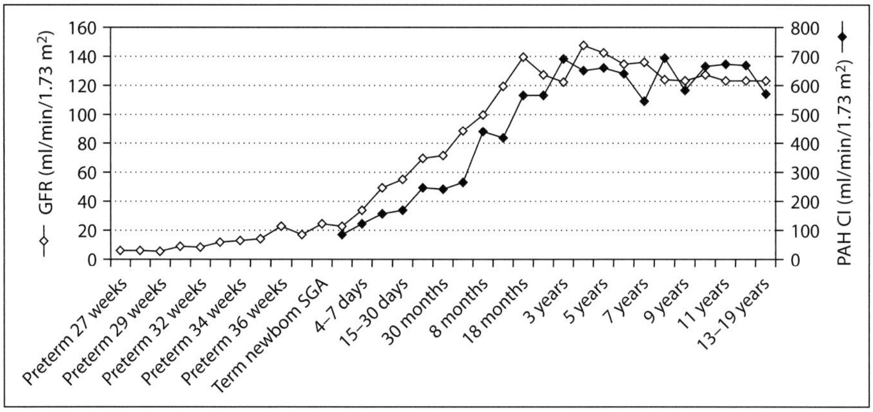


**Fig. 2.** Ontogeny of renal function. GFR = Glomerular filtration rate; PAH Cl = para-aminohippurate clearance; SGA = small for gestational age.

with information on the age and renal status of the child to whom the drug is administered [59, 60, 65–67]. Hence aminoglycoside plasma clearance in the neonate is delayed while that of the young child may exceed the observed clearance estimates reported in the adult population.

Proposed pharmacodynamic surrogates for aminoglycosides in TB treatment are generally associated with the ratio of $C_{max}$ to MIC. Proposed 2-hour serum concentrations of streptomycin, amikacin, kanamycin and capreomycin range from 35 to 45 µg/ml with daily dosing and from 65 to 80 µg/ml when utilizing thrice weekly dosing [30]. In children 6 months to 12 years of age, 30 mg/kg of streptomycin administered intramuscularly achieved $C_{max}$ values ranging from 85 to 95 µg/ml and 2-hour concentrations ranging from 57 to 84 µg/ml. Maximum concentrations following a 20 mg/kg intramuscular injection were approximately 28–30 µg/ml, and 2-hour serum concentrations fell below the recommended therapeutic target [66, 70]. This suggests that for streptomycin, a dose of 30 mg/kg should result in adequate serum concentrations if given daily but may be subtherapeutic in some children if administered less frequently [67].

When contemplating dividing the total daily aminoglycoside dose, consideration should be given to the fact that plasma $C_{max}$ achieved with twice/thrice daily dosing will be lower than those observed after a single daily dose. For example, amikacin dosed twice daily (7.5 mg/kg/dose i.v. every 12 h) in children resulted in an average $C_{max}$ of 19.5 µg/ml as compared with 37.7 µg/ml when the drug was administered as a once daily 15 mg/kg intravenous dose [67, 71, 72].

At recommended kanamycin doses (5–10 mg/kg), plasma $C_{max}$ ranged from 10 to 30 µg/ml in neonates and children [64, 73], a finding that is likely associated with a greater apparent volume of distribution and, in young children, higher plasma clearance. Consequently, higher weight-adjusted doses of this drug may be required in young children to achieve the putative pharmacodynamic targets described above.

Finally, the safety and efficacy of capreomycin have not been established in the paediatric population, and, thus, age-dependent pharmacokinetic data for the drug are not available for infants or children. However, a comparable disposition profile to the other aminoglycosides and a clearance profile that directly correlates with creatinine clearance suggest that the dose-exposure relationship for capreomycin should be similar to that of other aminoglycosides [74].

## Fluoroquinolones

The fluoroquinolones, as a class, possess a number of desirable pharmacokinetic and pharmacodynamic characteristics including excellent oral bioavailability, extensive tissue penetration and a broad antimicrobial spectrum. Paediatric pharmacokinetic data confirm that these drugs are well absorbed in children with the absolute bioavailability of ofloxacin and levofloxacin approaching 100% [75, 76]. Notably, a single paediatric pharmacokinetic study suggests that gatifloxacin administered in tablet formulation produces higher $C_{max}$ and earlier $t_{max}$ values when compared to a suspension formulation. Although this was not a crossover study, cohorts were similar for age. However, children receiving the suspension (i.e. a formulation with a higher drug concentration than the currently marketed drug product) experienced higher rates of nausea and vomiting which theoretically could have resulted in delayed gastric emptying [77].

With apparent distribution volumes in excess of 1–2 l/kg, development is not expected to have a significant impact on the distribution of fluoroquinolones. In contrast, differences in the clearance of selected fluoroquinolones are expected between children and adults. For example, gatifloxacin, levofloxacin and ofloxacin are primarily eliminated unchanged in urine. As both glomerular filtration rate and tubular excretion capacity mature through the first 6–12 months of life (fig. 2), it would be expected that their plasma clearance would be significantly reduced in neonates and young infants. This is confirmed when evaluating ciprofloxacin where the elimination rate constant is 2-fold slower and the AUC 3-fold higher in infants aged 5–14 weeks as compared with children aged 1–5 years [78]. Consistent with renal clearance capacity in young children that can exceed that of older children and adolescents, both levofloxacin and gatifloxacin demonstrate AUCs that are lower and elimination rates that are faster in young children as compared with older children [75, 77].

In contrast to the fluoroquinolones noted above, moxifloxacin undergoes a moderate degree of phase II biotransformation mediated by the UDP glucuronosyl transferases (UGT) and sulphotransferases. Though the primary UGT isoforms responsible for conjugating moxifloxacin in vivo are not well described, in vitro data demonstrate that several UGT isoforms (e.g. UGT1A1, UGT1A3, UGT1A7 and UGT1A9) are capable of glucuronidating this drug [79]. Limited ontogenic data suggest that hepatic transcript expression of UGT1A1 in children 6 months of age is comparable to that of adults [80], suggesting that metabolic competence of moxifloxacin biotransformation is likely achieved during infancy.

Among the fluoroquinolones, levofloxacin, ofloxacin, gatifloxacin and moxifloxacin appear to be the most effective against *M. tuberculosis*; however, information is lacking on their desired pharmacodynamic targets. Both in vitro and in vivo data suggest that several fluoroquinolones are bactericidal against *M. tuberculosis* with MICs ranging from 0.5 to 1.0 μg/ml. Proposed pharmacodynamic surrogates include an AUC/MIC ratio of >100 and a $C_{max}$/MIC ratio of no less than 8–10 [81]. In children 6 months to 12 years of age receiving a 7 mg/kg oral dose of levofloxacin, a $C_{max}$ of 4.0–4.75 mg/l and an AUC of 26–41 mg/h•l were measured [75]. Similar levels were observed following a 10 mg/kg oral gatifloxacin dose in the same age group [77]. Thus, at the fluoroquinolone doses currently used in children, target AUC/MIC ratios would not be attained and target $C_{max}$/MIC ratios would only be achieved when MICs are below 0.5 μg/ml. Consequently, pharmacodynamic surrogates need to be confirmed and dosing recommendations for children reassessed accordingly.

### Para-Aminosalicylic Acid

Examination of pharmacokinetic data for para-aminosalicylic acid (PAS) poses a unique challenge given that 2 distinct formulations have been in clinical use. Many early pharmacokinetic studies evaluated a tablet formulation of the PAS salt which displayed characteristics compatible with an immediate-release formulation. The present day formulation of PAS is a modified granule formulation encased in an acid-resistant coating designed to ameliorate the gastrointestinal adverse effects experienced with the earlier tablet formulation [82, 83]. When compared to the immediate-release tablet form, the granules produce a lower $C_{max}$ and a delayed $t_{max}$ although they generate more sustained serum drug concentrations secondary to the prolonged rate of absorption [82, 84, 85].

Despite the fact that PAS was introduced into clinical practice in the mid-1940s, only a single paper describes the dose-exposure relationship of PAS in 3 children following administration of the earlier immediate-release formulation [84]. Consistent with data from adults, $t_{max}$ in this paediatric study ranged from 30 to 75 min. There appeared to be a slight trend toward higher $C_{max}$ values (normalized for milligram per kilogram dose) in the infant (9 months) and child (4 years) in this study as compared with the adolescent patient (12 years) although no definitive assessments can be made based upon this limited sample set. As the absorption profile of PAS in granule form is predominantly driven by the rate of release from the formulation, it is reasonable to assume that the granular formulation administered intact to children would result in delayed $t_{max}$ values consistent with those observed in adults. The only paediatric population wherein this assumption may not hold would be neonates where higher intragastric pH would be expected to alter the release characteristics of the coated tablet formulation.

With respect to PAS clearance, the drug is predominately metabolized by acetylation and glycine conjugation. Limited in vivo data suggest that the acetylated metabolite dominates at lower PAS doses (e.g. 4 g) while the glycine conjugate predominates at higher doses (e.g. 12 g) [86]. According to the manufacturer, the rate and extent of PAS acetylation do not appear to be genetically determined implying that enzymes other than NAT2 may be involved [83]. In the absence of additional data on PAS biotransformation, the impact of ontogeny on PAS elimination remains unknown.

The limited paediatric pharmacokinetic data suggest a terminal half-life of PAS ranging from 0.8 to 1.7 h; however, the reported terminal rate constant differed from the rate constant that could be calculated from the plasma concentration versus time profile data depicted in the paper making it difficult to draw any meaningful conclusions on PAS elimination in children from the data presented [84].

The suggested pharmacodynamic surrogate for PAS is to maintain serum concentrations above the *M. tuberculosis* MIC (1 μg/ml) for the majority of the dosing interval. In this context, factors influencing the absorption and clearance of PAS (as reviewed above) would be expected to have the greatest impact on achieving and sustaining therapeutic drug concentrations [85]. Additional factors relevant to PAS disposition in children include the co-administration of PAS with age-appropriate foodstuffs. Absorption of PAS does not appear to be compromised when taken with a meal, suggesting that dispersion of PAS granules in food for administration to children should not impair the bioavailability of the drug [82].

### Cycloserine (Seromycin) and Terizidone

Only limited pharmacokinetic data are available on cycloserine with no data for children. $C_{max}$ values following a single 500-mg dose of the immediate-release formulation in adults range from 12 to 19 μg/ml, while sustained-release formulations achieve concentrations approximately half those following the immediate-release formulation [87–89]. Importantly, cycloserine is only stable in alkaline environments suggesting that the solid oral dosage form cannot be compromised for the administration of fractional doses to children [87]. After oral absorption, cycloserine is widely distributed, and concentrations observed in the CNS approximate those seen in blood [90]. The relevant routes of metabolism for cycloserine have not been defined but these pathways account for only a minority of drug clearance with 65% of the drug eliminated unchanged in urine [90]. Consequently, knowledge on the acquisition of renal function (i.e. the ontogeny of glomerular filtration rate) can be used to estimate the impact of age on cycloserine clearance in infants and young children.

Though active against *M. tuberculosis* in vitro, optimal pharmacodynamic surrogates for cycloserine in TB management remain unknown. Importantly, the average MIC for this drug (25 μg/ml) is only slightly lower than serum concentrations previously associated with CNS toxicity (>30 μg/ml) [91, 92]. Given this narrow therapeutic index, the future role of cycloserine in treating multidrug-resistant TB is unclear. The excellent CNS penetration observed with this drug makes it a 'theoretical' candidate for the treatment of disseminated TB in children; however, the practicality of its use is likely limited in populations where the CNS is actively developing and where assessing/interpreting drug-induced CNS changes in non-verbal children is difficult.

Structurally, terizidone is comprised of 2 cycloserine molecules and 1 molecule of terephthalaldehyde. Terizidone demonstrates a slightly slower rate of absorption as compared to cycloserine, though this is unlikely to be clinically relevant as absorption of terizidone is almost complete. Terizidone demonstrates a comparable volume of distribution to cycloserine, a longer terminal elimination half-life and a lower propensity for ADR although the composition of ADRs that are observed are identical for both drugs (e.g. primarily neurological) [93]. To date, there are no published studies of the pharmacokinetics and/or safety-efficacy of terizidone in paediatric patients.

### Thioamides

Ethionamide and prothionamide represent the 2 agents in the thioamide class that are used interchangeably in TB management. The agents differ structurally by a singular methyl group present on prothionamide. Although the thioamides have a similar chemical structure and final pathway of action to that of INH, ethionamide and prothionamide are not activated by the same mycobacterial enzyme [94]. While optimal pharmacodynamic surrogates remain unknown for the thioamides, a $C_{max}$ between 1 and 5 μg/ml is recommended for ethionamide in the treatment of susceptible strains of *M. tuberculosis* (MIC of ≤1.25 μg/ml) [30]. As with many of the existing antitubercular agents, there are essentially no paediatric pharmacokinetic data for the thioamides. However, further evaluation of thioamide pharmacokinetics in children is warranted given the role of these drugs as second-line agents in multidrug-resistant TB treatment.

In adults, ethionamide is well absorbed following peroral administration, and bioavailability does not appear to be influenced by co-administration of food, antacids or juice [95]. Similarly, prothionamide absorption does not appear to be impacted by nutritional status [96]. Neither gender nor co-infection with HIV appears to impact serum concentrations of ethionamide [97]; however, delivery via rectal suppository results in delayed and incomplete absorption compared with oral dosing [98]. Nonetheless, rectal administration may be valuable in the paediatric patient who is unable to tolerate the gastrointestinal side effects accompanying oral dosing. Regarding the need for extemporaneous formulation of these drugs for infants and young children, crushing ethionamide or prothionamide does little to impair their absolute bioavailability in adults with both satisfying the FDA criteria for bioequivalence (based on the AUC) when compared with the intravenous formulation [99].

Ethionamide is not significantly bound to circulating serum proteins (30%) and the volume of distribution is large enough (1.3–2.5 l/kg) to suggest that developmental differences in body composition are unlikely to have a substantial impact on thioamide distribution. Though the thioamides undergo activation by the target bacteria, they are also metabolized by human flavin-containing monooxygenases (FMOs), a family of enzymes present in the liver, kidney and lung [100]. With respect to ontogeny, an FMO isoform switch appears to occur in the liver around the time of birth with FMO1 rapidly turned off and FMO3 expression turned on and increasing from infancy through adolescence [101]. However, postnatal expression of FMO1 persists in the kidney, and FMO2 appears to be expressed in the lung. Importantly both FMO2 and FMO3 are polymorphically expressed, the former seemingly absent in Caucasian populations but expressed in individuals of sub-Saharan African ancestry. Whether age or genetics are more relevant to the metabolism of the thioamides remains to be determined. Attempts to tease out ethionamide pharmacokinetic data in a single 6.7-year-old child represented in a pooled data analysis appeared to suggest that this child achieved a lower dose-normalized $C_{max}$ as compared with adults and a higher dose-normalized AUC [102]. Whether this finding is an artefact of an incomplete sampling scheme or the result of a legitimate age-dependent change in ethionamide disposition remains to be determined.

### Clofazimine (Lamprene, B663)

Clofazimine is currently indicated for the treatment of multibacillary forms of leprosy and erythema nodosum leprosum. While adequate drug concentrations required for efficacy against *M. tuberculosis* have not been determined, there are reports of its use in multidrug-resistant TB treatment. Thus, this agent may find more broad-based utility in the future as *M. tuberculosis* acquires resistance to other currently available drugs.

While clofazimine absorption was historically poor with earlier crystal-based formulations, bioavailability significantly improved when the currently marketed capsule formulation (micronized clofazimine suspension in an oil wax base) became available. Absorption of clofazimine appears capacity limited as the fraction of the dose absorbed is inversely proportional to dose size [103]. Whether this represents intralumenal clofazimine concentrations in excess of the concentration of half-maximal velocity (km) for an active influx transporter or lumenal bile salt concentrations below those necessary to achieve the critical micelle concentration is unclear, though either process can be influenced by development. Interestingly, exposure (both $C_{max}$ and AUC) more than doubles when clofazimine is administered with a high-fat meal [104], a finding which supports a theoretical role for the importance of lumenal bile salts in the bioavailability of the drug. Unfortunately, it is unclear whether extemporaneous alteration of the current formulation so as to enable its delivery to young children is feasible.

Given the highly lipophilic nature of clofazimine, the drug distributes at measurable concentrations into a number of tissues (e.g. adrenal, gall bladder, heart, liver, kidney, nerve, pancreas, skin) with relatively high concentrations observed in the spleen, lymph nodes and lung. Consistent with this finding is an apparent distribution volume exceeding 10 l/kg that reflects substantial tissue association/binding of the drug. With such a large apparent volume of distribution, it is possible that body composition changes in severely malnourished patients, and reduced fat stores in young infants could influence the total body burden of clofazimine. Despite its large apparent volume of distribution, clofazimine does not appear to penetrate the intact blood-brain barrier, limiting its therapeutic utility in children with CNS disease [105].

Finally, clofazimine is eliminated very slowly with a mean terminal elimination half-life of approximately 10 days following a single dose. Only 35% of dose was recovered in bile and faeces (as unchanged drug) during the first 72 h following dosing with less than 1% recovered in urine [106]. Without any additional information, it is difficult to speculate whether significant age-dependent differences in clofazimine clearance would be expected.

### Linezolid

Given that the disposition of linezolid in paediatric patients was included as part of the drug's development plan in the USA, much is known about the impact of age on linezolid pharmacokinetics and dose requirement [107]. Linezolid demonstrates excellent oral bioavailability, irrespective of feeding status, and this is not expected to differ substantially in pediatric patients [108]. Following absorption, the drug distributes into a space approximating total body water stores. As a consequence, the apparent volume of distribution for linezolid is higher, and the corresponding plasma $C_{max}$ values are lower, in young children as compared with adolescents and adults [109].

Linezolid is eliminated via renal and non-renal pathways with approximately 65% of a dose undergoing oxidative metabolism to the inactive amino-ethoxyacetic acid and hydroxyethyl glycine metabolites [110]. To date, the nature of the pathways responsible for the inactivation of linezolid is not completely understood. Fortunately, clinical pharmacokinetic investigations conducted along the continuum of age have facilitated our understanding of the impact that development has on linezolid disposition. In neonates under the age of 7 days, linezolid plasma clearance is low. Clearance increases dramatically after the first week of life (up to 12 years of age) to rates in excess of those observed in adults [109, 111]. Age-associated changes in linezolid clearance and apparent volume of distribution produce lower $C_{max}$ and AUC values in young children as compared to adults receiving identical weight-based doses.

These changes have significant implications for a drug whose pharmacodynamic activity is best characterized by the duration of time when plasma concentrations are above the MIC of the infecting pathogen. As a consequence, linezolid is dosed more frequently in children than it is in adults (i.e. every 8 h vs. every 12 h) so that desirable pharmacodynamic targets can be attained [111]. When pharmacodynamic targets for linezolid against *M. tuberculosis* are elucidated, simple in silico modeling should permit the identification of a suitable paediatric dose necessary to achieve target exposures comparable to those defined for adults.

## Thiacetazone (Amithiozone, Thioacetazone)

There have been no studies of thiacetazone pharmacokinetics in children and only a few studies examining its biodisposition in adults. Peak plasma concentrations occur 3–5 h after oral dose administration and average slightly over 1.5 μg/ml following a 150-mg dose [112–114]. Peak concentrations appear to be slightly delayed when larger doses are administered although this observation may be an artefact of the limited sampling scheme used in these studies [112]. Thiacetazone distributes into an apparent distribution volume of approximately 2 l/kg suggesting a low likelihood that distribution would be substantially altered with age [114]. Thiacetazone demonstrates a terminal half-life ranging from 13 to 17 h. Up to 25% of the drug is recovered in urine unchanged with the remainder of the dose metabolized. In vitro data suggest that the FMO family of enzymes may play a role in thiacetazone metabolism as the drug is a substrate for human FMO types 1, 2 and 3 [115]. As discussed above, both ontogeny and genetics influence the expression of FMOs making it difficult to estimate the impact of age on thiacetazone biodisposition. However, the severe and sometimes fatal ADRs observed with thiacetazone in TB patients co-infected with HIV would limit the use of this drug in such children.

## The Diarylquinoline TMC207 (R207910)

TMC207 is a first-in-class investigational diarylquinoline that offers a new approach for TB treatment via its unique mechanism of action (i.e. inhibition of mycobacterial ATP synthase). Although this agent is not yet commercially available, it is currently being studied in several adult phase I and II clinical trials, 5 of which have been completed and an additional 5 of which are ongoing [116]. Not surprisingly at this stage of development, there are no studies of TMC207 disposition in children. However, existing adult data provide some insight into expected disposition processes that may differ as a consequence of development.

In adults, TMC207 is well absorbed following peroral administration with peak serum concentrations occurring approximately 5 h after dosing [117]. Whether this delayed absorption is a consequence of delayed drug liberation from the oral solid dosage form, delayed translocation across the intestinal epithelium or selective absorption from distal segments of the intestines is unclear. However, if absorption of TMC207 is capacity limited, development could certainly be expected to play a role depending on the active transport processes involved. When TMC207 is administered in conjunction with food, a 2-fold increase in exposure is observed [118]. Consequently, higher exposures may be expected in neonates and young infants where the feeding frequency is greater than that of adults.

TMC207 demonstrates excellent tissue penetration with slow redistribution back into the plasma. Concentrations of TMC207 in the mouse lung are 22 times higher than those observed in plasma. Similarly, concentrations observed in other highly perfused tissues (e.g. liver, kidney, heart, spleen) also exceed plasma concentrations [117]. Though volume of distribution estimates have not been reported in humans, calculations from adult total body exposure data suggest an apparent distribution volume slightly in excess of total body water stores [119]. Consequently, it is conceivable that slightly larger apparent distribution volumes of TMC207 may be observed in infants and young children owing to the greater extracellular and total body water stores observed in this population (fig. 2).

TMC207 appears to be extensively metabolized and is converted to its N-desmethyl metabolite by cytochrome 3A4 [120]. The expression of this cytochrome P450 isoform demonstrates a clear ontogenic profile suggesting that TMC207 metabolism (in the liver or small bowel) is expected to be altered in very young infants. As a consequence, TMC207 may undergo less presystemic clearance in infants and young children although the rate of hepatic metabolism likely approximates that of adults by 1 year of age [121, 122]. The ultimate impact of these developmental changes on TMC207 elimination in children will depend on whether compensatory metabolic pathways are relevant in its biotransformation and whether absorption or elimination represents the rate-limiting disposition process in humans.

## Considerations for Paediatric Drug Development and Prospective Study Design

As evidenced by the paucity of paediatric pharmacokinetic data for many of the antitubercular agents discussed above, children have been poorly represented in the drug development process. Understandably, the involvement of children in outcome-based phase III clinical trials is complicated by the fact that the *M. tuberculosis* disease process in young children is more difficult to characterize and efficacy-based end points are more difficult to measure than in their adult counterparts. As a result, clinicians are left with little to no data to guide paediatric dose selection for many antitubercular agents. The reality, however, is that these drugs will eventually be used in children with formulation modifications that have not been evaluated and doses that have not been established.

For innovators and investigators looking to integrate paediatrics into antitubercular drug development plans, the single most critical aspect to ensuring the success of their trial is to design the protocol with an eye toward developmental physiology and pharmacology. One of the most common mistakes sponsors make is adapting existing adult protocols for children by simply exchanging the word 'child' for 'adult' without any additional review by investigators skilled in paediatric pharmacology. In doing so, the best-case scenario is a protocol whose initiation is delayed while it is reviewed and modified by paediatric institutional review boards. Worst-case scenarios range from trials into which investigators cannot enroll, trials that generate data which are uninformative or unusable and even to trials that can potentially harm the participant child. With a little attention to paediatric-specific elements during protocol development, paediatric trials can be easily conducted generating highly valuable data. Although we have reviewed paediatric clinical trial considerations in greater detail in an earlier publication, some key points are summarized below [123].

### *Are the Population Composition and Size Adequate to Answer the Study Question?*

Drug disposition and the resultant pharmacokinetic parameters of interest can vary owing to a number of factors including race, gender, ethnicity, genetics and underlying health status. In addition to accounting for the factors that influence normal interindividual variability in a population where anatomical and physiological development is complete (i.e. adults), sample size calculations for paediatric clinical trials need to take into consideration the variability introduced by ongoing maturation of tissue composition and end organ function across the continuum of ages being studied. The trials need also to consider transient temporal changes occurring in their paediatric population of interest that can alter drug disposition (e.g. prenatal and perinatal events in newborns, changing circulating hormone profiles in adolescents). Failure to appreciate the magnitude of intersubject variability contributed by virtue of the cohort's age can result in sample sizes that lack the statistical power to answer the research questions.

### *Do You Have a Paediatric-Specific Formulation or Will You Be Using the Adult Dosage Form?*

If the only available formulation is an adult solid oral dosage form, it must be established whether it can be effectively titrated to administer an acceptable, accurate dose to children in a 'real-world' situation. For example, it does no good to conduct a single-dose pharmacokinetic study in children capable of swallowing a tablet if the dosage form will be extemporaneously compounded in the field. If an extemporaneous formulation is to be used in the clinical trial, careful assessment of formulation impact on relative bioavailability is necessary (e.g. reduced RIF concentrations when tablets are crushed and/or formulated in suspension, reduced INH absorption when administered with various foodstuffs, reduced palatability of fluoroquinolones when crushed). A priori identification of these potential problems is essential to insure integrity of the study results.

*Do You Need to Adjust Your Sampling Strategy to Account for Normal Developmental Changes in Body Composition and End Organ Function?*

When designing a paediatric pharmacokinetic study, the degree to which developmental physiology must be considered is driven in large part by the nature of the analytical assay being used to support the study. If the assay can accommodate small sample volumes, classical pharmacokinetic studies become very feasible in even the youngest of populations. If, however, larger sample volumes are required, alternative sampling strategies (e.g. sparse sampling, population pharmacokinetics) need to be considered and weighed against the less than robust pharmacokinetic parameter estimates that these strategies sometimes generate. The upper and lower limits of quantitation for the assay also need to be considered when designing paediatric studies. If expanded distribution volumes are expected (owing to an increase in body water stores), the entire plasma concentration versus time profile can shift downward resulting in concentrations that fall below the lower limit of quantitation. With too few values on the ascending or descending phases of the profile, variables defining the absorption rate and elimination rate may be inaccurate or unquantifiable. Similarly, developmental changes that increase the elimination rate can yield terminal samples that fall below the lower limit of quantitation. In contrast, volume contraction can result in peak plasma concentrations that exceed the upper limit of quantitation, necessitating reanalysis of the sample if a sufficient residual volume is available. When development alters the rate of absorption, plasma $C_{max}$ can be altogether missed if a limited sampling scheme extrapolated from adult profiles is utilized. Importantly, many of these developmental changes often occur together and, thus, must be considered in a multifactorial context.

*Are Safety/Tolerability Monitoring Criteria Age Appropriate?*

Successfully monitoring tolerability and safety may require strategies that consider aspects unique to the paediatric population. The assessment of many subjective ADRs is challenging in non-verbal children or in circumstances where the education/training of health care workers is insufficient to objectively evaluate a potential drug-related adverse event. Consequently, ADRs relating to pain or discomfort often go underreported. Assessing objective ADRs that impact vision or hearing require physical maturation, abstract thinking and the cognitive capacity to comprehend what is being requested of them (e.g. use of a Snellen chart requires that the child has learned the alphabet, traditional audiometry testing requires that the participant performs a task in response to hearing a test signal). Paediatric considerations extend to monitoring devices (e.g. blood pressure cuffs need to be age appropriate), third-party evaluation (e.g. adult vs. paediatric cardiologist interpretations of an electrocardiogram) and centralization of safety laboratory monitoring (e.g. external laboratories set up for small sample volumes). Providing the appropriate degree of attention to trial design represents an invaluable investment to insure validity of the results and their ultimate applicability to clinical care/practice. Failure to consider trial elements unique to the paediatric population can result in an unpleasant experience for the participants, their parents and the investigator/sponsor. It can also result in data that are insufficient to define age-appropriate doses and potentially lead to the dissemination of data that inadequately characterize drug biodisposition in the paediatric population. In contrast, well-designed trials contribute to a positive experience for all involved and produce generalizable knowledge that benefits children as a whole. Recognition of these facts is imperative given the WHO-based recommendations to develop new, age-appropriate 'fixed-dose' formulations of drugs for paediatric patients with TB [31], products which must be evaluated in the target population before they are put into general clinical use.

## Conclusions

As illustrated above, a firm knowledge of human development must be incorporated in the processes of discovery, development and deployment of drugs for the treatment of TB in infants and children. This includes new drugs, new formulations of 'old' drugs and drugs being repurposed for use in TB treatment. Relatively speaking, the obtainment of pharmacokinetic data for either the purpose of guiding therapy (e.g. therapeutic drug monitoring) or characterizing the impact of age and/or disease on drug disposition represents the 'low-hanging fruit' as the enabling technology (e.g. sensitive micro-analytical techniques for drug analysis, genotyping, population-based methods for pharmacokinetic analysis) exists in developed countries and, increasingly, the developing world. In contrast, the characterization of pharmacodynamic properties in infants and children remains a vexing challenge for the drugs used to treat TB, especially when age and/or disease status make paediatric patients markedly different from adults, the population where 'target exposure' data associated with drug efficacy have been described. Expanded development and utilization of applicable technologies (e.g. biomarkers that can serve as surrogate pharmacodynamic end points) that will enable integrated pharmacokinetic-pharmacodynamic evaluation of antitubercular drugs in paediatric patients should be actively explored. Only in this fashion can age-specific optimization of drug therapy be achieved.

## References


1 Marais BJ, Gupta A, Starke JR, El-Sony A: Tuberculosis in women and children. Lancet 2010;375:2057–2059.
2 Mukherjee A, Lodha R, Kabra SK: Changing trends in childhood tuberculosis. Indian J Pediatr 2011;78:328–333.
3 Graham SM: Treatment of paediatric TB: revised WHO guidelines. Paediatr Respir Rev 2011;12:22–26.
4 Kearns GL, Abdel-Rahman SM, Alander SW, Blowey DL, Leeder JS, Kauffman RE: Developmental pharmacology – drug disposition, action, and therapy in infants and children. N Engl J Med 2003;349:1157–1167.
5 Thee S, Detjen AA, Wahn U, Magdorf K: Isoniazid pharmacokinetic studies of the 1960s: considering a higher isoniazid dose in childhood tuberculosis. Scand J Infect Dis 2010;42:294–298.
6 Seth V, Beotra A, Seth SD, Semwal OP, Kabra S, Jain Y, Mukhopadhya S: Serum concentrations of rifampicin and isoniazid in tuberculosis. Indian Pediatr 1993;30:1091–1098.
7 Roy V, Gupta D, Gupta P, Sethi GR, Mishra TK: Pharmacokinetics of isoniazid in moderately malnourished children with tuberculosis. Int J Tuberc Lung Dis 2010;14:374–376.
8 Peloquin CA, Namdar R, Dodge AA, Nix DE: Pharmacokinetics of isoniazid under fasting conditions, with food, and with antacids. Int J Tuberc Lung Dis 1999;3:703–710.
9 Schaaf HS, Parkin DP, Seifart HI, Werely CJ, Hesseling PB, van Helden PD, Maritz JS, Donald PR: Isoniazid pharmacokinetics in children treated for respiratory tuberculosis. Arch Dis Child 2005;90:614–618.
10 Notterman DA, Nardi M, Saslow JG: Effect of dose formulation on isoniazid absorption in two young children. Pediatrics 1986;77:850–852.
11 Donald PR, Gent WL, Seifart HI, Lamprecht JH, Parkin DP: Cerebrospinal fluid isoniazid concentrations in children with tuberculous meningitis: the influence of dosage and acetylation status. Pediatrics 1992;89:247–250.
12 Pariente-Khayat A, Rey E, Gendrel D, Vauzelle-Kervroedan F, Cremier O, d'Athis P, Badoual J, Olive G, Pons G: Isoniazid acetylation metabolic ratio during maturation in children. Clin Pharmacol Ther 1997;62:377–383.
13 Parkin DP, Vandenplas S, Botha FJ, Vandenplas ML, Seifart HI, van Helden PD, van der Walt BJ, Donald PR, van Jaarsveld PP: Trimodality of isoniazid elimination phenotype and genotype in patients with tuberculosis. Am J Respir Crit Care Med 1997;155:1717–1722.
14 Pariente-Khayat A, Pons G, Rey E, Richard MO, d'Athis P, Moran C, Badoual J, Olive G: Caffeine acetylator phenotyping during maturation in infants. Pediatr Res 1991;29:492–495.
15 Donald PR, Parkin DP, Seifart HI, Schaaf HS, van Helden PD, Werely CJ, Sirgel FA, Venter A, Maritz JS: The influence of dose and N-acetyltransferase-2 (NAT2) genotype and phenotype on the pharmacokinetics and pharmacodynamics of isoniazid. Eur J Clin Pharmacol 2007;63:633–639.
16 Peloquin CA: Therapeutic drug monitoring in the treatment of tuberculosis. Drugs 2002;62:2169–2183.
17 McIlleron H, Willemse M, Werely CJ, Hussey GD, Schaaf HS, Smith PJ, Donald PR: Isoniazid plasma concentrations in a cohort of South African children with tuberculosis: implications for international pediatric dosing guidelines. Clin Infect Dis 2009;48:1547–1553.
18 Nakajo MM, Rao M, Steiner P: Incidence of hepatotoxicity in children receiving isoniazid chemoprophylaxis. Pediatr Infect Dis J 1989;8:649–650.
19 Gumbo T, Louie A, Deziel MR, Liu W, Parsons LM, Salfinger M, Drusano GL: Concentration-dependent *Mycobacterium tuberculosis* killing and prevention of resistance by rifampin. Antimicrob Agents Chemother 2007;51:3781–3788.
20 Nahata MC, Morosco RS, Hipple TF: Effect of preparation method and storage on rifampin concentration in suspensions. Ann Pharmacother 1994;28:182–185.
21 Koup JR, Williams-Warren J, Viswanathan CT, Weber A, Smith AL: Pharmacokinetics of rifampin in children. II. Oral bioavailability. Ther Drug Monit 1986;8:17–22.
22 Tan TQ, Mason EO, Ou CN, Kaplan SL: Use of intravenous rifampin in neonates with persistent staphylococcal bacteremia. Antimicrob Agents Chemother 1993;37:2401–2406.
23 Acocella G: Clinical pharmacokinetics of rifampicin. Clin Pharmacokinet 1978;3:108–127.
24 Thee S, Detjen A, Wahn U, Magdorf K: Rifampicin serum levels in childhood tuberculosis. Int J Tuberc Lung Dis 2009;13:1106–1111.
25 Hussels H, Kroening U, Magdorf K: Ethambutol and rifampicin serum levels in children: second report on the combined administration of ethambutol and rifampicin. Pneumonologie 1973;149:31–38.
26 McCracken GH, Ginsburg CM, Zweighaft TC, Clahsen J: Pharmacokinetics of rifampin in infants and children: relevance to prophylaxis against *Haemophilus influenzae* type b disease. Pediatrics 1980;66:17–21.
27 Koup JR, Williams-Warren J, Weber A, Smith AL: Pharmacokinetics of rifampin in children. I. Multiple dose intravenous infusion. Ther Drug Monit 1986;8:11–16.
28 Holdiness MR: Clinical pharmacokinetics of the antiberculosis drugs. Clin Pharmacokinet 1984;9:511–544.
29 Nahata MC, Fan-Harvard P, Barson WJ, Bartkowski HM, Kosnik EJ: Pharmacokinetics, cerebrospinal fluid concentration, and safety of intravenous rifampin in pediatric patients undergoing shunt placements. Eur J Clin Pharmacol 1990;38:515–517.
30 Peloquin CA: Therapeutic drug monitoring: principles and application in mycobacterial infections. Drug Ther 1992;22:31–36.
31 World Health Organization: Pharmacokinetic analyses of fixed-dose drug combinations for pediatric tuberculosis. 2009. http://www.who.int/selection_medicines/committees/expert/17/application/TB_Children.pdf (accessed January 3, 2011).
32 Blake MJ, Abdel-Rahman SM, Jacobs RF, Lowery NK, Sterling TR, Kearns GL: Pharmacokinetics of rifapentine in children. Pediatr Infect Dis J 2006;25:405–409.
33 Marshall JD, Abdel-Rahman S, Johnson K, Kauffman RE, Kearns GL: Rifapentine pharmacokinetics in adolescents. Pediatr Infect Dis J 1999;18:882–888.
34 Gonzalez-Montaner LJ, Natal S, Yongchaiyud P, Olliaro P: Rifabutin for the treatment of newly-diagnosed pulmonary tuberculosis: a multinational, randomized, comparative study versus rifampicin. Rifabutin Study Group. Tuberc Lung Dis 1994;75:341–347.
35 Skinner MH, Hsieh M, Torseth J, Pauloin D, Bhatia G, Harkonen S, Merigan TC, Blaschke TF: Pharmacokinetics of rifabutin. Antimicrob Agents Chemother 1989;33:1237–1241.
36 Mycobutin – rifaputin capsules (package insert). New York, Pharmacia & Upjohn, 2010.
37 Skinner MH, Blaschke TF: Clinical pharmacokinetics of rifabutin. Clin Pharmacokinet 1995;28:115–125.
38 Peloquin CA, Jaresko GS, Yong CL, Keung AC, Bulpitt AE, Jelliffe RW: Population pharmacokinetics modeling of isoniazid, rifampin, and pyrazinamide. Antimicrob Agents Chemother 1997;41;2670–2679.
39 Thee S, Detjen A, Wahn U, Magdorf K: Pyrazinamide serum levels in childhood tuberculosis. Int J Tuberc Lung Dis 2008;12:1099–1101.

40 Gupta P, Roy V, Sethi GR, Mishra TK: Pyrazinamide blood concentrations in children suffering from tuberculosis: a comparative study at two doses. Br J Clin Pharmacol 2007;65:423–427.
41 Lacroix C, Hoang TP, Nouveau J, Guyonnaud C, Laine G, Duwoos H, Lafont O: Pharmacokinetics of pyrazinamide and its metabolites in healthy subjects. Eur J Clin Pharmacol 1989;36:395–400.
42 Donald PR, Seifart H: Cerebrospinal fluid pyrazinamide concentrations in children with tuberculous meningitis. Pediatr Infect Dis J 1988;7:469–471.
43 Pyrazinamide tablets (package insert). Mumbai, Macleods Pharmaceuticals Ltd, 2007.
44 Graham SM, Bell DJ, Nyirongo S, Hartkoorn R, Ward SA, Molyneux EM: Low levels of pyrazinamide and ethambutol in children with tuberculosis and impact of age, nutritional status, and human immunodeficiency virus infection. Antimicrob Agents Chemother 2006;50:407–413.
45 Arya DS, Ojha SK, Semwal OP, Nandave M: Pharmacokinetics of pyrazinamide in children with primary progressive disease of lungs. Indian J Med Res 2008;128:611–615.
46 Roy V, Tekur U, Chopra K: Pharmacokinetics of pyrazinamide in children suffering from pulmonary tuberculosis. Int J Tuberc Lung Dis 1999;3:133–137.
47 Zhu M, Starke JR, Burman WJ, Steiner P, Stambaugh JJ, Ashkin D, Bulpitt AE, Berning SE, Peloquin CA: Population pharmacokinetic modeling of pyrazinamide in children and adults with tuberculosis. Pharmacotherapy 2002;22:686–695.
48 US Public Health Service: Hepatic toxicity of pyrazinamide used with isoniazid in tuberculous patients. Am Rev Respir Dis 1969;59:13.
49 Zhu M, Burman WJ, Starke JR, Stambaugh JJ, Steiner P, Bulpitt AE, Ashkin D, Auclair B, Berning SE, Jelliffe RW, Jaresko GS, Peloquin CA: Pharmacokinetics of ethambutol in children and adults with tuberculosis. Int J Tuberc Lung Dis 2004;8:1360–1367.
50 Thee S, Detjen A, Quarcoo D, Wahn U, Magdorf K: Ethambutol in paediatric tuberculosis: aspects of ethambutol serum concentration, efficacy and toxicity in children. Int J Tuber Lung Dis 2007;11:965–971.
51 Peloquin CA, Bulpitt AE, Jaresko GS, Jelliffe RW, Childs JM, Nix DE: Pharmacokinetics of ethambutol under fasting conditions, with food, and with antacids. Antimicrob Agents Chemother 1999;43:568–572.
52 Jusko WJ, Gretch M: Plasma and tissue protein binding of drugs in pharmacokinetics. Drug Metab Rev 1976;5:43–140.
53 Place VA, Peets EA, Buyske DA: Metabolic and special studies of ethambutol in normal volunteers and tuberculous patients. Ann NY Acad Sci 1966;135:775–795.
54 Lee CS, Gambertoglio JG, Brater DC, Benet LZ: Kinetics of oral ethambutol in the normal subject. Clin Pharmacol Ther 1977;22:615–621.
55 John, TR, Moore WM, Jeffries JE (eds): Children Are Different: Developmental Physiology, ed 2. columbus, Ross Laboratories, 1978.
56 Benkert K, Blaha H, Petersen KF, Schmid PC: Tagesprofile und Profilverlaufskontrollen von Ethambutol bei Kindern. Med Klin 1974;69:1808–1813.
57 Adcock JD, Hettig RA: Absorption, distribution and excretion of streptomycin. Arch Med Intern 1946;77:179–195.
58 Briedis DJ, Robson HG: Cerebrospinal fluid penetration of amikacin. Antimicrob Agents Chemother 1978;13:1042–1043.
59 Padovani EM, Pistolesi C, Fanos V, Messori A, Martini N: Pharmacokinetics of amikacin in neonates. Dev Pharmacol Ther 1993;20:167–173.
60 Assael BM, Parini R, Rusconi F, Cavanna G: Influence of intrauterine maturation on the pharmacokinetics of amikacin in the neonatal period. Pediatr Res 1982;16:810–815.
61 Marik PE, Havlik I, Monteagudo FS, Lipman J: The pharmacokinetics of amikcacin in critically ill adult and paediatric patients: comparison of once- versus twice-daily dosing regimens. J Antimicrob Chemother 1991;27(suppl C):81–89.
62 Beachler CW, Speer ME, Mason EO, Yow MD: Pharmacology of kanamycin in the newborn. South Med J 1982;75:301–305.
63 Howard JB, McCracken GH: Reappraisal of kanamycin usage in neonates. J Pediatr 1975;86:949–956.
64 Hieber JP, Nelson JD: Reevaluation of kanamycin dosage in infants and children. Antimicrob Agents Chemother 1976;9:899–902.
65 Herngren L, Boreus LO, Jalling B, Lagercrantz R: Pharmacokinetic aspects of streptomycin treatment of neonatal septicemia. Scand J Infect Dis 1977;9:301–308.
66 Bolme P, Eriksson M, Habte D, Paalzow L: Pharmacokinetics of streptomycin in Ethiopian children with tuberculosis of different nutritional status. Eur J Clin Pharmacol 1988;33:647–649.
67 Zhu M, Burman WJ, Jaresko GS, Berning SE, Jelliffe RW, Peloquin CA: Population pharmacokinetics of intravenous and intramuscular streptomycin in patients with tuberculosis. Pharmacotherapy 2001;21:1037–1045.
68 Doluisio JT, Dittert LW, La Piana JC: Pharmacokinetics of kanamycin following intramuscular administration. J Pharmacokinet Biopharm1973;1:253–265.
69 Plantier J, Forrey AW, O'Neill MA, Blair AD, Christopher TG, Cutler RE: Pharmacokinetics of amikacin in patients with normal or impaired renal function: radioenzymatic acetylation assay. J Infect Dis 1976;134(suppl):S323–S330.
70 Eriksson M, Bolme P, Habte D, Paalzow L: INH and streptomycin in Ethiopian children with tuberculosis and different nutritional status. Acta Paediatr Scand 1988;77:890–894.
71 Hendricks MK, van der Bijl P, Parkin DP, Donald PR: Pharmacokinetics of amikacin in children with kwashiorkor. Ann Trop Paediatr 1995;15:295–298.
72 Forsyth NB, Botha JH, Hadley GP: A comparison of two amikacin dosing regimens in paediatric surgical patients. Ann Trop Paediatr 1997;17:253–261.
73 McCracken GH, Threlkeld N, Thomas ML: Intravenous administration of kanamycin and gentamicin in newborn infants. Pediatrics 1977;60:463–466.
74 Black HR, Griffith RS, Peabody AM: Absorption, excretion and metabolism of capreomycin in normal and diseased states. Ann NY Acad Sci 1966;135:974–982.
75 Chien S, Wells TG, Blumer JL, Kearns GL, Bradley JS, Bocchini JA, Natarajan J, Maldonado S, Noel GJ: Levofloxacin pharmacokinetics in children. J Clin Pharmacol 2005;45:153–160.
76 Bethell DB, Day NP, Dung NM, McMullin C, Loan HT, Tam DT, Minh LT, Linh NT, Dung NQ, Vinh H, MacGowan AP, White LO, White NJ: Pharmacokinetics of oral and intravenous ofloxacin in children with multidrug-resistant typhoid fever. Antimicrob Agents Chemother 1996;40:2167–2172.
77 Capparelli EV, Reed MD, Bradley JS, Kearns GL, Jacobs RF, Damle BD, Blumer JL, Grasela DM: Pharmacokinetics of gatifloxacin in infants and children. Antimicrob Agents Chemother 2005;49:1106–1112.
78 Peltola H, Vaarala M, Renkonen OV, Neuvonen PJ: Pharmacokinetics of single-dose oral ciprofloxacin in infants and small children. Antimicrob Agents Chemother 1992;36:1086–1090.
79 Tachibana M, Tanaka M, Masubuchi Y, Horie T: Acyl glucuronidation of fluoroquinolone antibiotics by the UDP-glucuronosyltransferase 1A subfamily in human liver microsomes. Drug Metab Dispos 2005;33:803–811.
80 Strassburg CP, Strassburg A, Kneip S, Barut A, Tukey RH, Rodeck B, Manns MP: Developmental aspects of human hepatic drug glucuronidation in young children and adults. Gut 2002;50:259–265.
81 Johnson JL, Hadad DJ, Boom WH, Daley CL, Peloquin CA, Eisenach KD, Jankus DD, Debanne SM, Charlebois ED, Maciel E, Palaci M, Dietze R: Early and extended early bactericidal activity of levofloxacin, gatifloxacin and moxifloxacin in pulmonary tuberculosis. Int J Tuberc Lung Dis 2006;10:605–612.
82 Peloquin CA, Zhu M, Adam RD, Singleton MD, Nix DE: Pharmacokinetics of para-aminosalicylic acid granules under four dosing conditions. Ann Pharmacother 2001;35:1332–1338.
83 Paser aminosalicylic acid granules delayed release (package insert). Princeton, Jacobus Pharmaceutical Company Inc, 1996.
84 Soderhjelm L: Serum para-aminosalicylic acid following oral ingestion in children. Tex Rep Biol Med 1949;7:471–479.
85 Way EL, Smith PK, Howie DL, Weiss R, Swanson R: The absorption, distribution, excretion and fate of para-aminosalicylic acid. J Pharmacol Exp Ther 1948;93:368–382.
86 Lehmann J: The role of the metabolism of *p*-aminosalicylic acid (PAS) in the treatment of tuberculosis: interaction with the metabolism of isonicotinic acid hydrazide (INH) and the synthesis of cholesterol. Scand J Respir Dis 1969;50:169–185.

87 Zhu M, Nix DE, Adam RD, Childs JM, Peloquin CA: Pharmacokinetics of cycloserine under fasting conditions and with high-fat meal, orange juice, and antacids. Pharmacotherapy 2001;21:891–897.
88 Zitkova L, Tousek J: Pharmacokinetics of cycloserine and terizidone. Chemotherapy 1974;20:18–28.
89 Niemisto M: The influence of sustained release tablets effect on cycloserine concentration in serum. Scand J Respir Dis Suppl 1970;71:64–67.
90 Curci C: Pharmacological considerations on cycloserine. Scand J Respir Dis Suppl 1970;71:51–60.
91 Seromycin cycloserine capsule (package insert). Indianapolis, Eli Lilly & Co, 2005.
92 Conte JE, Barriere SL: Manual of Antibiotics and Infectious Diseases, ed 5. Philadelphia, Lea & Febiger, 1984.
93 Arbex MA, Varella MCL, de Siqueira HR, de Mello FA: Antituberculosis drugs: drug interactions, adverse effects, and use in special situations. 2. Second line drugs. J Bras Pneumol 2010;36:641–656.
94 Wang F, Langley R, Gulten G, Dover LG, Besra GS, Jacobs WR, Sacchettini JC: Mechanism of thioamide drug action against tuberculosis and leprosy. J Exp Med 2007;204:73–78.
95 Auclair B, Nix DE, Adam RD, James GT, Peloquin CA: Pharmacokinetics of ethionamide administered under fasting conditions or with orange juice, food or antacids. Antimicrob Agents Chemother 2001;45:810–814.
96 Lee HW, Kim DW, Park JH, Kim SD, Lim MS, Phapale PB, Kim EH, Park SK, Yoon YR: Pharmacokinetics of prothionamide in patients with multidrug-resistant tuberculosis. Int J Tuberc Lung Dis 2009;13:1161–1166.
97 Conte JE, Golden JA, McQuitty M, Kipps J, Lin ET, Zurlinden E: Effects of AIDS and gender on steady-state plasma and intrapulmonary ethionamide concentrations. Antimicrob Agents Chemother 2000;44:1337–1341.
98 Peloquin CA, James GT, McCarthy E, Goble M: Pharmacokinetic evaluation of ethionamide suppositories. Pharmacotherapy 1991;11:359–363.
99 Jenner PJ, Smith SE: Plasma levels of ethionamide and prothionamide in a volunteer following intravenous and oral dosages. Lepr Rev 1987;58:31–37.
100 Henderson MC, Siddens LK, Morre JT, Krueger SK, Williams DE: Metabolism of the antituberculosis drug ethionamide by mouse and human FMO1, FMO2 and FMO3 and mouse and human lung microsomes. Toxicol Appl Pharmacol 2008;233:420–427.
101 Koukouritaki SB, Simpson P, Yeung CK, Rettie AE, Hines RN: Human hepatic flavin-containing monooxygenases 1 (FMO1) and 3 (FMO3) developmental expression. Pediatr Res 2002;51:236–243.
102 Zhu M, Namdar R, Stambaugh JJ, Starke JR, Bulpitt AE, Berning SE, Peloquin CA: Population pharmacokinetics of ethionamide in patients with tuberculosis. Tuberculosis 2002;82:91–96.
103 Mathur A, Venkatesan K, Bharadwaj VP, Ramu G: Evaluation of effectiveness of clofazimine therapy. I. Monitoring of absorption of clofazimine from gastrointestinal tract. Indian J Lepr 1985;57:146–148.
104 Nix DE, Adam RD, Auclair B, Krueger TS, Godo PG, Peloquin CA: Pharmacokinetics and relative bioavailability of clofazimine in relation to food, orange juice and antacid. Tuberculosis 2004;84:365–373.
105 Mansfield RE: Tissue concentrations of clofazimine (B663) in man. Am J Trop Med Hyg 1974;23:1116–1119.
106 Schaad-Lanyi Z, Dieterle W, Dubois JP, Theobald W, Vischer W: Pharmacokinetics of clofazimine in healthy volunteers. Int J Lepr Other Mycobacter Dis 1987;55:9–15.
107 Abdel-Rahman SM, Kearns GL: An update on the oxazolidinone antibiotics. Pediatr Infect Dis J 1999;18:1101–1102.
108 Stalker DJ, Jungbluth GL: Clinical pharmacokinetics of linezolid, a novel oxazolidinone antibacterial. Clin Pharmacokinet 2003;42:1129–1140.
109 Kearns GL, Jungbluth GL, Abdel-Rahman SM, Hopkins NK, Welshman IR, Grzebyk RP, Bruss JB, van den Anker JN, Pediatric Pharmacology Research Unit Network: Impact of ontogeny on linezolid disposition in neonates and infants. Clin Pharmacol Ther 2003;74:413–422.
110 Moellering RC: Linezolid: the first oxazolidinone antimicrobial. Ann Intern Med 2003;138:135–142.
111 Jungbluth GL, Welshman IR, Hopkins NK: Linezolid pharmacokinetics in pediatric patients: an overview. Pediatr Infect Dis J 2003;22(suppl):S153–S157.
112 Ellard GA, Dickinson JM, Gammon PT, Mitchison DA: Serum concentrations and antituberculosis activity of thiacetazone. Tubercle 1974;55:41–54.
113 Jenner PJ, Ellard GA, Swai OB: A study of thiacetazone blood levels and urinary excretion in man, using high performance liquid chromatography. Lepr Rev 1984;55:121–128.
114 Peloquin CA, Nitta AT, Berning SE, Iseman MD, James GT: Pharmacokinetic evaluation of thiacetazone. Pharmacotherapy 1996;16:735–741.
115 François AA, Nishida CR, de Montellano PR, Phillips IR, Shephard EA: Human flavin-containing monooxygenase 2.1 catalyzes oxygenation of the antitubercular drugs thiacetazone and ethionamide. Drug Metab Dispos 2009;37:178–186.
116 US National Institutes of Health clinical trials web site. www.clinicaltrials.gov/ct2/results?term=TMC207 (accessed April 11, 2010).
117 Andries K, Verhasselt P, Guillemont J, Göhlmann HW, Neefs JM, Winkler H, van Gestel J, Timmerman P, Zhu M, Lee E, Williams P, de Chaffoy D, Huitric E, Hoffner S, Cambau E, Truffot-Pernot C, Lounis N, Jarlier V: A diarylquinoline drug active on the ATP synthase of *Mycobacterium tuberculosis*. Science 2005;307:223–227.
118 McNeeley DF: Update on the clinical development programme of TMC207 (R207910). Open Forum, London, UK, December 12–13, 2006. http://www.kaisernetwork.org/health_cast/uploaded_files/McNeeley,_David_(12-12)_TMC207.pdf.
119 Van Heeswijk R, Lachaert R, Leopold L, De Beule K, McNeeley D, Hoetelmans R: The effect of CYP3A4 inhibition on the clinical pharmacokinetics of TMC207 (poster PS-71358-11). 38th Union World Conf Lung Health, Cape Town, November 2007.
120 Matteelli A, Carvalho AC, Dooley KE, Kritski A: TMC207: the first compound of a new class of potent anti-tuberculosis drugs. Future Microbiol 2010;5:849–858.
121 Johnson TN, Tanner MS, Taylor CJ, Tucker GT: Enterocytic CYP3A4 in a paediatric population: developmental changes and the effect of coeliac disease and cystic fibrosis. Br J Clin Pharmacol 2001;51:451–460.
122 Lacroix D, Sonnier M, Moncion A, Cheron G, Cresteil T: Expression of CYP3A in the human liver – evidence that the shift between CYP3A7 and CYP3A4 occurs immediately after birth. Eur J Biochem 1997;247:625–634.
123 Abdel-Rahman SM, Reed MD, Wells TG, Kearns GL: Considerations in the rational design and conduct of phase I/II pediatric clinical trials: avoiding the problems and pitfalls. Clin Pharmacol Ther 2007;81:483–494.



Susan Abdel-Rahman, Pharm D, Professor of Pediatrics
Division of Clinical Pharmacology and Medical Toxicology
Children's Mercy Hospitals and Clinics, 2401 Gillham Road
Kansas City, MO 64108 (USA)
Tel. +1 816 234 3059, E-Mail srahman@cmh.edu

Donald PR, van Helden PD (eds): Antituberculosis Chemotherapy.
Prog Respir Res. Basel, Karger, 2011, vol 40, pp 176–190

# Pharmacogenetics of Antituberculosis Drugs

Rob Aarnoutse

Department of Pharmacy, Radboud University Nijmegen Medical Centre, Nijmegen, The Netherlands

**Abstract**

Pharmacogenetics can be defined as the study of genetic factors affecting (desirable or undesirable) drug responses. The genetic polymorphism in the acetylation of isoniazid was one of the earliest described pharmacogenetic traits. Trimodality in isoniazid elimination has been demonstrated, resulting in homozygous fast, heterozygous fast (or intermediate) and slow metabolizers. This 'acetylator status' can be assessed by phenotyping or genotyping. Exposure to isoniazid is considerably lower in homozygous fast than in intermediate or slow acetylators, but the acetylator status is only relevant with highly intermittent once weekly isoniazid-containing regimens, with fast acetylators performing less well than slow acetylators. The majority of genotyping studies suggest that slow acetylation and genetic polymorphisms in CYP2E1 and glutathione S-transferase are associated with an increased risk for isoniazid-induced hepatotoxicity, caused by hepatotoxic metabolites. Few studies have addressed the pharmacogenetics of other antituberculosis (anti-TB) drugs. The interindividual variability in exposure to rifampicin is clinically relevant and can be explained to a large extent by polymorphism in genes for organic anion-transporting polypeptides. Clinical application of pharmacogenetics in TB treatment is still in its infancy and warrants more clinical studies, evaluation of cost-effectiveness and overcoming of hurdles associated with implementation of this new approach in clinical practice.

Copyright © 2011 S. Karger AG, Basel

Pharmacogenetics can be defined as the study of genetic factors affecting drug response [1, 2]. The ultimate goal of pharmacogenetics is to identify patients, or groups of patients within populations, in whom treatment adjustments could be made, based on their genetic make-up, to enhance drug efficacy and safety [2] (fig. 1). In this way pharmacogenetics offers the opportunity to tailor therapy to individuals and groups.

There is considerable overlap between pharmacogenetics and the newer discipline of pharmacogenomics. Pharmacogenomics is sometimes described as the whole-genome application of pharmacogenetics, which has traditionally been considered to be concerned with single-gene effects [1]. The terms pharmacogenetics and pharmacogenomics are often used interchangeably. In this chapter, the term pharmacogenetics is used.

The response to tuberculosis (TB) treatment in relation to the genetic make-up of individuals has been a focus of interest since the early days of the development of the currently available TB treatment. Already during the 1950s, reports on drug-specific pharmacogenetic observations appeared concerning isoniazid, which was introduced as a new anti-TB drug in that era. Variation between individuals in urinary excretion [4] and shortly afterwards an association between isoniazid's metabolic profile and the incidence of an adverse reaction, peripheral neuritis, were reported [5]. Further studies led to recognition of a genetic polymorphism in the acetylation of isoniazid as one of the earliest described pharmacogenetic traits [6–8]. In the following decades, many studies focussed on the pharmacogenetics of isoniazid, and very few addressed other anti-TB drugs.

The study and consideration of factors that determine the response to TB chemotherapy is still a timely topic of the highest priority, considering the major problems with currently available TB treatment, including the high

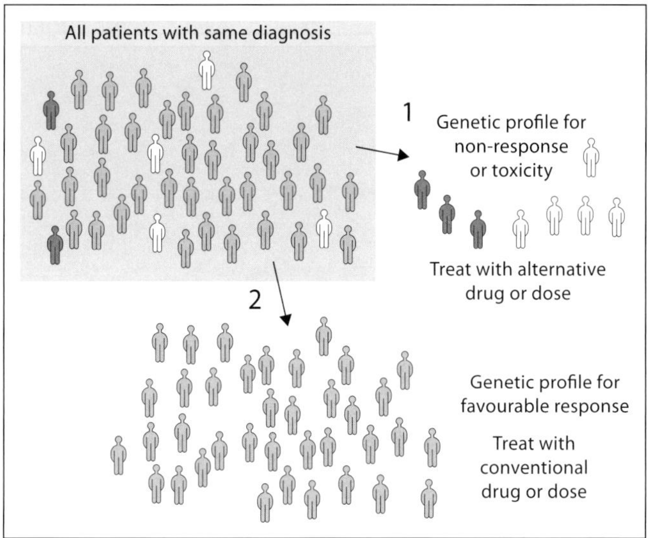


**Fig. 1.** The concept of pharmacogenetics at a glance (modified after McLeod and Evans [3]).

incidence of adverse effects that affect adherence to TB treatment and the suboptimal response (treatment failure, relapse and the emergence of resistance) to drug therapy [9]. The goal of this chapter is to present an overview of pharmacogenetic studies related to TB treatment and to discuss how pharmacogenetics could be applied to improve the response to TB drugs.

## Basic Concepts in Pharmacogenetics

Part of the differences in response to a drug can be explained by differences in genetic profile (DNA). A gene is a fragment of the DNA that contains information for one specific hereditary property [1, 2, 10]. It usually consists of 2 alleles, which are each located on one of the chromosomes of a chromosome pair. As a result of genetic variation due to mutations, slightly different alleles exist. The most common allele in a population is designated as the wild type, the others are called variant alleles. Variant alleles are often denoted with the so-called star notation, e.g. CYP2D6*4. An individual may carry a pair of identical alleles (homozygotes, e.g. CYP2D6*4/CYP2D6*4) or 2 different allelic forms of the gene (heterozygotes, e.g. CYP2D6*1/CYPD6*4).

Mutations are termed polymorphisms if they are transferred to subsequent generations and if they occur with a frequency of at least 1% [1, 2]. Thus, mutations in the DNA of somatic cells are not considered to be polymorphic because they are not transferred to offspring. All human genes are subject to extensive genetic polymorphisms, with many of these polymorphisms resulting in functionally significant effects. Three major types of genetic mutations exist: single-nucleotide polymorphisms (SNPs), variable number of tandem repeats and base insertions/deletions of one or more nucleotides [2]. The term SNP relates to a difference between alleles in just 1 single nucleotide. Up to the present, much research in pharmacogenetics has considered SNPs in relation to drug response, but it is increasingly recognized that such approaches are often inadequate. Instead groups of SNPs present in the same general chromosome region, known as haplotypes, may need to be analysed in order to better account for pharmacogenetic variation [2].

The term 'genotype' refers to the particular alleles of a specific gene that are present in each cell of the organism. In contrast, the 'phenotype' is the observed effect of the genotype in combination with endogenous (e.g. age, comorbidity) and environmental (e.g. concomitant drug use) factors [2]. Genotyping is only clinically relevant to the degree with which it predicts phenotype.

## Mechanisms for Genetic Variation to Affect Drug Response

Pharmacogenetics considers the impact of genetic variation on both the *pharmacokinetics* and *pharmacodynamics* of drugs. In addition, the pharmacogenetics of *idiosyncratic adverse drug reactions* is sometimes distinguished as a separate third class of gene-drug interactions [1, 10].

The *pharmacokinetics* of a drug relate to the processes of absorption, distribution, metabolism, excretion and transport. Genetic variations at the level of each of these processes may lead to changes in plasma concentrations and changes in (desirable or undesirable) responses. These are by far the best studied polymorphisms, especially those in genes relevant to phase I metabolism [2]. Based on polymorphisms in cytochrome (CYP) P450 enzymes (e.g. in CYP2D6, CYP2C19, CYP2E1), 4 phenotypes can be distinguished: fast (ultrarapid) metabolizers, normal (extensive), intermediate and slow (poor) metabolizers. Functionally significant polymorphisms have also been described in genes encoding other enzymes of phase I metabolism, including esterases and dehydrogenases.

In phase II conjugation reactions, drugs and chemicals of intermediate polarity undergo further biotransformation to generate products that are readily excreted in urine and faeces. Pharmacogenetic variation in phase II enzymes (e.g. in

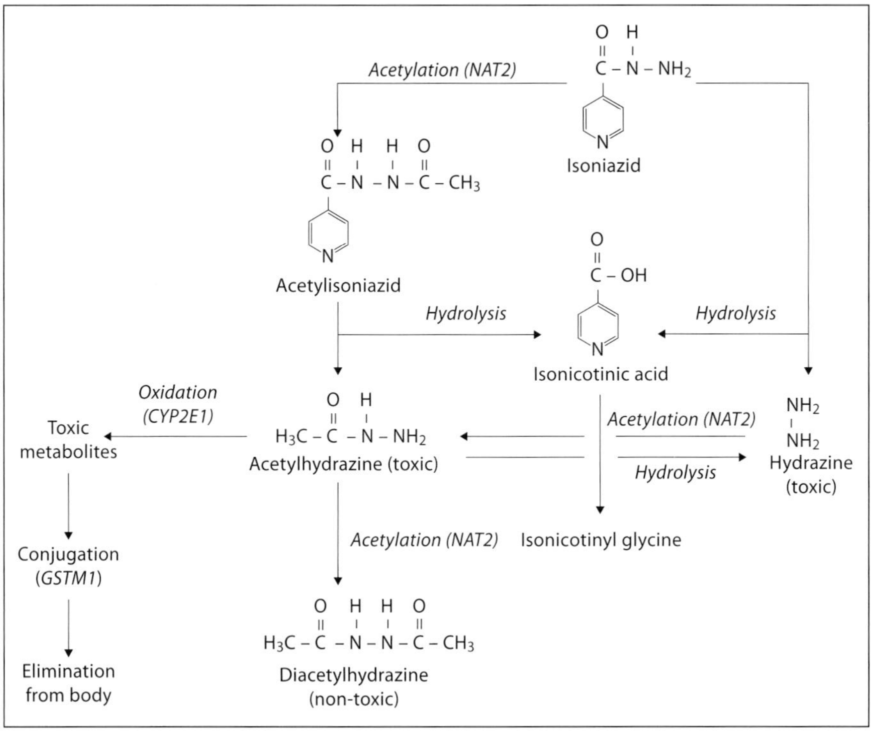


**Fig. 2.** The metabolism of isoniazid (modified after Tostmann et al. [12]).

acetylation by N-acetyltransferase 2, NAT2) may affect drug clearance, and other phase II enzymes (e.g. glutathione-S-transferases, GSTs) have important protective roles against reactive intermediates and toxic metabolites generated.

As to drug transporters, polymorphisms have been described for outward drug transporters that are mainly members of the ATP-binding cassette transporter family, including P-glycoprotein. Drug transporters of the SLCO/OATP (solute carrier organic anion transporter/organic anion-transporting polypeptide) family, which are mainly concerned with the inward transport of drugs into cells, have also been the subject of pharmacogenetic analysis [1].

*Pharmacodynamics* relates to the pharmacological effects of a drug by coupling to a receptor, enzyme or ion channel. An example of a gene-pharmacodynamic interaction is the variable presence of a certain receptor as a result of genetic make-up, or the occurrence of polymorphisms in receptors and target enzymes [1].

*Idiosyncratic reactions*, also referred to as type B adverse drug reactions, are not directly predictable from drug concentrations. It is suggested that reactive metabolites, rather than the parent drug, are responsible for most idiosyncratic reactions [11]. Isoniazid-induced hepatotoxicity is an example of such an idiosyncratic reaction probably related to toxic metabolites.

## Pharmacogenetics of Antituberculosis Drugs: Isoniazid

Pharmacogenetic studies with anti-TB drugs mainly relate to isoniazid and to polymorphisms in the metabolism of this drug. The genetic polymorphism in NAT2 has been related to response to isoniazid in the context of multidrug treatment, and genetic polymorphisms in NAT2, CYP2E1 and GST have been associated with anti-TB drug-induced hepatotoxicity.

*Metabolism of Isoniazid*

To understand the effects of genetic polymorphisms on the response to isoniazid, its metabolism should be clear (fig. 2) [13–16].

The predominant metabolic pathway of isoniazid metabolism is acetylation by NAT2. The acetylated isoniazid exhibits at least 500 times less activity in vitro and 100 times less activity in vivo against *Mycobacterium tuberculosis* than the parent compound [14, 16]. Acetylisoniazid is further hydrolysed into acetylhydrazine (probably toxic) and isonicotinic acid. In turn, acetylhydrazine is either hydrolysed into hydrazine (probably toxic) or acetylated into diacetylhydrazine (harmless). Furthermore, acetylhydrazine is oxidized by CYP2E1, probably into toxic intermediates such as acetyldiazene, acetylonium ion, acetyl radical or ketene.

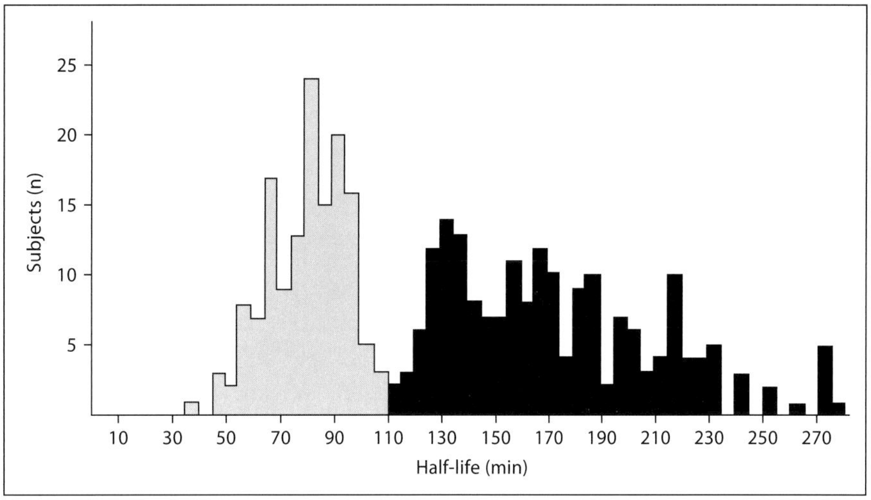


**Fig. 3.** Distribution of isoniazid half-lives among 336 Finnish subjects. Five subjects with isoniazid half-lives of 291, 295, 316 and 344 min have been excluded to avoid widening the figure excessively (from Tiitiinen [20]).

These hepatotoxins could be detoxified by GSTs in the liver. Isonicotinic acid is conjugated with glycine and excreted by the kidneys.

Importantly, a part of isoniazid is also directly hydrolysed (without involvement of an acetylation step) into isonicotinic acid and hydrazine (fig. 2, right side). The quantitative significance of this pathway is strongly dependent on the genetic polymorphism in NAT2.

*The Genetic Polymorphism in N-Acetyltransferase: Effect on Isoniazid Plasma Concentrations and Epidemiology*

As described above, observations in the 1950s on the occurrence of peripheral neuritis led to the recognition that subjects differ in their rate of acetylation of isoniazid [4–8]. Based on their 'acetylator status', fast and slow metabolizers were initially distinguished. It was soon shown that slow acetylation of isoniazid, resulting in higher plasma concentrations of isoniazid and slower elimination of the drug, is a genetically determined homozygous recessive trait [8]. However, it appeared that the gene that controls fast isoniazid acetylation is not completely dominant over that controlling slow acetylation: two groups of fast acetylators could be distinguished based on isoniazid plasma levels [15]. Indeed trimodality in isoniazid elimination has been demonstrated genotypically as well [17], resulting in homozygous fast (or 'rapid') metabolizers, who are also called fast metabolizers, heterozygous fast metabolizers, who are also designated as 'intermediate' metabolizers, and slow metabolizers. In children, maturation of isoniazid acetylation (i.e expression of the genotype) occurs over the first 4 years of life, reflected in an increase with age in the percentage of children with a fast acetylator phenotype [18]. A recent study showed a genotype-dependent enzyme maturation, demonstrated as an increase in the isoniazid clearance between 3 and 24 months of age in children with the fast and intermediate genotypes and no change in the genotypically slow metabolizers [19].

The differences in acetylation rate between the three types of metabolizers are large. The mean acetylation rate in heterozygous fast metabolizers and fast metabolizers is about 5 and 10 times that of the slow metabolizers, respectively [15]. As a result, it was shown in early studies that fast acetylators have a significantly shorter isoniazid elimination half-life than slow acetylators (fig. 3) [20]. In accordance with this, isoniazid concentrations in fast acetylators are considerably lower than those in intermediate and slow acetylators. For example, a roughly 3-fold difference between fast and slow acetylators in exposure to isoniazid at the regular dose of 5 mg/kg was demonstrated in South African patients [21]. Another study showed a linear relationship between isoniazid clearance and the number of slow acetylating alleles in NAT2 (fig. 4) [22].

The proportions of fast, intermediate and slow acetylators vary substantially between populations. About 50–60% of subjects from European (Caucasian), African and Indian origin are slow metabolizers (showing a relatively high mean exposure to isoniazid), whereas a minority varying from 5 to 25% among populations from Asian origin (Chinese, Japanese, Eskimos) consists of slow metabolizers (resulting in a relatively low mean exposure to isoniazid) [15, 16].

*Methods of Classifying Fast, Intermediate an Slow Acetylators: Phenotyping and Genotyping*

An assessment of the acetylator status of subjects is required for studies focussing on the pharmacokinetics of isoniazid, the epidemiology of the acetylator status and

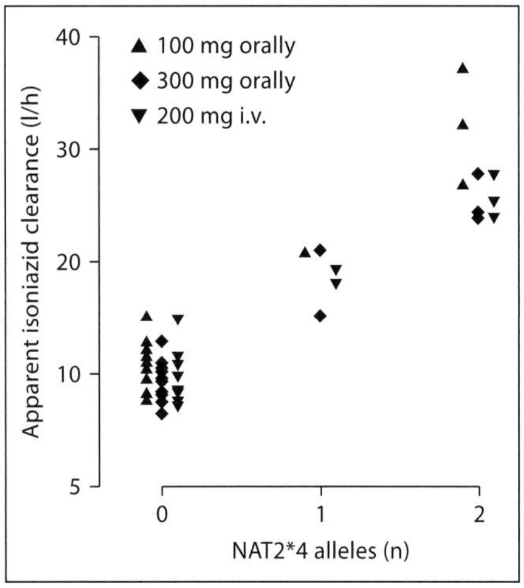


**Fig. 4.** Individual clearance of isoniazid in relation to the number of NAT2*4 alleles after administration of isoniazid in various doses. Values are slightly shifted along the x-axis to improve clarity (from Kinzig-Schippers et al. [22]).

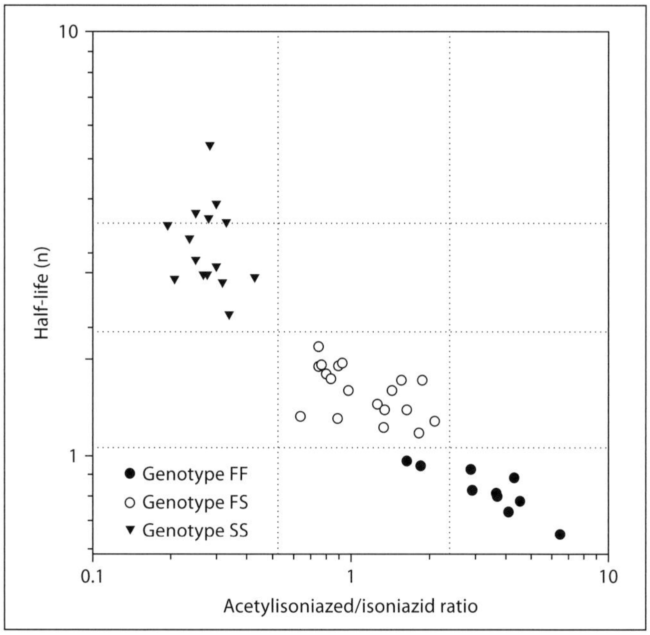


**Fig. 5.** Scatter plot of the metabolic ratio of acetylisoniazid and isoniazid in plasma (x-axis, log scale; 3 h after dose) against the genotype (FF: homozygous fast acetylators, FS: heterozygous fast or intermediate acetylators, SS: homozygous slow acetylators). Antimodes were drawn to distinguish between the groups that were phenotyped as slow, intermediate and fast, from left to right. Note the two discrepant FF patients that were wrongly phenotyped as intermediate (FS) acetylators. The more labour-intensive determination of isoniazid half-life (y-axis) predicted the genotype perfectly (from Seifart et al. [24]).

the effect of pharmacogenetic variation on the response to, and adverse effects of, isoniazid (see below). The acetylator status can be assessed by using phenotypic or genotypic methods.

Assessment of acetylator status by phenotyping has taken place by determining the plasma or serum half-life of isoniazid, by assessing the isoniazid plasma or serum concentration 6 h after oral dosage or by determining the ratio of the urinary excretion of acetylisoniazid to isoniazid at appropriate times after oral, intravenous or intramuscular administration of the drug (reviewed in Ellard [15]). A very sensitive yet relatively simple phenotypic method is the concentration ratio (or metabolic ratio) of acetylisoniazid to isoniazid in plasma at a fixed time after dosing. In one study there was complete agreement in classification of subjects as fast or slow acetylators between this single sample test and determination of the half-life of isoniazid, which requires withdrawal of multiple blood samples over a 6- to 8-hour period and is thus less convenient for patients and more labour intensive [23]. In a South African population, plasma metabolic ratios 3 h after dose were even able to reveal the trimodal distribution in NAT2 phenotype and were almost as reliable as isoniazid elimination half-life (fig. 5) [24]). In this study, the 2-hour metabolic ratio data only discriminated between the fast and other phenotypes, whereas the 6 hour metabolic ratio data only discriminated between the slow and other phenotypes. Measurement of isoniazid concentrations (rather than metabolic ratios) 6 h after dose, an alternative simple phenotyping method, also classified the study group as bimodal [24]. Therefore, assessment of the metabolic ratio of isoniazid 3 h after dose seems the best compromise between reliability and convenience for phenotypic assessment of the acetylator status. The optimal 3-hour sampling point is in accordance with that assessed in other studies [25, 26]. Assessment of the isoniazid metabolic ratio (and elimination half-life) for prediction of phenotype can also be performed with saliva [27, 28], which is especially convenient for children. However, use of isoniazid for phenotyping has certain disadvantages, including the extreme instability of isoniazid requiring immediate centrifugation and freezing of plasma at –80°C, and the limited availability of acetylisoniazid as raw material. Acetylisoniazid can be prepared by organic chemistry [29] or possibly be isolated from urine by preparative high-performance liquid chromatography. Apart from isoniazid, other so-called probe drugs (all substrates for NAT2) have been used extensively to assess the acetylator status, including sulphamethazine (sulphadimidine) [15], dapsone and caffeine [30].

The acetylator status can be assessed *genotypically* by extracting DNA from the patients' peripheral white blood cells and by performing polymerase chain reaction restriction fragment length polymorphism [16]. Genotyping at several SNPs at the NAT2 locus is needed to determine the proper acetylation status of an individual in a population. At present, most investigators study 7 or fewer SNPs at nucleotide positions 191 (G/A), 282 (C/T), 341 (T→C), 481 (C→T), 590 (G→A), 803 (A→G) and 857 (G→A) at exon 2 on the NAT2 locus [16]. Instead of analysing the genotype data at these polymorphic sites separately, the genotypes are generally expressed as alleles/haplotypes such as NAT2*4, NAT2*5, NAT2*6, NAT2*7, NAT2*12, depending on the specific arrangements of nucleotides at the polymorphic sites mentioned above [16]. The common allele, i.e. NAT2*4, is having common nucleotides at all polymorphic sites and is known as the NAT2 rapid acetylating allele. Individuals carrying two NAT2*4 alleles in the pair of chromosomes are homozygous fast acetylators; those carrying one slow and one fast acetylating allele are intermediate or heterozygous fast acetylators, and those carrying two slow acetylating alleles are slow acetylators. Clearly, genotyping of NAT2 and other enzymes involved in the metabolism of isoniazid (see below) requires involvement of experts to prevent pitfalls in methodology, terminology and specific mutations to be checked dependent on the population studied [16, 31].

Phenotype and genotype are generally concordant [24, 32, 33], but do not always correlate. Discrepancies are explained by endogenous and/or environmental factors that affect the phenotype but not the genotype.

*Impact of Acetylator Status on the Therapeutic Response to Isoniazid*

Obviously, the recognition of genetic polymorphism in NAT2 and the related differences in exposure to isoniazid have led to clinical studies to investigate whether the response to isoniazid-containing anti-TB regimens is dependent on acetylator status.

Isoniazid is known to be very active against rapidly multiplying bacilli that are present in the initial phase of TB treatment. Studies have evaluated whether the acetylator status affects the so-called early bactericidal activity (EBA) of isoniazid. This EBA is the rate at which a TB drug kills *M. tuberculosis* in the cavities of pulmonary TB during the first 2 days of therapy [34]. It is measured as the decline in log10 colony-forming unit counts in sputum of smear-positive patients. Indeed the EBA of homozygous slow acetylators appeared to be higher than that of the heterozygous fast or homozygous fast acetylators, but there was no significant difference in EBA between the homozygous and heterozygous fast acetylators [35]. Of note, isoniazid has an EBA greater than any other anti-TB drug, and even in fast acetylators, a relatively high EBA is still attained [35]: the fast acetylators' relative deficiency in killing of actively metabolizing bacilli over the first 2 days of treatment is probably unimportant. However, TB treatment as a whole takes at least 6 months, and the question is whether a lower exposure to isoniazid over such a long period is clinically relevant.

The potential clinical relevance of the isoniazid acetylator phenotype in long-term TB treatment (rather than response in the first days of treatment) has been extensively reviewed [15]. As to *daily* administered isoniazid-containing regimens, there is clear evidence that the acetylator phenotype of pulmonary TB patients is without prognostic significance, even when isoniazid is combined with only a single bacteriostatic drug such as thiacetazone or para-aminosalicylic acid (PAS) [15]. A review of 9 studies of various *twice weekly* isoniazid-containing regimens revealed no clear evidence that fast acetylators fared significantly worse than slow acetylators, and the therapeutic significance of the polymorphism in NAT2 for twice weekly TB regimens was considered to be of doubtful significance [15]. However, results of controlled clinical trials of *once weekly* isoniazid -containing regimens clearly showed that fast acetylators performed less well than slow acetylators [15]. The response to intermittent therapy is often explained by a postantibiotic effect, i.e. an antibiotic effect that is still present although the drug itself has disappeared from the site of action. The length of this postantibiotic effect is thought to be dependent on the dose of or exposure to the drug. Apparently, the postantibiotic effect of the applied isoniazid dose is not strong enough to conceal the therapeutic disadvantage of rapid acetylators over a 1-week period [36]. This means that once weekly regimens of isoniazid are not suitable, especially not for patients from races with predominantly fast acetylators.

More recently, once weekly isoniazid-based regimens were re-evaluated, now with rifapentine, an analogue to rifampicin, but with a longer elimination half-life. In 3 randomized trials, once weekly isoniazid/rifapentine was less effective than twice or thrice weekly isoniazid/rifampicin in the last 4 weeks of treatment of active TB [37]. In an in-depth analysis of one of these studies, low plasma concentrations of isoniazid were associated with failure/relapse with once weekly isoniazid-rifapentine, but not with twice weekly isoniazid-rifampicin [37]. Furthermore, isoniazid acetylator status determined by NAT2 genotype was associated with outcome in once weekly isoniazid-rifapentine, but not twice weekly isoniazid-rifampicin. Finally, patients who relapsed with rifamycin monoresistance had low concentrations of isoniazid. These findings confirm that the pharmacokinetics of isoniazid and the therapeutic deficiencies of fast acetylators become relevant in once weekly treatment.

Of note, highly intermittent treatment such as once weekly administration of anti-TB drugs can be considered as a model for non-adherence [21, 35]. Therefore non-adherence may be another risk factor that reveals or accentuates the therapeutic disadvantage of fast acetylators.

Apart from once weekly intermittent therapy and non-adherence, advanced HIV infection may be another risk factor that exposes the additional risk of fast acetylators. In a trial with isoniazid and rifabutin (another rifamycin) among TB/HIV-co-infected patients, acquired rifamycin resistance occurred despite twice weekly directly observed administration of the regimen. In this study, the median exposure to isoniazid for all patients appeared to be lower than that for HIV-negative patients in other studies. In addition, an even lower exposure to isoniazid in a subset of patients was associated with failure or relapse related to acquired rifamycin resistance [38]. The lower exposure to isoniazid in this study may be explained by the decreased levels of antituberculosis drugs often associated with HIV infection [39–41]. In addition, the acetylator status of patients may have contributed to the lowest exposures to isoniazid and may have contributed to selection of rifamycin resistance, but this is not clear from the results of this study. In any case, lower isoniazid drug levels probably interacted with an ineffective cellular immune function in HIV/AIDS to enable the emergence of resistance [38]. Further research is needed to assess whether HIV infection may reinforce the relative disadvantage of fast acetylators.

*Impact of Pharmacogenetic Variation on Adverse Effects to Isoniazid: Hepatotoxicity*

Hepatotoxicity is the most serious of adverse effects to isoniazid [12, 16, 42]. Apart from isoniazid, rifampicin and pyrazinamide are also hepatotoxic, and hepatoxicity to this anti-TB drug combination has been termed anti-TB drug-induced hepatotoxicity (ATDH) [41]. ATDH manifests itself as a treatment-emergent increase in serum alanine aminotransferase, and clinical features include jaundice, abdominal pain, nausea and vomiting. ATDH may cause non-adherence and interruption of TB treatment and thereby contributes to treatment failure, relapse or the emergence of resistance to TB treatment. Unfortunately, many definitions for drug-induced hepatotoxicity in general, and for ATDH more specifically, have been used in many studies. These definitions differ in the extent to which liver function parameters are raised and the use (or absence) of a proper assessment of drugs as causal factors for hepatotoxicity (e.g. by evaluating the response to re-administration of a drug, i.e. 'rechallenge') [12]. Partly because of this heterogeneity in definition, the incidence of ATDH during standard multidrug TB treatment has been variably reported as between 2 and 28% [12]. Risk factors for ATDH include genetic risk factors related to the metabolism of isoniazid, a higher age (above 60 years), female sex, low body mass index or malnutrition, HIV/AIDS, pre-existent liver diseases, alcoholism and use of other hepatotoxic drugs, including certain antiretroviral drugs [12, 43]. Hepatotoxicity associated with isoniazid has been related to genetic polymorphisms in NAT2, CYP2E1 and GST.

*Hepatotoxicity and Genetic Polymorphism in NAT2*

Based on the above, the study of isoniazid-induced hepatotoxicity and its potential relationship to genetic variation is a topic of major interest which is also complex to evaluate given the heterogeneity in the definition of ATDH, the use of other anti-TB drugs and the multiple other factors that may contribute to hepatoxicity. Most attention has been focussed on the relevance of the acetylator phenotype of patients, and this has been a topic of debate and controversy in the past decades. Initially, fast acetylators appeared to be more susceptible to ATDH. It was postulated that a reactive derivative of acetylhydrazine would mediate the isoniazid-induced hepatoxicity [44] (fig. 2). It was argued that fast acetylators would be more prone to isoniazid-induced hepatotoxicity, since fast acetylators form acetylisoniazid and hence acetylhydrazine more rapidly than slow acetylators. However, the pharmacological basis of this hypothesis was undermined by the demonstration that the disposal of acetylhydrazine also depends on further acetylation by NAT2 to form the non-toxic diacetylhydrazine (fig. 2), a metabolic route which is more rapid in fast acetylators [14, 15]. Since then only 1 study found fast acetylators to be specifically prone to isoniazid-induced elevated transaminases or hepatotoxicity [45], several studies showed no difference in risk between fast and slow metabolizers [46–49] (including a very large and influential study among nearly 3,000 patients in India [50]), and several studies showed that slow (phenotypic) acetylators are at a greater risk [51–54]. As the rationale for slow acetylators having an increased risk, it is postulated that most isoniazid cannot be acetylated in slow acetylators, but is directly hydrolysed to toxic hydrazine (fig. 2, right side). The concurrent administration of rifampicin causes an induction of the hydrolysis to hydrazine, which is one of the explanations for the increased risk of hepatotoxicity when isoniazid and rifampicin are combined [55]. In contrast, isoniazid would be rapidly converted to non-toxic diacetylhydrazine in rapid acetylators, which makes them less susceptible to ATDH (fig. 2, left side). In addition, it is argued that acetylhydrazine cannot be acetylated to non-toxic diacetylhydrazine in slow acetylators, but is oxidized into toxic products (fig. 2). In any case, it seems that the many *phenotyping* studies (mostly distinguishing between fast and slow acetylators, i.e. a bimodal distribution) have shown that there is either a higher risk of hepatoxicity for slow acetylators or that no such difference exists. The discrepancy between studies could be explained by differences in dose and frequency of administration of isoniazid, the inclusion or exclusion of patients with other predisposing factors, the definition of hepatoxicity, the use of different study designs, intra-individual variability in acetylation activity and use of different phenotyping methods [43, 56].

Genotyping may alleviate some of the concerns of phenotyping and may be more reliable, reproducible and feasible for mass survey [43]. More recent studies since the year 2000 have studied the influence of NAT2 *genotypes* on the susceptibility to ATDH. In Japanese pulmonary TB patients, the relative risk for hepatotoxicity was 4.0 for intermediate metabolizers and 28.0 for slow metabolizers compared to fast metabolizers [56]. Likewise, among Taiwanese patients, the risk of having ATDH was significantly higher in slow versus fast metabolizers (26.4 vs. 11.1%, odds ratio 2.87) [43]. Importantly, these and other studies used relatively mild transaminase increases as criterion for hepatotoxicity (aspartate or alanine aminotransferase more than twice the level before administration and 1.5–2 times the laboratories' upper limit of normal), resulting in a high incidence of hepatotoxicity (18.2% in the Japanese patients and 14.7% among the Taiwanese). In the Japanese study, it was stated that such criteria may be clinically useful for finding hepatic reactions earlier and for preventing the development of overt hepatitis [56]. A study in a Korean population also observed that NAT2 slow acetylators had a significantly (3.8-fold) higher risk of ATDH [57]. No association between NAT2 genotype and ATDH could be shown in an Indian population [58], but the authors mention that no conclusions can be drawn from this study as not all mutations at the NAT2 locus were screened. Genotyping in a mixed population of Caucasians, Hispanics, Africans, South Americans and Asians showed no association between genotype and ATDH either [59]. A study in a highly heterogeneous population found a trend for increasing hepatotoxicity across the fast, intermediate and slow acetylator groups ($p = 0.08$) [60] – this study was probably underpowered [61].

Nevertheless, the majority of studies with NAT2 genotyping suggest that slow acetylators are at an increased risk for hepatotoxicity. More studies with large sample sizes from different populations and with genotyping at appropriate polymorphic sites are still warranted to further substantiate the association between NAT2 acetylation status and isoniazid-induced hepatoxicity [16].

*Hepatotoxicity and Genetic Polymorphism in CYP2E1*

CYP2E1 may convert acetylhydrazine into toxic metabolites (fig. 2). Rifampicin is an inducer of CYP2E1 and can thus upregulate the production of toxic metabolites, one of the explanations for the increased risk of hepatotoxicity when isoniazid and rifampicin are combined [16]. In a study among Taiwanese TB patients, patients with homozygous wild genotype CYP2E1 c1/c1 had a higher risk of hepatotoxicity (20%) than those with mutant allele c2 (CYP2E1 c1/c2 or c2/c2, 9% risk, odds ratio 2.52) [61]. If the CYP2E1 c1/c2 or c2/c2 genotype combined with fast acetylator status was regarded as the reference group, the risk of hepatotoxicity increased from 3.94 for CYP2E1 c1/c1 with fast acetylator status to 7.43 for CYP2E1 c1/c1 with slow acetylator status. In the same study, this CYP2E c1/c1 genotype was also associated with a higher CYP2E1 activity, which concurs with the generation of more toxic metabolites from acetylhydrazine (fig. 2). Other studies in Indian patients [63] and in a mixed population of Caucasians, Hispanics, Africans, South Americans and Asians [59] also observed that the common c1 (currently also known as *1A [16]) allele at CYP2E1 was associated with ATDH. A study in Koreans did not find such an association [57] and, similarly, a study in a highly heterogeneous population found no association between CYP2E1 polymorphism and hepatotoxicity [60], although this study was criticized for its methodology and lack of statistical power [61].

*Hepatotoxicity and Genetic Polymorphism in GST*

Glutathione plays an important role as an intracellular scavenger by conjugating with toxic reactive substances that are generated from biotransformation of drugs and xenobiotics. GSTs catalyse these conjugation reactions. These enzymes are coded by at least 5 different loci, of which GSTM1 and GSTT1 have been investigated in TB hepatotoxicity studies. Homozygous deletion at GSTM1 and GSTT1 results in complete loss of enzymatic activity, but individuals who carry one or both of the functional alleles possess enzymatic activity [16]. Frequencies of these GSTM1 and GSTT1 homozygous deletion genotypes in healthy individuals have been reported for different populations [16]. Deficiency in GST activity, because of homozygous null mutations at GSTM1, increased the risk of ATDH in Indian [58] and Taiwanese patients [43] with odds ratios of 2.13 and 2.23, respectively. The GSTT1 homozygous deletion did not affect the risk for ATDH.

*Hepatotoxicity and Other Genetic Polymorphisms*
Manganese superoxide dismutase is an enzyme involved in the reduction of reactive oxygen species that could cause hepatic injury. Among patients with drug-induced liver injury, subjects with a mutant C allele (T/C or C/C genotype) of manganese superoxide dismutase had a higher risk of drug-induced hepatotoxicity than those with the manganese superoxide dismutase T/T genotype, both in patients who had not used anti-TB drugs and in the subcategory of those exposed to anti-TB drugs (odds ratio 2.5) [64].

Specific human leucocyte antigen (HLA) alleles have been associated with the development of pulmonary tuberculosis in various populations. In a study to investigate the role of these genes in the development of drug-induced hepatotoxicity in TB patients, the presence of HLA-DQB1*0201 and absence of HLA-DQA1*0102 were found to be significant risk factors for the development of drug-induced hepatotoxicity [65].

*Interplay between Genetic Risk Factors for Hepatotoxicity*
In the studies described thus far, the interplay between the various genetic risk factors relevant to ATDH has not been studied extensively. One study evaluated the effect of polymorphisms of NAT2, CYP2E1 and GST in Japanese TB patients on the generation of hydrazine as a proxy for hepatotoxicity [66]. The serum concentration of hydrazine was significantly higher in slow acetylators than in rapid acetylators of NAT2, the effect of CYP2E1 gene polymorphisms on the serum concentration of hydrazine was rarely observed, while that of GST gene polymorphism was observed in intermediate acetylators of NAT2. Hydrazine tended to accumulate in patients with the GSTM1 null genotype. Of note, higher concentrations of rifampicin were also associated with high serum concentrations of hydrazine [66].

Another study compared genotype distributions in 7 drug-metabolizing enzyme genes (NAT2, CYP2C9, CYP2C19, CYP2D6, CYP2E1, NAT2, UGT1A1 and UGT1A3) between 67 cases with TB drug-induced hepatitis and 159 controls. Only NAT2 polymorphism was associated with hepatitis, and no essential role for genetic mutation of the other metabolizing enzymes in the development of hepatitis could be shown [67].

More studies evaluating the simultaneous effects of genetic polymorphisms as well as interactions between genetic and exogenous risk factors for TB drug-induced hepatotoxicity are warranted.

*Other Adverse Effects to Isoniazid*
Peripheral neuropathy is uncommon (less than 0.2%) at the normal dose of isoniazid. The risk is increased in persons with other conditions that may be associated with neuropathy, including nutritional deficiency, diabetes mellitus, HIV infection, renal failure, alcoholism, pregnancy and breastfeeding [68]. Peripheral neuropathy is related to the polymorphism in NAT2, with slow acetylators being more susceptible [5, 69]. This is probably related to the higher exposure (area under the curve) to isoniazid in slow acetylators [15]. Somehow this relates to isoniazid competitively inhibiting the action of pyridoxine (vitamin $B_6$), as supplementation of at least 6 mg pyridoxine/day [15] (but usually more, 20–25 mg/day [68]) can be given for prevention of peripheral neuropathy.

A study among Japanese patients who used isoniazid but no rifampicin showed an association between NAT2 genotype and the incidence of other serious adverse events to isoniazid, i.e nausea and vomiting, fever, visual impairment and peripheral neuritis. Six out of 102 patients developed these adverse events, and 5 of them were slow acetylators [70].

In one study in a very small (n = 25) Latin American population of the use of prophylactic isoniazid, only 2 individuals experienced adverse events (gastric intolerance): both were slow acetylators [29].

## Other First-Line Antituberculosis Drugs

Very few studies have focussed on the pharmacogenetics of anti-TB drugs other than isoniazid. The pivotal anti-TB drug rifampicin is metabolized in the liver by desacetylation resulting in a more polar compound with increased capacity for biliary excretion [71, 72]. In a separate metabolic pathway, hydrolysis yields a 3-formylrifampicin which is present only in urine [71, 72]. About 15–20% of rifampicin is glucuronized [73], and rifampicin is a substrate for OATPs [74]. Interindividual variability in rifampicin plasma concentrations is large and relevant, considering that the current dose of rifampicin is at the lower end of the dose-response curve [75]. Low plasma concentrations of rifamycins have been associated with delayed sputum conversion, treatment failure, relapse and acquired rifamycin resistance [38, 76, 77], although other studies have not found such associations

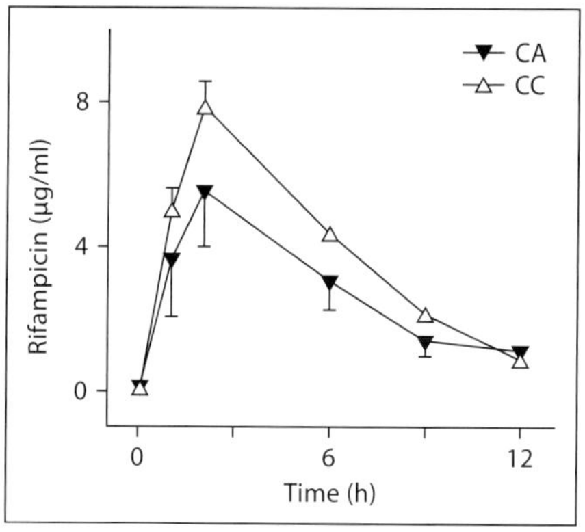


**Fig. 6.** Plasma rifampicin concentrations versus time in patients with *SLCO1B1* c.463CA genotype (closed triangles) versus *SLCO1B1* c.463CC genotypes (open triangles), resulting in a 36% lower adjusted exposure ($AUC_{0-24\,h}$) of rifampicin in the former genotype (arithmetic means, standard errors in vertical bars; from Weiner et al. [80]).

between concentrations and effect [78, 79]. A recent study found that the exposure to rifampicin ($AUC_{0-24\ h}$) was affected by polymorphism in the *SLCO1B1* gene, which codes for OATPs [80]. The adjusted rifampicin $AUC_{0-24\,h}$ was 36% lower among participants with the *SLCO1B1* genotype c.463CA than among other participants with the *SLCO1B1* genotype c.463CC (fig. 6). Of note, subjects of black race were 2.4-fold more likely than Caucasians to have the polymorphism associated with lower rifampicin exposure. The *SLCOB1* c.521T→C polymorphism did not affect the pharmacokinetics of rifampicin in this [80] and another study [81]. Polymorphism in MDR1 (coding for the transporter P-glycoprotein) was not associated with rifampicin pharmacokinetics either [80]. More research is warranted to explain variability in exposure to rifampicin, e.g. by investigating the polymorphism in esterases that catalyze the desacetylation of this drug. No relevant polymorphisms are known for the pharmacokinetics of pyrazinamide and ethambutol.

## Second-Line Anti-TB Drugs

There appear to be few pharmacogenetic data for second-line anti-TB drugs (designated as groups 2–5 in the WHO classification of anti-TB drugs [82]) that are used in multidrug-resistant (MDR) TB and in case of adverse effects to the first-line anti-TB drugs (group 1).

The injectable agents (aminoglycosides and capreomycin, group 2) and the most widely used fluoroquinolones in TB treatment (ofloxacin and levofloxacin, group 3) are primarily excreted unchanged in the urine. Moxifloxacin is probably the fluoroquinolone most active against *M. tuberculosis*. It is used for MDR-TB in developed countries where it is available, and it is currently being investigated for its potential to shorten TB treatment in drug-susceptible TB [9]. About 50% of moxifloxacin is metabolized by phase II metabolism only (glucuronidation and sulphation). In one study, polymorphisms in the *MDR1* gene coding for the transporter P-glycoprotein, for which the fluoroquinolones are a substrate, had no effect on the exposure to moxifloxacin [83]. In vitro [84] and murine data [85] suggest that the current dose and exposure to moxifloxacin should be increased to achieve optimal response, but the possibility of QT interval prolongation with this drug should be considered although this is rarely seen in the usual dose [86]. QT interval prolongation can be considered as another form of idiosyncratic adverse drug reaction [1]. Current knowledge of the genetic basis for QT interval prolongation is limited, but a range of rare polymorphisms and mutations in ion channels appear to be associated with increased risk [1, 87]. For example, a polymorphism in *KCNE1*, coding for a voltage-gated potassium channel, is more common in individuals who have suffered drug-induced QT prolongation [88].

Among the TB drugs in group 4, ethionamide and probably the structurally related prothionamide are metabolized by sulphoxidation, desulphuration and deamination, followed by demethylation [89]. Cycloserine (group 4) is largely excreted unchanged by glomerular filtration. PAS (group 4) is metabolized by N-acetyltransferase 1 (NAT1) to acetyl-PAS, which is subsequently cleared renally. Historically, NAT1 was considered to be monomorphic in nature, but NAT1 activity appears to be bimodally distributed in slow and fast acetylators, and base substitutions associated with the slow acetylator status have been assessed [90]. PAS has been used as a phenotyping probe for NAT1 activity [91]. As PAS may bioactivate several carcinogens, the polymorphism in NAT1 may be relevant for cancer risk in individual subjects [90], but its relevance in TB treatment is unknown. Anti-TB drugs in group 5 have unclear efficacy, are generally not recommended and are not described here.

## New Anti-TB Drugs in Development

Several new potential TB drugs are in the clinical phase of drug development [9]: moxifloxacin, gatifloxacin, TMC207, PA-824, delamanid, SQ109 and LL3858. At present there are no pharmacogenetic data on these drugs. The metabolism and elimination of most of these compounds has

| Development phase | Problems |
|---|---|
| Phase I: basic biomedical research<br>Aim: proof of principle | |
| Phase II: clinical research<br>Aim: proof of efficacy<br>Aim: proof of cost-effectiveness | Lack of randomized controlled trials proving efficacy<br>Lack of well-designed studies to prove cost-effectiveness |
| Phase III: clinical practice<br>Aim: implementation | Lack of knowledge of physician, pharmacist and patient<br>Lack of guidelines on interpreting pharmacogenetic tests<br>Lack of regulatory approval for pharmacogenetic tests<br>Lack of reimbursement for pharmacogenetic tests |

**Fig. 7.** Consecutive phases and problems on the road to clinical implementation of pharmacogenetics (modified after Swen et al. [10, 97]).

been described [9], but their modes of transport are largely unknown. Moxifloxacin (approved as second-line anti-TB drug, but not for drug-susceptible TB) is furthest on the road in phase III of clinical development and some pharmacogenetic considerations are described above. One of the other new compounds, SQ-109, an ethambutol analogue with 1,2-diamine pharmacophore, is metabolized by CYP2D6 and CYP2C19 [9]. Both of these metabolic enzymes have well-described polymorphisms that are relevant for many drugs [1, 2], but the implications for response to SQ-109 are unknown at present.

## Application of Pharmacogenetics in Clinical Practice and Barriers to Its Application

In TB treatment, the most obvious and best-founded application for pharmacogenetics would be to perform NAT2 genotyping or phenotyping before starting treatment. According to the acetylator status, isoniazid dosage is then individualized, thereby ensuring a minimal probability of toxicity, but, nonetheless, reaching adequate isoniazid concentrations to ensure adequate bactericidal activity. Based on data available, the recommended standard daily dose of isoniazid of 5 mg/kg in adults, which is probably balanced for the best benefit-risk ratio for all NAT2 genotypes, could be individualized to 2.5, 5.0 and 7.5 mg/kg for subjects with none (slow acetylators), 1 (intermediate acetylators) or 2 (fast acetylators) NAT2*4 alleles [22]. Others have suggested a dose of 3 mg/kg in slow acetylators and at least 6 mg/kg in fast acetylators [24]. However, this practice of individualizing isoniazid therapy is rarely used in TB treatment. In a limited number of centres across the world, dosing of isoniazid and other anti-TB drugs is individualized, but based on measurement of drug concentrations in plasma (therapeutic drug monitoring) rather than pharmacogenetic analyses [92–96]. It could be argued though that pharmacogenetics is performed at a population basis, considering that the 4–6 mg/kg range in the isoniazid dose allowed by the WHO enables national programmes to adapt their fixed dose based on the expected proportion of fast and slow acetylators in their country [21].

Clearly, in case of TB treatment, the limited application of pharmacogenetics can be explained by the epidemiology of this disease, with large numbers of patients needing treatment in TB control programmes with limited resources. In TB treatment, individualized and expensive treatment guided by pharmacogenetics is simply not feasible at this moment. However, pharmacogenetics is not applied in TB treatment in developed countries either. In general, the clinical application of pharmacogenetics for many other drugs remains in its infancy, despite predictions that pharmacogenetics would be one of the first applications from the human genome project [1, 97]. To understand the reasons for the limited application of pharmacogenetics in general, the course of translation of biomedical discoveries into clinically relevant testing modalities may be considered (fig. 7) [10, 97], and this course is also relevant for the future application of pharmacogenetics in TB treatment. First, fundamental biomedical research should provide the 'proof of principle' for the technique in question. Second, clinical research in pharmacogenetics is performed in limited numbers of patients, to demonstrate the efficacy and cost-effectiveness of the technique. In the third phase, the technique is implemented for widespread use in clinical practice. For pharmacogenetics, an important limitation is the amount of scientific evidence demonstrating that its application leads to improved patient outcome [10, 97]. The number of original scientific publications is relatively limited, many original studies involve a small specific study population, administer single doses and use healthy volunteers rather than patients. Most studies

**Table 1.** Pharmacogenetics of anti-TB drugs: key points

- Pharmacogenetics can be defined as the study of genetic factors affecting (desirable or undesirable) drug responses
- Pharmacogenetics considers the impact of genetic variation on both the pharmacokinetics and pharmacodynamics of drugs; the pharmacogenetics of idiosyncratic adverse drug reactions is distinguished as a third class of gene-drug interactions
- Slow acetylation of isoniazid is a genetically determined homozygous recessive trait
- Trimodality in isoniazid elimination has been demonstrated, resulting in homozygous fast, heterozygous fast (or intermediate) and slow metabolizers
- The proportions of fast, intermediate and slow acetylators vary substantially between populations; about 50–60% of subjects from European (Caucasian), African and Indian origin are slow metabolizers, whereas a minority varying from 5 to 25% among populations from Asian origin consists of slow metabolizers
- Assessment of the acetylisoniazid/isoniazid (metabolic) ratio of isoniazid 3 h after dose is the best compromise between reliability and convenience for the phenotypic assessment of the acetylator status
- Genotyping of NAT2 and other enzymes requires involvement of experts to prevent pitfalls in methodology and terminology and to check for specific mutations dependent on the population studied
- Exposure to isoniazid is considerably lower in fast acetylators than in intermediate or slow acetylators
- The EBA of homozygous slow acetylators is higher than that of the heterozygous fast or homozygous fast acetylators, but probably not to a clinically relevant extent
- The acetylator phenotype of pulmonary TB patients is without prognostic significance in *daily* isoniazid-containing regimens, is of doubtful significance in *twice weekly* regimens, but is relevant in *once weekly* isoniazid-containing regimens, with fast acetylators performing less well than slow acetylators
- Non-adherence and advanced HIV infection may be other risk factors that expose the therapeutic disadvantage of fast acetylators
- The majority of genotyping studies suggest that slow acetylators are at an increased risk for isoniazid-induced hepatotoxicity
- Genetic polymorphisms in CYP2E1 and GST are associated with an increased risk for isoniazid-induced hepatotoxicity
- Slow acetylators are more susceptible to peripheral neuropathy to isoniazid, but this can be prevented by giving pyridoxine
- The interindividual variability in exposure to rifampicin is clinically relevant and can be explained to a large extent by polymorphism in genes for OATPs
- Polymorphisms in ion channels may be relevant for the risk of QT interval prolongation, a dose-limiting adverse effect of the promising anti-TB drug moxifloxacin
- Clinical application of pharmacogenetics is still in its infancy and warrants more clinical studies, evaluation of cost-effectiveness and overcoming of hurdles associated with implementation of this new approach in clinical practice
- Genome-wide association studies will be used increasingly to understand the simultaneous effects of multiple genes on drug response

are retrospective and are not aiming at the evaluation of a pharmacogenetic intervention [97]. Cost-effectiveness has been convincingly demonstrated for only a limited number of pharmacogenetic tests [10, 97, 98], and such research has not been performed in the context of TB treatment so far. An important barrier in the implementation phase (fig. 7) is the lack of education and knowledge of pharmacogenetics amongst physicians and pharmacists [10, 99]. If individual physicians are aware of the potential of pharmacogenetics, they may not understand how to manage a patient on the basis of a test result, and guidelines in this respect are scarce [10, 99]. In addition, there is a complex and evolving regulatory environment for submission and clearance of pharmacogenetic devices by national regulatory instances [99]. If there is no regulatory clearance of a test, this promotes an additional barrier to clinical implementation: reimbursement. Many insurers will not reimburse pharmacogenetic testing at this moment, on the grounds that it is still experimental or investigational [10, 99].

## Conclusions and Future Perspectives

In the past decades, genetic factors that affect drug response to TB drugs have been studied extensively, with a strong emphasis on isoniazid. Based on this chapter, several key points can be formulated (table 1). However, the ultimate goal of pharmacogenetics to individualize and tailor drug therapy, rather than to apply a 'one size fits all' and 'trial and error' approach in drug prescribing and dosing, has not been met for TB treatment at all. This relates to the scientific evidence for such an approach as well as to the poverty-related character of TB with many patients to be treated with limited resources. In addition, it is clear that specific hurdles need to be cleared, related to implementation of a new technique in clinical practice.

Pharmacogenetics will continue to develop in the years to come. The focus of research will turn more and more from understanding of single gene effects to the study of the simultaneous effects of multiple genes. In this respect, another type of research, i.e. genome-wide association studies, will be used increasingly [1]. These studies involve genotyping disease cases and unaffected controls for typically between 500,000 and 1,000,000 SNPs. Apparently positive associations related to response or toxicity need to be replicated in a second independent set of cases and controls. Genome-wide association studies have a completely open approach, allowing the detection of simultaneous effects of multiple different genes as well as associations that are not directly predictable from existing knowledge.

New anti-TB drugs will hopefully be introduced in the near future and will probably be used in a traditional way, using a fixed rather than personalized dose based on pharmacogenetic approaches. Pharmacogenetic studies will inevitably be performed on these drugs as well. It seems that we are just at the beginning of a new era of more personalized medicine and that the future of pharmacogenetics is still full of promise for patient care.

## References


1 Daly AK: Pharmacogenetics and human genetic polymorphisms. Biochem J 2010;429:435–449.
2 Crettol S, Petrovic N, Murray M: Pharmacogenetics of phase I and phase II drug metabolism. Curr Pharm Des 2010;16:204–219.
3 McLeod HL, Evans WE: Pharmacogenomics: unlocking the human genome for better drug therapy. Annu Rev Pharmacol Toxicol 2001;41:101–121.
4 Hughes HB: On the metabolic fate of isoniazid. J Pharmacol Exp Ther 1953;109:444–452.
5 Hughes HB, Biehl JP, Jones AP, Schmidt LH: Metabolism of isoniazid in man as related to the occurrence of peripheral neuritis. Am Rev Tuberc 1954;70:266–273.
6 Mitchell RS, Bell JC: Clinical implications of isoniazid, PAS and streptomycin blood levels in pulmonary tuberculosis. Trans Am Clin Climatol Assoc 1957;69:98–102.
7 Harris HW, Knight RA, Selin MJ: Comparison of isoniazid concentrations in the blood of people of Japanese and European descent: therapeutic and genetic implications. Am Rev Tuberc 1958;78:944–948.
8 Evans DA, Manley KA, McKusick VA: Genetic control of isoniazid metabolism in man. Br Med J 1960;2:485–491.
9 Van den Boogaard J, Kibiki GS, Kisanga ER, Boeree MJ, Aarnoutse RE: New drugs against tuberculosis: problems, progress, and evaluation of agents in clinical development. Antimicrob Agents Chemother 2009;53:849–862.
10 Swen JJ, Wessels JAM, Guchelaar HJ: Farmacogenetica: van abstract begrip naar klinische praktijk (in Dutch). Geneesmiddelenbulletin 2010;44:97–103.
11 Knowles SR, Uetrecht J, Shear NH: Idiosyncratic drug reactions: the reactive metabolite syndromes. Lancet 2000;356:1587–1591.
12 Tostmann A, Boeree MJ, Aarnoutse RE, de Lange WC, van der Ven AJAM, Dekhuijzen R: Antituberculosis drug-induced hepatotoxicity: concise up-to-date review. J Gastroenterol Hepatol 2008;23:192–202.
13 Mitchell JR, Zimmerman HJ, Ishak KG, Thorgeirsson UP, Timbrell JA, Snodgrass WR, Nelson SD: Isoniazid liver injury: clinical spectrum, pathology, and probable pathogenesis. Ann Intern Med 1976;84:181–192.
14 Ellard GA, Gammon PT: Pharmacokinetics of isoniazid metabolism in man. J Pharmacokinet Biopharm 1976;4:83–113.
15 Ellard GA: The potential clinical significance of the isoniazid acetylator phenotype in the treatment of pulmonary tuberculosis. Tubercle 1984;65:211–227.
16 Roy PD, Majumder M, Roy B: Pharmacogenomics of anti-TB drugs-related hepatotoxicity. Pharmacogenomics 2008;9:311–321.
17 Parkin DP, Vandenplas S, Botha FJ, Vandenplas ML, Seifart HI, van Helden PD, van der Walt BJ, Donald PR, van Jaarsveld PP: Trimodality of isoniazid elimination: phenotype and genotype in patients with tuberculosis. Am J Respir Crit Care Med 1997;155:1717–1722.
18 Pariente-Khayat A, Rey E, Gendrel D, Vauzelle-Kervroëdan F, Crémier O, d'Athis P, Badoual J, Olive G, Pons G: Isoniazid acetylation metabolic ratio during maturation in children. Clin Pharmacol Ther 1997;62:377–383.
19 Zhu R, Kiser JJ, Seifart HI, Werely CJ, Mitchell CD, D'Argenio DZ, Fletcher CV: The pharmacogenetics of NAT2 enzyme maturation in perinatally HIV exposed infants receiving isoniazid. J Clin Pharmacol 2011, E-pub ahead of print.
20 Tiitinen H: Isoniazid and ethionamide serum levels and inactivation in Finnish subjects. Scand J Respir Dis 1969;50:110–124.
21 Donald PR, Parkin DP, Seifart HI, Schaaf HS, van Helden PD, Werely CJ, Sirgel FA, Venter A, Maritz JS: The influence of dose and N-acetyltransferase-2 (NAT2) genotype and phenotype on the pharmacokinetics and pharmacodynamics of isoniazid. Eur J Clin Pharmacol 2007;63:633–639.
22 Kinzig-Schippers M, Tomalik-Scharte D, Jetter A, Scheidel B, Jacob V, Rodamer M, Cascorbi I, Doroshyenko O, Sorgel F, Fuhr U: Should we use N-acetyltransferase type 2 genotyping to personalize isoniazid doses? Antimicrob Agents Chemother 2005;49:1733–1738.
23 Hutchings A, Routledge PA: A simple method for determining acetylator phenotype using isoniazid. Br J Clin Pharmacol 1986;22:343–345.
24 Seifart HI, Parkin DP, Botha FJ, Donald PR, van der Walt BJ: Population screening for isoniazid acetylator phenotype. Pharmacoepidemiol Drug Saf 2001;10:127–134.
25 Mashimo M, Suzuki T, Abe M, Deguchi T: Molecular genotyping of N-acetylation polymorphism to predict phenotype. Hum Genet 1992;90:139–143.
26 Smith CA, Wadelius M, Gough AC, Harrison DJ, Wolf CR, Rane A: A simplified assay for the arylamine N-acetyltransferase 2 polymorphism validated by phenotyping with isoniazid. J Med Genet 1997;34:758–760.
27 Hutchings AD, Monie RD, Spragg BP, Routledge PA: Saliva and plasma concentrations of isoniazid and acetylisoniazid in man. Br J Clin Pharmacol 1988;25:585–589.
28 Hutchings AD, Routledge PA: A single sample saliva test to determine acetylator phenotype. Br J Clin Pharmacol 1996;42:635–637.
29 Diaz-Molina R, Cornejo-Bravo JM, Ramos-Ibarra MA, Estrada-Guzmán JD, Morales-Arango O, Reyes-Báez R, Robinson-Navarro OM, Soria-Rodríguez CG: Genotype and phenotype of NAT2 and the occurrence of adverse drug reactions in Mexican individuals to an isoniazid-based prophylactic chemotherapy for tuberculosis. Mol Med Rep 2008;1:875–879.
30 Rane A: Phenotyping of drug metabolism in infants and children: potentials and problems. Pediatrics 1999;104:640–643.
31 Cascorbi I, Roots I: Pitfalls in N-acetyltransferase 2 genotyping. Pharmacogenetics 1999;9:123–127.

32 Cascorbi I, Drakoulis N, Brockmoller J, Maurer A, Sperling K, Roots I: Arylamine N-acetyltransferase (NAT2) mutations and their allelic linkage in unrelated Caucasian individuals: correlation with phenotypic activity. Am J Hum Genet 1995;57:581–592.
33 Gross M, Kruisselbrink T, Anderson K, Lang N, McGovern P, Delongchamp R, Kadlubar F: Distribution and concordance of N-acetyltransferase genotype and phenotype in an American population. Cancer Epidemiol Biomarkers Prev 1999;8:683–692.
34 Jindani A, Aber VR, Edwards EA, Mitchison DA: The early bactericidal activity of drugs in patients with pulmonary tuberculosis. Am Rev Respir Dis 1980;121:939–949.
35 Donald PR, Sirgel FA, Venter A, Parkin DP, Seifart HI, van de Wal BW, Werely C, van Helden PD, Maritz JS: The influence of human N-acetyltransferase genotype on the early bactericidal activity of isoniazid. Clin Infect Dis 2004;39:1425–1430.
36 Donald PR, Sirgel FA, Botha FJ, Seifart HI, Parkin DP, Vandenplas ML, Van de Wal BW, Maritz JS, Mitchison DA: The early bactericidal activity of isoniazid related to its dose size in pulmonary tuberculosis. Am J Respir Crit Care Med 1997;156:895–900.
37 Weiner M, Burman W, Vernon A, Benator D, Peloquin CA, Khan A, Weis S, King B, Shah N, Hodge T, Tuberculosis Trials Consortium: Low isoniazid concentrations and outcome of tuberculosis treatment with once-weekly isoniazid and rifapentine. Am J Respir Crit Care Med 2003;167:1341–1347.
38 Weiner M, Benator D, Burman W Peloquin CA, Khan A, Vernon A, Jones B, Silva-Trigo C, Zhao Z, Hodge T, Tuberculosis Trials Consortium: Association between acquired rifamycin resistance and the pharmacokinetics of rifabutin and isoniazid among patients with HIV and tuberculosis. Clin Infect Dis 2005;40:1481–1491.
39 Sahai J, Gallicano K, Swick L, Tailor S, Garber G, Seguin I, Oliveras L, Walker S, Rachlis A, Cameron DW: Reduced plasma concentrations of antituberculosis drugs in patients with HIV infection. Ann Intern Med 1997;127:289–293.
40 Gurumurthy P, Ramachandran G, Hemanth Kumar AK, Rajasekaran S, Padmapriyadarsini C, Swaminathan S, Bhagavathy S, Venkatesan P, Sekar L, Mahilmaran A, Ravichandran N, Paramesh P: Decreased bioavailability of rifampin and other antituberculosis drugs in patients with advanced human immunodeficiency virus disease. Antimicrob Agents Chemother 2004;48:4473–4475.
41 McIlleron H, Wash P, Burger A, Norman J, Folb PI, Smith P: Determinants of rifampin, isoniazid, pyrazinamide, and ethambutol pharmacokinetics in a cohort of tuberculosis patients. Antimicrob Agents Chemother 2006;50:1170–1177.
42 Saukkonen JJ, Cohn DL, Jasmer RM, Schenker S, Jereb JA, Nolan CM, Peloquin CA, Gordin FM, Nunes D, Strader DB, Bernardo J, Venkataramanan R, Sterling TR, ATS (American Thoracic Society) Hepatotoxicity of Antituberculosis Therapy Subcommittee: An official ATS statement: hepatotoxicity of antituberculosis therapy. Am J Respir Crit Care Med 2006;174:935–952.
43 Huang YS, Chern HD, Su WJ, Wu JC, Lai SL, Yang SY, Chang FY, Lee SD: Polymorphism of the N-acetyltransferase 2 gene as a susceptibility risk factor for antituberculosis drug-induced hepatitis. Hepatology 2002;35:883–889.
44 Mitchell JR, Thorgeirsson UP, Black M, Timbrell JA, Snodgrass WR, Potter WZ, Jollow HR, Keiser HR: Increased incidence of isoniazid hepatitis in rapid acetylators: possible relation to hydranize metabolites. Clin Pharmacol Ther 1975;18:70–79.
45 Yamamoto T, Suou T, Hirayama C: Elevated serum aminotransferase induced by isoniazid in relation to isoniazid acetylator phenotype. Hepatology 1986;6:295–298.
46 Ellard GA, Mitchison DA, Girling DJ, Nunn AJ, Fox W: The hepatic toxicity of isoniazid among rapid and slow acetylators of the drug. Am Rev Respir Dis 1978;118:628–629.
47 Ellard GA, Girling DJ, Nunn AJ: The hepatotoxicity of isoniazid among the three acetylator phenotypes. Am Rev Respir Dis 1981;123:568–570.
48 Singh J, Garg PK, Thakur VS, Tandon RK: Antitubercular treatment induced hepatotoxicity: does acetylator status matter? Indian J Physiol Pharmacol 1995;39:43–46.
49 Hwang SJ, Wu JC, Lee CN, Yen FS, Lu CL, Lin TP, Lee SD: A prospective clinical study of isoniazid-rifampicin-pyrazinamide-induced liver injury in an area endemic for hepatitis B. J Gastroenterol Hepatol 1997;12:87–91.
50 Gurumurthy P, Krishnamurthy MS, Nazareth O, Parthasarathy R, Sarma GR, Somasundaram PR, Tripathy SP, Ellard GA: Lack of relationship between hepatic toxicity and acetylator phenotype in three thousand South Indian patients during treatment with isoniazid for tuberculosis. Am Rev Respir Dis 1984;129:58–61.
51 Gronhagen-Riska C, Hellstrom PE, Froseth B: Predisposing factors in hepatitis induced by isoniazid-rifampin treatment of tuberculosis. Am Rev Respir Dis 1978;118:461–466.
52 Dickinson DS, Bailey WC, Hirschowitz BI, Soong SJ, Eidus L, Hodgkin MM: Risk factors for isoniazid (NIH)-induced liver dysfunction. J Clin Gastroenterol 1981;3:271–279.
53 Parthasarathy R, Sarma GR, Janardhanam B Ramachandran P, Santha T, Sivasubramanian S, Somasundaram PR, Tripathy SP: Hepatic toxicity in South Indian patients during treatment of tuberculosis with short-course regimens containing isoniazid, rifampicin and pyrazinamide. Tubercle 1986;67:99–108.
54 Pande JN, Singh SP, Khilnani GC, Khilnani S, Tandon RK: Risk factors for hepatotoxicity from antituberculosis drugs: a case-control study. Thorax 1996;51:132–136.
55 Sarma GR, Immanuel C, Kailasam S, Narayana AS, Venkatesan P: Rifampin-induced release of hydrazine from isoniazid: a possible cause of hepatitis during treatment of tuberculosis with regimens containing isoniazid and rifampin. Am Rev Respir Dis 1986;133:1072–1075.
56 Ohno M, Yamaguchi I, Yamamoto I Fukuda T, Yokota S, Maekura R, Ito M, Yamamoto Y, Ogura T, Maeda K, Komuta K, Igarashi T, Azuma J: Slow N-acetyltransferase 2 genotype affects the incidence of isoniazid and rifampicin-induced hepatotoxicity. Int J Tuberc Lung Dis 2000;4:256–261.
57 Cho HJ, Koh WJ, Ryu YJ, Ki CS, Nam MH, Kim JW, Lee SY: Genetic polymorphisms of NAT2 and CYP2E1 associated with antituberculosis drug-induced hepatotoxicity in Korean patients with pulmonary tuberculosis. Tuberculosis (Edinb) 2007;87:551–556.
58 Roy B, Chowdhury A, Kundu S Santra A, Dey B, Chakraborty M, Majumder PP: Increased risk of antituberculosis drug-induced hepatotoxicity in individuals with glutathione S-transferase M1 'null' mutation. J Gastroenterol Hepatol 2001;16:1033–1037.
59 Vuilleumier N, Rossier MF, Chiappe A Degoumois F, Dayer P, Mermillod B, Nicod L, Desmeules J, Hochstrasser D: CYP2E1 genotype and isoniazid-induced hepatotoxicity in patients treated for latent tuberculosis. Eur J Clin Pharmacol 2006;62:423–429.
60 Yamada S, Tang M, Richardson K Halaschek-Wiener J, Chan M, Cook VJ, Fitzgerald JM, Elwood RK, Brooks-Wilson A, Marra F: Genetic variations of NAT2 and CYP2E1 and isoniazid hepatotoxicity in a diverse population. Pharmacogenomics 2009;10:1433–1445.
61 Leiro-Fernandez V, Valverde D, Vazquez-Gallardo R, Constenla L, Fernandez-Villar A: Genetic variations of NAT2 and CYP2E1 and isoniazid hepatotoxicity in a diverse population. Pharmacogenomics 2010;11:1205–1206.
62 Huang YS, Chern HD, Su WJ, Wu JC, Chang SC, Chiang CH, Chang FY, Lee SD: Cytochrome P450 2E1 genotype and the susceptibility to antituberculosis drug-induced hepatitis. Hepatology 2003;37:924–930.
63 Roy B, Ghosh SK, Sutradhar D, Sikdar N, Mazumder S, Barman S: Predisposition of antituberculosis drug induced hepatotoxicity by cytochrome P450 2E1 genotype and haplotype in pediatric patients. J Gastroenterol Hepatol 2006;21:784–786.
64 Huang YS, Su WJ, Huang YH, Chen CY, Chang FY, Lin HC, Lee SD: Genetic polymorphisms of manganese superoxide dismutase, NAD(P)H:quinone oxidoreductase, glutathione S-transferase M1 and T1, and the susceptibility to drug-induced liver injury. J Hepatol 2007;47:128–134.
65 Sharma SK, Balamurugan A, Saha PK, Pandey RM, Mehra NK: Evaluation of clinical and immunogenetic risk factors for the development of hepatotoxicity during antituberculosis treatment. Am J Respir Crit Care Med 2002;166:916–919.

66 Fukino K, Sasaki Y, Hirai S, Nakamura T, Hashimoto M, Yamagishi F, Ueno K: Effects of N-acetyltransferase 2 (NAT2), CYP2E1 and glutathione-S-transferase (GST) genotypes on the serum concentrations of isoniazid and metabolites in tuberculosis patients. J Toxicol Sci 2008;33:187–195.
67 Kim SH, Kim SH, Bahn JW, Kim YK, Chang YS, Shin ES, Kim YS, Park JS, Kim BH, Jang IJ, Song J, Kim SH, Park HS, Min KU, Jee YK: Genetic polymorphisms of drug-metabolizing enzymes and anti-TB drug-induced hepatitis. Pharmacogenomics 2009;10:1767–1779.
68 Blumberg HM, Burman WJ, Chaisson RE, Daley CL, Etkind SC, Friedman LN, Fujiwara P, Grzemska M, Hopewell PC, Iseman MD, Jasmer RM, Koppaka V, Menzies RI, O'Brien RJ, Reves RR, Reichman LB, Simone PM, Starke JR, Vernon AA, American Thoracic Society, Centers for Disease Control and Prevention and the Infectious Diseases Society: American Thoracic Society/Centers for Disease Control and Prevention/Infectious Diseases Society of America: treatment of tuberculosis. Am J Respir Crit Care Med 2003;167:603–662.
69 Goel UC, Bajaj S, Gupta OP, Dwivedi NC, Dubey AL: Isoniazid induced neuropathy in slow versus rapid acetylators: an electrophysiological study. J Assoc Physicians India 1992;40:671–672.
70 Hiratsuka M, Kishikawa Y, Takekuma Y, Matsuura M, Narahara K, Inoue T, Hamdy SI, Endo N, Goto J, Mizugaki M: Genotyping of the N-acetyltransferase 2 polymorphism in the prediction of adverse drug reactions to isoniazid in Japanese patients. Drug Metab Pharmacokinet 2002;17:357–362.
71 Acocella G: Clinical pharmacokinetics of rifampicin. Clin Pharmacokinet 1978;3:108–127.
72 Kenny MT, Strates B: Metabolism and pharmacokinetics of the antibiotic rifampin. Drug Metab Rev 1981;12:159–218.
73 Holdiness MR: Clinical pharmacokinetics of the antituberculosis drugs. Clin.Pharmacokinet 1984;9:511–544.
74 Konig J, Seithel A, Gradhand U, Fromm MF: Pharmacogenomics of human OATP transporters. Naunyn Schmiedebergs Arch Pharmacol 2006;372:432–443.
75 Van Ingen J, Aarnoutse RE, Donald PR, Diacon AH, Dawson R, Plemper van Balen G, Gillespie SH, Boeree MJ: Why do we use 600 mg of rifampicin in tuberculosis treatment? Clin Infect Dis 2011;52:e194-e199.
76 Kimerling ME, Phillips P, Patterson P, Hall M, Robinson CA, Dunlap NE: Low serum antimycobacterial drug levels in non-HIV-infected tuberculosis patients. Chest 1998;113:1178–1183.
77 Mehta JB, Shantaveerapa H, Byrd RP Jr, Morton SE, Fountain F, Roy TM: Utility of rifampin blood levels in the treatment and follow-up of active pulmonary tuberculosis in patients who were slow to respond to routine directly observed therapy. Chest 2001;120:1520–1524.
78 Chang KC, Leung CC, Yew WW, Kam KM, Yip CW, Ma CH, Tam CM, Leung EC, Law WS, Leung WM: Peak plasma rifampicin level in tuberculosis patients with slow culture conversion. Eur J Clin Microbiol Infect Dis 2008;27:467–472.
79 Narita M, Hisada M, Thimmappa B, Stambaugh J, Ibrahim E, Hollender E, Ashkin D: Tuberculosis recurrence: multivariate analysis of serum levels of tuberculosis drugs, human immunodeficiency virus status, and other risk factors. Clin Infect Dis 2001;32:515–517.
80 Weiner M, Peloquin C, Burman W, Luo CC, Engle M, Prihoda TJ, MacKenzie WR, Bliven-Sizemore E, Johnson JL, Vernon A: Effects of tuberculosis, race, and human gene *SLCO1B1* polymorphisms on rifampin concentrations. Antimicrob Agents Chemother 2010;54:4192–4200.
81 He YJ, Zhang W, Chen Y, Guo D, Tu JH, Xu LY, Tan ZR, Chen BL, Li Z, Zhou G, Yu BN, Kirchheiner J, Zhou HH: Rifampicin alters atorvastatin plasma concentration on the basis of *SLCO1B1* 521T→C polymorphism. Clin Chim Acta 2009;405:49–52.
82 WHO: Guidelines for the programmatic management of drug-resistant tuberculosis. Emergency update 2008. 2010. www.who.int.
83 Weiner M, Burman W, Luo CC, Peloquin CA, Engle M, Goldberg S, Agarwal V, Vernon A: Effects of rifampin and multidrug resistance gene polymorphism on concentrations of moxifloxacin. Antimicrob Agents Chemother 2007;51:2861–2866.
84 Gumbo T, Louie A, Deziel MR, Parsons LM, Salfinger M, Drusano GL: Selection of a moxifloxacin dose that suppresses drug resistance in *Mycobacterium tuberculosis*, by use of an in vitro pharmacodynamic infection model and mathematical modeling. J Infect Dis 2004;190:1642–1651.
85 Almeida D, Nuermberger E, Tyagi S, Bishai WR, Grosset J: In vivo validation of the mutant selection window hypothesis with moxifloxacin in a murine model of tuberculosis. Antimicrob Agents Chemother 2007;51:4261–4266.
86 Pranger AD, van Altena R, Aarnoutse RE, van Soolingen D, Uges DR, Kosterink JG, van der Werf TS, Alffenaar JW: Evaluation of moxifloxacin for the treatment of tuberculosis: 3 years of experience. Eur Respir J 2011, E-pub ahead of print.
87 Kannankeril PJ, Roden DM: Drug-induced long QT and torsade de pointes: recent advances. Curr Opin Cardiol 2007;22:39–43.
88 Nishio Y, Makiyama T, Itoh H, Sakaguchi T, Ohno S, Gong YZ, Yamamoto S, Ozawa T, Ding WG, Toyoda F, Kawamura M, Akao M, Matsuura H, Kimura T, Kita T, Horie M: D85N, a KCNE1 polymorphism, is a disease-causing gene variant in long QT syndrome. J Am Coll Cardiol 2009;54:812–819.
89 Coyne KM, Pozniak AL, Lamorde M, Boffito M: Pharmacology of second-line antituberculosis drugs and potential for interactions with antiretroviral agents. AIDS 2009;23:437–446.
90 Butcher NJ, Ilett KF, Minchin RF: Functional polymorphism of the human arylamine N-acetyltransferase type 1 gene caused by C190T and G560A mutations. Pharmacogenetics 1998;8:67–72.
91 Hughes NC, Janezic SA, McQueen KL, Jewett MA, Castranio T, Bell DA, Grant DM: Identification and characterization of variant alleles of human acetyltransferase NAT1 with defective function using *p*-aminosalicylate as an in-vivo and in-vitro probe. Pharmacogenetics 1998;8:55–66.
92 Yew WW: Therapeutic drug monitoring in antituberculosis chemotherapy. Ther Drug Monit 1998;20:469–472.
93 Peloquin CA: Therapeutic drug monitoring in the treatment of tuberculosis. Drugs 2002;62:2169–2183.
94 Ray J, Gardiner I, Marriott D: Managing antituberculosis drug therapy by therapeutic drug monitoring of rifampicin and isoniazid. Intern Med J 2003;33:229–234.
95 Holland DP, Hamilton CD, Weintrob AC, Engemann JJ, Fortenberry ER, Peloquin CA, Stout JE: Therapeutic drug monitoring of antimycobacterial drugs in patients with both tuberculosis and advanced human immunodeficiency virus infection. Pharmacotherapy 2009;29:503–510.
96 Heysell SK, Moore JL, Keller SJ, Houpt ER: Therapeutic drug monitoring for slow response to tuberculosis treatment in a state control program, Virginia, USA. Emerg Infect Dis 2010;16:1546–1553.
97 Swen JJ, Huizinga TW, Gelderblom H, de Vries EG, Assendelft WJ, Kirchheiner J, Guchelaar HJ: Translating pharmacogenomics: challenges on the road to the clinic. PLoS Med 2007;4:e209.
98 Phillips KA, Van Bebber S: A systematic review of cost-effectiveness analyses of pharmacogenomic interventions. Pharmacogenomics 2004;5:1139–1149.
99 Baudhuin LM, Langman LJ, O'Kane DJ: Translation of pharmacogenetics into clinically relevant testing modalities. Clin Pharmacol Ther 2007;82:373–376.

Rob Aarnoutse, PharmD, PhD
Department of Pharmacy, Radboud University Nijmegen Medical Centre
PO Box 9101, Internal postal code 864
NL–6500 HB Nijmegen (The Netherlands)
Tel. +31 24 3616405, E-Mail R.Aarnoutse@akf.umcn.nl

Donald PR, van Helden PD (eds): Antituberculosis Chemotherapy.
Prog Respir Res. Basel, Karger, 2011, vol 40, pp 191–202

# Interactions between Antituberculosis and Antiretroviral Agents

Helen McIlleron[a] · Saye H. Khoo[b]

[a]Division of Clinical Pharmacology, Department of Medicine, University of Cape Town, Cape Town, South Africa;
[b]Department of Pharmacology, Institute of Translational Medicine, University of Liverpool, Liverpool, UK

**Abstract**

The potential for interactions between antituberculosis and antiretroviral regimens is considerable. This review focuses on the pharmacokinetics, safety and effectiveness of combined antituberculosis treatment and antiretroviral therapy, particularly in settings with high tuberculosis and HIV burdens. Efavirenz plus 2 nucleoside reverse-transcriptase inhibitors is compatible with rifampicin-based short-course antituberculosis treatment; standard twice daily doses of nevirapine provide an acceptable alternative for adults with contraindications to efavirenz. However, combination regimens that are safe, effective and feasible to implement have yet to be defined for patients requiring second-line antiretroviral regimens, and for young children. Overlapping toxicities threaten adherence, may lead to treatment interruption and are a particular concern in HIV-infected patients treated with the poorly tolerated second-line regimens for drug-resistant tuberculosis. An expanded formulary of suitable drug regimens and formulations is needed for adults and children in settings where tuberculosis and HIV are prevalent.

Copyright © 2011 S. Karger AG, Basel

Tuberculosis is the commonest cause of death amongst people infected with HIV. An estimated 1.4 million HIV-infected persons developed tuberculosis in 2008, the vast majority in Africa (78%) and South-East Asia (13%); 0.5 million patients with HIV-associated tuberculosis died in the same year [1]. In high-burden countries, up to 60% of tuberculosis patients have HIV co-infection and in some settings more than 30% of patients commencing antiretroviral therapy (ART) have tuberculosis [2]. The early introduction of effective ART amongst patients with advanced immunosuppression who present with HIV-associated tuberculosis results in an enormous improvement in survival [3]. Such patients should commence ART as soon as possible after starting antituberculosis treatment [4, 5]. However, combined therapy is complicated by drug-drug interactions, overlapping toxicity, a very high pill burden and development of the immune reconstitution inflammatory syndrome. These complications threaten the durability of regimens due to reduced efficacy or treatment-limiting side effects. Most evidence regarding the risks and benefits of combined treatment arises from studies amongst patients with relatively advanced immunosuppression presenting with tuberculosis and started on standard short-course chemotherapy for tuberculosis (SCC; rifampicin and isoniazid for 6 months with pyrazinamide and ethambutol for the first 2 months) before ART comprising efavirenz or nevirapine with 2 nucleoside reverse-transcriptase inhibitors (NRTIs). Adherence and tolerability in patients with well-preserved immunity need further evaluation. In high-burden settings the risk of incident tuberculosis in patients established on ART remains high in those with less than 500 CD4+ lymphocytes/$mm^3$ [6]. As antiretroviral programmes mature and patients move onto second-line regimens, a steep increase in the use of protease inhibitors (PIs) is anticipated. The interactions between PIs and the rifamycins are more extensive and require dose adjustments. There is a critical need for evidence to inform optimal treatment, dosing and monitoring strategies for tuberculosis patients requiring PI-based regimens. Studies are urgently required to inform treatment approaches for young children with HIV-associated tuberculosis, and suitable formulations need to be developed. ART improves survival amongst HIV-infected patients with drug-resistant tuberculosis [7] and should be introduced at an early stage.

However, treatment-limiting side effects are common amongst HIV-infected and uninfected patients treated with second-line antituberculosis drugs. Standardized monitoring and reporting of adverse events, drug exposures and other factors predisposing to toxicity are necessary to ascertain the tolerability of different drug combinations. The provision of combined antituberculosis therapy and ART is particularly challenging in high-burden settings where there is a tendency to rely on standardized therapy and the use of fixed-dose combination products, where drug formularies are frequently restricted, and there is usually limited access to laboratory-based monitoring. Thus, health care services are often not equipped to provide complex individualized care. Compatible regimens that have enduring efficacy and are well tolerated are required.

## Pharmacokinetic Interactions

Rifampicin, a key component of SCC, is a potent activator of the pregnane X receptor (PXR). PXR is a nuclear receptor regulating transcription of multiple drug-metabolizing enzymes including phase I enzymes such as cytochrome P450 (CYP) 2B6, 2B9, 2C8, 2C9, 3A4 and 3A7, phase II enzymes such as the glutathione-S-transferases, UDP glucuronosyltransferases (UGTs) and sulphotransferases and transporters such as P-glycoprotein, multidrug resistance protein 2, multidrug resistance-associated protein 2 and the organic anion transporter polypeptide 2 [8]. Hence rifampicin reduces the concentrations of many concomitantly administered drug substrates including the non-nucleoside reverse-transcriptase inhibitors (NNRTIs) metabolized by CYP2B6 and CYP3A4, PIs and maraviroc which are substrates of P-glycoprotein and CYP3A4, and raltegavir, a UGT1A1 substrate. Induction of the activity of these enzymes and transporters takes several days to weeks to reach a maximum and declines gradually after exposure to the activator has ceased. Rifapentine is thought to be a less potent activator of PXR than rifampicin but data quantifying its impact on concentrations of concomitantly administered antiretroviral agents are lacking. Rifabutin does not reduce the concentrations of NNRTIs or ritonavir-boosted PIs; however, the rifabutin dose needs adjustment when given with PIs or efavirenz [9]. Peptide mimetic PIs including ritonavir are moderate activators of PXR; efavirenz and nevirapine also induce expression of CYP3A4 and 2B6, largely via activation of the constitutive androstane receptor.

Ritonavir is a promiscuous mechanism-based inhibitor. It potently inhibits CYP3A4 and P-glycoprotein and is used in low doses to boost concentrations of PIs. Higher doses of ritonavir counteract the effect of rifampicin on P-glycoprotein and CYP3A4. This approach has been used to maintain saquinavir and lopinavir concentrations during rifampicin therapy but is associated with hepatotoxicity. Antituberculosis drugs known to inhibit drug-metabolizing enzymes include isoniazid (CYP1A2, 2A6, 2C19 and 3A4), clarithromycin (P-glycoprotein and CYP3A) and clofazamine (a weak CYP450 enzyme inhibitor). Inhibition reactions are rapid in onset and last hours to days depending on the half-lives of the inhibitor and target protein, and the affinity between them.

Dietary, environmental and genetic factors affect the intrinsic activity of metabolizing enzymes, transporters and their transcriptional regulators [8] and thus contribute to considerable variability in the magnitude of changes in drug concentrations due to induction or inhibition interactions. In addition to regulating intestinal absorption and clearance via the liver and kidneys, transmembrane drug transporters control concentrations of substrates within cells and across cellular barriers. Hence, induction of efflux transporters such as P-glycoprotein by rifampicin potentially further reduces concentrations of substrates such as PIs in crucial sites including the brain, testes and lymphocytes. Drug-drug interaction mechanisms other than those mediated by metabolic enzymes or transporters can be important. Magnesium, aluminium and iron cations tend to bind to fluoroquinolones, thus preventing absorption. Therefore the administration of fluoroquinolones should be separated from buffered drugs such as didanosine. Similarly, zidovudine concentrations are reduced when it is administered at the same time as clarithromycin. Many potential pharmacokinetic interactions between antituberculosis and antiretroviral drugs have not been evaluated. The metabolic pathways of some of the drugs are incompletely described; hence, unanticipated interactions might occur. Moreover the clinical relevance of drug interactions needs to be established in studies evaluating efficacy and safety. Table 1 summarizes pharmacokinetic interactions described between antituberculosis drugs and antiretroviral agents.

## Antituberculosis Drug Concentrations in Patients Infected with the Human Immunodeficiency Virus

Antituberculosis drug concentrations vary widely between patients and study populations. Reductions in the bioavailability of rifampicin of 32–50% have been ascribed to HIV infection [10–12]. Pyrazinamide and ethambutol

**Table 1.** Selected pharmacokinetic interactions involving antituberculosis drugs in patients with HIV-associated tuberculosis

| | |
|---|---|
| Rifampicin | Poorly defined disposition pathways: a substrate of microsomal β-esterases, PGP, OATP1B1; potent PXR-mediated action on CYP2B6, 2B9, 2C8, 2C9, 3A4, 3A7, GSTs, UGTs, SULTs, PGP, MDR2, OATP2, MRP2, and likely other enzymes and transporters to be defined; reduces trough concentrations of ritonavir-boosted PIs >90%; reduces exposure to NNRTIs (delavirdine > nevirapine > efavirenz), abacavir, zidovudine, maraviroc (60–70%), raltegravir (40%), linezolid (32%), moxifloxacin (approx. 30%) and rifampicin itself |
| Rifapentine | Like rifampicin, primarily metabolized by esterases and undergoes auto-induction; it has similar but less potent pharmacokinetic interactions compared to those of rifampicin; induces CYP3A4 and CYP2C8/9 |
| Rifabutin | Undergoes auto-induction but does not reduce PI concentrations; exposure is increased by inhibitors such as PIs (approx. 4-fold increase with ritonavir-boosted PIs, and even greater increases in the active metabolite 25-O-desacetylrifabutin) and clarithromycin |
| Isoniazid | Metabolized in the liver and intestine primarily by acetylation (NAT2 substrate) and dehydrazination; inhibits CYP1A2, 2A6, 2C19, 3A4 and MAO; induces CYP2E1 |
| Ethionamide | Undergoes extensive intestinal and hepatic metabolism by enzymes including FMOs; potential interactions have not been characterized |
| Fluoroquinolones | Absorption is reduced by $Mg^{2+}$, $Al^{3+}$ and $Fe^{2+}$ ions; hence, administration of buffered didanosine and antacids should be separated by several hours; moxifloxacin and sparfloxacin are UGT substrates: exposure may be increased with inhibitors such as atazanavir and lopinavir |
| Linezolid | PGP substrate, MAO inhibitor; concentrations increased by clarithromycin and reduced by rifampicin |
| Clarithromycin | Substrate and potent inhibitor of CYP3A4 and PGP; concentrations increased by ritonavir, other PIs (including atazanavir, darunavir and lopinavir) and delavirdine; a reduced dose of maraviroc is advised; efavirenz, nevirapine and etravirine reduce clarithromycin concentrations while increasing its 14-hydroxy metabolite, which is associated with rashes, and combination should be avoided, zidovudine reduces absorption |
| Clofazimine | Weak inhibitor of CYP3A4 |
| PAS | Reduces absorption of digoxin and vitamin $B_{12}$ |
| Trimethoprim/ sulphamethoxazole | Reduces clearance of lamivudine and potentially other NRTIs such as stavudine and zidovudine |

PGP = P-glycoprotein; OATP = organic anion transporter polypeptide; GSTs = glutathione-S-transferases; SULTs = sulphotransferases; MDR = multidrug resistance protein; MRP = multidrug resistance-associated protein; NAT2 = N-acetyltransferase; MAO = mono-amine oxidase; FMO = flavin-containing mono-oxygenase; PAS = para-aminosalicylic acid.

concentrations may also be reduced amongst patients with HIV infection compared to those without HIV. Similar trends have been described for isoniazid in association with diarrhoea. Should these findings be confirmed, higher doses of the antituberculosis drugs should be considered amongst HIV infected patients who have an increased risk of relapse, notably when less robust regimens are used, treatment duration is shorter or dosing intermittent. There is concern that patients with advanced HIV infection may have more extensive malabsorption of antituberculosis drugs due to HIV-associated enteropathy and increased susceptibility to enteric infections, and that reduced antituberculosis drug exposure amongst these patients might contribute to their increased risk of tuberculosis recurrence and acquisition of drug resistance [13, 14]. Reassuringly, a recent study amongst patients with HIV-associated tuberculosis (CD4+ lymphocyte count 12–500/$mm^3$) found that the level of immunosuppression and concomitant ART (including efavirenz, zidovudine and lamivudine) had minimal impact on concentrations of the first-line antituberculosis drugs, although patients with very low CD4+ lymphocyte counts (<50/$mm^3$) were not well represented [15]. Other factors such as weight, dose per kilogram of body weight, sex, nutrition, formulation and genetic polymorphisms have been associated with altered concentrations of the first-line antituberculosis drug concentrations in patients. Population-modelling methods pooling data across different populations could provide an improved basis for understanding the contributions of various factors to pharmacokinetic variability.

### Pharmacokinetics in Children

Young children are prone to severe forms of tuberculosis and rapid progression to active disease; they should therefore receive regimens at least as effective as those used in adults. However, a growing body of evidence indicates that current international dosing recommendations result in the systematic underdosing of antituberculosis drugs in children. Any additional effect of HIV infection on antituberculosis drug concentrations in children has not been adequately evaluated. Moreover, there is very limited information about the pharmacokinetics of antituberculosis drugs and many of the antiretroviral drugs in neonates and infants who experience rapid changes in enzyme maturation, growth and development. Administration of accurate doses in young children is complicated by a paucity of suitable drug formulations. Very few studies have evaluated the pharmacokinetic interactions, safety and efficacy of combined antituberculosis and ART regimens in children. Greater reductions in nevirapine concentrations were shown amongst young children (median age 1.6 years) during tuberculosis treatment compared to the reductions reported in adults [16], and whilst doubling the standard dose of lopinavir/ritonavir (LPV/r) overcame the induction of rifampicin amongst adult HIV-infected and uninfected volunteers without tuberculosis [17, 18], this approach was not successful amongst young children (median age 1.25 years) during SCC [19]. Hence the findings of studies conducted in adults should not be assumed to apply to children in whom additional studies are required.

### Toxicity

Toxicity profiles of antituberculosis drugs and antiretroviral agents overlap considerably (table 2). HIV-infected patients receiving SCC regimens commonly experience peripheral neuropathy, rash and gastrointestinal events, and frequently have raised transaminases. Few studies in patients with HIV-associated tuberculosis have included a detailed comparison of safety end points in those starting ART during tuberculosis treatment versus those with ART deferred until after antituberculosis treatment. Interestingly, rashes may be more frequent amongst patients not receiving concomitant efavirenz or nevirapine with 2 NRTIs [20]. NNRTI-based ART is generally well tolerated in patients under antituberculosis treatment in comparison to people without tuberculosis. However, the impact of overlapping toxicity and high pill burdens on treatment adherence are insufficiently characterized for patients with well-preserved immunity and in operational settings. Ongoing controlled studies in patients with less advanced immunosuppression will shed more light on the risks attributable to the addition of antiretroviral agents.

Hepatotoxicity is a serious complication of antituberculosis regimens containing rifampicin, isoniazid and pyrazinamide. There is inconsistent evidence about the added risk of hepatitis due to antituberculosis treatment amongst patients started on ART. Amongst South Africans and Indians under efavirenz-based ART, the hepatitis risk was increased severalfold in patients treated for tuberculosis [21, 22]. Similarly, a study in Botswana found that patients under efavirenz- or nevirapine-based ART with antituberculosis therapy had a rate of hepatitis about 3 times that in patients under ART alone [23]. However, these findings could be due to confounding by underlying risk factors such as chronic viral hepatitis, as other studies have found a similar tolerability of NNRTI-based regimens with and without antituberculosis therapy [24–26]. The use of adjusted doses of the PIs with rifampicin-containing regimens is limited by concerns about hepatotoxicity. Hepatotoxicity resulted in the termination of 3 studies investigating adjusted doses of ritonavir-boosted lopinavir, saquinavir and atazanavir in healthy subjects pre-induced with rifampicin [27–29]. Although evidence of safety in the relevant patient populations is inadequate, serious hepatotoxicity seems less frequent in patients (grade 3 and 4 elevations of approximately 15 and 25% in children and adults, respectively) [30–32]. Nonetheless, limited evidence suggests that nausea and vomiting results in high rates of treatment discontinuation amongst adults treated with adjusted doses of lopinavir or saquinavir with ritonavir during SCC [30, 31]. The hepatotoxicity risk appears lower when treatment with PIs precedes the introduction of rifampicin [17, 18, 27]. It has been hypothesized that pre-induction of the liver enzymes by rifampicin leads to increased formation of a toxic intermediate metabolite when PIs are introduced [29].

Isoniazid-induced neuropathy is related to pyridoxine depletion and associated with age, slow acetylator type, isoniazid dose and treatment duration. Peripheral neuropathy is common amongst HIV-infected patients given antuberculosis treatment: prophylactic pyridoxine supplementation

**Table 2.** Overlapping syndromes and combined toxicity

| | |
|---|---|
| Febrile, generally unwell | IRIS, paradoxical IRIS, MDR-TB |
| Rash | Isoniazid, pyrazinamide, rifampicin, PAS, abacavir, nevirapine, efavirenz, stavudine, others, HIV; thiacetazone is contraindicated in HIV-infected patients due to severe reactions |
| Hepatotoxicity | Isoniazid, ethionamide, prothionamide, rifampicin, pyrazinamide, thiacetazone, nevirapine, efavirenz, ritonavir and other PIs, NRTIs, paradoxical IRIS, hepatitis virus 'flares'; rarely: fluoroquinolones, PAS |
| Neuropathy | Isoniazid, linezolid, ethionamide, cycloserine, terizidone, stavudine, didanosine, zalcitabine, HIV |
| Eye problems | Ethambutol, rifabutin, linezolid, ethionamide, prothionamide, didanosine |
| CNS | Efavirenz, cycloserine, terizidone, ethionamide, prothionamide, isoniazid |
| QT interval prolongation | Lopinavir, atazanavir, moxifloxacin, gatifloxacin, levofloxacin, clarithromycin |
| Arthropathies/arthralgia | Pyrazinamide, fluoroquinolones, PAS, HIV |
| Gastrointestinal disturbance/ abdominal pain | Ethionamide, prothionamide, PAS, clofazimine, isoniazid, ethambutol, pyrazinamide, ritonavir, stavudine, nevirapine, others |
| Pancreatitis | Stavudine, didanosine, zalcitabine, linezolid |
| Lactic acidosis | Stavudine, didanosine, zidovudine, linezolid |
| Renal impairment, electrolyte disturbance | Aminoglycosides, capreomycin, tenofovir, HIV |
| Haematological abnormalities | Linezolid, rifabutin, rifampicin, isoniazid, zidovudine, trimethoprim/sulphamethoxazole, HIV, tuberculosis |
| Hypothyroidism | Ethionamide, prothionamide, PAS, stavudine, HIV |
| Dysglycaemia | Protease inhibitors, fluoroquinolones, ethionamide, prothionamide, isoniazid |

IRIS = Immune reconstitution inflammatory syndrome; MDR-TB = multidrug-resistant tuberculosis; PAS = para-aminosalicylic acid.

should be used. Stavudine continues to play a critical role in the scaling up of ART in resource-limited settings, but in combination with isoniazid as part of SCC is associated with particularly high rates of peripheral neuropathy. Stavudine-sparing regimens should be considered in patients with concurrent or prior tuberculosis treatment due to a heightened risk of peripheral neuropathy when commencing stavudine-containing ART [33, 34].

There is a rapid expansion of access to second-line antituberculosis drugs for treatment of drug-resistant tuberculosis. These regimens are poorly tolerated, and in many instances patients may be predisposed to adverse effects due to long-standing illness, nutritional depletion and comorbid conditions. Amongst patients treated for multidrug-resistant tuberculosis, 23–56% require permanent discontinuation of a second-line agent [35–38]. Given high mortality rates among patients with resistant tuberculosis and HIV co-infection, early initiation of ART is recommended to prevent early mortality. Antiretroviral drugs share many of the adverse effects associated with second-line antituberculosis drugs (table 2); however, there are scant data evaluating the risks of combined regimens. High rates of neuropathy, hypokalaemia, hypothyroidism and marked renal impairment have been reported in cohorts with multidrug-resistant tuberculosis and a high proportion of HIV-infected patients [39, 40]. Poor clinical status and malnutrition are common amongst patients with HIV-associated and drug-resistant tuberculosis in resource-poor settings, and there is an urgent need for evidence to guide optimal drug combinations in these populations.

Large prospective studies are needed to characterize the risks attributable to first- and second-line antituberculosis and antiretroviral drug combinations as well as potential confounding factors such as the extent of immunosuppression, comorbid diseases such as chronic viral hepatitis and diabetes, concomitant medication or toxins and nutritional status.

## First-Line Antiretroviral Therapy Regimens

Efavirenz is metabolized almost exclusively by CYP2B6. A wide range of efavirenz concentrations is observed between patients receiving standard doses. Much of the variability is explained by genetic polymorphisms encoding CYP2B6, but dose, weight and sex also play a role [41–44]. In keeping with induction of CYP2B6 by rifampicin, a retrospective analysis of a therapeutic drug-monitoring database found efavirenz concentrations reduced by 35% in patients concomitantly prescribed rifampicin [44]. However, studies in Spanish, South African, Indian and Thai patients have not found reduced efavirenz concentrations during SCC [45–49]. Although some clinicians recommend increasing the dose of efavirenz from 600 to 800 mg in patients weighing >60 kg [9], similar concentrations were reported in patients randomized to a 600- or 800-mg dose during antituberculosis treatment [50]. Moreover, excellent virological, immunological and clinical responses are reported in patients treated concomitantly with standard doses of efavirenz- and rifampicin-containing regimens in comparison to patients without tuberculosis [21, 24, 51]. Intriguingly, interindividual variability in efavirenz concentrations tends to be increased during antituberculosis treatment; contrary to expectation, patients with high (>4 mg/l) concentrations of efavirenz during SCC tend to have reduced concentrations on cessation of the rifampicin-containing regimen [47, 49, 52]. Conceivably, inhibition of accessory metabolic pathways by SCC might account for this phenomenon. Indeed, in vitro studies show that isoniazid inhibits CYP2A6 which has a critical role in limiting drug accumulation in individuals characterized as CYP2B6 slow metabolizers [53]. Since the G516T polymorphism which is associated with reduced CYP2B6 activity is more prevalent in people of African or Asian origin, such an interaction would be more frequent in these regions where the tuberculosis and HIV burdens are greatest. The clinical implications of this finding should be investigated since high efavirenz concentrations are associated with central nervous system side effects, and tolerability might be reduced amongst slow metabolizers prescribed isoniazid-containing regimens for the prevention or treatment of tuberculosis.

CYP2B6 contributes to nevirapine metabolism, but CYP3A4 is the predominant metabolic pathway. An in vitro experiment found that the expression of CYP3A4 mRNA was increased approximately 6-fold more than CYP2B6 mRNA in primary human hepatocytes exposed to rifampicin [54]. Accordingly, nevirapine concentrations are more markedly reduced than efavirenz during SCC. Reductions in trough concentrations of 7–40% are reported in tuberculosis patients established on maintenance doses of nevirapine, such that 14–40% of patients have trough concentrations <3 mg/l (the lower limit of the target range [55]) during antituberculosis treatment [26, 56–59]. The proportion of patients with low nevirapine concentrations varies considerably between different studies with fewer low concentrations reported from Malawi, Mozambique and Thailand than from Burkina Faso and South Africa. Increasing the dose of nevirapine by 50% would overcome the effect of rifampicin [60, 61]; however, the safety of this approach is a concern [62] and needs further evaluation. Studies in Thailand and Botswana evaluating patients treated with nevirapine-based ART have not found a difference in virological or immunological outcomes between those with and without concomitant SCC [23, 26]. Neither were virological or immunological outcomes different in Thai patients randomized to start efavirenz- or nevirapine-based ART during SCC [51]. However, analysis of a large South African cohort found that nevirapine-based ART was associated with a higher risk of virological failure in patients concomitantly treated with SCC compared to patients without tuberculosis, and compared to patients, with or without tuberculosis, treated with efavirenz [24]. Nonetheless, as more than 80% of patients treated for tuberculosis during nevirapine-based ART achieved viral suppression at 6 months, nevirapine provides an acceptable alternative first-line regimen for patients in whom efavirenz cannot be used. Interestingly, patients established on full doses of nevirapine before initiation of SCC were not more likely to have virological failure than those without tuberculosis. This suggests that, in patients started on SCC first, subtherapeutic concentrations of nevirapine during the14-day period of lead-in dosing may contribute to the increased risk of failure. Hence it may be prudent to omit lead-in dosing in patients established on rifampicin when ART is introduced as the majority of patients have subtherapeutic nevirapine concentrations during the 14-day lead-in phase when nevirapine 200 mg is given just once a day [62–64]. In contrast to a small study in Thailand [62], preliminary results from the CARINEMO study in Mozambique suggest that this approach is well tolerated [65].

## Second-Line Antiretroviral Therapy Regimens

Rifampicin reduces systemic exposure to ritonavir-boosted PIs by more than 75%, and adjusting the doses of PIs to overcome the effect of rifampicin is associated with concerns of serious toxicity. Hence, CDC guidelines state that rifampicin should not be co-administered with PIs and that rifabutin should be used [9]. However, ritonavir-boosted PIs increase exposure to rifabutin by approximately 4-fold and cause even greater increases in plasma concentrations of the active metabolite 25-O-desacetylrifabutin. Rifabutin doses need to be reduced accordingly, but a safe, effective dose in combination with PIs has not been defined: rifabutin 150 mg thrice weekly in combination with LPV/r-based ART may result in insufficient rifabutin concentrations [66, 67]; case reports raise concern that rifamycin resistance is readily acquired in patients with severe immunosuppression and low rifabutin concentrations [66, 68], as has been found with twice weekly doses [69]; on the other hand higher doses might increase toxicity [70, 71] including neutropenia, leucopenia, elevations of hepatic enzymes, rash, gastrointestinal symptoms and uveitis. Toxicity may be a greater hazard in resource-limited or overburdened health care systems where individualized monitoring is limited. Rifabutin use is further complicated by a lack of suitable formulations: a once daily dose that could be incorporated in a fixed-dose combination would be easier to implement in tuberculosis control programmes, and formulations suitable for children are not available. Although access is improving, rifabutin is not currently available in many countries. SCC and PI-based ART (usually with LPV/r) are frequently the only effective regimens available to treat patients with tuberculosis who have failed NNRTI-based regimens. Rifampicin reduces trough concentrations of lopinavir by more than 90% when LPV/r is administered in standard doses [17]. Adding extra ritonavir to LPV/r ('superboosted' lopinavir; lopinavir/ritonavir ratio = 1:1), or doubling the dose of LPV/r achieves adequate lopinavir concentrations in adults given concomitant rifampicin [17, 18]. There are inadequate data about treatment outcomes associated with these approaches and, as outlined above, tolerability is an important concern. Patients should be monitored closely and, if available, therapeutic drug concentration monitoring should be performed as lopinavir concentrations are highly variable. There is an urgent need for safe and effective approaches that are suited to high-burden settings to treat the expanding number of patients who are failing first-line ART regimens or established on second-line regimens when they develop tuberculosis. Studies evaluating the pharmacokinetic interactions, safety and efficacy of currently available approaches and alternative approaches are obligatory.

## Alternative Regimens

Triple nucleoside regimens are less potent than NNRTI- or PI-based regimens [72]. Few studies have evaluated triple nucleoside regimens in tuberculosis patients [73, 74]. However, in spite of the potential for rifampicin to reduce zidovudine and abacavir concentrations by induction of UGTs, a small study found that 76% of Ugandan tuberculosis patients with CD4+ lymphocyte counts >350/mm$^3$ who were started on ART comprising abacavir, lamivudine and zidovudine achieved virological suppression (HIV RNA <50 copies/ml) after 24 weeks [73]. A subsequent study in Tanzania described satisfactory virological responses amongst patients starting the same regimen 2 or 8 weeks after commencing SCC for pulmonary tuberculosis (90% were suppressed to <400 copies/ml and 61% to <50 copies/ml 48 weeks after starting ART) [74]. Hence triple nucleoside regimens may provide an acceptable alternative regimen for patients who have not failed an ART regimen and in whom efavirenz is not recommended; however, the results should be confirmed in larger controlled studies.

The roles of newer antiretroviral drugs such as integrase inhibitors and CCR5 antagonists in antiretroviral treatment programmes of high-burden countries are unclear, and current pricing precludes their use in resource-limited settings. Rifampicin reduces systemic exposure to raltegravir and maraviroc by approximately 40 and 60%, respectively, and increased doses are recommended. As reported clinical experience of these combinations is limited, patients should be carefully monitored. Doubled doses of raltegravir with rifampicin were generally well tolerated in 14 healthy subjects and in 2 patients during antituberculosis treatment [75, 76]. Much hope for improved antituberculosis treatments is invested in several agents currently in development which have shown promise of excellent sterilizing activity. Hence potent rifamycin-sparing regimens might be available in the future, conceivably providing effective antituberculosis treatment that is more compatible with a range of antiretroviral agents. Certainly there is an urgent need for such regimens particularly for patients requiring second-line ART.

## Regimens for Children

ART options are limited for young children with HIV-associated tuberculosis, especially those under 3 years of age in whom efavirenz cannot be used. Rifabutin is not suitably formulated for children and data guiding dosing are lacking. Although guidelines recommend triple NRTI regimens in under 2-year-olds with tuberculosis previously exposed to nevirapine [77], triple NRTI regimens are associated with high rates of NRTI mutations and virological failure in children [78, 79]. Consequently, only 2 ART regimens are available: an NNRTI or a boosted PI, typically LPV/r, given with 2 NRTIs.

In children older than 3 years, efavirenz and 2 NRTIs are preferred during antituberculosis treatment [77]. Like adults, children display wide interindividual variation of efavirenz concentrations [80, 81]. Using recommended doses, younger children are at an increased risk of low concentrations although limited data are available for infants [80–83]. Few studies have evaluated efavirenz concentrations amongst children during antituberculosis therapy. Fifteen South African children (median age 6.3 years) with tuberculosis [47] had similar efavirenz concentrations during versus after SCC with 9 (60%) and 8 (53%), respectively, having a predicted trough concentration <1 mg/l (the lower limit of the recommended target range [55]). Thus, concomitant rifampicin-based antitubercular treatment does not appear to be an important predictor of underexposure to efavirenz in children; however, larger studies are needed. Given the lack of suitable ART alternatives for children with concurrent tuberculosis, optimization of efavirenz doses in young children should be investigated.

In many resource-limited settings, relatively expensive drugs like efavirenz, PIs and abacavir are not available. Worldwide there are still large numbers of children with tuberculosis who can only access ART comprising nevirapine with 2 NRTIs. There are scant data describing the impact of rifampicin-containing antituberculosis treatment on nevirapine pharmacokinetics in children. Eight Thai children, with a median age of 9.7 years, who were dosed according to the WHO simplified weight band-based guidelines with a median 171 $mg/m^2$/dose, had median nevirapine trough concentrations of 6.48 mg/l (range: 3.03–13.66) [84]. In contrast, 11 of 21 (52%) young Zambian children (median age 1.55 years), dosed according to the same guidelines (median 177 $mg/m^2$/dose) [16], had trough nevirapine concentrations <3 mg/l (the lower limit of the target range [55]). The median trough concentration was half that of children from the same population with similar weights and ages, but without tuberculosis. The high proportion of children with low nevirapine concentrations was not anticipated since nevirapine concentrations in children dosed according to the WHO simplified weight-based guidelines are generally higher than those in adults [85]. Thus, there is concern that nevirapine concentrations may be disproportionately reduced in young children during SCC compared to their adult counterparts and it is imperative to establish the pharmacokinetics of nevirapine amongst children receiving rifampin based antituberculosis treatment across a range of ages and in different population groups.

The use of NNRTIs for the prevention of mother-to-child transmission further complicate tuberculosis and HIV treatment in children as prevention of mother-to-child transmission regimens result in a high prevalence of NNRTI resistance mutations in infected infants [86, 87]. The preferred first-line ART regimen for infants with prior exposure to NNRTIs is LPV/r with 2 NRTIs [77]. Hence the use of LPV/r in children is expanding in many settings. Acceptable concentrations of lopinavir were achieved in >85% of children during SCC, when extra ritonavir was added to standard doses of LPV/r [88]. However, implementation of 'superboosted' lopinavir is impractical as it is complex to administer, ritonavir solution has a short shelf life (up to 30 days at <25°C) resulting in frequent stock-outs at clinics, and provision of lopinavir and ritonavir separately further complicates the logistics of correct ART provision to clinics. Contrary to the findings in adults, double doses of coformulated LPV/r resulted in inadequate lopinavir concentrations in young children treated concurrently with SCC [19]. A recently reported retrospective South African study provides compelling evidence that these pharmacokinetic findings influence outcomes: the proportion of children achieving viral suppression at 6 months was lower in children given double doses of LPV/r during SCC for tuberculosis compared to controls without tuberculosis on standard doses of LPV/r, whereas children with tuberculosis on superboosted lopinavir regimens achieved similar virological outcomes compared to controls. A population pharmacokinetic model estimating the doses of coformulated LPV/r required to maintain lopinavir concentrations >1 mg/l in at least 95% of children predicted that smaller children (weighing 4–6 kg) would require 50 mg/kg of lopinavir in LPV/r (more than 4 times the standard dose of LPV/r) to achieve the target using 12-hourly doses. However, more feasible doses were predicted with an 8-hourly dosing schedule: respective lopinavir doses of 25, 22, 21 and 18 mg/kg to achieve the target in children weighing 4–6, 6–8, 8–12 and 12–18 kg [89]. This approach has yet to be validated ex silico; moreover, safety of rifampicin with LPV/r in relatively high doses is a concern.

## Conclusions

ART enormously improves survival amongst patients with HIV-associated tuberculosis. NNRTI-based ART provides excellent virological outcomes and is well tolerated amongst tuberculosis patients with CD4+ lymphocyte counts <350 cells/$mm^3$. There is an obligation to research and institute effective and safe combined treatment approaches for tuberculosis patients failing NNRTI-based ART regimens, those on PI-containing regimens who develop incident tuberculosis, and for young children with tuberculosis. Ensuring optimal efficacy and safety of regimens is particularly critical as treatment options for both tuberculosis and HIV are restricted, and individualized monitoring is limited. A wider formulary of drugs is needed in resource-limited settings to combine the most effective treatment regimens and avoid drug toxicities. Recent guidelines recommending that all HIV-infected patients with tuberculosis should be started on ART provide a considerable challenge to health care systems in resource-constrained settings. Suitable formulations are required to simplify drug supply, dispensing and administration within the HIV and tuberculosis control programmes, and child-friendly formulations that are palatable and do not require refrigeration are essential. Lastly, emerging antituberculosis agents offer hope for potent antituberculosis regimens compatible with a wide range of antiretroviral agents, and it is imperative that such regimens are evaluated in children at an early stage.

## Acknowledgements

H.M. received partial support from the European and Developing Countries Clinical Trials Partnership and training through grants from the Fogarty International Center (U2RTW007370/3 and 5U2RTW007373).

## References


1 Global tuberculosis control: a short update to the 2009 report. World Health Organization, 2009, WHO/HTM/TB/2009.426.
2 Lawn SD, Kranzer K, Edwards DJ, McNally M, Bekker LG, Wood R: Tuberculosis during the first year of antiretroviral therapy in a South African cohort using an intensive pretreatment screening strategy. AIDS 2010;24:1323–1328.
3 Manosuthi W, Chottanapand S, Thongyen S, Chaovavanich A, Sungkanuparph S: Survival rate and risk factors of mortality among HIV/tuberculosis-coinfected patients with and without antiretroviral therapy. J Acquir Immune Defic Syndr 2006;43:42–46.
4 Blanc F, Sok T, Laureillard D, Borand L, Rekacewicz C, Nerrienet E, Madec Y, Marcy O, Chan S, Prak N, et al: Significant enhancement in survival with early (2 weeks) vs late (8 weeks) initiation of highly active antiretroviral treatment (HAART) in severely immunosuppressed HIV-infected adults with newly diagnosed tuberculosis (abstract THLBB106). 18th Int AIDS Conf, Vienna, July 2010.
5 Antiretroviral therapy for HIV infection in adults and adolescents: recommendations for a public health approach. 2010 revision. Geneva, World Health Organization, 2010.
6 Lawn SD, Myer L, Edwards D, Bekker LG, Wood R: Short-term and long-term risk of tuberculosis associated with CD4 cell recovery during antiretroviral therapy in South Africa. AIDS 2009;23:1717–1725.
7 Dheda K, Shean K, Zumla A, Badri M, Streicher EM, Page-Shipp L, Willcox P, John MA, Reubenson G, Govindasamy D, et al: Early treatment outcomes and HIV status of patients with extensively drug-resistant tuberculosis in South Africa: a retrospective cohort study. Lancet 2010;375:1798–1807.
8 Zhang B, Xie W, Krasowski MD: PXR: a xenobiotic receptor of diverse function implicated in pharmacogenetics. Pharmacogenomics 2008;9:1695–1709.
9 Panel on Antiretroviral Guidelines for Adults and Adolescents: Guidelines for the use of antiretroviral agents in HIV-1-infected adults and adolescents. Department of Health and Human Services, December 1, 2009, pp 1–161. http://wwwaidsinfonihgov/ContentFiles/AdultandAdolescentGLpdf (accessed November 7, 2010).
10 McIlleron H, Wash P, Burger A, Norman J, Folb PI, Smith P: Determinants of rifampin, isoniazid, pyrazinamide, and ethambutol pharmacokinetics in a cohort of tuberculosis patients. Antimicrob Agents Chemother 2006;50:1170–1177.
11 Gurumurthy P, Ramachandran G, Hemanth Kumar AK, Rajasekaran S, Padmapriyadarsini C, Swaminathan S, Bhagavathy S, Venkatesan P, Sekar L, Mahilmaran A, et al: Decreased bioavailability of rifampin and other antituberculosis drugs in patients with advanced human immunodeficiency virus disease. Antimicrob Agents Chemother 2004;48:4473–4475.
12 Sahai J, Gallicano K, Swick L, Tailor S, Garber G, Seguin I, Oliveras L, Walker S, Rachlis A, Cameron DW: Reduced plasma concentrations of antituberculosis drugs in patients with HIV infection. Ann Intern Med 1997;127:289–293.
13 Vernon A, Burman W, Benator D, Khan A, Bozeman L: Acquired rifamycin monoresistance in patients with HIV-related tuberculosis treated with once-weekly rifapentine and isoniazid. Tuberculosis Trials Consortium. Lancet 1999;353:1843–1847.
14 Nettles RE, Mazo D, Alwood K, Gachuhi R, Maltas G, Wendel K, Cronin W, Hooper N, Bishai W, Sterling TR: Risk factors for relapse and acquired rifamycin resistance after directly observed tuberculosis treatment: a comparison by HIV serostatus and rifamycin use. Clin Infect Dis 2004;38:731–736.
15 McIlleron H, Rustomjee R, Vahedi M, Mthiyane T, Denti P, Connolly C, Rida W, Pym A, Smith P, Onyebujoh PC: Weight and sex are important determinants of antituberculosis drug concentrations in patients with HIV associated tuberculosis (abstract O_10). 3rd Int Workshop Clin Pharmacol Tuberculosis Drugs, Boston, September 2010.
16 Oudijk JM, McIlleron H, Mulenga V, Chintu C, Merry C, Gibb D, Burger D: PKs of nevirapine in young children during combined ART and rifampicin-containing anti-TB treatment (abstract LBPEB10). 5th IAS Conf Pathogen Treat Prev, Cape Town, July 2009.
17 La Porte CJ, Colbers EP, Bertz R, Voncken DS, Wikstrom K, Boeree MJ, Koopmans PP, Hekster YA, Burger DM: Pharmacokinetics of adjusted-dose lopinavir-ritonavir combined with rifampin in healthy volunteers. Antimicrob Agents Chemother 2004;48:1553–1560.
18 Decloedt EH, McIlleron H, Smith P, Merry C, Orrell C, Maartens G: The pharmacokinetics of lopinavir in HIV-infected adults receiving rifampicin with adjusted doses of lopinavir/ritonavir tablets. Antimicrob Agents Chemother 2011, in press.
19 McIlleron H, Ren Y, Nuttall J, Fairlie L, Rabie H, Cotton M, Eley B, Meyers T, Smith PJ, Merry C, et al: Lopinavir exposure is insufficient in children given double doses of lopinavir/ritonavir during rifampicin-based treatment for tuberculosis. Antivir Ther 2011;16:417–421.
20 Varma JK, Nateniyom S, Akksilp S, Mankatittham W, Sirinak C, Sattayawuthipong W, Burapat C, Kittikraisak W, Monkongdee P, Cain KP, et al: HIV care and treatment factors associated with improved survival during TB treatment in Thailand: an observational study. BMC Infect Dis 2009;9:42.

21 Patel A, Patel K, Patel J, Shah N, Patel B, Rani S: Safety and antiretroviral effectiveness of concomitant use of rifampicin and efavirenz for antiretroviral-naive patients in India who are coinfected with tuberculosis and HIV-1. J Acquir Immune Defic Syndr 2004;37:1166–1169.

22 Hoffmann CJ, Charalambous S, Thio CL, Martin DJ, Pemba L, Fielding KL, Churchyard GJ, Chaisson RE, Grant AD: Hepatotoxicity in an African antiretroviral therapy cohort: the effect of tuberculosis and hepatitis B. AIDS 2007;21:1301–1308.

23 Shipton LK, Wester CW, Stock S, Ndwapi N, Gaolathe T, Thior I, Avalos A, Moffat HJ, Mboya JJ, Widenfelt E, et al: Safety and efficacy of nevirapine- and efavirenz-based antiretroviral treatment in adults treated for TB-HIV co-infection in Botswana. Int J Tuberc Lung Dis 2009;13:360–366.

24 Boulle A, Van Cutsem G, Cohen K, Hilderbrand K, Mathee S, Abrahams M, Goemaere E, Coetzee D, Maartens G: Outcomes of nevirapine- and efavirenz-based antiretroviral therapy when coadministered with rifampicin-based antitubercular therapy. JAMA 2008;300:530–539.

25 Chu KM, Boulle AM, Ford N, Goemaere E, Asselman V, Van Cutsem G: Nevirapine-associated early hepatotoxicity: incidence, risk factors, and associated mortality in a primary care ART programme in South Africa. PLoS One 2010;5:e9183.

26 Manosuthi W, Ruxrungtham K, Likanonsakul S, Prasithsirikul W, Inthong Y, Phoorisri T, Sungkanuparph S: Nevirapine levels after discontinuation of rifampicin therapy and 60-week efficacy of nevirapine-based antiretroviral therapy in HIV-infected patients with tuberculosis. Clin Infect Dis 2007;44:141–144.

27 Grange S, Schutz M, Schmitt C, Riek M, Gaudeul-Ehrhart E: Unexpected hepatotoxicity observed in a healthy volunteer study on the effects of multiple dose rifampicin on the steady-state pharmacokinetics of ritonavir-boosted saquinavir and vice versa (abstract 35). 6th Int Workshop Clin Pharmacol HIV Ther, Quebec City, 30 April 2005.

28 Nijland HM, L'Homme RF, Rongen GA, van Uden P, van Crevel R, Boeree MJ, Aarnoutse RE, Koopmans PP, Burger DM: High incidence of adverse events in healthy volunteers receiving rifampicin and adjusted doses of lopinavir/ritonavir tablets. AIDS 2008;22:931–935.

29 Haas DW, Koletar SL, Laughlin L, Kendall MA, Suckow C, Gerber JG, Zolopa AR, Bertz R, Child MJ, Hosey L, et al: Hepatotoxicity and gastrointestinal intolerance when healthy volunteers taking rifampin add twice-daily atazanavir and ritonavir. J Acquir Immune Defic Syndr 2009;50:290–293.

30 Rolla VC, da Silva Vieira MA, Pereira Pinto D, Lourenco MC, de Jesus Cda S, Goncalves Morgado M, Ferreira Filho M, Werneck-Barroso E: Safety, efficacy and pharmacokinetics of ritonavir 400 mg/saquinavir 400 mg twice daily plus rifampicin combined therapy in HIV patients with tuberculosis. Clin Drug Invest 2006;26:469–479.

31 L'Homme RF, Nijland HM, Gras L, Aarnoutse RE, van Crevel R, Boeree M, Brinkman K, Prins JM, Juttmann JR, Burger DM: Clinical experience with the combined use of lopinavir/ritonavir and rifampicin. AIDS 2009;23:863–865.

32 Frohoff C, Moodley M, Fairlie L, Coovadia A, Moultrie H, Kuhn L, Meyers T: Antiretroviral therapy outcomes in HIV-infected children after adjusting protease inhibitor dosing during tuberculosis treatment. PLoS One 2011;6:e17273.

33 Westreich DJ, Sanne I, Maskew M, Malope-Kgokong B, Conradie F, Majuba P, Funk MJ, Kaufman JS, Van Rie A, Macphail P: Tuberculosis treatment and risk of stavudine substitution in first-line antiretroviral therapy. Clin Infect Dis 2009;48:1617–1623.

34 Maritz JBM, Dave JA, Harrison TB, Badri M, Levitt NS, Heckmann JM: HIV neuropathy in South Africans: frequency, characteristics, and risk factors. Muscle Nerve 2010;41:599–606.

35 Chan ED, Laurel V, Strand MJ, Chan JF, Huynh ML, Goble M, Iseman MD: Treatment and outcome analysis of 205 patients with multidrug-resistant tuberculosis. Am J Respir Crit Care Med 2004;169:1103–1109.

36 Palmero DJ, Ambroggi M, Brea A, De Lucas M, Fulgenzi A, Martinez D, Mosca C, Musella R, Natiello M, Gonzalez C, et al: Treatment and follow-up of HIV-negative multidrug-resistant tuberculosis patients in an infectious diseases reference hospital, Buenos Aires, Argentina. Int J Tuberc Lung Dis 2004;8:778–784.

37 Cox HS, Kalon S, Allamuratova S, Sizaire V, Tigay ZN, Rusch-Gerdes S, Karimovich HA, Kebede Y, Mills C: Multidrug-resistant tuberculosis treatment outcomes in Karakalpakstan, Uzbekistan: treatment complexity and XDR-TB among treatment failures. PLoS One 2007;2:e1126.

38 Bloss E, Kuksa L, Holtz TH, Riekstina V, Skripconoka V, Kammerer S, Leimane V: Adverse events related to multidrug-resistant tuberculosis treatment, Latvia, 2000–2004. Int J Tuberc Lung Dis 2010;14:275–281.

39 Seung KJ, Omatayo DB, Keshavjee S, Furin JJ, Farmer PE, Satti H: Early outcomes of MDR-TB treatment in a high HIV-prevalence setting in Southern Africa. PLoS One 2009;4:e7186.

40 Huerga H, Arnold A, Chikwanha I, Muller M, Oucho N, Odongo A, Varaine F: MDR-TB treatment in Kenya: cohort description from the first program (abstract PC-100347-14). 41st Union World Conf Lung Health, Berlin, November 2010.

41 Arab-Alameddine M, Di Iulio J, Buclin T, Rotger M, Lubomirov R, Cavassini M, Fayet A, Decosterd LA, Eap CB, Biollaz J, et al: Pharmacogenetics-based population pharmacokinetic analysis of efavirenz in HIV-1-infected individuals. Clin Pharmacol Ther 2009;85:485–494.

42 Mukonzo JK, Roshammar D, Waako P, Andersson M, Fukasawa T, Milani L, Svensson JO, Ogwal-Okeng J, Gustafsson LL, Aklillu E: A novel polymorphism in ABCB1 gene, CYP2B6*6 and sex predict single-dose efavirenz population pharmacokinetics in Ugandans. Br J Clin Pharmacol 2009;68:690–699.

43 Burger D, van der Heiden I, la Porte C, van der Ende M, Groeneveld P, Richter C, Koopmans P, Kroon F, Sprenger H, Lindemans J, et al: Interpatient variability in the pharmacokinetics of the HIV non-nucleoside reverse transcriptase inhibitor efavirenz: the effect of gender, race, and CYP2B6 polymorphism. Br J Clin Pharmacol 2006;61:148–154.

44 Stohr W, Back D, Dunn D, Sabin C, Winston A, Gilson R, Pillay D, Hill T, Ainsworth J, Pozniak A, et al: Factors influencing efavirenz and nevirapine plasma concentration: effect of ethnicity, weight and co-medication. Antivir Ther 2008;13:675–685.

45 Lopez-Cortes LF, Ruiz-Valderas R, Viciana P, Alarcon-Gonzalez A, Gomez-Mateos J, Leon-Jimenez E, Sarasanacenta M, Lopez-Pua Y, Pachon J: Pharmacokinetic interactions between efavirenz and rifampicin in HIV-infected patients with tuberculosis. Clin Pharmacokinet 2002;41:681–690.

46 Cohen K, Grant A, Dandara C, McIlleron H, Pemba L, Fielding K, Charalombous S, Churchyard G, Smith P, Maartens G: Effect of rifampicin-based antitubercular therapy and the cytochrome P450 2B6 516G→T polymorphism on efavirenz concentrations in adults in South Africa. Antivir Ther 2009;14:687–695.

47 Ren Y, Nuttall JJ, Eley BS, Meyers TM, Smith PJ, Maartens G, McIlleron HM: Effect of rifampicin on efavirenz pharmacokinetics in HIV-infected children with tuberculosis. J Acquir Immune Defic Syndr 2009;50:439–443.

48 Ramachandran G, Hemanth Kumar AK, Rajasekaran S, Kumar P, Ramesh K, Anitha S, Narendran G, Menon P, Gomathi C, Swaminathan S: CYP2B6 G516T polymorphism but not rifampin coadministration influences steady-state pharmacokinetics of efavirenz in human immunodeficiency virus-infected patients in South India. Antimicrob Agents Chemother 2009;53:863–868.

49 Uttayamakul S, Likanonsakul S, Manosuthi W, Wichukchinda N, Kalambaheti T, Nakayama EE, Shioda T, Khusmith S: Effects of CYP2B6 G516T polymorphisms on plasma efavirenz and nevirapine levels when co-administered with rifampicin in HIV/TB co-infected Thai adults. AIDS Res Ther 2010;7:8.

50 Manosuthi W, Kiertiburanakul S, Sungkanuparph S, Ruxrungtham K, Vibhagool A, Rattanasiri S, Thakkinstian A: Efavirenz 600 mg/day versus efavirenz 800 mg/day in HIV-infected patients with tuberculosis receiving rifampicin: 48 weeks results. AIDS 2006;20:131–132.

51 Manosuthi W, Sungkanuparph S, Tantanathip P, Lueangniyomkul A, Mankatitham W, Prasithsirskul W, Burapatarawong S, Thongyen S, Likanonsakul S, Thawornwa U, et al: A randomized trial comparing plasma drug concentrations and efficacies between 2 nonnucleoside reverse-transcriptase inhibitor-based regimens in HIV-infected patients receiving rifampicin: the N2R Study. Clin Infect Dis 2009;48:1752–1759.
52 Friedland G, Khoo S, Jack C, Lalloo U: Administration of efavirenz (600 mg/day) with rifampicin results in highly variable levels but excellent clinical outcomes in patients treated for tuberculosis and HIV. J Antimicrob Chemother 2006;58:1299–1302.
53 Di Iulio J, Fayet A, Arab-Alameddine M, Rotger M, Lubomirov R, Cavassini M, Furrer H, Günthard HF, Colombo S, Csajka C, et al: In vivo analysis of efavirenz metabolism in individuals with impaired CYP2A6 function. Pharmacogenet Genomics 2009;19:300–309.
54 Rae JM, Johnson MD, Lippman ME, Flockhart DA: Rifampin is a selective, pleiotropic inducer of drug metabolism genes in human hepatocytes: studies with cDNA and oligonucleotide expression arrays. J Pharmacol Exp Ther 2001;299:849–857.
55 La Porte CJL, Back DJ, Blaschke T, Boucher CAB, Fletcher CV, Flexner C, Gerber JG, Kashuba ADM, Schapiro J, Burger D: Updated guideline to perform therapeutic drug monitoring for antiretroviral agents. Rev Antiviral Ther 2006;3:4–14.
56 Cohen K, van Cutsem G, Boulle A, McIlleron H, Goemaere E, Smith PJ, Maartens G: Effect of rifampicin-based antitubercular therapy on nevirapine plasma concentrations in South African adults with HIV-associated tuberculosis. J Antimicrob Chemother 2008;61:389–393.
57 Ribera E, Pou L, Lopez RM, Crespo M, Falco V, Ocana I, Ruiz I, Pahissa A: Pharmacokinetic interaction between nevirapine and rifampicin in HIV-infected patients with tuberculosis. J Acquir Immune Defic Syndr 2001;28:450–453.
58 Autar RS, Wit FW, Sankote J, Mahanontharit A, Anekthananon T, Mootsikapun P, Sujaikaew K, Cooper DA, Lange JM, Phanuphak P, et al: Nevirapine plasma concentrations and concomitant use of rifampin in patients coinfected with HIV-1 and tuberculosis. Antivir Ther 2005;10:937–943.
59 Matteelli A, Saleri N, Villani P, Bonkoungou V, Carvalho AC, Kouanda S, Sanou MJ, Simpore J, Monno L, Carosi G, et al: Reversible reduction of nevirapine plasma concentrations during rifampicin treatment in patients coinfected with HIV-1 and tuberculosis. J Acquir Immune Defic Syndr 2009;52:64–69.
60 Elsherbiny D, Cohen K, Jansson B, Smith P, McIlleron H, Simonsson US: Population pharmacokinetics of nevirapine in combination with rifampicin-based short course chemotherapy in HIV- and tuberculosis-infected South African patients. Eur J Clin Pharmacol 2009;65:71–80.
61 Ramachandran G, Hemanthkumar AK, Rajasekaran S, Padmapriyadarsini C, Narendran G, Sukumar B, Sathishnarayan S, Raja K, Kumaraswami V, Swaminathan S: Increasing nevirapine dose can overcome reduced bioavailability due to rifampicin coadministration. J Acquir Immune Defic Syndr 2006;42:36–41.
62 Avihingsanon A, Manosuthi W, Kantipong P, Chuchotaworn C, Moolphate S, Sakornjun W, Gorowara M, Yamada N, Yanai H, Mitarai S, et al: Pharmacokinetics and 48-week efficacy of nevirapine: 400 mg versus 600 mg per day in HIV-tuberculosis coinfection receiving rifampicin. Antivir Ther 2008;13:529–536.
63 Van Oosterhout JJ, Kumwenda JJ, Beadsworth M, Mateyu G, Longwe T, Burger DM, Zijlstra EE: Nevirapine-based antiretroviral therapy started early in the course of tuberculosis treatment in adult Malawians. Antivir Ther 2007;12:515–521.
64 Lamorde M, Byakika-Kibwika P, Okaba-Kayom V, Ryan M, Coakley P, Boffito M, Namakula R, Kalemeera F, Colebunders R, Back D, et al: Nevirapine pharmacokinetics when initiated at 200 mg or 400 mg daily in HIV-1 and tuberculosis co-infected Ugandan adults on rifampicin. J Antimicrob Chemother 2011;66:180–183.
65 Bonnet M, Bhatt NB, Jani IV, Slawuski A, Silva C, Rouzioux R, Calmy A, Barrail-Tran A, Furlan V, Taburet A-M, et al: Pharmacokinetic (pk) parameters of nevirapine (NVP) when initiated without 2-weeks leading dose in tuberculosis (TB)-HIV co-infected patients receiving rifampicin (RMP): substudy of the CARINEMO-ANRS 12146 trial in Maputo (Mozambique) (abstract MOPEB032). 5th IAS Conf Pathogen Treat Prev, Cape Town, July 2009.
66 Boulanger C, Hollender E, Farrell K, Stambaugh JJ, Maasen D, Ashkin D, Symes S, Espinoza LA, Rivero RO, Graham JJ, et al: Pharmacokinetic evaluation of rifabutin in combination with lopinavir-ritonavir in patients with HIV infection and active tuberculosis. Clin Infect Dis 2009;49:1305–1311.
67 Khachi H, O'Connell R, Ladenheim D, Orkin C: Pharmacokinetic interactions between rifabutin and lopinavir/ritonavir in HIV-infected patients with mycobacterial co-infection. J Antimicrob Chemother 2009;64:871–873.
68 Jenny-Avital ER, Joseph K: Rifamycin-resistant *Mycobacterium tuberculosis* in the highly active antiretroviral therapy era: a report of 3 relapses with acquired rifampin resistance following alternate-day rifabutin and boosted protease inhibitor therapy. Clin Infect Dis 2009;48:1471–1474.
69 Weiner M, Benator D, Burman W, Peloquin CA, Khan A, Vernon A, Jones B, Silva-Trigo C, Zhao Z, Hodge T: Association between acquired rifamycin resistance and the pharmacokinetics of rifabutin and isoniazid among patients with HIV and tuberculosis. Clin Infect Dis 2005;40:1481–1491.
70 Ng J, Nada A, Freeman S, Chiu Y-L, Cohen D, Bernstein B, Awni W, Klein C: Pharmacokinetics of RIFABUTIN 150 mg tiw plus lopinavir/ritonavir (LPV/r) 400/100 mg bid administered in healthy adult subjects (abstract O_21). 10th Int Workshop Clin Pharmacol HIV Ther, Amsterdam, April 2009.
71 Sekar V, Lavreys L, van de Casteele T, Berckmans C, Spinosa-Guzman S, Vangeneugden T, De Pauw M, Hoetelmans R: Pharmacokinetics of darunavir/ritonavir and rifabutin coadministered in HIV-negative healthy volunteers. Antimicrob Agents Chemother 2010;54:4440–4445.
72 Gulick RM, Ribaudo HJ, Shikuma CM, Lustgarten S, Squires KE, Meyer WA 3rd, Acosta EP, Schackman BR, Pilcher CD, Murphy RL, et al: Triple-nucleoside regimens versus efavirenz-containing regimens for the initial treatment of HIV-1 infection. N Engl J Med 2004;350:1850–1861.
73 Srikantiah P, Walusimbi MN, Kayanja HK, Mayanja-Kizza H, Mugerwa RD, Lin R, Charlebois ED, Boom WH, Whalen CC, Havlir DV: Early virological response of zidovudine/lamivudine/abacavir for patients co-infected with HIV and tuberculosis in Uganda. AIDS 2007;21:1972–1974.
74 Shao HJ, Crump JA, Ramadhani HO, Uiso LO, Ole-Nguyaine S, Moon AM, Kiwera RA, Woods CW, Shao JF, Bartlett JA, et al: Early versus delayed fixed dose combination abacavir/lamivudine/zidovudine in patients with HIV and tuberculosis in Tanzania. AIDS Res Hum Retroviruses 2009;25:1277–1285.
75 Burger DM, Magis-Escurra C, van den Berk GE, Gelinck LB: Pharmacokinetics of double-dose raltegravir in two patients with HIV infection and tuberculosis. AIDS 2010;24:328–330.
76 Wenning LA, Hanley WD, Brainard DM, Petry AS, Ghosh K, Jin B, Mangin E, Marbury TC, Berg JK, Chodakewitz JA, et al: Effect of rifampin, a potent inducer of drug-metabolizing enzymes, on the pharmacokinetics of raltegravir. Antimicrob Agents Chemother 2009;53:2852–2856.
77 Antiretroviral therapy of HIV infection in infants and children: towards universal access: recommendations for a public health approach – 2010 revision. Geneva, World Health Organization, 2010. http://www.who. int/hiv/pub/paediatric/paed-prelim-summary.pdf (accessed June 30, 2010).
78 Neely M, Rutstein R, del Bianco G, Heresi G, Barton T, Wheeling J, Wiegand R, Bohannon B, Dominguez K, Wiznia A, et al: Safety and efficacy of NRTI-only antiretroviral regimens in HIV-infected children (abstract 879). 17th Conf Retroviruses Opportunistic Infect, San Francisco, February 2010.
79 Bobat R, Kiepiela P, Kindra G, Reddy S, Esterhuizen T, Pillay V, Jeena P, Adhikari M, Coovadia H, Morris L: Resistance in ART-naïve paediatric subjects with chronic HIV-1 infection: experiences from a pilot study (abstract TUBEB053). 4th IAS Conf HIV Pathogen Treat Prev, Sydney, July 2007.

80 Ren Y, Nuttall JJ, Egbers C, Eley BS, Meyers TM, Smith PJ, Maartens G, McIlleron HM: High prevalence of subtherapeutic plasma concentrations of efavirenz in children. J Acquir Immune Defic Syndr 2007;45:133–136.
81 Hirt D, Urien S, Olivier M, Peyriere H, Nacro B, Diagbouga S, Zoure E, Rouet F, Hien H, Msellati P, et al: Is the recommended dose of efavirenz optimal in young West African human immunodeficiency virus-infected children? Antimicrob Agents Chemother 2009;53:4407–4413.
82 Bakeera-Kitaka S, Natukunda E, Kendall L, Q. F, Kekitiinwa A, Tumusiime C, Mugyenyi P, Walker AS, Gibb D, Burger D, et al: Pharmacokinetics of efavirenz dosed according to the WHO weight-bands in children in Uganda (abstract 878). 17th Conf Retroviruses Opportunistic Infect, San Francisco, February 2010.
83 Capparelli EV, Robbins B, Rathmore M, Britto P, Weinberg A, Browning R, Hazra R, Graham B, McKinney JR: Pediatric population pharmacokinetics of efavirenz (EFV) – high dose requirements in infants likely due to reduced absorption (abstract A1-2008). 50th Intersci Conf Antimicrob Agents Chemother, Boston, September 2010.
84 Prasitsuebsai W, Cressey T, Capparelli E, Vanprapar N, Lapphra K, Chearskul P, Chokephaibulkit K: Pharmacokinetics of nevirapine when co-administered with rifampin in HIV-infected Thai children with TB (abstract 908). 16th Conf Retroviruses Opportunistic Infect, Montreal, February 2009.
85 L'Homme RF, Kabamba D, Ewings FM, Mulenga V, Kankasa C, Thomason MJ, Walker AS, Chintu C, Burger DM, Gibb DM: Nevirapine, stavudine and lamivudine pharmacokinetics in African children on paediatric fixed-dose combination tablets. AIDS 2008;22:557–565.
86 Arrive E, Newell ML, Ekouevi DK, Chaix ML, Thiebaut R, Masquelier B, Leroy V, Perre PV, Rouzioux C, Dabis F: Prevalence of resistance to nevirapine in mothers and children after single-dose exposure to prevent vertical transmission of HIV-1: a meta-analysis. Int J Epidemiol 2007;36:1009–1021.
87 Moorthy A, Gupta A, Bhosale R, Tripathy S, Sastry J, Kulkarni S, Thakar M, Bharadwaj R, Kagal A, Bhore AV, et al: Nevirapine resistance and breast-milk HIV transmission: effects of single and extended-dose nevirapine prophylaxis in subtype C HIV-infected infants. PLoS One 2009;4:e4096.
88 Ren Y, Nuttall JJ, Egbers C, Eley BS, Meyers TM, Smith PJ, Maartens G, McIlleron HM: Effect of rifampicin on lopinavir pharmacokinetics in HIV-infected children with tuberculosis. J Acquir Immune Defic Syndr 2008;47:566–569.
89 Zhang C, McIlleron H, Ren Y, van der Walt JS, Karlsson MO, Simonsson USH, Denti P: Population pharmacokinetics of lopinavir and ritonavir in combination with rifampicin-based antitubercular treatment in HIV-infected children. Antivir Ther, in press.

Dr. Helen McIlleron
Division of Clinical Pharmacology, University of Cape Town
K-45 Old Main Building, Groote Schuur Hospital
Observatory 7925, Cape Town (South Africa)
Tel. +27 21 406 6292, E-Mail helen.mcilleron@uct.ac.za

Chapter 20
Donald PR, van Helden PD (eds): Antituberculosis Chemotherapy.
Prog Respir Res. Basel, Karger, 2011, vol 40, pp 203–212

# Diabetes Mellitus and Tuberculosis Treatment

Rovina Ruslami[a] · Reinout van Crevel[b]

[a]Faculty of Medicine, University of Padjadjaran/Hasan Sadikin Hospital, Bandung, Indonesia; [b]Department of Medicine, Radboud University Nijmegen Medical Centre, Nijmegen, The Netherlands

**Abstract**

Diabetes mellitus (DM) not only increases the risk of active tuberculosis (TB) 3- to 5-fold, it also puts patients at an increased risk for poor treatment outcomes. The global epidemic of DM thus has serious implications for control and treatment of TB. DM in TB patients often goes unnoticed, but as many as 10–30% of TB patients may have concurrent DM. With regard to treatment, rifampicin hampers glycaemic control by increasing the metabolism of most oral antidiabetic drugs, while DM has been associated with failure of TB treatment. Some data suggest that plasma rifampicin concentrations are lower in patients with DM. Although sometimes advocated, TB prophylaxis has not been implemented widely among patients with DM. Prospective studies are needed to improve prevention, early detection and treatment of concomitant DM and TB, especially in developing countries.

Copyright © 2011 S. Karger AG, Basel

In the era before insulin therapy, patients with type 1 diabetes in the western world appeared doomed to die of pulmonary tuberculosis (TB) if they survived diabetic coma [1]. With the introduction of insulin in 1922, this picture changed, although the risk of developing TB remained high, especially in lean diabetic patients [2]. The risk correlated with duration of diabetes and with the extent of hyperglycaemia [2]. Once diagnosed, TB often ran a rapid, progressive course in diabetes patients. Among 2,010 patients treated between 1930 and 1953, 1,061 (53%) died, the majority within 1 year [3]. Following the introduction of the first antituberculous drugs, streptomycin (1945), para-aminosalicylic acid (1949) and isoniazid (INH; 1952), the prognosis of diabetic patients with TB improved dramatically. Although mortality was not as high as before, according to most studies, diabetes still enhanced the severity of TB, with more pulmonary cavities and a higher bacterial load [3].

In the second half of the 20th century, the association between TB and diabetes mellitus (DM) was neglected. In recent years, with the current global growth of DM, the link between the 2 diseases is being rediscovered. The epidemic growth of DM occurs especially in developing countries, where TB is highly endemic. As a result, DM and TB will increasingly present together, and this calls for renewed interest in this topic. In this chapter we will focus on combined TB and DM, and on TB prophylaxis for DM patients.

## Diabetes Mellitus and Tuberculosis – Epidemiology

Both type 1 and type 2 DM are associated with an increased risk of TB; among TB patients type 2 DM is often undiagnosed. Given its worldwide prevalence, DM contributes significantly to the TB problem, especially in areas with a low HIV prevalence. Because DM is emerging rapidly, especially in TB-endemic countries, the effect of DM on the global TB epidemic will increase in the near future.

Globally, an estimated 285 million people live with DM, a number expected to grow to at least 438 million by the year 2030 when more than 80% of adult cases will live in low- or middle-income countries [4]. At present, 12–16 million people live with TB disease, and 1.2–1.4 million people die from TB every year [5]. With regard to DM, Asia is considered as the epicentre of the current diabetes pandemic; India, China, Indonesia and Pakistan (the 4 most populous

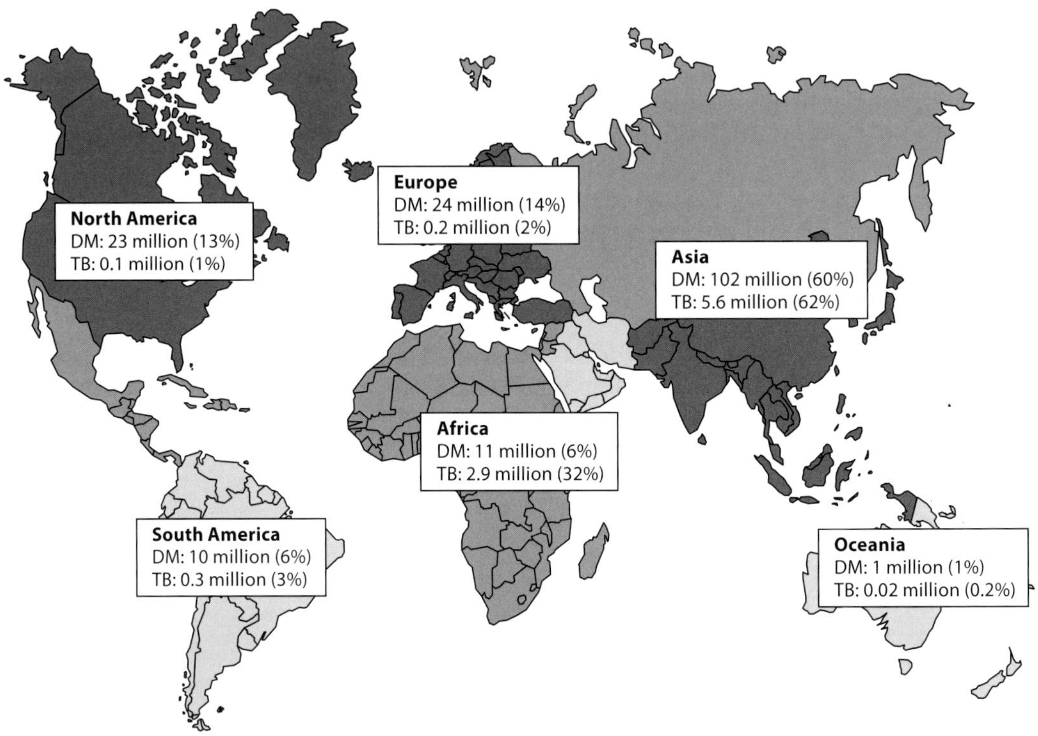


**Fig. 1.** Epidemiological picture of TB and DM.

countries of Asia) harbour more than 60% of all patients with diabetes worldwide [4], and although the incidence of TB is higher in many African countries, the greatest burden of TB is in Asia, with more than 50% of TB cases found in those same 5 countries (fig. 1) [4, 5].

At first sight one might assume that these 2 epidemics will largely remain separate, as TB is associated with malnutrition, while type 2 diabetes is linked to obesity. However, studies from different parts of the world have shown that as many as 5–30% of TB patients present with concomitant DM [6], and available evidence indicates that DM acts as risk factor for the development of TB. Studies from the 1930s showed that patients with DM had a 3- to 4-fold increased risk of developing TB [2, 3], and this association was confirmed in more recent studies.

In a study in Mexico [49] the prevalence of DM was 29.6% among TB patients, which was 6.8-fold higher than the background prevalence of DM in the study area. In contrast, in our study in Indonesia, which has the fifth highest number of TB patients worldwide and the fourth highest number of people with DM, DM was present in 13.3% of TB patients versus 3.2% of age-matched controls [24]. Similar studies have appeared worldwide, and in 2008 a meta-analysis assessed that people with DM had a 3.11 times higher risk of getting TB (95% confidence interval, CI, 2.27–4.26) compared to people without DM [7]. Although HIV is by far the strongest risk factor for TB, DM may be equally or more important in countries with a low HIV prevalence [6].

Few studies specified whether diabetic TB patients had type 1 or type 2 DM. Type 2 DM is more prevalent, but type 1 DM is associated with a higher TB risk. Studies from Ethiopia, Tanzania and Chile showed that type 1 DM patients had a 3- to 5-fold higher risk of developing TB than type 2 DM patients. It seems that long duration of illness and poor glucose control increase the TB risk [6].

Type 2 DM among TB patients is often unrecognized. Studies in Tanzania and in Indonesia found that 61–73% of DM was newly diagnosed [6]. One might postulate that TB may trigger the development of hyperglycaemia, e.g. by inflammation-associated insulin resistance [8]. Transient glucose intolerance has been described in TB patients, but in a recent study from Indonesia, only 3.7% of hyperglycaemia in TB patients was transient [24].

Socio-economic and lifestyle changes in developing countries lead to increased DM, especially type 2 DM. We recently estimated the contribution of DM to the TB epidemic in 10 countries with the highest number of new TB cases. Based on the prevalence of DM, the incidence of TB and the relative risk to develop TB associated with DM, we estimated that almost half a million, or 7.6% (95% CI 5.5–10.4%) of TB cases in 2003 were due to DM in these 10 countries [6]. As the total number of people with DM worldwide will more than double in the coming 20 years and, similarly to the situation now, an estimated 80% of diabetic patients in 2030 will live in TB-endemic countries [4], the proportion of TB cases attributable to DM will increase sharply in coming decades.

## Diabetes Mellitus and Tuberculosis – Clinical Presentation

DM does not seem to have a major impact on the severity and presentation of TB, and it remains uncertain whether DM is associated with specific chest X-ray abnormalities. Almost all of the published studies lack detail regarding the diagnosis, possible complications and regulation of DM.

From recent studies it seems that DM has no major effect on the clinical manifestation of TB. Several studies showed a similar occurrence and duration of symptoms between diabetic and non-diabetic TB patients [6]. A study from Turkey reported that more sputum smear-negative cases were among hospitalized TB patients with DM compared to age- and sex-matched non-patients without concurrent DM (19.2 vs. 0.7%, $p < 0.01$) [9]. In contrast, a recent retrospective study from Texas showed a higher rate of smear positivity among TB patients with self-reported DM than among patients without DM (odds ratio, OR, 1.8; 95% CI 1.3–2.4) [10]. With regard to disease localization, recent studies in Malaysia, Turkey and Guinea did not find a clear association between DM and extrapulmonary involvement [6].

Much has been written about putative effects of DM on the radiological appearance of TB. Some studies have reported a higher frequency of pulmonary cavities, but this has been challenged by others [6]. A higher frequency of 'atypical' images with lower lung lesions and fewer cavities has also been reported [9], but this finding may be confounded by age; older age is associated with more cases of lower lung involvement in TB and fewer pulmonary cavities. Based on the available literature therefore, uncertainty remains with regard to the radiological appearance of TB in DM patients, but the conflict is possibly caused by differences between study populations, e.g. with respect to severity of DM. An overview of studies evaluating the relation between DM and the radiological appearance of TB is provided in table 1.

One difference is however consistently found: TB patients with DM are usually 10–20 years older and mostly have a higher body weight than those without DM [6]. This seems logical, as type 2 diabetes is associated with obesity and older age. Therefore, as expected, compared to non-DM patients, TB patients with DM usually have a higher body weight before start of treatment, and even more so after treatment. A study from West Africa [50] showed that 23% of TB-DM patients were obese (BMI >30), compared with 3% of non-diabetic patients (OR 10.1; 95% CI 3.1–21.2), while in Indonesia, 53% of TB patients with DM were above 50 kg of weight before treatment started, compared to only 16.5% of non-diabetic patients ($p < 0.01$; fig. 2) [24]. Of course, one has to take into account that this finding is biased by the fact that both uncontrolled DM and active TB are associated with significant weight loss. However, some DM TB patients in this study were overtly undernourished, and faced with DM in these lean individuals, we asked ourselves if this was caused by insulin deficiency or insulin resistance. In a subset of patients, fasting insulin was measured. No absolute insulin deficiency was found, and median fasting plasma insulin concentrations indicated that diabetic TB patients and age- and gender-matched type 2 DM patients had similar levels of insulin resistance [Stalenhoef J., unpubl. data]. These data support the general conclusion that DM among TB patients in less-developed settings is mostly type 2 diabetes, which is often unrecognized and which may be found in non-obese individuals. It is important to realize that differences in body weight between DM patients with and without concurrent TB may have implications for the dosing of TB drugs.

## Combined Treatment of Diabetes Mellitus and Tuberculosis

*Diabetes Treatment*

By induction of the hepatic metabolism of many antidiabetic drugs, rifampicin hampers glycaemic control. This calls for more frequent monitoring and use of higher doses of sulphonylureas and thiazolidine diones, or other hypoglycaemic drugs, which do not have an interaction with rifampicin, most notably insulin or metformin.

Combining antituberculous drugs with other medication has a potential for drug interactions. The concentrations of antituberculous drugs are generally not prone to be influenced by other drugs [25]. On the other hand, TB drugs, especially rifampicin, may enhance the metabolism of antidiabetic drugs and distort glucose homeostasis.

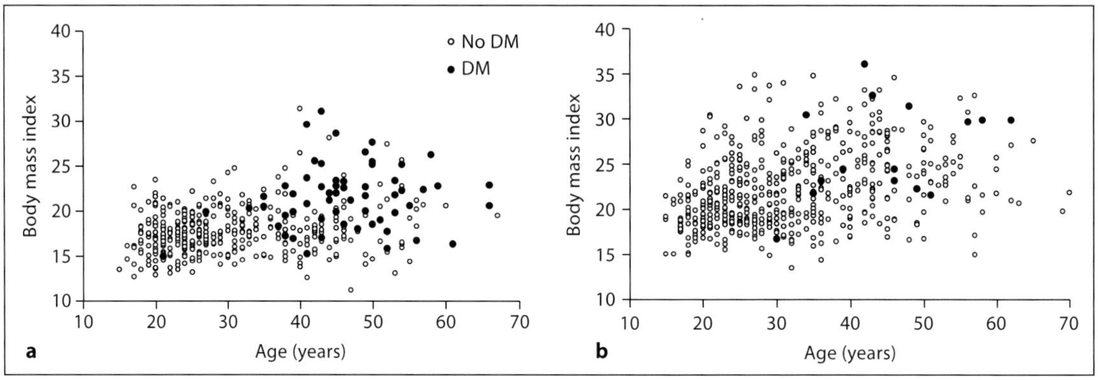


**Fig. 2.** Clinical picture (body mass index and age of TB and DM [Alisjahbana, unpubl. data]. **a** TB patients. **b** Control subjects.

**Table 1.** Effect of DM on radiological appearance of TB [6]

| Country, year | TB patients, n | | Radiological findings | | Reference |
|---|---|---|---|---|---|
| | diabetic | non-diabetic | more lower lobe involvement in DM | more cavitations/other lesions in DM | |
| USA, 1974 | 20 | 182 | yes | n.a. | Weaver [11], 1974 |
| South Africa, 1980 | 9 | 427 | yes (29 vs. 5%) | n.a. | Marais [12], 1980 |
| UK, 1983 | 43 | 31 | no difference | yes (22 vs. 6%) | Hendy and Stableforth [13], 1983 |
| Japan, 1992 | 39 | 71 | no (18 vs. 17%) | yes (44 vs. 21%) | Ikezoe et al. [14], 1992 |
| USA, 1992 | 20 | 20 | no difference | no difference | Morris et al. [15], 1992 |
| Turkey, 1994 | 37 | 37 | more multilobar involvement in DM | yes | Umut et al. [16], 1994 |
| Saudi Arabia, 1997 | 28 | 38 | no difference | no difference | Al-Wabel et al. [17], 1997 |
| Turkey, 2001 | 92 | 92 | no difference | no difference in cavities; fewer reticulonodular lesions (13 vs. 30%) | Bacakoglu et al. [9], 2001 |
| Mexico, 2000–2001 | 192 | 130 | yes (19 vs. 7%) | yes (82 vs. 59%); more lower lung cavities (29 vs. 3%) | Perez-Guzman et al. [18, 19], 2000 and 2001 |
| Saudi Arabia, 2003 | 187 | 505 | yes (23 vs .2.4%) | yes (51 vs. 39%) | Shaikh et al. [20], 2003 |
| Malaysia, 2005 | 230 | 1226 | yes (11 vs. 9%), n.s. | no (63 vs. 73%; n.s.) | Nissapatorn et al. [21], 2005 |
| Taiwan, 2005 | 99 | 362 | no (n.s.) | yes (19 vs. 10%) | Wang et al. [22], 2005 |
| Texas, 2007 | 401 | 1040 | – | yes (60 vs. 48%) | Restrepo et al. [10], 2007 |
| Taiwan, 2009 | 74 | 143 | yes (27 vs. 15.4%) | yes (45.9 vs. 30.8%) | Wang et al. [23], 2009 |

n.a. = Not available; n.s. = not significant.

**Table 2.** Effect of rifampicin on the exposure to antidiabetic drugs [6]

| Antidiabetic drug | Change in exposure (AUC) | Enzyme induction | Reference |
|---|---|---|---|
| Insulin | no effect anticipated | | no studies published |
| Sulphonylureas | | | |
| Tolbutamide | strong decrease | | Zilly et al. [26], 1975; Syvälahti et al. [27], 1976 |
| Glibenclamide (Glyburide) | –39% | CYP2C9 | Niemi et al. [28], 2001 |
| Gliclazide | –70% | CYP2C9 | Park et al. [29], 2003 |
| Glimepiride | –34% | CYP2C9 | Niemi et al. [30], 2000 |
| Glipizide | –22% | CYP2C9 | Niemi et al. [28], 2001 |
| Biguanides | | | |
| Metformin | no effect anticipated | | no studies published |
| Meglitinide analogues | | | |
| Repaglinide | –57%, –31%, –50% | CYP3A4, CYP2C8 | Niemi et al. [31], 2000; Hatorp et al. [32], 2003; Bidstrup et al. [33], 2004 |
| Nateglinide | –24% | CYP2C9, CYP3A4 | Niemi et al. [34], 2003 |
| Thiazolidine diones | | | |
| Rosiglitazone | –54%, –65% | CYP2C8 | Park et al. [35], 2004 |
| Pioglitazone | –54% | CYP2C8 | Jaakkola et al. [36], 2006 |

AUC = Area under the concentration-time curve.

Many antidiabetic drugs are currently available. The most important ones are classified as insulin secretagogue (sulphonylureas and metiglinides), biguanide (metformin), thiazolidine diones and insulin. Among them, sulphonylureas, the new meglitinide derivatives and thiazolidine diones are metabolized by cytochrome (CYP) P450 enzymes in the liver. Rifampicin is a very potent CYP P450 enzyme inducer, and as such plasma levels of these antidiabetic drugs are significantly lower when co-administered with rifampicin (table 2) [6]. INH is an inhibitor (rather than an inducer) of some of the enzymes that are induced by rifampicin, most notably CYP2C9 which is relevant to the metabolism of sulphonylureas. However, the inductive effect of rifampicin generally outweighs the inhibitory effect of INH on the same enzyme so that the overall effect of INH + rifampicin is a decrease in the concentrations of other drugs [25].

The biguanide drug metformin can be used as an alternative drug, as it is not likely that rifampicin and/or INH will affect its pharmacokinetics, as this antidiabetic agent is not metabolized in the liver. However, this has not been investigated. Metformin has become a first-choice drug for type 2 DM [37] as it has several mechanisms to control hyperglycaemia and does not lead to hypoglycaemia. Metformin is relatively cheap, widely available and associated with less weight increase compared to other oral antidiabetic drugs. The disadvantage of metformin when combined with antituberculous drugs is that patients could experience gastrointestinal side effects, possibly leading to non-adherence and poor treatment outcome.

Nothing is known about the effect of rifampicin and INH on insulin metabolism, but it is unlikely to be significant as insulin is mostly degraded in the liver by hydrolysis of disulphide connections between the A and B chains through the action of insulin-degrading enzyme. It is unlikely that other first-line TB drugs (pyrazinamide and ethambutol) interact with any antidiabetic drugs, but fluoroquinolones, especially gatifloxacin, are associated with hyper- and hypoglycaemia [6]. Full induction of drug-metabolizing enzymes is reached after approximately 1 week of rifampicin treatment and induction dissipates in roughly 2 weeks after discontinuing rifampicin [34]. Based on the above, blood glucose levels should be monitored after start and discontinuation of rifampicin in patients using oral antidiabetic drugs.

*Tuberculosis Treatment*

There is accumulating evidence that TB treatment is less effective when DM is present. Earlier studies reported an association between DM and drug-resistant TB, but this could not be confirmed in several recent studies. An alternative explanation may lie in impaired immunity associated with DM, but it may also have to do with altered pharmacokinetics of TB drugs in diabetic TB patients.

TB patients with DM should receive standard TB treatment, consisting of 4 different antituberculous drugs for 2 months (rifampicin, INH, pyrazinamide and ethambutol), followed by 2 drugs (rifampicin and INH) for another 4 months. Rifampicin is the cornerstone for TB treatment. Its action is concentration dependent, and the recommended dose of rifampicin is 10 mg/kg body weight [38] which might be at the lower end of the dose-response curve. Higher daily doses are probably more effective and may reduce treatment duration [39]. In practice most guidelines advise 450 mg/day for patients below 50 kg and 600 mg/day for patients above 50 kg. Considering that patients with DM are usually heavier and gain more weight during TB treatment, adjustment of drug dose, especially in the later phase of treatment, seems indicated. Besides adjustment for body weight, no further adjustment is needed; antidiabetic drugs do not affect the concentrations of antituberculous drugs [25].

An important question is whether DM affects TB treatment outcome. As mentioned above, DM had a dramatic effect on TB outcome before the introduction of insulin, and later antituberculous drugs. With effective treatment available for both diseases, diabetes may have no or only mild effects on the outcome of TB treatment. Recently, this issue has been addressed in a number of publications. Studies in Malaysia and in Saudi Arabia showed that treatment outcome between diabetic and non-diabetic patients was similar [6]. In a retrospective study involving 5,049 TB patients along the Texan-Mexican border, patients with self-reported DM (19.9%) remained sputum smear positive significantly longer during the first 2 months of treatment [10]. However, no 6-month results were reported for this study, and none of the above studies has reported sputum culture results. This may be relevant: in a cohort of 634 Indonesian TB patients, DM patients had a significantly higher rate of positive sputum cultures at 6 months (adjusted OR 7.65, $p = 0.004$) [40]. It should be noted however that in this study a much smaller proportion of DM patients still had a productive cough after 6 months of TB treatment compared to non-diabetic patients (28.7 vs. 61.6%). As a result, although the proportion of sputum samples which were culture positive was much higher among DM patients, this was no longer the case when the data were analysed according to 'intention to treat' (6.4 vs. 5.9%). Finally, in a recent report from Taiwan, 1-year mortality was higher among TB patients with DM than among those without (17.6 vs. 7.7%; adjusted OR 5.5, 95% CI 2.3–13.4) [41].

If DM indeed has a negative effect on TB treatment, what could be the possible mechanism(s)? Non-adherence to TB treatment and drug resistance of *M. tuberculosis* are the most important risk factors for treatment failure and TB relapse [42]. Adherence to TB treatment among DM patients seems similar or better than among non-diabetic TB patients [24]. With regard to drug resistance, the results of some studies are indistinct; some reported a higher rate of drug resistance among diabetic TB patients while others have found the opposite [6]. It is unclear why diabetic TB patients might have a higher risk of becoming infected with a drug-resistant strain. Another possible explanation may be that diabetic TB patients have impaired cellular immunity interfering with effective eradication of mycobacteria. However, studies have met with conflicting results. Altered pharmacokinetics of TB drugs in DM patients might be an alternative explanation, as explained in the next section.

## Pharmacokinetics of Tuberculosis Drugs in Patients with Diabetes Mellitus

So far only 2 studies, both performed in Indonesia, have evaluated whether altered pharmacokinetics of TB drugs might contribute to the higher risk of a poor treatment outcome among patients with diabetes. Their findings suggest that diabetes per se is not associated with altered pharmacokinetics of TB drugs in the intensive phase, but that a higher body weight, especially in the continuation phase, may account for lower rifampicin levels in patients with diabetes during the continuation phase of TB treatment.

It has been shown that diabetes patients have lower plasma concentrations of certain drugs. If this also applies to antituberculous drugs, this might explain a reduced response to tuberculosis treatment, as lower plasma concentrations of antituberculous drugs have been associated with clinical failure and acquired drug resistance [9]. As far as we know, only 2 studies (both from our group) have evaluated a possible role of altered pharmacokinetics. For rifampicin, a key drug in TB treatment, available evidence suggests that its efficacy is dependent on exposure to the drug or to the maximum drug concentrations achieved. We have evaluated if patients with diabetes have reduced plasma concentrations of rifampicin. In the first study, exposure ($AUC_{0-6\,h}$) to rifampicin in

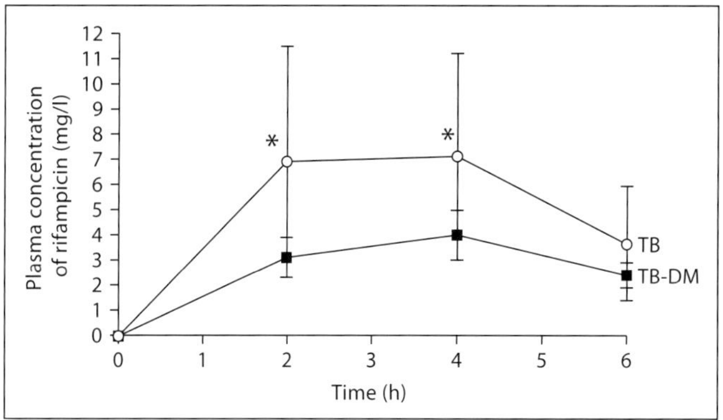


**Fig. 3.** Pharmacokinetics of rifampicin in diabetic versus non-diabetic TB patients in the continuation phase of treatment [43].

the continuation phase of treatment was 2-fold lower in TB patients with DM compared to patients without DM (fig. 3) [43]. Similar differences were found for the maximal plasma concentrations of rifampicin: the maximal plasma concentration of rifampicin was above the target concentration of 8 mg/l in 6% of TB patients with DM, as compared to 47% of patients without DM. Regression analysis showed that both higher body weight and the presence of DM accounted for the differences found. Interestingly, more profound hyperglycaemia correlated significantly with rifampicin exposure ($p = 0.016$).

To exclude a major effect from differences in body weight (the body weight of diabetes patients in the first study was on average 20% higher), we matched patients with and without diabetes for gender and body weight in a second study [44]. Intensive pharmacokinetic sampling was performed for rifampicin, pyrazinamide and ethambutol during the intensive phase of TB treatment. Rifampicin bioavailability was determined by comparing rifampicin exposure after oral and intravenous administration. Pharmacokinetic assessments were repeated in 10 diabetic TB patients after glycaemic control. Somewhat to our surprise, no differences were found in pharmacokinetics of rifampicin, pyrazinamide and ethambutol. Exposure to TB drugs as well as their maximal plasma concentrations were not correlated with blood glucose level or glucose control, and oral bioavailability, absorption, metabolism and clearance of rifampicin, pyrazinamide and ethambutol were similar in both groups (fig. 4).

What factors can explain the contrasting results of the 2 studies? The study setting and study drugs were exactly the same, and disease severity was similar. The different pharmacokinetics were not due to more intensive sampling in the present study either (limited time point analysis from the second study led to similar results), and samples from both studies were processed, transferred and analysed with the same validated methods. Therefore, from all the possible explanations we feel that only 2 may have had a significant role. First, as noted above, diabetic TB patients had a 20% higher body weight than non-diabetic TB patients in the first study, and a higher body weight results in a more than dose-proportional decrease in the mean $AUC_{0-24\ h}$, consistent with the non-linear pharmacokinetics of rifampicin [45]. That is why we matched for body weight in the second study. Timing of pharmacokinetic sampling may also have affected the results, because the second study was performed in the intensive phase and the first study in the continuation phase of treatment, with rifampicin taken thrice weekly without pyrazinamide and ethambutol. Our studies in Indonesian patients have shown lower plasma rifampicin concentrations during the continuation phase than the intensive phase of treatment [44]. On the one hand this seems counterintuitive because higher induction of liver CYPs with daily use of rifampicin and co-administration of pyrazinamide will lower rifampicin concentrations in the intensive phase. On the other hand, a higher body weight might decrease rifampicin concentrations during the continuation phase. Clearly, further study is needed to confirm these findings, to examine possible other causes of treatment failure among patients with DM, and to evaluate if diabetic TB patients should receive prolonged or dose-adjusted TB treatment.

## Tuberculosis Screening and Prophylactic Treatment for Diabetes Patients

In the light of the expanding epidemic of type 2 diabetes in TB-endemic settings, screening of TB patients for the presence of DM and vice versa will help control and treatment of both diseases in developing countries. However, screening is not routinely performed or investigated, and recent studies evaluating tuberculosis prophylaxis for diabetes patients are lacking.

Active screening leads to detection of TB among DM patients and DM among TB patients. However, although often advocated, such screening is no routine, and data on its effectiveness and costs are mostly lacking. Obviously, the yield of screening TB patients for DM is higher in areas with a high background prevalence of diabetes as seen in a study in Mexico, and the chance of finding DM is higher among older patients (i.e. above 35 years of age) as shown in a study in Indonesia [6]. A recent systematic review concluded that in some areas screening as few as 2–10 TB patients would

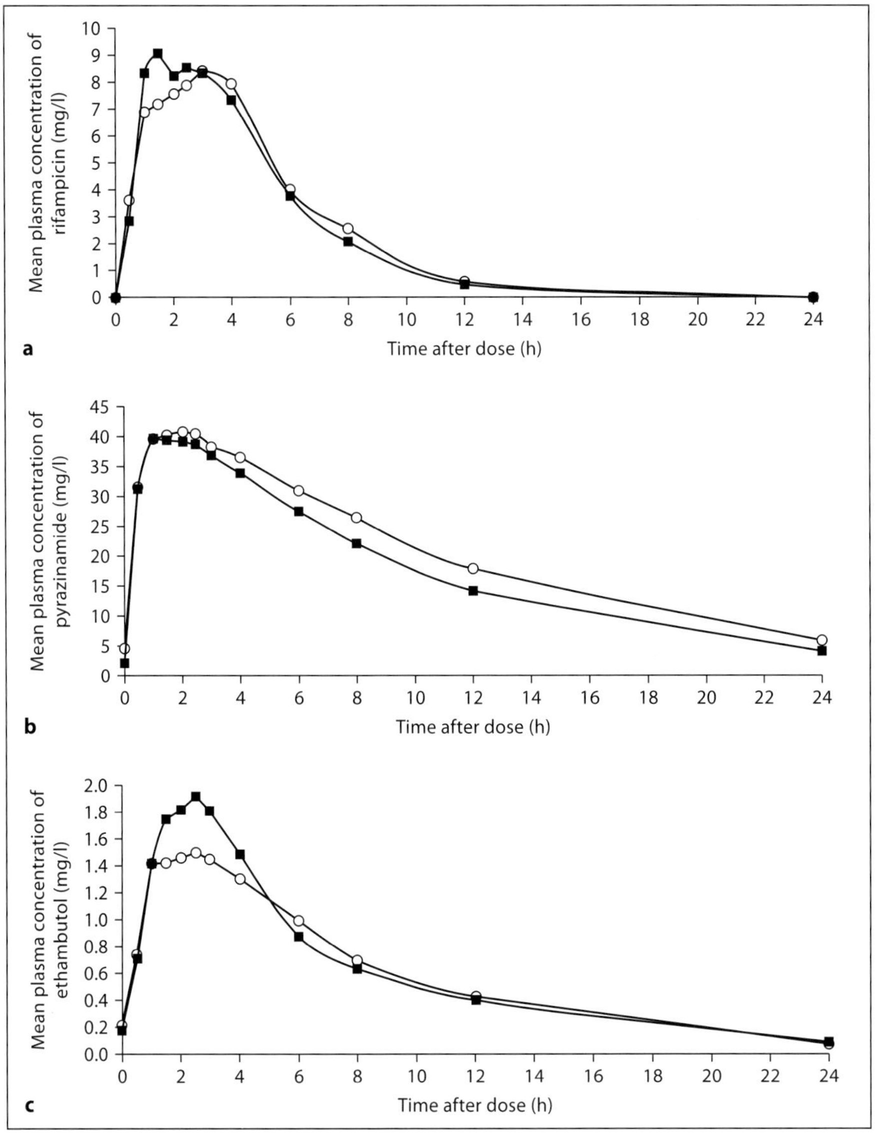


**Fig. 4.** Pharmacokinetics of antituberculous drugs (rifampicin, pyrazinamide and ethambutol) in diabetic versus non-diabetic tuberculosis patients [43]. Mean steady-state plasma concentration-time profiles of rifampicin (**a**, n = 17), pyrazinamide (**b**, n = 18) and ethambutol (**c**, n = 17) in TB patients with (■) and without (○) DM.

lead to the detection of 1 case of diabetes [46]. The number of diabetes patients which need to be screened to detect 1 case of TB is much higher. According to the same review, more than 1,000 DM patients would need to be screened to find 1 additional case of TB if the prevalence of TB is below 25/100,000. However, in a country like India with a 10-fold higher prevalence of TB, approximately 100 patients would need to be screened [46]. This will even be less among those with long-standing DM, with insulin dependence or with more poorly controlled DM [46].

Very little is known about the role of TB prophylaxis. INH preventive therapy reduced the incidence of TB in 2 observational studies. In a study conducted in Germany [47] in the 1950s, no TB relapse occurred in a small group of 63 patients with diabetes who were treated with INH for 6–24 months after completion of a full course of treatment for active TB, while 11% of patients from a group of patients with DM who did not receive INH prophylaxis after TB treatment had recurrent TB within 2 years. Primary prophylaxis with an analogue of INH was evaluated among diabetes patients in Russia in the 1960s [48]. Roughly 2,000 DM patients who received prophylaxis showed a 2–3 times lower incidence of TB during a follow-up period of 5 years compared with 236 control patients who did not receive prophylaxis. Both studies lack detail in terms of raw numbers of TB cases, specification of follow-up and selection of controls. Since then, no systematic evaluation of TB prophylaxis among DM patients has been reported.

## Conclusions

The association of DM and TB is epidemiologically important in the light of the expanding epidemic of type 2 DM in TB-endemic settings. DM is associated with higher age and body weight, but data regarding the effect of DM on clinical presentation are conflicting. With regard to treatment, rifampicin increases the metabolism of most oral antidiabetic drugs, complicating glycaemic control during TB treatment. The tolerability and effectiveness of metformin for glucose control is unknown when combined with TB drugs. At the same time, TB treatment failure and death may be common among patients with diabetes. However, these findings need further confirmation, and the underlying mechanisms should be explored. Most importantly, long-term follow-up data of combined treatment are lacking, and neither cohort studies nor controlled trials have compared standard treatment with intensified or prolonged TB treatment. Finally, it seems rational to screen for TB in patients with DM and vice versa, as this will have implications for control and treatment of both diseases in developing countries. Cost analysis of such interventions on a large scale will help us in the comprehensive management of both diseases. This is an important area of future research. Also, DM, TB and HIV might be a deadly threesome, but this has not been studied either.

Weaknesses in the current scientific literature, which is mostly cross-sectional and retrospective, contribute to the lack of good data. We therefore call for more interest and well-designed studies (e.g. clinical trials or prospective cohort studies), which will help to improve prevention and treatment of concomitant DM and TB, especially in developing countries.

## References


1 Root HF: The association of diabetes and tuberculosis: epidemiology, pathology, treatment and prognosis. N Engl J Med 1934;210:1–13.
2 Boucot KR, Dillon ES, Cooper DA, Meier P, Richardson R: Tuberculosis among diabetics: the Philadelphia survey. Am Rev Tuberc 1952;65:1–50.
3 Luntz GR: Management of the tuberculosis diabetic: follow-up of 84 cases for one year. Br Med J 1957;i:1082–1086.
4 http://www.eatlas.idf.org/prevalence/index (accessed December 2, 2010).
5 World Health Organization: WHO Report 2010: Global Tuberculosis Control. WHO/HTM/TB/2010.7. Geneva, WHO, 2010.
6 Ruslami R, Aarnoutse RA, Alisjahbana B, van der Ven A, van Crevel R: Implications of global increase of diabetes for tuberculosis control and patient care. Trop Med Int Health 2010;15:1289–1299.
7 Jeon CY, Murray MB: Diabetes mellitus increases the risk of active tuberculosis: a systematic review of 13 observational studies. PLoS Med 2008;5:e152.
8 Bloomgarden ZT: Inflammation and insulin resistance. Diabetes Care 2003;26:1922–1926.
9 Bacakoglu F, Basoglu OK, Cok G, Sayiner A, Ates M: Pulmonary tuberculosis in patients with diabetes mellitus. Respiration 2001;68:595–600.
10 Restrepo BI, Fisher-Hoch SP, Crespo JG, Whitney E, Perez A, Smith B, McCormick JB, Nuevo Santander Tuberculosis Trackers: Type 2 diabetes and tuberculosis in a dynamic bi-national border population. Epidemiol Infect 2007;135:483–491.
11 Weaver R: Unusual radiographic presentation of pulmonary tuberculosis in diabetic patients. Am Rev Respir Dis 1974;109:162–163.
12 Marais RM: Diabetes mellitus in black and colored tuberculosis patients. S Afr Med J 1980;57:483–484.
13 Hendy HH, Stableforth D: The effect of established diabetes mellitus on the presentation of infiltrative pulmonary tuberculosis in the immigrant Asian community of an inner city area of the United Kingdom. Br J Dis Chest 1983;77:87–90.
14 Ikezoe J, Takeuchi N, Johkoh T, Kohno N, Tomiyama N, Kozuka T, Noma K, Ueda T: CT appearance of pulmonary tuberculosis in diabetic and immunocompromised patients: comparison with patients who had no underlying disease. Am J Roentgenol 1992;159:1175–1179.
15 Morris JT, Seaworth BJ, McAllister CK: Pulmonary tuberculosis in diabetics. Chest 1992;102:539–541.
16 Umut S, Tosun GA, Yildirim N: Radiographic location of pulmonary tuberculosis in diabetic patients. Chest 1994;106:326.
17 Al-Wabel AH, Teklu B, Mahfouz AA, al-Ghamdi AS, el-Amin OB, Khan AS: Symptomatology and chest roentgenographic changes of pulmonary tuberculosis among diabetics. East Afr Med J 1997;74:62–64.
18 Perez-Guzman C, Torres-Cruz A, Villareal-Velarde H, Vargas MH: Progressive age-related changes in pulmonary tuberculosis images and the effect of diabetes. Am J Respir Crit Care Med 2000;162:1738–1780.
19 Perez-Guzman C, Torres-Cruz A Villareal-Velarde H, Salazar-Lezama MA, Vargas MH: Atypical radiological images of pulmonary tuberculosis in 192 diabetic patients: a comparative study. Int J Tuberc Lung Dis 2001;5:455–461.
20 Shaikh MA, Singla R, Khan NB, Sharif NS, Saigh MO: Does diabetes alter the radiological presentation of pulmonary tuberculosis? Saudi Med J 2003;24:278–281.
21 Nissapatorn V, Kuppusamy I, Jamaiah I, Fong MY, Rohela M, Anuar AK: Tuberculosis in diabetic patients: a clinical perspective. Southeast Asian J Trop Med Public Health 2005;36(suppl 4):213–220.
22 Wang JY, Lee LN, Hsueh PR: Factors changing the manifestation of pulmonary tuberculosis. Int J Tuberc Lung Dis 2005;9:777–783.
23 Wang CS, Chen HC, Yang CJ, Chen HC, Chuang SH, Chong IW, Hwang JJ, Huang MS: Impact of type 2 diabetes on manifestations and treatment outcome of pulmonary tuberculosis. Epidemiol Infect 2009;137:203–210.
24 Alisjahbana B, van Crevel R, Sahiratmadja E, den Heijer M, Maya A, Istriana E, Danusantoso H, Ottenhoff TH, Nelwan RH, van der Meer JW: Diabetes mellitus is strongly associated with tuberculosis in Indonesia. Int J Tuberc Lung Dis 2006;10:696–700.
25 Venkatesan K: Pharmacokinetic drug interactions with rifampicin. Clin Pharmacokinet 1992;22:47–65.

26 Zilly W, Breimer DD, Richter E: Induction of drug metabolism in man after rifampicin treatment measured by increased hexobarbital and tolbutamide clearance. Eur J Clin Pharmacol 1975;9:219–227.
27 Syvälahti E, Pihlajamäki K, Iisalo E: Effect of tuberculostatic agents on the response of serum growth hormone and immunoreactive insulin to intravenous tolbutamide, and on the half-life of tolbutamide. Int J Clin Pharmacol Biopharm 1976;13:83–89.
28 Niemi M, Backman JT, Neuvonen M, Neuvonen PJ, Kivisto KT: Effects of rifampin on the pharmacokinetics and pharmacodynamics of glyburide and glipizide. Clin Pharmacol Ther 2001;69:400–406.
29 Park JY, Kim KA, Park PW, Park CW, Shin JG: Effect of rifampin on the pharmacokinetics and pharmacodynamics of gliclazide. Clin Pharmacol Ther 2003;74:334–340.
30 Niemi M, Kivisto KT, Backman JT, Neuvonen PJ: Effect of rifampicin on the pharmacokinetics and pharmacodynamics of glimepiride. Br J Clin Pharmacol 2000;50:591–595.
31 Niemi M, Backman JT, Neuvonen M, Neuvonen PJ, Kivisto KT: Rifampin decreases the plasma concentrations and effects of repaglinide. Clin Pharmacol Ther 2000;68:495–500.
32 Hatorp V, Hansen KT, Thomsen MS: Influence of drugs interacting with CYP3A4 on the pharmacokinetics, pharmacodynamics and safety of the prandial glucose regulator repaglinide. J Clin Pharmacol 2003;43:649–660.
33 Bidstrup TB, Stilling N, Damkier P, Scharling B, Thomsen MS, Brosen K: Rifampicin seems to act as both an inducer and an inhibitor of the metabolism of repaglinide. Eur J Clin Pharmacol 2004;60:109–114.
34 Niemi M, Backman JT, Fromm MF, Neuvonen PJ, Kivisto KT: Pharmacokinetic interactions with rifampicin: clinical relevance. Clin Pharmacokinet 2003;42:819–850.
35 Park JY, Kim KA, Kang MH, Kim SL, Shin JG: Effect of rifampin on the pharmacokinetics of rosiglitazone in healthy subjects. Clin Pharmacol Ther 2004;75:157–162.
36 Jaakkola T, Backman JT, Neuvonen M, Laitila J, Neuvonen PJ: Effect of rifampicin on the pharmacokinetics of pioglitazone. Br J Clin Pharmacol 2006;61:70–78.
37 Nathan DM, Buse JB, Davidson M, Ferrannini E, Holman RR, Sherwin R, Zinman B: Management of hyperglycemia in type 2 diabetes: a consensus algorithm for the initiation and adjustment of therapy: a consensus statement from the American Diabetes Association and the European Association for the Study of Diabetes. Diabetes Care 2009;23:193–203.
38 Blumberg HM, Burman WJ, Chaisson RE, Daley CL, Etkind SC, Friedman LN, Fujiwara P, Grzemska M, Hopewell PC, Iseman MD, Jasmer RM, Koppaka V, Menzies RI, O'Brien RJ, Reves RR, Reichman LB, Simone PM, Starke JR, Vernon AA: American Thoracic Society/Centers for Disease Control and Prevention/Infectious Diseases Society of America: treatment of tuberculosis. Am J Respir Crit Care Med 2003;167:603–662.
39 Mitchison DA: Role of individual drugs in the chemotherapy of tuberculosis. Int J Tuberc Lung Dis 2000;4:796–806.
40 Alisjahbana B, Sahiratmadja E, Nelwan EJ, Purwa AM, Ahmad Y, Ottenhoff TH, Nelwan RH, Parwati I, van der Meer JW, van Crevel R: The effect of type 2 diabetes mellitus on the presentation and treatment response of pulmonary tuberculosis. Clin Infect Dis 2007;45:428–435.
41 Wang CS, Chen HC, Yang CJ, Wang WY, Chong IW, Hwang JJ, Huang MS: The impact of age on the demographic, clinical, radiographic characteristics and treatment outcomes of pulmonary tuberculosis patients in Taiwan. Infection 2008;36:335–340.
42 Ridzon R, Whitney CG, McKenna MT, Taylor JP, Ashkar SH, Nitta AT, Harvey SM, Valway S, Woodley C, Cooksey R, Onorato IM: Risk factors for rifampin mono-resistant tuberculosis. Am J Respir Crit Care Med 1998;157:1881–1884.
43 Nijland HM, Ruslami R, Stalenhoef JE, Nelwan EJ, Alisjahbana B, Nelwan RH, van der Ven AJ, Danusantoso H, Aarnoutse RE, van Crevel R: Exposure to rifampicin is strongly reduced in patients with tuberculosis and type 2 diabetes. Clin Infect Dis 2006;43:848–854.
44 Ruslami R, Nijland HM, Adhiarta IG, Kariadi SH, Alisjahbana B, Aarnoutse RE, van Crevel R: Pharmacokinetics of antituberculosis drugs in pulmonary tuberculosis patients with type 2 diabetes. Antimicrob Agents Chemother 2010;54:1068–1074.
45 Burman WJ, Gallicano K, Peloquin C: Comparative pharmacokinetics and pharmacodynamics of the rifamycin antibacterials. Clin Pharmacokinet 2001;40:327–341.
46 Harries AD, Murray MB, Jeon CY, Ottmani SE, Lonnroth K, Barreto ML, Billo N, Brostrom R, Bygbjerg IC, Fisher-Hoch S, Mori T, Ramaiya K, Roglic G, Strandgaard H, Unwin N, Viswanathan V, Whiting D, Kapur A: Defining the research agenda to reduce the joint burden of disease from diabetes mellitus and tuberculosis. Trop Med Int Health 2010;15:659–663.
47 Pfaffenberg R, Jahler H: Isoniazid and recurrence of tuberculosis in diabetics. Z Tuberk 1958;111:167–173.
48 Lesnichii AV, Karpina LZ: Experience with the chemoprophylaxis of pulmonary tuberculosis in diabetes mellitus patients. Probl Tuberk 1969;47:1–3.
49 Ponce-de-Leon A, Garcia-Garcia ML, Garcia-Sancho MC, et al: Tuberculosis and diabetes in southern Mexico. Diabetes Care 2004;27:1584–1590.
50 Balde NM, Camara A, Camara LM, Diallo MM, Kake A, Bah-Sow OY: Associated tuberculosis and diabetes in Conakry, Guinea: prevalence and clinical characteristics. Int J Tuberc Lung Dis 2006;10:1036–1040.

Reinout van Crevel, MD, PhD
Department of Internal Medicine
Radboud University Nijmegen Medical Centre
NL–6500 HB Nijmegen (The Netherlands)
Tel. +31 243 618 822, E-Mail r.vancrevel@aig.umcn.nl

Donald PR, van Helden PD (eds): Antituberculosis Chemotherapy.
Prog Respir Res. Basel, Karger, 2011, vol 40, pp 213–219

# Early Bactericidal Activity of Antituberculosis Agents

Andreas H. Diacon[a] · J. Stefan Maritz[b] · Peter R. Donald[c]

DST/NRF Centre of Excellence for Biomedical TB Research/MRC Centre for Molecular and Cellular Biology, [a]Division of Molecular Biology and Human Genetics, [b]Division of Physiology, [c]Department of Paediatrics and Child Health, Faculty of Health Sciences, Stellenbosch University, Cape Town, South Africa

**Abstract**

The assessment of the early bactericidal activity (EBA) of antituberculosis agents by measurement of viable colony-forming units (CFU) of *Mycobacterium tuberculosis* in sputum of patients with smear-positive pulmonary tuberculosis is now an established methodology for the early clinical evaluation of a new antituberculosis agent. EBA establishes the daily rate at which a specific dose of a new agent reduces the number of viable bacilli present in sputum during the first 14 days of treatment. Simultaneous study of pharmacokinetics offers the opportunity to evaluate the relationship between dosage, serum concentration, efficacy and specific host or mycobacterial factors relevant to the agent under investigation. Recently the clinical efficacy of several new classes of antituberculosis agents has been confirmed by EBA studies, and these have shown these agents to have a relatively slow onset of detectable activity; by contrast, the newer fluoroquinolones have an EBA over days 0–2 comparable to that of isoniazid and may prove valuable in the prevention of resistance amongst companion drugs. Recent experience has shown that time to detection of metabolic activity in liquid media reflects drug activity in a manner comparable to that of CFU counting and needs further exploration.

Copyright © 2011 S. Karger AG, Basel

In 1980, Jindani et al. [1] published details of an assessment of the early bactericidal activity (EBA) of antituberculosis agents by measurement of the decline in viable colony-forming units (CFU) of *Mycobacterium tuberculosis* in the sputum of patients with sputum microscopy smear-positive pulmonary tuberculosis. During this study nearly all of the available antituberculosis agents were studied, either alone or in combination, during the first 14 days of therapy. A considerable amount of valuable information was generated which contributed to a better understanding of the actions of antituberculosis agents during early therapy. During the next 30 years, the technique has been refined and, in particular, relationships between the pharmacokinetics and pharmacodynamics of antituberculosis agents have been explored. This paper reviews the experience with EBA studies in the clinical assessment of new antituberculosis agents, in particular regarding the relationship between pharmacokinetics, pharmacogenetics and bactericidal activity. The results of the various EBA studies are expressed as the fall in $\log_{10}$ CFU per millilitre sputum per day with the number of days over which the study was conducted indicated as a postscript.

The most notable finding of the Jindani study was that the greatest difference between the activity of various drugs was evident during the first 2 days of treatment. During this period, for example, the EBA over 0–2 days ($EBA_{0-2}$) of isoniazid (INH) in a dose of 300 mg was 0.72, compared to those of ethambutol 25 mg/kg, rifampicin (RIF) 10 mg/kg and para-aminosalicylic acid 300 mg/kg which were 0.24, 0.19 and 0.26, respectively, while streptomycin and thiacetazone had values less than 0.10. During the period days 2–14, bactericidal activity continued at a slower rate for most drugs; a notable exception was pyrazinamide (PZA), where no activity was detected during the first 2–4 days of treatment but thereafter its activity was unrelenting leading to a total decrease in counts of 1.56 $\log_{10}$ CFU over the 14 days. One of the consequences of this finding was that most subsequent EBA studies were carried out over a 2-day treatment period. The second important finding was that, in the case of RIF and ethambutol, a dosage related response was evident, suggesting that the EBA technique could be used to select the most appropriate dosage of a drug for further evaluation and clinical use. In 1 patient receiving 150 mg INH, resistance to INH emerged on day 14; in no subsequent EBA study, whether conducted over 2, 7 or 14 days, has the emergence of resistance to a study drug been documented.

### Pharmacokinetics and Pharmacodynamics

Pharmacokinetics were not evaluated in this early study, but several later studies were coupled to an exploration of the pharmacokinetics of the relevant drug, and this is now an integral part of any EBA study of a new antituberculosis agent. In a Hong Kong study of the $EBA_{0-2}$ of RIF and rifabutin, RIF doses of 150, 300 and 600 mg were associated with mean 2-hour RIF serum concentrations of 1.96, 3.21 and 9.25 μg/ml, respectively, on the first day of the study [2]. RIF serum concentrations were also determined during a study in South Africa [3]. The same RIF doses yielded maximum concentration ($C_{max}$) values of 2.53, 3.19 and 13.0 μg/ml, respectively, on day 1 of treatment and by day 5, following induction of RIF metabolism, $C_{max}$ concentrations of 1.49, 2.89 and 9.53 μg/ml. The associated EBA results showed no activity at a dose of 150 mg, but for a dose of 300 mg an EBA of 0.16 in Hong Kong and 0.12 in South Africa and for a dose of 600 mg EBAs of 0.29 and 0.22, respectively. Thus, although a detectable EBA is associated with RIF serum $C_{max}$ values of approximately 3 μg/ml, a much higher EBA is associated with concentrations of approximately 9 μg/ml; this value falls within the suggested range of 8–24 μg/ml for desirable 2-hour RIF concentrations derived from experience with healthy volunteers and tuberculosis patients [4]. A recent EBA study explored the use of a RIF dose of 20 mg/kg [5]; the $C_{max}$ on the first day of treatment was 14.0 (SD 4.7) μg/ml, which was not significantly higher than that found previously after a RIF dose of 12 mg/kg [3]; however, the area under the curve $AUC_{0-\infty}$ on the first treatment day increased significantly from 100.1 (SEM 7.5) to 171(SD 56) μg/ml•h and the $EBA_{0-2}$ from approximately 0.22 to 0.44 (SD ±0.22) indicating that the currently recommended RIF dose range of 8–12 mg/kg may not offer optimal efficacy; further dose-ranging EBA, and other studies, with higher RIF doses are indicated.

Similar studies of the $EBA_{0-2}$ of INH in conjunction with pharmacokinetics and pharmacogenetics highlighted the potential importance of pharmacogenetics in response to antituberculosis drugs [6]. Determination of the N-acetyltransferase 2 genotype in conjunction with dose-ranging EBA studies showed that at a dose as low as 37.5 mg homozygous slow acetylators of INH still maintained an EBA of 0.11, while that of heterozygous and homozygous rapid acetylators was 0.01 and –0.09, respectively; at a dose of 75 mg homozygous slow acetylators had an EBA of 0.38 and heterozygous and homozygous rapid acetylators had 0.29 and 0.30, respectively. It was also noteworthy that no increase in EBA occurred above 2-hour serum concentrations (fig. 1) of approximately 2.5 μg/ml but that 50% of homozygous rapid acetylators of INH receiving an INH dose of 300 mg did not reach this concentration. In a later analysis of these data, it was shown that homozygous slow acetylators of INH receiving an INH dose of 3 mg/kg all reached a 2-hour INH serum concentration of 2.19 (SE 0.68) μg/ml associated with an EBA 90% of the mean maximum EBA ($EBA_{90}$) but that a dosage of 6 mg/kg was needed for homozygous rapid acetylators to reach $EBA_{90}$ [7].

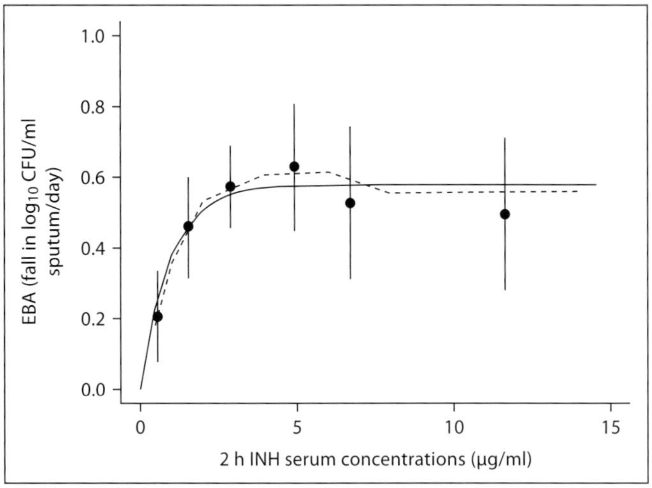


**Fig. 1.** An exponential regression illustrating the relationship between the 2-hour post-dose serum concentrations of INH and EBA on days 0–2.

The $EBA_{0-7}$ of the new fluoroquinolones moxifloxacin, gatifloxacin and levofloxacin and their associated pharmacokinetics were assessed in comparison to that of INH, but at only 1 dosage [8]. The results of this study are summarized in table 1. The relationship $AUC_{0-24}$/minimum inhibitory concentration (MIC) was also assessed and was positively correlated with $EBA_{0-2}$ for gatifloxacin, but not for levofloxacin and moxifloxacin, and no correlation was observed for the $EBA_{2-7}$. When the treatment groups were ranged according to AUC/MIC in order of magnitude, however, the

**Table 1.** The EBA and pharmacokinetics of 3 fluoroquinolones in patients with sputum smear-positive pulmonary tuberculosis

| Drug | Dose mg | Median $C_{max}$ µg/ml | $AUC_{0-24}$ µg/ml•h | $EBA_{0-2}$ $log_{10}$ CFU/ml/day | $EBA_{2-7}$ $log_{10}$ CFU/ml/day | Mean CFU slope on days 2–7 |
|---|---|---|---|---|---|---|
| LFX | 1,000 | 15.6 (8.6–43.0) | 129.1 (103.4–358.3) | 0.45 (0.45) | 0.18 (0.13) | 0.24 (0.12) |
| GFX | 400 | 4.8 (3.8–6.4) | 42.8 (31.7–51.0) | 0.35 (0.27) | 0.17 (0.13) | 0.27 (0.10) |
| MFX | 400 | 6.1 (4.5–9.0) | 55.3 (36.0–79.1) | 0.33 (0.39) | 0.17 (0.09) | 0.24 (0.17) |

Adapted from Johnson et al. [8]. Figures in parentheses are ranges or standard deviations. LFX = Levofloxacin; GFX = gatifloxacin; MFX = moxifloxacin.

same ranking was found for $EBA_{0-2}$ (INH < levofloxacin < moxifloxacin < gatifloxacin). In an interesting approach, the mean rates of fall (slopes of CFU counts) for the period 2–7 days were also calculated and although neither the $EBA_{2-7}$ nor the rates of fall in CFU differed, the rate for all of the quinolones pooled was greater than that for INH. This study has confirmed that the quinolones are thus far the only drug group to have an EBA comparable to that of INH.

### New Classes of Antituberculosis Agents

In 2005 the first new chemical class of antituberculosis agents introduced for more than 4 decades entered clinical evaluation; TMC207 is a diarylquinoline that inhibits ATP synthase, thus causing bacterial death [9]. TMC207 was used at 3 dosages in an EBA study conducted over 7 days, and its action was compared to that of INH and RIF [10]. Interestingly the bactericidal activity of TMC207, like that of PZA, became apparent only on treatment day 4, but thereafter matched that of INH and RIF; while the fall in CFU counts from baseline values was not significant for the lower 25-mg and 100-mg doses, that for the 400-mg dose was significant from day 4 onwards resulting in a total fall of 0.77 $log_{10}$ CFU. The pharmacokinetic data showed that TMC exposure was linearly related to dosage, but that steady state was not reached within the 7-day study period. The results of this study stimulated a reconsideration of the duration of EBA studies, and a number of subsequent studies have been conducted over 14 days.

PA-824 is a promising nitro-imidazo-oxazine that during in vitro and in vivo animal studies showed good antituberculosis activity and characteristics that suggested that it might contribute to early sterilization of tuberculosis lesions and thus treatment shortening. During a 14-day EBA study doses of 200, 600, 1,000 and 1,200 mg were evaluated, and surprisingly all showed a similar bactericidal activity [11]. Also, as was the case with TMC207, activity did not become significant until day 3. Thus the $EBA_{0-2}$ was only 0.047 (SD 0.37), but for days 2–14 it was 0.106 (SD 0.077). Pharmacokinetics were also examined during this study and showed a dose-linear, but less than dose-proportional increase in serum concentrations at doses from 200 to 1,000 mg, but with no additional drug exposure after the 1,200 mg dose in comparison to the 1,000 mg dose. This result implies that it may be possible to use a relatively low dose of PA-824 associated with lower costs and less risk of toxicity; lower doses of PA-824 are now being studied to determine the dose to take forward into further clinical evaluation.

Delamanid (DLM), previously known as OPC-67683, is a nitro-dihydro-imidazo-oxazole derivative that inhibits mycolic acid synthesis; it has a very low minimum inhibitory concentration (range 0.006–0.024 µg/ml) and good activity against intracellular *M. tuberculosis* [12]. In murine experiments DLM in combination with RIF and PZA caused a much more rapid sterilization of lung tissue (within 3 months) than the standard regimen of INH, RIF, PZA and ethambutol. During an EBA study, DLM, as with PZA, TMC207 and PA-824, had a delayed onset of action, but satisfactory bactericidal activity thereafter [13].

In another recent study the $EBA_{0-7}$ of the oxazolidinone linezolid (LZD) given as 600 mg once or twice daily was compared to that of INH 300 mg [14]. The mean $EBA_{0-2}$ of INH (0.67, SD 0.35) was greater than that of LZD once daily (0.18, SD 0.27) or twice daily (0.26, SD 0.42). The $EBA_{2-7}$ for INH was 0.16 (SD 0.11) and that for LZD once or twice daily 0.09 (SD 0.17) and 0.04 (SD 0.11), and the relevant slopes of fall in CFU on days 2–7, 0.13 (SD 0.16), 0.06 (SD 0.16) and 0.06 (SD 0.08), respectively. The authors comment that although the study suggests that once daily LZD dosing may be sufficient for the treatment of tuberculosis this

**Table 2.** Culture positivity for *M. tuberculosis* in sputum specimens following culture on solid media or liquid media

| Authors | Culture media | n | Smear+, % | | n | Smear–, % | | Contamination, % | |
|---|---|---|---|---|---|---|---|---|---|
| | | | L | S | | L | S | L | S |
| Anargyros et al. [15], 1990 | BACTEC TB | 46 | 98 | | 16 | 88 | | 5 | |
| | LJ | | | 67 | | | 69 | | 3.3 |
| Abe et al. [16], 1992 | BACTEC | 37 | 97.3 | | 12 | 91.7 | | 0.8 | |
| | MB check | | 100 | | | 83.3 | | 0.4 | |
| | Ogawa | | | 89.2 | | | 50 | | 5.3 |
| Badak et al. [17], 1996 | MGIT | 93 | 94.6 | | 85 | 75.2 | | 5.6 | |
| | BACTEC | | 95.7 | | | 72.9 | | 3.9 | |
| | LJ | | | 93.5 | | | 58.8 | | 6.7 |
| Pfyffer et al. [18], 1997 | MGIT | 70 | 88.6 | | 110 | 68.2 | | 2.0–13.8 | |
| | BACTEC | | 95.7 | | | 82.7 | | 2.4–12.4 | |
| | LJ | | | 85.7 | | | 59.1 | | 8–9.2 |
| Chew et al. [19], 1998 | MGIT | 46 | 93 | | 15 | 87 | | 4.1 | |
| | BACTEC | | 98 | | | 93 | | 3.0 | |
| | LJ | | | 100 | | | 80 | | 4.1 |
| Somskövi and Magyar [20], 1999 | MGIT | 22 | 100 | | 90 | 76.6 | | 4.3 | |
| | MB Redox | | 95.5 | | | 66.6 | | 3.9 | |
| | LJ | | | 95.5 | | | 56.6 | | 2.1 |
| | Middlebrook | | | 95.5 | | | 52.2 | | 2.7 |

L = Liquid culture; LJ = Löwenstein-Jensen; S = solid medium; MGIT = mycobacteria growth indicator tube.

would not necessarily prevent the development of peripheral neuropathy.

## Alternative Methodologies to Evaluate Bactericidal Activity

Quantification of sputum CFU is now established as a method for evaluating the activity of a new antituberculosis drug; nonetheless the method is labour intensive, and requires the use of specialized laboratory facilities and experienced, qualified staff. With the accelerating availability of new antituberculosis agents there is a need for a methodology that could also be used in less sophisticated environments where tuberculosis patients can be more readily recruited for appropriate studies. There is thus considerable interest in alternative methodologies that might reflect the bactericidal activity of an agent in the same manner as sputum-viable CFU counting.

Liquid medium has become an increasingly popular means for culture of *M. tuberculosis* from clinical specimens. In the case of sputum a number of studies, summarized in table 2, have shown it to be more sensitive than solid medium culture, and this relatively greater sensitivity is especially evident in sputum microscopy smear-negative specimens. Several studies have demonstrated that time to detection (TTD) of critical metabolic activity correlates with outcome in pulmonary tuberculosis patients [21, 22] and is also correlated with CFU counts [23].

Against this background it has been hypothesized that there are 4 populations of mycobacteria within tuberculosis lesions that vary in the speed with which they grow and metabolize [24]. These populations are:

(A) a large population of rapidly metabolizing bacilli found in the walls of cavities that is killed mainly by INH; as the growth rate of surviving bacilli slows, so does the efficacy of INH;

(B) a population of more slowly metabolizing organisms found in an acid environment that are specifically killed by PZA;

(C) a population of intermittently metabolizing bacilli that are preferentially killed by the rapid onset of the action of RIF;

(D) a population of dormant organisms that are not killed by any existing drug.

It has also been demonstrated that in vitro bacilli gradually exposed to increasingly micro-aerophilic conditions undergo several phases of shift-down to a non-replicating form that enables them to persist dormant, but still viable within a tuberculosis lesion [25]. A further hypothesis proposes that at least 3 subpopulations of bacilli can be found within 100-day-old cultures exposed to conditions that mimic those within the necrotic lesions of pulmonary tuberculosis [26].

(A) The largest population (approx. $4 \times 10^7$/ml) cannot grow on solid media but can grow in liquid media. These bacilli are also susceptible to RIF, and it was proposed that this population forms part of the heterogeneous populations present in sputum at the start of chemotherapy and to an increasing extent later into therapy and that this would account 'for the greater sensitivity of liquid medium than that of solid medium in culture of sputum'.

(B) A population of approximately $7 \times 10^5$/ml is able to grow on solid media and is killed by RIF faster than by INH.

(C) A small population of $1 \times 10^3$/ml is unable to grow on solid media and can survive exposure to RIF.

Following chronic 10-month infections in the mouse, the same group of researchers [27] identified a large population of bacilli that grew only in broth cultures and not on 7H11 solid agar medium. This population was likened to the majority of mycobacteria present in old stationary phase cultures that will grow in broth cultures, but not on solid media. It is proposed that the proportion of the bacilli that have gone into a dormant or slowly replicating phase might be measured as the proportion of a population that will grow in broth but not on plates.

It is unclear how the above hypotheses and the increased sensitivity of liquid media in the face of more indolent mycobacterial cultures might impact on the measurement of EBA compared to the standard CFU counting on solid media. It is also likely that liquid media will remain culture positive longer into treatment. With ongoing duration of treatment, however, the bacterial populations present in sputum will tend to be less actively metabolizing and grow less well on solid culture media, but more readily in liquid culture.

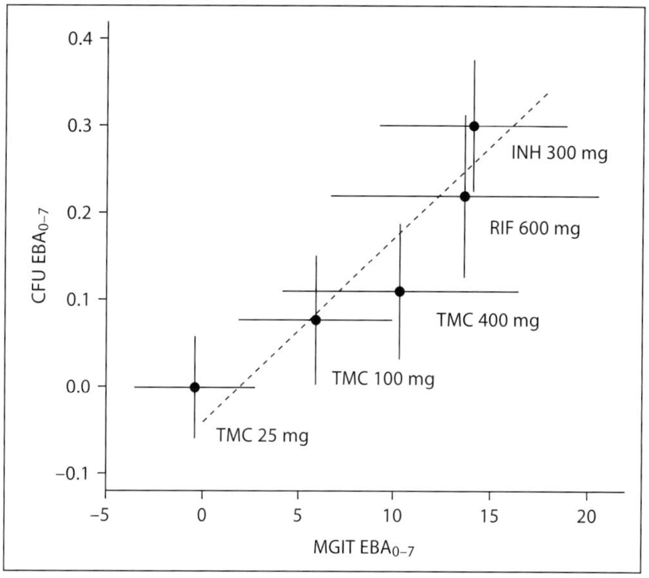


**Fig. 2.** The mean early bactericidal activity (EBA) of the investigational drug TMC207 (TMC), isoniazid (INH) and rifampicin (RIF) measured over days 0-7 of treatment by the daily fall in logCFU/mL sputum/day plotted against mean EBA measured by prolongation of time in hours to detection (TTD) of critical metabolic activity in MGIT with ±1.4(SE) limits. For illustration, a line is drawn at a perfect correlation of r=1. A value below that line suggests a higher EBA value when measured in liquid media in MGIT by TTD for that group; values above that line suggest a higher EBA value when measured on solid media by the fall in logCFU counts. CFU = Colony forming units; MGIT = mycobacteria growth indicator tube.

Since 2004 several EBA studies have been conducted with mycobacterial activity measured by TTD as well as conventional CFU counting [10, 28]. Amongst a subgroup of patients participating in a 7-day EBA study with different doses of the investigational agent TMC207, as well as INH and RIF as positive controls, there was a significant linear correlation between diminishing individual log CFU (from solid media) and increasing TTD (in liquid media) [28]. Figure 2 shows that the $EBA_{0-7}$ ranking of the agents by both methodologies is similar. The figure also illustrates the reason why assessing both log CFU on solid media as well as TTD in liquid media might be an interesting measurement in EBA studies. The straight line inserted theoretically separates groups above it, with higher EBA when measured with log CFU (solid media), or below it with higher EBA when measured with TTD (liquid media). In the example shown all confidence intervals intersect the line, which indicates that this differentiation has no statistical significance in this example; both methods measure a similar degree of activity of the compounds tested. However, the number of patients in this subanalysis was relatively small, and it is too early to state with certainty what roles assessment by TTD and log CFU can have for the determination of EBA. The similar ranking of the different agents and doses in this substudy is encouraging.

Several molecular markers of response to treatment have been evaluated and shown promise of augmenting or replacing CFU counting. These include the polymerase chain reaction (PCR) [29], measurement of sputum *M. tuberculosis* messenger RNA (mRNA) [30, 31] and monitoring of the induction of *M. tuberculosis* antigen 85 [32]. While PCR has had some success as a means of diagnosing tuberculosis after treatment initiation, PCR may be positive in sputum a considerable period after sputum cultures become negative. mRNA by contrast is a marker of cell viability and quantitative assay of gene targets, such as that for the glyoxylate cycle enzyme isocitrate lyase, has documented a decline in response to antituberculosis chemotherapy that parallels that of the decline in sputum CFU and may well prove useful in drug evaluation [31].

## Conclusion

The determination of EBA is now established as a first step in the clinical evaluation of a new antituberculosis agent; enrolling a relatively small number of patients with smear-positive pulmonary tuberculosis it confirms that the new agent is actually killing mycobacteria as reflected in the fall in CFU in sputum; it enables the evaluation of the efficacy of a new agent in relation to dosage and pharmacokinetics and pharmacogenetics and thus aids the selection of an appropriate dose to take forward to the next stage of clinical evaluation; finally it offers the opportunity for a close, intensive evaluation of toxicity in a small group of hospitalized patients. The value and place of other simultaneous investigations remains uncertain. Determination of TTD probably provides much the same information as CFU counting, but this must still be shown in a greater number of patients, before TTD can replace sputum CFU counting; TTD may also augment CFU counting if it can be shown that the use of TTD will reveal the killing of a specific population of bacilli that will grow only in liquid media and which might reflect the sterilizing capacity of a new agent.

## References


1 Jindani A, Aber V, Edwards EA, Mitchison DA: The early bactericidal activity of drugs in patients with pulmonary tuberculosis. Am Rev Respir Dis 1980;121; 939–949.

2 Chan SL, Yew WW, Ma WK, Girling DJ, Aber VR, Felmingham D, Allen BW, Mitchison DA: The early bactericidal activity of rifabutin measured by sputum viable counts in Hong Kong patients with pulmonary tuberculosis. Tuber Lung Dis 1992;73:33–38.

3 Sirgel FA, Fourie PB, Donald PR, Padayatchi N, Rustomjee R, Levin J, Roscigno G, Norman J, McIlleron H, Mitchison DA, Rifapentine EBA Collaborative Study Group: The early bactericidal activities of rifampin and rifapentine in pulmonary tuberculosis. Am J Respir Crit Care Med 2005;172:128–135.

4 Peloquin CA: Therapeutic drug monitoring: principles and application in mycobacterial infections. Drug Ther 1992;22:31–36.

5 Diacon AH, Patientia RF, Venter A, van Helden PD, Smith PJ, McIlleron H: Early bactericidal activity of high dose rifampin in patients with pulmonary tuberculosis evidenced by positive sputum smears. Antimicrob Agents Chemother 2007;51:2994–2996.

6 Donald PR, Sirgel FA, Venter A, Parkin DP, Seifart HI, van de Wal BW, Werely C, van Helden PD, Maritz JS: The influence of human N-acetyltransferase genotype on the early bactericidal activity of isoniazid. Clin Infect Dis 2004;39:1425–1430.

7 Donald PR, Parkin DP, Seifart HI, Schaaf HS, van Helden PD, Werely CJ, Sirgel FA, Venter A, Maritz JS: The influence of dose and N-acetyltransferase-2 (NAT2) genotype and phenotype on the pharmacokinetics and pharmacodynamics of isoniazid. Eur J Clin Pharmacol 2007;63:633–639.

8 Johnson JL, Hadad DJ, Boom WH, Daley CL, Peloquin CA, Eisenach KD, Jankus DD, Debanne SM, Charlebois ED, Maciel E, Palaci M, Dietze R: Early and extended bactericidal activity of levofloxacin, gatifloxacin and moxifloxacin in pulmonary tuberculosis. Int J Tuberc Lung Dis 2006;10:605–612.

9 Andries K, Verhasselt P, Guillemont J, Göhlmann HW, Neefs JM, Winkler H, van Gestel J, Timmerman P, Zhu M, Lee E, Williams P, de Chaffoy D, Huitric E, Hoffner S, Cambau E, Truffot-Pernot C, Lounis N, Jarlier V: A diarylquinoline drug active on the ATP synthase of *Mycobacterium tuberculosis*. Science 2005;307:223–227.

10 Rustomjee R, Diacon AH, Allen J, Venter A, Reddy C, Patientia RF, Mthiyane TC, de Marez T, van Heeswijk R, Kerstens R, Koul A, de Beule K, Donald PR, McNeeley DF: Early bactericidal activity and pharmacokinetics of the diarylquinoline TMC207 in treatment of pulmonary tuberculosis. Antimicrob Agents Chemother 2008;52:2831–2835.

11 Diacon AH, Dawson R, Hanekom M, Narunsky K, Maritz SJ, Venter A, Donald PR, van Niekerk C, Whitney K, Rouse DJ, Laurenzi MW, Ginsberg AM, Spigelman MK: Early bactericidal activity and pharmacokinetics of PA-824 in smear-positive tuberculosis patients. Antimicrob Agents Chemother 2010;54:3402–3407.

12 Matsumoto M, Hashizume H, Tomishige T, Kawasaki M, Tsubouchi H, Sasaki H, Shimokawa Y, Komatsu M: OPC-67683, a nitro-dihydro-imidazooxazole derivative with promising action against tuberculosis in vitro and in mice. PLoS Med 2006;3:e466.

13 Diacon AH, Dawson R, Hanekom M, Narunsky K, Venter A, Hittel N, Geiter LJ, Wells C, Paccaly AJ, Donald PR: Early bactericidal activity of delamanid (OPC-67683) in smear-positive pulmonary tuberculosis patients. Int J Tuberc Lung Dis, in press.

14 Dietze R, Hadad DJ, McGee B, Molino LP, Maciel EL, Peloquin CA, Johnson DF, Debanne SM, Eisenach K, Boom WH, Palaci M, Johnson JL: Early and extended bactericidal activity of linezolid in pulmonary tuberculosis. Am J Respir Crit Care Med 2008;178:1180–1185.
15 Anargyros P, Astill DSJ, Lim ISL: Comparison of improved BACTEC and Lowenstein-Jensen media for culture of mycobacteria from clinical specimens. J Clin Microbiol 1990;28:1288–1291.
16 Abe C, Hosojima S, Fukasawa Y, Kazumi Y, Takahashi M, Hirano K, Mori T: Comparison of MB-Check BACTEC and egg-based media for recovery of mycobacteria. J Clin Micobiol 1992;30:878–881.
17 Badak FZ, Kiska DL, Setterquist S, Hartley C, O'Connel MA, Hopfer RL: Comparison of mycobacteria growth indicator tube with BACTEC 460 for detection and recovery of mycobacteria from clinical specimens. J Clin Microbiol 1996;34:2236–2239.
18 Pfyffer GE, Wlescher H-M, Kissling P, Cieslak C, Casal MJ, Gutierrez J, Rüsch-Gerdes S: Comparison of the mycobacteria growth indicator tube (MGIT) with radiometric and solid culture for recovery of acid-fast bacilli. J Microbiol 1997;35:364–368.
19 Chew WK, Lasaitis RM, Schio FA, Gilbert GL: Clinical evaluation of the mycobacterial growth indicator tube (MGIT) compared with radiometric (BACTEC) and solid media for isolation of *Mycobacterium* species. J Med Microbiol 1998;47:821–827.
20 Somskövi Á, Magyar P: Comparison of the mycobacteria growth indicator tube with MB Redox, Löwenstein-Jensen and Mddlebrook 7H11 media for recovery of mycobacteria in clinical specimens. J Clin Microbiol 1999;37:1366–1369.
21 Hesseling AC, Walzl G, Enarson DA, Carroll NM, Duncan K, Lukey PT, Lombard C, Donald PR, Lawrence KA, Gie RP, van Helden PD, Beyers N: Baseline sputum time to detection predicts month two culture conversion and relapse in non-HIV-infected patients. Int J Tuberc Lung Dis 2010;14:560–570.
22 Epstein MD, Schluger NW, Davidow AL, Bonk S, Rom WN, Hanna B: Time to detection of *Mycobacterium tuberculosis* in sputum culture correlates with outcome in patients receiving treatment for pulmonary tuberculosis. Chest 1998;113:379- 386.
23 Pheiffer C, Carrol NM, Beyers N, Donald P, Duncan K, Uys P, van Helden P: Time to detection of *Mycobacterium tuberculosis* in BACTEC systems as a viable alternative to colony counting. Int J Tuberc Lung Dis 2008;12:792–798.
24 Mitchison DA: Basic mechanisms of chemotherapy. Chest 1979;76(suppl): 771–781.
25 Wayne LG, Hayes LG: An in vitro model for sequential study of shiftdown of *Mycobacterium tuberculosis* through two stages of nonreplicating persistence. Infect Immun 1996;64:2062–2069.
26 Mitchison DA, Coates ARM: Predictive in vitro models of the sterilizing activity of antituberculosis drugs. Curr Pharm Des 2004;10:3285–3295.
27 Dhillon J, Lowrie DB, Mitchison DA: *Mycobacterium tuberculosis* from chronic murine infection grows in liquid but not on solid media. BMC Infect Dis 2004;4:51.
28 Diacon AH, Maritz JS, Venter A, van Helden PD, Andries K, McNeeley DF, Donald PR: Time to detection of the growth of *Mycobacterium tuberculosis* in MGIT 960 for determining the early bactericidal activity of antituberculosis agents. Eur J Microbiol Clin Med 2010;29:1561–1565.
29 Kennedy N, Gillespie SH, Saruni AOS, Kisyombe G, McNerney R, Ngowi FI, Wilson S: Polymerase chain reaction for assessing treatment response in patients with pulmonary tuberculosis. J Infect Dis 1994;170:713–716.
30 Desjardin LE, Perkins MD, Wolski K, Haun S, Teixeira L, Chen Y, Johnson JL, Ellner JJ, Dietze R, Bates J, Cave D, Eisenach KD: Measurement of sputum *Mycobacterium tuberculosis* messenger RNA as a surrogate for response to chemotherapy. Am J Respir Crit Care Med 1999;160:203–210.
31 Li L, Mahan CS, Palaci M, Horter L, Loeffelholz L, Johnson JL, Dietze R, Debanne SM, Joloba ML, Okwera A, Boom WH, Eisenach KD: Sputum *Mycobacterium tuberculosis* mRNA as a marker of bacteriologic clearance in response to antituberculosis therapy. J Clin Microbiol 2010;48:46–51.
32 Wallis RS, Phillips M, Johnson JL, Teixeira L, Rocha LM, Maciel E, Rose L, Wells C, Palaci M, Dietze R, Eisenach K, Ellner JJ: Inhibition of isoniazid-induced expression of *Mycobacterium tuberculosis* antigen 85 in sputum: potential surrogate marker in tuberculosis chemotherapy trials. Antimicrob Agents Chemother 2001;45:1302–1304.

Prof. P.R. Donald
Paediatrics and Child Health
Faculty of Health Sciences
Stellenbosch University
PO Box 19063, Tygerberg 7505 (South Africa)
Tel. +27 21 9389 592, E-Mail prd@sun.ac.za

Donald PR, van Helden PD (eds): Antituberculosis Chemotherapy.
Prog Respir Res. Basel, Karger, 2011, vol 40, pp 220–226

# Assessment of Whole-Blood Bactericidal Activity in the Evaluation of New Antituberculosis Drugs

Robert S. Wallis

Pfizer, Groton, Conn., USA

## Abstract

Intracellular mycobacterial subpopulations with altered metabolism and reduced replication arise in vivo as a result of pressure from host immune mechanisms. These subpopulations, which show altered susceptibility to the action of antituberculosis (anti-TB) drugs, play an important role in mycobacterial persistence and TB relapse. This paper describes the use of whole-blood cultures infected ex vivo with *Mycobacterium tuberculosis* to assess the effectiveness of administered anti-TB treatment against non-replicating persisters. Studies in TB patients have shown that cumulative whole-blood bactericidal activity is indirectly linked to outcome, and that drug activity in the ex vivo cultures is modulated by the intracellular immune milieu. Three studies in healthy volunteers have used the method for dose selection and regimen optimization. Further research in TB patients is warranted to explore the potential role of this method in accelerating the development of new TB drugs and regimens.

Copyright © 2011 S. Karger AG, Basel

Distinct subpopulations of *Mycobacterium tuberculosis* exist in patients with active tuberculosis (TB). These organisms differ in metabolism, gene expression profiles, rates of replication and other functional characteristics. Although these subpopulations can arise at random in small numbers in otherwise uniform bacterial populations, their numbers increase greatly in response to specific stresses created by the host immune response, often in distinct anatomical locations. These adaptations facilitate specific stages of the mycobacterial life cycle. For example, large numbers of metabolically active, replicating bacilli within caseous material in cavities are required for efficient aerosolization and transmission, whereas semidormant bacilli sequestered in hypoxic granulomas make possible persistence, reactivation and relapse. Current TB drugs act differentially on these subpopulations [1]. Isoniazid, for example, acts primarily on replicating, aerobic, extracellular bacilli, whereas rifampicin appears equally active against both replicating and semidormant bacilli. Pyrazinamide requires low pH, found within granulomas and in macrophages after phagosome-lysosomal fusion, for its activity to be expressed [2]. Certain subpopulations can also emerge in response to specific stresses induced by drug treatments. Thus, the critical unit in TB is an unusually complex triad that includes host, pathogen and therapy-related elements.

The existence of sequestered mycobacterial subpopulations poses a challenge for drug developers and clinicians who wish to meaningfully assess the therapeutic potential of a new drug or regimen. Monitoring tissue sterilization and predicting relapse risk can presently be accomplished only by measuring either rates of relapse after completion of therapy or by proportions with sputum culture conversion after 2 months of treatment [3]. These end points have relatively large sample size requirements, and in most circumstances cannot be used to study single new drugs. Measurement of serial sputum colony counts during the first several weeks of therapy has been proposed as an alternative end point, based on a retrospective analysis of 34 subjects enrolled in separate trials of isoniazid/rifampicin/ethambutol/pyrazinamide and streptomycin/isoniazid [4]. These 2 regimens, which differ substantially in the duration of treatment required for cure (6 vs. 18 months), differed significantly in their effects on log colony counts from days 2 to 28 (–0.163 vs. –0.095 log/day). The serial sputum colony count was measured prospectively in the OFLOTUB phase II study, which found moxifloxacin- and gatifloxacin-containing regimens to be superior to standard therapy (–0.169 and –0.166 log/day, respectively, vs. –0.134) [5]. The effects of moxifloxacin and gatifloxacin on 2-month conversion and relapse rates remain to be determined, as studies to date have been contradictory [5–8]. These observations indicate an urgent need for other methods that can be used to efficiently evaluate the sterilizing activity of new compounds and regimens in early clinical trials.

## Rationale

The ex vivo whole-blood model is an alternative strategy to measure drug effects on otherwise elusive but critical microbial subpopulations that arise in the context of the host immune response. The approach benefits from the simplicity of whole-blood culture to study cellular immune function. Whole-blood cultures consist of blood collected in a heparinized tube that is diluted with an equal volume of tissue culture medium, to which a microbe or other immune stimulus is added. Mycobacteria added to the cultures rapidly undergo essentially complete phagocytosis by neutrophils and monocytes [9, 10]. Mycobacterial antigens are processed, expressed and recognized by CD4, CD8, natural killer, γδ and other lymphocytes. Cytokines, adhesion ligands, activation markers and effector molecules are expressed, resulting in restriction of mycobacterial replication. The extent of mycobacterial growth or killing in whole-blood culture therefore reflects the balance between microbial pathogenicity and host immune mechanisms. In healthy donors negative for the tuberculin skin test, for example, the time required for doubling of *M. tuberculosis* H37Rv is increased to over 34 h from the usual 18–20 h in simple broth culture. Superior restriction of growth is evident in blood of subjects positive for the tuberculin skin test. The balance between host and pathogen can be shifted by removal of CD4 or CD8 T cells, addition of prednisolone, tumour necrosis factor antibodies or dihydroxyvitamin D [9–12]. Growth inhibition in whole-blood culture has improved in clinical trials in which patients were vaccinated with bacille Calmette-Guérin or given oral vitamin D supplementation, or in AIDS patients following initiation of antiretroviral therapy [13–15].

Of greatest relevance to this review is the finding that whole-blood cultures of patients with newly diagnosed active TB are capable of full restriction of growth of virulent clinical isolates, including the patient's own strain [16, 17]. This presumably reflects the influence of antigen-driven in vivo expansion and activation of *M. tuberculosis*-reactive T cells. The resulting bacteriostasis can therefore serve to model the killing of non-replicating *M. tuberculosis* by a single drug or by drug combinations in vitro as it occurs in granulomas in vivo. This differs fundamentally from simple macrophage cultures, which are generally very permissive of intracellular mycobacterial replication.

Drug levels in whole-blood culture reflect those in the blood at the time of phlebotomy. By collecting blood samples at various intervals before and after dosing, the full magnitude of therapeutic effects can be determined as drug concentrations rise and fall due to absorption, distribution, metabolism and elimination. The parameter of greatest interest is therefore the area under the curve over 24 h of dosing.

## Technical Aspects

Fresh blood with viable cells is required. Blood can be collected in heparin-containing Vacutainers (BD) or similar prefilled tubes. Sodium heparin is preferred, though lithium may be acceptable. Other anticoagulants such as acid-citrate-dextrose adversely affect cell function and should not be used. A total volume of approximately 1 ml blood per time point is sufficient. The specific times and number of time points depend on the kinetics of the drugs to be studied, but generally at least 4 and even better 5 are preferred. Sampling at the same time points for assessment of pharmacokinetics is desirable, as it facilitates additional analyses of the pharmacokinetic/pharmacodynamic relationship. Practical considerations favour reserving samples for transport as a batch to the laboratory for processing by mid-afternoon. For drugs administered once daily in the morning, this can be facilitated by collecting specimens for later time points the prior evening. While awaiting transport, tubes are maintained at room temperature with slow constant rotation. Variability was increased in baseline (pretreatment) samples in 1 study in which samples were stored on a table top without mixing. Sixteen hours is the maximum recommended duration of such temporary storage.

Cultures are performed in sealed 2-ml tubes that are rotated slowly during incubation. The slow mixing enhances immune restriction of mycobacterial growth. At the conclusion of the period of incubation (usually 72 h), cells are pelleted. The supernatant is removed and may be reserved for analysis of induced cytokines. Sterile distilled water is added to lyse red blood cells. The cells are pelleted again, and the liquid phase is again removed. The remaining pellet is resuspended in a small volume of 7H9 broth and added to a mycobacterial growth indicator tube (MGIT, Becton Dickinson). MGIT time to positivity (TTP) is recorded. In early studies, BACTEC culture bottles were used instead. Mycobacterial growth in BACTEC bottles is measured daily as production of $^{14}CO_2$ from radiolabelled palmitic acid. A subsequent study has shown a high correlation between TTP in BACTEC and MGIT. The disadvantages of the BACTEC system are its requirements that $^{14}CO_2$ production by each culture must be measured daily, and that each completed culture must be disposed of in a manner appropriate for low-level radioisotopes.

The MGIT 960 system has largely replaced BACTEC in clinical mycobacteriology laboratories. MGIT tubes contain Middlebrook 7H9 liquid media plus an oxygen-quenched fluorochrome (tris-4,7-diphenyl-1,10-phenonthroline ruthenium chloride pentahydrate) embedded in silicone at the bottom of the tube. Bacterial growth within the tube results in depletion of free oxygen, which in turn results in fluorescence within the MGIT tube when visualized under UV light. The intensity of fluorescence is directly proportional to the extent of oxygen depletion. MGIT tubes placed in an MGIT 960 instrument are maintained at 37°C and monitored every 60 min for increasing fluorescence. The instrument declares a culture positive if either it reaches a predetermined level of fluorescence or if it shows a rapid rate of increase in fluorescence. Cultures of *M. tuberculosis* generally have $10^5$–$10^6$ CFU/ ml medium at the time they are declared positive, although cultures with large inocula may be declared positive earlier. MGIT TTP is highly inversely related to the CFU count of the inoculum (fig. 1). The main advantage of the MGIT system (aside from its automation) is that results are not affected by bacterial clumping and therefore show reduced variability. A secondary advantage is that the read-out has a wide dynamic range (at least $10^5$) such that measurement of serially diluted specimens is not necessary.

Haemoglobin can interfere with detection of growth in the MGIT, both by increasing the starting oxygen content in the culture tube and by interfering with UV light transmission. However, the starting volume of blood in each whole-blood culture is small (300 μl), and a sufficient proportion of haemoglobin is removed by the red blood cell lysis step to prevent its interference with the MGIT system. The lysis step also reduces the amount of drug carried over from the completed whole-blood culture into the MGIT tube.

MGIT tubes are also used to prepare the inoculum and determine the appropriate volume for inoculation of whole-blood cultures. This has the advantage that cultures are at

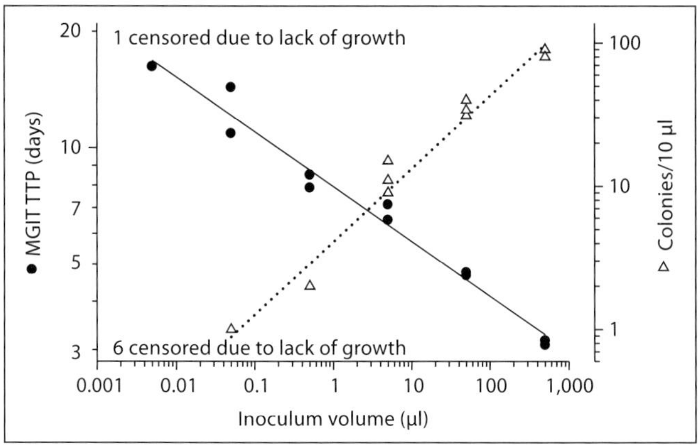


**Fig. 1.** Relationship between MGIT TTP and CFU count.

a relatively early stage of growth when harvested, resulting in reduced bacterial clumping. In one study, this method reduced the variability among replicate cultures by half. The approach also facilitates the study of killing of unique patient isolates if desired. The inoculum size is specified as that calculated to be positive in 4.5 or 5.5 days in various experiments, based on the titration curve. In one experiment, changes as much as 50-fold in inoculum size had no effect on the extent of bactericidal activity [10].

## Data Analysis

Logarithmic change in viability in each whole-blood culture is calculated as log(final) – log(initial), where 'final' and 'initial' are the volumes corresponding to TTP of the completed culture and its inoculum, respectively, based on a titration curve of the mycobacterial stock. Results are expressed on a log scale, with zero indicating bacteriostasis, and negative values killing. In recent studies, results have been calculated as log change per day of whole-blood culture. In early studies, results were expressed simply as log change for the entire 3-day duration of culture. Those results here have been divided by 3 days for consistency in presentation.

Bactericidal activity in vivo varies as drug concentration rise and fall during the dosing interval. These changes are not mirrored in individual whole-blood cultures, each of which reflects levels in blood at the moment of phlebotomy. To better understand the total extent of killing throughout dosing, static values are integrated over time to determine the cumulative or total extent of killing throughout a 24-hour interval, equal to the area under the curve over 24 h.

The units of this parameter are Δlog/day • day or simply log change. These data may be presented in tabular form or illustrated as they evolve during the dosing interval, in which case they have the appearance of a dynamic time-kill curve. The data differ from a typical dynamic time-kill experiment, however, in that postantibiotic effects (PAEs) are not represented. PAEs can delay the resumption of bacterial growth in vivo as drug concentrations fall. The lack of a PAE in the whole-blood model would be expected to result in underestimation of the cumulative whole-blood bactericidal activity (WBA) of drugs with long PAEs such as the rifamycins, but would be anticipated to have little or no effect on the measurement of activity of others such as linezolid with short PAEs [18, 19].

### Studies in Tuberculosis Patients

One WBA trial has been conducted to date in patients with pulmonary tuberculosis [16]. In that study, WBA was evaluated in 36 patients with fully drug-sensitive disease treated with daily standard 4-drug therapy (isoniazid/rifampicin/ethambutol/pyrazinamide). Each patient was studied with his or her own isolate, in week 8 (during the intensive 4-drug phase of treatment) and in week 12 (during the continuation phase). Blood was sampled for WBA determination 0, 2 and 6 h after dose. Bactericidal activity was present throughout the dosing interval during both the intensive and continuation phases. Peak activity was evident 2 h after dose (–1.6 to –2.0 log/day), when plasma drug concentrations were maximal. Minimal bactericidal activity was detected immediately before dose during the continuation phase; this time point was superior during the intensive phase (–0.25 vs. –0.08 log/day), presumably reflecting the long intracellular half-life of pyrazinamide.

Cumulative WBA for the 24-hour dosing interval was calculated assuming that at steady state values at 0 and 24 h were equal. Cumulative WBA was greater during the intensive versus the continuation phases (–0.77 ± 0.27 vs. –0.56 ± 0.30, $p < 0.001$ by paired t test). Since ethambutol exerts only a bacteriostatic effect in the whole-blood model, the difference between these 2 phases of therapy mainly reflects the activity of pyrazinamide. Cumulative activity throughout treatment, calculated as the weighted average of the 2 phases, was superior in patients whose sputum cultures converted by month 2 (–0.63 ± 0.26 vs. –0.46 ± 0.27, $p = 0.04$). Cumulative WBA also correlated with the rate of decline of log sputum CFU counts during the first month of treatment ($R = 0.39$, $p = 0.018$).

Patients in that study were also all tested against a single clinical isolate. In that case, variability among patients was reduced, but the extent of correlation with clinical microbiology was also reduced, indicating that strain characteristics – other than resistance, which was excluded by study entry criteria – contribute to outcome. This is consistent with other observations that differences among strains in phenotypic drug tolerance unrelated to the minimal inhibitory concentration (MIC) contribute to persistence and relapse in TB [20]. Thus, differences in efficacy among treatments may be most efficiently measured when patients are tested using a single isolate, whereas clinical or microbiological outcomes may be best predicted when patients are studied using their own isolates.

One study has directly compared bactericidal activity in patients and healthy volunteers [21]. In that report, whole-blood cultures of *M. tuberculosis* H37Rv were prepared with and without ofloxacin, added directly to the cultures at 1 μg/ml. Ofloxacin was highly active in the blood of healthy volunteers, in whom +0.21 log/day (growth) versus –0.13 log/day (killing) was evident in cultures in the absence and presence of ofloxacin (net effect, –0.34 ± 0.08). In contrast, TB patients exerted full bacteriostasis in baseline cultures (–0.17 log/day) and showed a markedly reduced additional effect when drug was added (–0.09 ± 0.04, $p < 0.001$). This is consistent with a recent study by Sala et al. [22] indicating that ofloxacin lacks activity against non-replicating *M. tuberculosis*. These findings underscore the importance of the immunological milieu as a modifier of drug activity during treatment of intracellular *M. tuberculosis* infection.

### Studies in Healthy Volunteers

The first publication of the whole-blood method described the activity of various drugs and drug combinations in 3 healthy volunteers [10]. Amoxicillin/sulbactam was inactive; ethambutol was bacteriostatic. The rank order of bactericidal activity was pyrazinamide < fluoroquinolones < isoniazid < rifampicin. The cumulative WBA of standard therapy (isoniazid/rifampicin/ethambutol/pyrazinamide) was approximately 3 times that of a fluoroquinolone-based regimen for multidrug-resistant (MDR) TB, consistent with their respective required durations of curative treatment. Standard therapy was inactive against MDR strains.

One study conducted in 10 healthy volunteers compared the activity of orally administered clofazimine 200 mg q.d. versus ofloxacin 600 mg q.d., when given alone and when combined with standard doses of pyrazinamide and ethambutol. The total dose of clofazimine administered during the study was 2 g. Whole-blood cultures were inoculated with *M. tuberculosis* H37Rv. The objective was to determine the potential activity of a clofazimine-based regimen against MDR-TB. WBA was measured 0, 2 and 6 h after dose on days 5 (monotherapy) and 10 (combination therapy). The study found clofazimine to be inactive at concentrations reached by oral dosing, and inferior to ofloxacin with regard to cumulative WBA (+0.15 ± 0.07 vs. –0.12 ± 0.10, $p < 0.001$). A trend toward inferiority of clofazimine persisted when combined with pyrazinamide and ethambutol (–0.01 ± 0.07 vs. –0.15 ± 0.13, $p = 0.067$). The basis of the lack of activity of clofazimine was examined further by directly adding it to whole-blood culture. The MIC of clofazimine against *M. tuberculosis* H37Rv has been reported as 0.1 μg/ml. Clofazimine accumulates in phagocytes during treatment. However, as indicated in figure 2, extracellular concentrations of 100 μg/ml were required to produce a bactericidal effect of –0.6 log/day against intracellular *M. tuberculosis* infection. These appear not to be achieved after short-term oral administration of moderate clofazimine doses.

Two studies have been reported in which the whole-blood model was used during early development of PNU-100480 [23, 24], a linezolid analogue that shows superior efficacy in the mouse TB model [25, 26]. Linezolid 300 mg q.d. served as a comparator, based on 1 report that this dose may be adequately tolerated during treatment of MDR-TB [27]. The studies found that both drugs showed concentration-independent killing that reached 90% of maximal effect at approximately twice the MIC, but that the maximal effect of PNU-100480 (approx. –0.42 log/day) was more than twice that of linezolid (–0.16 log/day, fig. 3). The cumulative WBA of PNU-100480 600 mg b.i.d. was –0.316 ± 0.04 vs. –0.072 ± 0.05 for linezolid 300 mg q.d. ($p < 0.001$). The activity of PNU-100480 was further enhanced to –0.420 ± 0.06 ($p = 0.002$) when administered together with pyrazinamide. These findings confirmed 2 key findings of PNU-100480 in the mouse model: superiority versus linezolid, and synergy with pyrazinamide.

These 2 studies also illustrate the statistical power of the whole-blood method. The multidose trial, for example, included 4 cohorts of 8 subjects dosed at 0, 100, 300, and 600 mg twice daily. Statistical analysis revealed highly significant differences among the cohorts by ANOVA ($p < 0.001$) and significant differences in all post hoc paired comparisons (all $p < 0.05$). In contrast, a study of the early bactericidal activity of linezolid 600 mg given b.i.d. and q.d. in a total of 19 subjects was unable to distinguish changes in log sputum

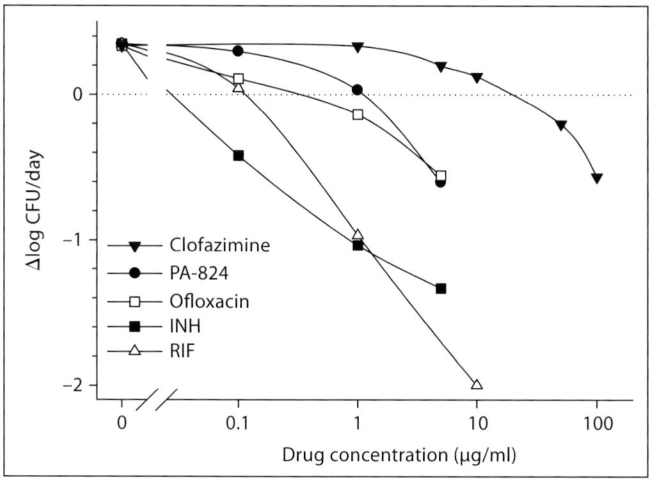


**Fig. 2.** Relationship between drug concentration and bactericidal activity against *M. tuberculosis* H37Rv in blood of healthy volunteers. INH = Isoniazid; RIF = rifampicin.

CFU counts of the 2 treatments from each other or from zero [28]. This indicates the strong potential of the whole-blood method to rapidly evaluate new drugs and regimens in small, short trials.

## Questions for Future Research

The body of evidence supporting a relationship of cumulative WBA to a clinical TB outcome is presently modest and comparable to that for serial CFU counts. For this reason, the method may be best described as an emerging candidate biomarker requiring validation. Further studies are warranted to determine the prognostic value of WBA for treatment arms in TB clinical trials and for individual TB patients.

Perhaps the most interesting and innovative use of the whole-blood model may be in the sequential evaluation of new TB regimens tested in TB patients in a double crossover manner. The use of within-subject (paired) comparisons would further reduce sample size requirements and permit rapid evaluation of multiple candidate regimens in as few as 5–6 subjects. Subsequent conventional trials would examine effects on 2-month sputum culture conversion, thus creating a highly efficient path to accelerated approval.

Modifications of the method may be of benefit in specific circumstances. For example, TMC207 shows a delay of up to several days in the time to onset of its bactericidal activity [29]. Whole-blood cultures of longer duration may be required to accurately reflect its activity. It may be possible

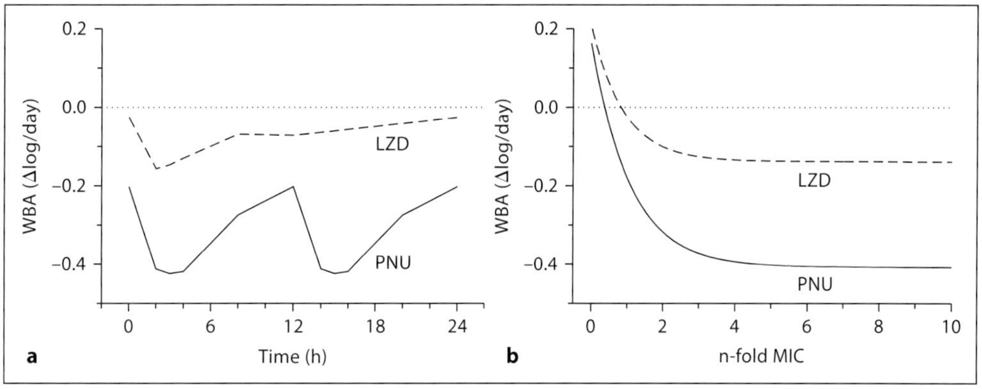


**Fig. 3.** WBA of linezolid (LZD) and PNU-100480 (PNU) against *M. tuberculosis* H37Rv after oral administration to healthy volunteers. **a** Mean WBA at steady state in subjects dosed with either linezolid 300 mg q.d. or PNU-100480 600 mg b.i.d. **b** Regression curves describing the relationship between drug concentration and WBA for linezolid and PNU-100480. PNU-100480 concentrations represent summed MIC ratios for PNU-100480 and its metabolites.

to modify culture conditions of whole-blood cultures of healthy volunteers to make them more like those in TB granulomas, by altering pH, nutrient availability and oxygen tension. Lastly, it may be possible to simplify aspects of the method to facilitate the study of patients with their own isolate, by reducing or eliminating the titration curve and simplifying the selection of the inoculum volume. This may ultimately result in a simple single assay with important prognostic value beyond that presently conferred by rifampicin resistance testing that may be incorporated into routine clinical care.

## References


1 Mitchison DA: The action of antituberculosis drugs in short-course chemotherapy. Tubercle 1985;66:219–225.

2 Zhang Y, Mitchison D: The curious characteristics of pyrazinamide: a review. Int J Tuberc Lung Dis 2003;7:6–21.

3 Wallis RS, Wang C, Doherty TM, Onyebujoh P, Vahedi M, Laang H, Olesen O, Parida S, Zumla A: Biomarkers for tuberculosis disease activity, cure, and relapse. Lancet Infect Dis 2010;10:68–69.

4 Jindani A, Dore CJ, Mitchison DA: Bactericidal and sterilizing activities of antituberculosis drugs during the first 14 days. Am J Respir Crit Care Med 2003;167:1348–1354.

5 Rustomjee R, Lienhardt C, Kanyok T, Davies GR, Levin J, Mthiyane T, Reddy C, Sturm AW, Sirgel FA, Allen J, Coleman DJ, Fourie B, Mitchison DA: A phase II study of the sterilising activities of ofloxacin, gatifloxacin and moxifloxacin in pulmonary tuberculosis. Int J Tuberc Lung Dis 2008;12:128–138.

6 Burman WJ, Goldberg S, Johnson JL, Muzanye G, Engle M, Mosher AW, Choudhri S, Daley CL, Munsiff SS, Zhao Z, Vernon A, Chaisson RE: Moxifloxacin versus ethambutol in the first two months of treatment for pulmonary tuberculosis. Am J Respir Crit Care Med 2006;174:331–338.

7 Conde MB, Efron A, Loredo C, De Souza GR, Graca NP, Cezar MC, Ram M, Chaudhary MA, Bishai WR, Kritski AL, Chaisson RE: Moxifloxacin versus ethambutol in the initial treatment of tuberculosis: a double-blind, randomised, controlled phase II trial. Lancet 2009;373:1183–1189.

8 Dorman SE, Johnson JL, Goldberg S, Muzanye G, Padayatchi N, Bozeman L, Heilig CM, Bernardo J, Choudhri S, Grosset JH, Guy E, Guyadeen P, Leus MC, Maltas G, Menzies D, Nuermberger EL, Villarino M, Vernon A, Chaisson RE: Substitution of moxifloxacin for isoniazid during intensive phase treatment of pulmonary tuberculosis. Am J Respir Crit Care Med 2009;180:273–280.

9 Janulionis E, Sofer C, Schwander S, Simmons D, Kreiswirth B, Shashkina E, Wallis RS: Survival and replication of clinical *Mycobacterium tuberculosis* isolates in the context of human innate immunity. Infect Immun 2005;73:2595–2601.

10 Wallis RS, Palaci M, Vinhas S, Hise AG, Ribeiro FC, Landen K, Cheon SH, Song HY, Phillips M, Dietze R, Ellner JJ: A whole blood bactericidal assay for tuberculosis. J Infect Dis 2001;183:1300–1303.

11 Cheon SH, Kampmann B, Hise AG, Phillips M, Song HY, Landen K, Li Q, Larkin R, Ellner JJ, Silver RF, Hoft DF, Wallis RS: Bactericidal activity in whole blood as a potential surrogate marker of immunity after vaccination against tuberculosis. Clin Diagn Lab Immunol 2002;9:901–907.

12 Saliu O, Sofer C, Stein DS, Schwander SK, Wallis RS: Tumor necrosis factor blockers: differential effects on mycobacterial immunity. J Infect Dis 2006;194:486–492.

13 Hoft DF, Worku S, Kampmann B, Whalen CC, Ellner JJ, Hirsch CS, Brown RB, Larkin R, Li Q, Yun H, Silver RF: Investigation of the relationships between immune-mediated inhibition of mycobacterial growth and other potential surrogate markers of protective *Mycobacterium tuberculosis* immunity. J Infect Dis 2002;186:1448–1457.

14 Kampmann B, Tena-Coki GN, Nicol M, Levin M, Eley B: Reconstitution of antimycobacterial immune responses in HIV-infected children receiving HAART. AIDS 2006;20:1011–1018.

15 Martineau AR, Wilkinson RJ, Wilkinson KA, Newton SM, Kampmann B, Hall BM, Packe GE, Davidson RN, Eldridge SM, Maunsell ZJ, Rainbow SJ, Berry JL, Griffiths CJ: A single dose of vitamin D enhances immunity to mycobacteria. Am J Respir Crit Care Med 2007;176:208–213.
16 Wallis RS, Vinhas SA, Johnson JL, Ribeiro FC, Palaci M, Peres RL, Sa RT, Dietze R, Chiunda A, Eisenach K, Ellner JJ: Whole blood bactericidal activity during treatment of pulmonary tuberculosis. J Infect Dis 2003;187:270–278.
17 Wallis RS, Vinhas S, Janulionis E: Strain specificity of antimycobacterial immunity in whole blood culture after cure of tuberculosis. Tuberculosis (Edinb) 2009;89:221–224.
18 Wallis RS, Weyer K, Fourie PB: Acquired rifamycin resistance: pharmacology and biology. Expert Rev Anti Infect Ther 2008;6:223–230.
19 Hui M, Au-Yeang C, Wong KT, Chan CY, Yew WW, Leung CC: Post-antibiotic effects of linezolid and other agents against *Mycobacterium tuberculosis.* Int J Antimicrob Agents 2008;31:395–396.
20 Wallis RS, Patil S, Cheon SH, Edmonds K, Phillips M, Perkins MD, Joloba M, Namale A, Johnson JL, Teixeira L, Dietze R, Siddiqi S, Mugerwa RD, Eisenach K, Ellner JJ: Drug tolerance in *Mycobacterium tuberculosis.* Antimicrob Agents Chemother 1999;43:2600–2606.
21 Wallis RS, Song HY, Whalen C, Okwera A: TB chemotherapy: antagonism between immunity and sterilization. Am J Respir Crit Care Med 2004;169:771–772.
22 Sala C, Dhar N, Hartkoorn RC, Zhang M, Ha YH, Schneider P, Cole ST: A simple model for testing drugs against non-replicating *Mycobacterium tuberculosis.* Antimicrob Agents Chemother 2010;54:4150–4158.
23 Wallis RS, Kumar V, Jakubiec W, Silvia AM, Paige D, Bedarida G, Mitton-Fry M, Miller PF: Safety, tolerability, PK, and WBA of multiple ascending doses of PNU-100480 (abstract A1-030a). ICAAC, Boston, September 2010.
24 Wallis RS, Jakubiec W, Kumar V, Silvia AM, Paige D, Dimitrova D, Li X, Ladutko L, Campbell S, Friedland G, Mitton-Fry M, Miller PF: Pharmacokinetics and whole blood bactericidal activity against *Mycobacterium tuberculosis* of single ascending doses of PNU-100480 in healthy volunteers. J Infect Dis 2010;202:745–751.
25 Williams KN, Stover CK, Zhu T, Tasneen R, Tyagi S, Grosset JH, Nuermberger E: Promising antituberculosis activity of the oxazolidinone PNU-100480 relative to linezolid in the murine model. Antimicrob Agents Chemother 2008;53:1314–1319.
26 Williams KN, Brickner SJ, Stover CK, Zhu T, Ogden A, Tasneen R, Tyagi S, Grosset JH, Nuermberger EL: Addition of PNU-100480 to first-line drugs shortens the time needed to cure murine tuberculosis. Am J Respir Crit Care Med 2009;180:371–376.
27 Koh WJ, Kwon OJ, Gwak H, Chung JW, Cho SN, Kim WS, Shim TS: Daily 300 mg dose of linezolid for the treatment of intractable multidrug-resistant and extensively drug-resistant tuberculosis. J Antimicrob Chemother 2009;64:388–391.
28 Dietze R, Hadad DJ, McGee B, Molino LP, Maciel EL, Peloquin CA, Johnson DF, Debanne SM, Eisenach K, Boom WH, Palaci M, Johnson JL: Early and extended early bactericidal activity of linezolid in pulmonary tuberculosis. Am J Respir Crit Care Med 2008;178:1180–1185.
29 Rustomjee R, Diacon AH, Allen J, Venter A, Reddy C, Patientia RF, Mthiyane TC, De Marez T, van Heeswijk R, Kerstens R, Koul A, De Beule K, Donald PR, McNeeley DF: Early bactericidal activity and pharmacokinetics of the diarylquinoline TMC207 in pulmonary tuberculosis. Antimicrob Agents Chemother 2008;52:2831–2835.

Robert S. Wallis, MD, FIDSA
Pfizer
445 Eastern Point Rd.
MS 8260–2516
Groton, CT 06340 (USA)
Tel. +1 860 441 5417, E-Mail robert.wallis@pfizer.com

Donald PR, van Helden PD (eds): Antituberculosis Chemotherapy.
Prog Respir Res. Basel, Karger, 2011, vol 40, pp 227–234

# Serial Sputum Colony Counting in Drug Development

Derek Sloan · Geraint Davies

Department of Pharmacology and Therapeutics, University of Liverpool, Liverpool, UK

**Abstract**

In order to effectively optimize and evaluate new potentially treatment-shortening strategies for tuberculosis, there is an urgent need to develop reliable surrogate end points of the sterilizing activity of antituberculosis drugs in vivo. Serial sputum colony counting can be used to directly quantify changes in sputum bacillary load during treatment and, with appropriate statistical modelling, can demonstrate the distinct phases of pharmacodynamic response which may reflect effects on putative subpopulations of *Mycobacterium tuberculosis*. These characteristics may allow this technique to efficiently compare the sterilizing activity of different multidrug regimens during the intensive phase of therapy, as suggested by existing studies in diverse settings. This methodology could be used to select the best drug doses and combinations to take forward into phase III clinical trials.

Copyright © 2011 S. Karger AG, Basel

Recent progress in antituberculosis drug development has generated considerable hope for delivery of more effective patient treatment [1]. Major research aims include reducing the duration of first-line and improving the efficacy of second-line therapy as reflected in treatment failure and relapse rates [2, 3]. In drug-susceptible disease, using a non-inferiority design with current short-course chemotherapy as the comparator, a phase III trial of any new approach based on these clinical end points would require approximately 500 patients per arm on study for 18–30 months [4]. Global mobilization of the research capacity necessary for such studies will be a major undertaking [5] and suggests an urgent need to carefully screen and select candidate combination regimens for such trials.

The key factor in any treatment-shortening strategy is likely to be enhancing 'sterilizing activity'. This concept is based on the hypothesis that clinical *Mycobacterium tuberculosis* infection comprises multiple bacillary subpopulations, demanding a spectrum of distinct pharmacodynamic properties from a combination regimen [6]. Potent bactericidal compounds (e.g. isoniazid) deal effectively and quickly with actively replicating organisms [7, 8] but metabolically quiescent bacilli exhibit broad phenotypic drug tolerance and may only be killed slowly by particular classes of drugs such as rifamycins. Although imprecisely defined, the ability of a regimen to eliminate this putative persister population is typically referred to as its 'sterilizing activity' [9]. The main sterilizing drugs in current short-course chemotherapy are pyrazinamide during the first 2 months and rifampicin over the whole 6 months of treatment. The fourth British Medical Research Council clinical trial demonstrated the critical importance of rifampicin for sterilization: increased posttreatment relapse was observed when the duration of administration of this drug was reduced below 6 months [10]. An early biomarker of sterilizing activity would be invaluable in tuberculosis pharmacology research, particularly if it could act as a surrogate end point in relatively small phase IIb clinical studies of short duration for selection and optimization of new combination regimens in advance of expensive and difficult phase III trials.

Serial sputum colony counting (SSCC) is a candidate approach to developing such a surrogate end point. We will review the arguments for bacteriological biomarkers of sterilization based on sputum culture, the methodological and statistical issues in the evolution of SSCC and evidence from recent experience with the technique, in order to assess its limitations and potential future applications.

## Bacteriological Biomarkers as Surrogates of Sterilizing Activity

A practically useful surrogate end point requires a biologically plausible relationship with the definitive clinical end point (relapse), useful statistical properties and must successfully undergo appropriate evaluation against the clinical end point. For tuberculosis treatment, the primary pharmacodynamic activity of current regimens is destruction of *M. tuberculosis* organisms, so the prima facie plausibility of bacteriological end points is strong. Furthermore, recent re-evaluation of 12 historical clinical trials conducted by the British Medical Research Council in Africa and East Asia in a modern meta-analytical framework confirms a moderately strong empirical correlation between 2- and 3-month sputum culture conversion and rates of relapse [11].

However, selection of a surrogate end point based on 'positive' or 'negative' culture at an arbitrarily selected stage of treatment is problematic for 2 reasons. Firstly, the power of this binary end point depends on the proportion of culture conversion in the comparator arm and as this is currently high even at 2 months, a relatively large sample or effect size is needed to make such trials practically feasible. Simulation studies confirm the expected theoretical result that prioritization of binary end points incurs a significant penalty in terms of sample size [12].

Secondly, measurement of outcome at a fixed time point does not efficiently capture information about the effect of treatment over the entire period of culture positivity. This generates uncertainty about which time point should be prioritized; the choice of the optimal time point may even vary between regimens based on their differing pharmacodynamic properties.

These difficulties have been brought into focus by the conflicting results obtained in recent phase IIb trials examining substitution of 8-methoxyquinolones for ethambutol [13]. Though it is not yet known whether these agents are truly capable of shortening therapy, much debate has centred on the differing designs of these studies. Those employing more intensive bacteriological sampling and time-to-event or hierarchical regression analysis appear to support an improved sterilizing activity [14, 15] whereas those using fewer samples and analysis based on proportions at fixed time points do not, even with much larger study cohorts.

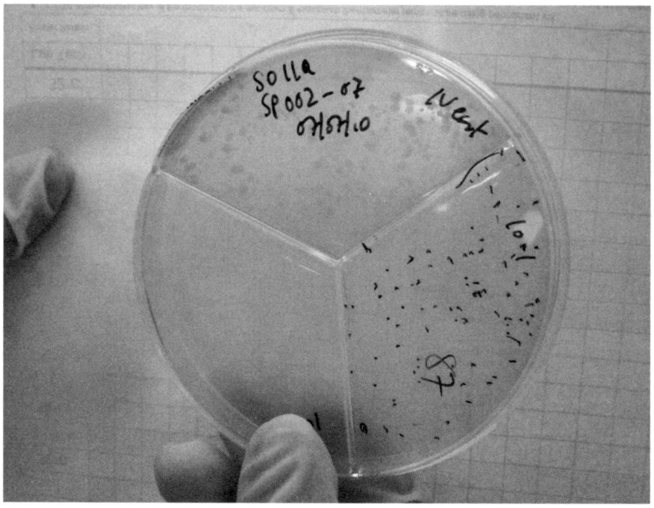


**Fig. 1.** A selective Middlebook 7H10 SSCC plate. One millilitre of neat sputum was homogenized with an equal volume of dithiothreitol, and 50 µl of serial 10-fold dilutions were plated into compartments of compartmentalized Petri dishes. In this case, after incubation for 3 weeks at 37°C, 87 CFU/ml were counted from the $10^{-1}$ dilution (marked with black dots during counting). A back-titration calculation estimates that there were 34,800 CFU/ml ($\log_{10}$ 4.54 CFU/ml) in the original sample.

## Evolution of Quantitative Bacteriology

A directly quantitative method is necessary to precisely describe the decline in viable *M. tuberculosis* organisms in sputum over time. Such a standardized bacteriological technique was originally developed for use in studies of early bactericidal activity (EBA). When serial dilutions of homogenized overnight sputum collections from tuberculosis patients are plated onto Middlebrook 7H10 or 7H11 media supplemented with oleic acid-albumen-catalase and made selective by addition of antibiotics (typically polymyxin B, carbenicillin, trimethoprim and amphotericin B), single colony-forming units (CFUs) can be counted after incubation for 3–4 weeks at 37°C (fig. 1). A back-titration calculation from the number of CFUs visible at an easily countable dilution can be used to quantify sputum viable bacillary counts in the original sample, expressed as CFUs per millilitre [7, 8]. Plates are normally prepared in duplicates, and mean counts take to improve accuracy. Careful attention has also to be paid to the quality of sputum collection and transport procedures.

The first EBA studies used this approach to show that the fall in viable bacillary counts over days 0–2 (sometimes referred to as the 'standard EBA') varied between drug doses and regimens [7]. Subsequently, 'standard EBA' has been a useful tool to establish proof of concept and initial dose finding of many antituberculosis agents but the need to perform longer studies when assessing treatment efficacy has become apparent. Serial bacillary counting for 5 days was required to demonstrate that the activity of isoniazid drops to almost zero after day 3 whilst rifampicin remains active [8]. A 7-day EBA study was needed to show that the new drug TMC207 predominantly becomes active after day 4 [16]. Even analysis of bacillary elimination rates out to day 14 with pyrazinamide-containing regimens failed to convincingly demonstrate the considerable sterilizing capabilities of this drug [17], and, most importantly, no convincing statistical evaluation of the relationship between changes in viable bacillary counts over the first 2 weeks and treatment failure or relapse rates in clinical trials has been carried out or indeed seems feasible.

Overall, 2-month sputum culture conversion has an established correlation with the target clinical end point but lacks quantitative precision for use in phase II studies. EBA is quantitative but unsuitable as a surrogate marker of relapse perhaps because sampling has not been continued for long enough periods to accurately measure sterilizing activity. As it would generally be considered unethical to prolong treatment with monotherapy or limited drug combinations for more than 2 weeks, a tool needs to be found which is capable of measuring sterilizing activity in the context of combination therapy. SSCC is a proposed solution to this dilemma in so far as it aims to extend the quantitative bacteriological approach over the entire intensive phase of treatment.

## Recent Experience with Serial Sputum Colony Counting

To date, 4 clinical studies have adopted the SSCC approach described here: three involved drug-susceptible disease and a fourth patients with multidrug resistance [14, 18–20]. The design and analysis of these studies has evolved with time, and the lessons learned from each are discussed below.

A number of other studies have also used quantitative bacteriology to evaluate combination regimens during extended sputum sampling [21, 22], but in these, investigators decontaminated samples with sodium hydroxide (NaOH) prior to culture. Detailed description of this work has not been undertaken here as sputum decontamination is known to alter the profile of the measurable treatment response (see below). In the most notable of these studies, however, an antituberculous regimen comprising rifampicin, isoniazid and ciprofloxacin was compared to current standard therapy with rifampicin, isoniazid, pyrazinamide and ethambutol. This trial reported poorer sterilizing activity with rifampicin, isoniazid and ciprofloxacin, measurable by a smaller fall in $\log_{10}$ CFU per millilitre during weeks 3–8, a longer time to culture conversion and a higher 6-month culture-proven relapse rate [22, 23].

## The Nairobi Serial Sputum Colony Counting Study: Short Course and Standard Regimens

In 1989 and 1990 in Kenya, the first SSCC study employing a modern combination regimen and methods without sputum decontamination recruited 122 new patients to treatment with isoniazid and streptomycin supplemented with either thiacetazone or rifampicin and pyrazinamide. Viable sputum colony counts were done at 0, 2, 7, 14 and 28 days, and it was reported that, although baseline CFUs per millilitre were higher in HIV-positive than HIV-negative patients (6.95 and 6.23 $\log_{10}$ CFU/ml, respectively), there was no difference in treatment response attributable to HIV status in the first 28 days [18].

In 2001, this data set was revisited to assess whether reanalysis could detect differences between the 2 treatment regimens used [24]. Analyses of variance of summary statistics representing the slope of the decline in $\log_{10}$ CFUs per millilitre sputum over different time periods were calculated, and 2 main conclusions were drawn. First, elimination during days 0–2 was much faster than that from days 2 to 28, making it inappropriate to fit a single linear regression line through all the time points. Second, the difference in the slopes in the streptomycin/isoniazid/rifampicin/pyrazinamide and isoniazid/streptomycin/thiacetazone groups over days 2–28 was highly significant (–0.163 vs. –0.095, $p = 0.004$), indicating superiority of streptomycin/isoniazid/rifampicin/pyrazinamide. Taken together, these findings point to the presence of more than 1 bacillary subpopulation in sputum: a rapidly eliminated population vulnerable to the EBA of isoniazid and a more slowly eliminated 'persister' population susceptible to the 'sterilizing activity' of rifampicin and pyrazinamide. However, whether these are present initially or evolve during therapy remains unclear.

Further refinement of this approach was undertaken in 2006, using non-linear mixed effects analysis to fit a bi-exponential model to the data with the formula:

$$\log_{10} \text{CFU} = \log_{10}(e^{\theta_1} \times e^{-\text{day} \times e^{\theta_2}} + \times e^{\theta_3} \times e^{-\text{day} \times e^{\theta_4}})\ [25].$$

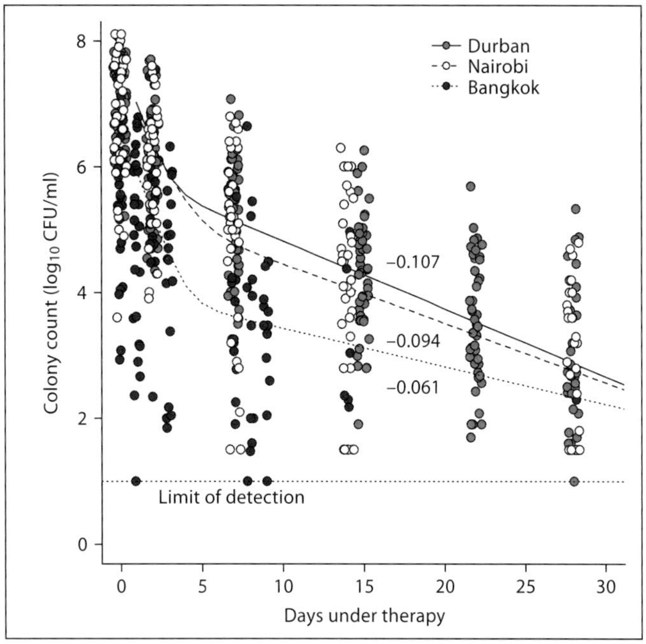


**Fig. 2.** Twenty-eight-day SSCC data from 3 clinical cohorts of patients with pulmonary tuberculosis. Serial viable bacillary counts are expressed as $log_{10}$ CFUs per millilitre, and data are modelled using non-linear mixed effects techniques to demonstrate the biphasic nature of treatment response and calculate regression coefficients for bacillary elimination during drug treatment.

This allows a flexible biphasic curve to be fitted to the aggregate effect of treatment on the 2 putative subpopulations based on the following parameters: $\theta_1$ and $\theta_3$ represent baseline bacillary loads of the fast and slow populations, whilst $\theta_2$ and $\theta_4$ represent their respective elimination rates on a log scale (fig. 2). When $\theta_4$ from non-linear mixed effects modelling was compared as a measure of sterilizing activity to the more straightforward day 2–28 linear regression coefficient, the linear statistic was found to overestimate the 'slow' bacillary elimination rate by 16–139%, probably reflecting the fact that the rapidly eliminated population is not completely eradicated by day 2 and so contaminates linear regression analysis starting at this time point. $\theta_4$ is therefore likely to be a more flexible and accurate measurement of sterilizing activity.

In addition, the ability of a mixed model to explicitly account for interindividual variability in the model parameters enhances its precision for treatment comparisons. Summary statistics unadjusted for baseline counts incorporate this source of variability, with a consequent loss of power. Another advantage of the regression modelling approach is that it can incorporate increasing intra-individual variability over time and account for missing observations, both of which may violate the assumptions of the simpler approach.

Subsequent simulation studies were performed using the findings from this study in order to identify the optimal number of sampling points per patient to maximize precision of the model-based approach. A scheme of between 5 and 11 time points based around a skeleton of sputum collections on days 0, 2, 7, 14 and 56 [26] was proposed. There are several reasons for frequent sampling: it increases overall precision in model parameters other than $\theta_4$, identifies correlation of parameter estimates for $\theta_3$ and $\theta_4$, can in principle detect simultaneous treatment effects of a new regimen on both $\theta_2$ and $\theta_4$ and protects against mis-specification of the model in future real-life studies. Extending the number of sampling points beyond 11, however, did not greatly improve precision and power.

Such intensive sampling schedules may appear impractical in some study settings but solutions may be possible; near-complete sampling can be done as essentially weekly sampling with an extra point in week 1 (day 2) or more imaginative schemes may be used (e.g. 1 baseline measurement followed by 2 balanced blocks of 5 points). Deliberately incomplete schemes can be accommodated using the modelling approach, though this may increase the sample size necessary for a clinical study by 20–40%.

Precision on $\theta_4$ is sensitive to location of later sampling points and, in general, is increased more by extending sampling duration than by performing more sputum collections. Clearly there is a tension between the desire to continue sampling for as long as possible and the progressive likelihood that later sputum samples may be unobtainable, be of poorer quality or be culture negative. In the only previous study to extend sampling beyond 2 months only 6% of subjects had detectable counts at 60 days and all cultures were negative at 90 days [21]. Simulations with the Kenyan data set predict that mean counts will fall below $log_{10}$ zero just after 56 days [25]. The need to recruit enough patients to generate sufficient data at later time points may put an absolute restriction on sample size but, even allowing for this, optimization of sample size calculations for a phase II SSCC superiority study using $\theta_4$ as a sterilization surrogate are likely to be less than a quarter of that required for a definitive phase III non-inferiority trial using relapse as the end point [25].

## The Durban Serial Sputum Colony Counting Cohort: Fluoroquinolones in Drug-Susceptible Disease

In 2004–2005, the OFLOTUB investigators in Kwa-Zulu Natal used SSCC methodology to compare substitution of ofloxacin, moxifloxacin and gatifloxacin for ethambutol in standard multidrug therapy [14]. Unlike prior clinical fluoroquinolone studies, statistical modelling of viable colony counts was used for the primary comparison of regimens. The estimates of $\theta_4$ derived from this model ranked moxifloxacin and gatifloxacin as superior sterilizing agents to ofloxacin or the control arm. Interestingly, this result was in agreement with the performance of the fluoroquinolones in preclinical models of sterilization [27]. More rapid bacillary elimination was also associated with decreasing age, HIV negativity and unilateral disease on chest radiographs, and adjustment for these covariates made the difference between the moxi-/gatifloxacin and ofloxacin/control arms more apparent (fig. 3). Survival analysis showed a similar effect but at a lower level of significance. Extension of the bacillary elimination rate from the late phase of the moxifloxacin arm of the OFLOTUB data beyond 8 weeks suggests that appropriate fluoroquinolone-containing regimens might allow treatment shortening of up to 30% but several factors could make this estimate unreliable including the absence of pyrazinamide in the continuation phase of therapy or the existence of further persister populations not detected by the SSCC technique.

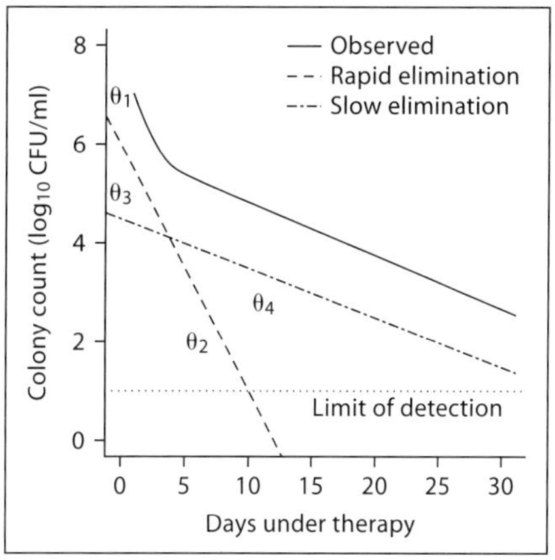


**Fig. 3.** Schematic illustration of bi-exponential model of response to treatment based on 2 distinct subpopulations of bacilli in sputum at baseline.

## The Bangkok Serial Sputum Colony Counting Cohort: Pharmacokinetic-Pharmacodynamic Analysis of First-Line Therapy

A factorial observational cohort study conducted in Bangkok, Thailand, in 2006–2007 employed the SSCC approach to examine the pharmacokinetic-pharmacodynamic relationships of first-line agents under conditions of combination chemotherapy in 86 patients [19]. The parameter estimates of the SSCC model were broadly similar to those of the African studies though the baseline bacillary load was lower, in agreement with previous multicentre studies of EBA. Using model-derived estimates of area under the curve for isoniazid, it was possible to reproduce previously described exposure-response relationships observed in dose-ranging EBA studies [28] over a narrower range of doses and in the presence of companion drugs. This encouraging result suggests that SSCC studies could facilitate at least limited dose-ranging in phase IIb studies. However, it was not possible to demonstrate similar relationships for either rifampicin or pyrazinamide during the late phase of elimination. This may have been due to the relatively small size of the study, limited pharmacogenetic variability of the sterilizing drugs or moderate shrinkage in the individual model-derived estimates of late-phase elimination, due to an unexpectedly high rate of culture conversion.

## Serial Sputum Colony Counting in the Assessment of TMC207 in Multidrug-Resistant Disease

In 2007–2008, a placebo-controlled phase II trial evaluated the benefit of adding the diarylquinoline ATP synthase inhibitor TMC207 to an optimized 5-drug treatment regimen for multidrug-resistant tuberculosis [20]. SSCC was used as a secondary end point in this study and was analysed by change in median $\log_{10}$ count of CFUs per millilitre at weekly time points rather than non-linear mixed effects modelling. The SSCC analysis concurred with the primary end point (time to conversion of sputum cultures grown in liquid media) that the TMC207 arm was superior. SSCC was also better able to profile different patterns of treatment response; bacillary elimination was only marginally higher in the TMC207 arm during week 1 but then appreciably increased compared to the placebo regimen for the next 3 weeks. This result is consistent with TMC207's proposed mode of action and its earlier performance in 7-day EBA studies [16] and further illustrates the benefit of direct viable colony counting methods to reveal qualitative differences in the pharmacodynamic responses of multidrug regimens.

## Current Limitations

Despite its potential advantages, there are several practical considerations and limitations associated with the SSCC methodology which may not make it suitable for all study settings. It requires intensive clinical follow-up with repeated patient visits and supervised sputum collection. However, this is likely to be economical in many settings since it requires recruitment of fewer patients overall. Patient selection is probably of great importance: strongly smear-positive patients producing copious amounts of sputum at baseline are preferred to maximize the period of culture positivity. Whilst increasing the likely precision of the results obtained, this homogenizes the study cohort and may potentially misrepresent treatment responses in the wider population. For the purposes of phase II development however, this is a secondary concern.

Strong laboratory support, supervision and training are also a necessity. This may stretch sample processing capacity or create biosafety concerns in inexperienced laboratories. Contamination of culture plates must be kept to a minimum. Modification of media to increase the antifungal concentration may be helpful [14] but constant supervision and control of laboratory technique are essential [29]. A common method of eliminating contaminants from sputum prior to other culture techniques is decontamination with NaOH, a procedure intended to destroy non-mycobacterial organisms. Unfortunately, however, this process is not entirely selective; NaOH treatment with concentrations as low as 1% are known to aversely influence *M. tuberculosis* recovery rates in liquid and solid culture systems [30], and in 1 EBA study decontamination dropped the sputum bacillary load by approximately 0.5–1 $\log_{10}$ [31]. It is unclear to what extent decontamination might affect metabolically distinct bacillary subpopulations but cohorts of extended sputum sampling which have used decontaminated samples have invariably reported monophasic elimination curves, suggesting that the pharmacodynamic profile has been distorted [21, 22]. The current bacteriological method cannot detect counts below 10–$10^3$ CFU/ml [32], and decontamination may further compromise the sensitivity of the assay. For these reasons, NaOH treatment is not an attractive general method for reducing contamination in SSCC studies.

Though the advanced statistical methods involved in SSCC modelling are well established theoretically and in other fields such as pharmacokinetics, expertise is not yet widespread among clinical trialists and there is continued conservatism regarding model-based approaches to early-phase clinical trials. They do however offer the opportunity to learn more effectively from phase II data and are gaining ground in other fields [33].

Ultimately, whilst the SSCC approach has greater prima facie plausibility than EBA and greater statistical power than 2-month culture conversion rates as a potential surrogate end point of sterilizing activity, it can only be fully evaluated in comparison with the clinical end point of relapse rate. It is critically important that future phase II studies using this and other methods make provision to study this relationship at both the individual (through prolonged follow-up of participants) and trial level (by comparison with subsequent phase III trials). Data to enable this analysis for both will increasingly emerge from clinical cohorts using SSCC in the near future.

## Future Applications

Despite the above concerns, SSCC is a tool with considerable potential in the development of new antituberculous treatment regimens. SSCC studies have been shown to be logistically feasible in diverse study settings with similar patterns of response, suggesting that the basic model is generally suitable (fig. 4). SSCC appears to represent in vivo pharmacodynamic responses more directly than other measurements, whilst eliminating some sources of bias and variability. It may clearly discriminate between the effects of treatment on different subpopulations of organisms, possibly allowing estimation of 'sterilizing activity' and is well suited to capture different patterns of response to different classes of drugs. For these reasons it could be used in the selection of new drugs and doses for multidrug treatment, and for regimen optimization prior to phase III trials. The relatively small sample sizes required open the way to efficient factorial evaluation of more than 1 drug and/or dose level in early clinical development, which could help to reduce current uncertainties regarding the predictions of both animal models and EBA studies.

SSCC could also be used in conjunction with other markers of treatment response to extend our understanding of persistence and possibly improve its surrogacy based on a better understanding of the underlying mechanisms. Liquid culture of sputum remains positive during treatment for much longer than colony counting plates [14, 21, 34], possibly because bacillary populations in different metabolic states respond differently to varied growth conditions and this makes the relationship between $\log_{10}$ CFUs per millilitre and characteristics of liquid culture systems pertinent to explore. Other biomarkers of treatment response are also

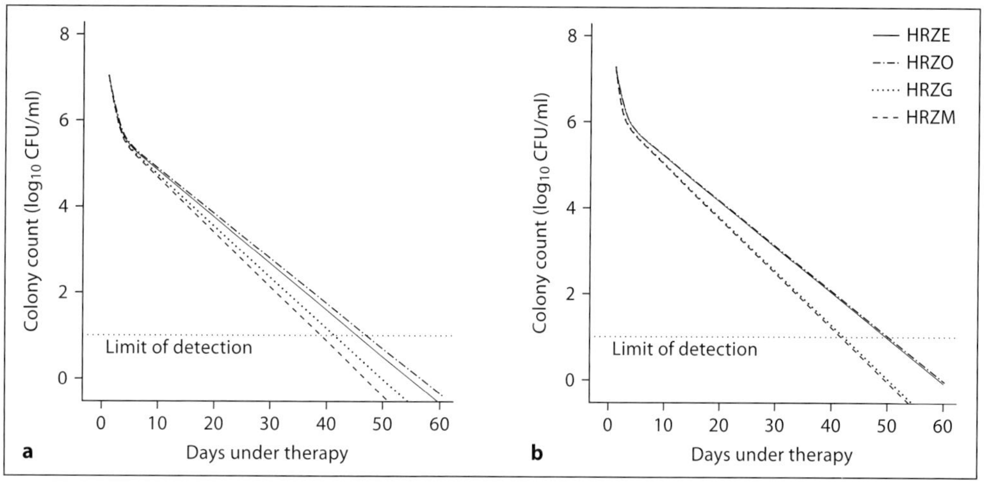


**Fig. 4.** Fitted bi-exponential curves for the 4 treatment series from the OFLOTUB data, using the non-linear mixed effects model. H = Isoniazid; R = rifampicin; Z = pyrazinamide; E = ethambutol; O = ofloxacin; G = gatifloxacin; M = moxifloxacin. Figure taken from Rustomjee et al. [14]. **a** Before adjustment for covariates. **b** After adjustment for covariates.

under development, including measurement of sputum *M. tuberculosis* mRNA [35] and enhancement of culture with resuscitation-promoting factors [36]. It is likely to be some years before these have been adequately evaluated but, once again, assessment of their relationship with bacteriological biomarkers such as SSCC, and perhaps a formal joint statistical modelling approach may potentially be worthwhile.

The SSCC approach is a potentially decisive tool at a critical stage of clinical development. Wider and more creative use of this and other allied quantitative methodologies could help to significantly accelerate the critical path to more effective antituberculosis regimens.

## References


1 Ginsberg AM, Spigelman M: Challenges in tuberculosis drug research and development. Nat Med 2007;13:290–294.
2 Global Alliance for Tuberculosis Drug Development: Scientific blueprint for tuberculosis drug development. Tuberculosis (Edinb) 2001;81(suppl 1):1–52.
3 Davies GR, Nuermberger EL: Pharmacokinetics and pharmacodynamics in the development of anti-tuberculosis drugs. Tuberculosis (Edinb) 2008;88(suppl 1:S65–S74.
4 Burman WJ: Rip Van Winkle wakes up: development of tuberculosis treatment in the 21st century. Clin Infect Dis 2010;50(suppl 3):S165–S172.
5 van Niekerk C, Ginsberg A: Assessment of global capacity to conduct tuberculosis drug development trials: do we have what it takes? Int J Tuberc Lung Dis 2009;13:1367–1372.
6 Mitchison DA: Basic mechanisms of chemotherapy. Chest 1979;76(suppl):771–781.
7 Jindani A, Aber VR, Edwards EA, Mitchison DA: The early bactericidal activity of drugs in patients with pulmonary tuberculosis. Am Rev Respir Dis 1980;121:939–949.
8 Sirgel FA, Donald PR, Odhiambo J, Githui W, Umapathy KC, Paramasivan CN, Tam CM, Kam KM, Lam CW, Sole KM, Mitchison DA: A multicentre study of the early bactericidal activity of anti-tuberculosis drugs. J Antimicrob Chemother 2000;45:859–870.
9 Davies GR: Early clinical development of anti-tuberculosis drugs: science, statistics and sterilizing activity. Tuberculosis (Edinb) 2010;90:171–176.
10 East African/British Medical Research Councils: Controlled clinical trial of five short-course (4-month) chemotherapy regimens in pulmonary tuberculosis. Second report of the 4th study. Am Rev Respir Dis 1981;123:165–170.
11 Phillips P, Fielding K: Surrogate markers for poor outcome to treatment for tuberculosis: results from extensive multi-trial analysis. Int J Tuberc Lung Dis 2008;12:S146–S147.
12 Fedorov V, Mannino F, Zhang R: Consequences of dichotomisation. Pharm Stat 2009;8:50–61.
13 Burman WJ, Goldberg S, Johnson JL, Muzanye G, Engle M, Mosher AW, Choudhri S, Daley CL, Munsiff SS, Zhao Z, Vernon A, Chaisson RE: Moxifloxacin versus ethambutol in the first 2 months of treatment for pulmonary tuberculosis. Am J Respir Crit Care Med 2006;174:331–338.
14 Rustomjee R, Lienhardt C, Kanyok T, Davies GR, Levin J, Mthiyane T, Reddy C, Sturm AW, Sirgel FA, Allen J, Coleman DJ, Fourie B, Mitchison DA: A phase II study of the sterilising activities of ofloxacin, gatifloxacin and moxifloxacin in pulmonary tuberculosis. Int J Tuberc Lung Dis 2008;12:128–138.
15 Conde MB, Efron A, Loredo C, De Souza GR, Graca NP, Cezar MC, Ram M, Chaudary MA, Bishai WR, Kritski AL, Chaisson RE: Moxifloxacin versus ethambutol in the initial treatment of tuberculosis: a double-blind randomised controlled phase II trial. Lancet 2009;373:1183–1189.
16 Rustomjee R, Diacon AH, Allen J, Venter A, Reddy C, Patientia RF, Mthiyane TC, De Marez T, van Heeswijk R, Kerstens R, Koul A, De Beule K, Donald PR, McNeeley DF: Early bactericidal activity and pharmacokinetics of the diarylquinoline TMC207 in treatment of pulmonary tuberculosis. Antimicrob Agents Chemother 2008;52:2831–2835.
17 Jindani A, Dore CJ, Mitchison DA: Bactericidal and sterilizing activities of antituberculosis drugs during the first 14 days. Am J Respir Crit Care Med 2003;167:1348–1354.
18 Brindle RJ, Nunn PP, Githui W, Allen BW, Gathua S, Waiyaki P: Quantitative bacillary response to treatment in HIV-associated pulmonary tuberculosis. Am Rev Respir Dis 1993;147:958–961.

19 Davies GR, Cheirakul N, Saguenwong N, Chaiprasert A, Chuchuttaworn C, Eompokalap B, Likanonsakul S, White NJ, Back DJ, Khoo SH: A factorial study of the effect of HIV, tuberculosis and pharmacogenetics on the pharmacokinetics and pharmacodynamics of anti-tuberculosis drugs (abstract 0-106). Conf Retroviruses Opportun Infect, Boston, 2008.

20 Diacon AH, Pym A, Grobusch M, Patientia R, Rustomjee R, Page-Shipp L, Pistorius C, Krause R, Bogoshi M, Churchyard G, Venter A, Allen J, Palomino JC, De Marez T, van Heeswijk RP, Lounis N, Meyvisch P, Verbeeck J, Parys W, de Beule K, Andries K, McNeeley DF: The diarylquinoline TMC207 for multidrug-resistant tuberculosis. N Engl J Med 2009;360:2397–2405.

21 Joloba ML, Johnson JL, Namale A, Morrissey A, Assegghai AE, Mugerwa RD, Ellner JJ, Eisenach KD: Quantitative sputum bacillary load during rifampin-containing short course chemotherapy in human immunodeficiency virus-infected and non-infected adults with pulmonary tuberculosis. Int J Tuberc Lung Dis 2000;4:528–536.

22 Kennedy N, Fox R, Kisyombe GM, Saruni AO, Uiso LO, Ramsay AR, Ngowi FI, Gillespie SH: Early bactericidal and sterilizing activities of ciprofloxacin in pulmonary tuberculosis. Am Rev Respir Dis 1993;148:1547–1551.

23 Kennedy N, Berger L, Curram J, Fox R, Gutmann J, Kisyombe GM, Ngowi FI, Ramsay AR, Saruni AO, Sam N, Tillotson G, Uiso LO, Yates M, Gillespie SH: Randomized controlled trial of a drug regimen that includes ciprofloxacin for the treatment of pulmonary tuberculosis. Clin Infect Dis 1996;22:827–833.

24 Brindle R, Odhiambo J, Mitchison D: Serial counts of *Mycobacterium tuberculosis* in sputum as surrogate markers of the sterilising activity of rifampicin and pyrazinamide in treating pulmonary tuberculosis. BMC Pulm Med 2001;1:2.

25 Davies GR, Brindle R, Khoo SH, Aarons LJ: Use of nonlinear mixed-effects analysis for improved precision of early pharmacodynamic measures in tuberculosis treatment. Antimicrob Agents Chemother 2006;50: 3154–3156.

26 Davies GR, Khoo SH, Aarons LJ: Optimal sampling strategies for early pharmacodynamic measures in tuberculosis. J Antimicrob Chemother 2006;58:594–600.

27 Hu Y, Coates AR, Mitchison DA: Sterilizing activities of fluoroquinolones against rifampin-tolerant populations of *Mycobacterium tuberculosis*. Antimicrob Agents Chemother 2003;47:653–657.

28 Donald PR, Parkin DP, Seifart HI, Schaaf HS, van Helden PD, Werely CJ, Sirgel FA, Venter A, Maritz JS: The influence of dose and N-acetyltransferase-2 (NAT2) genotype and phenotype on the pharmacokinetics and pharmacodynamics of isoniazid. Eur J Clin Pharmacol 2007;63:633–639.

29 Sirgel F, Venter A, Mitchison D: Sources of variation in studies of the early bactericidal activity of antituberculosis drugs. J Antimicrob Chemother 2001;47:177–182.

30 Peres RL, Maciel EL, Morais CG, Ribeiro FC, Vinhas SA, Pinheiro C, Dietze R, Johnson JL, Eisenach K, Palaci M: Comparison of two concentrations of NALC-NaOH for decontamination of sputum for mycobacterial culture. Int J Tuberc Lung Dis 2009;13:1572–1575.

31 Chambers HF, Kocagoz T, Sipit T, Turner J, Hopewell PC: Activity of amoxicillin/clavulanate in patients with tuberculosis. Clin Infect Dis 1998;26:874–877.

32 Burdz TV, Wolfe J, Kabani A: Evaluation of sputum decontamination methods for *Mycobacterium tuberculosis* using viable colony counts and flow cytometry. Diagn Microbiol Infect Dis 2003;47:503–509.

33 Zhang L, Sinha V, Fogue Sl: Model-based drug development : the road to quantitative pharmacology. J Pharmacokin Pharmacodyn 2006;33:369–393.

34 Diacon AH, Maritz JS, Venter A, van Helden PD, Andries K, McNeeley DF, Donald PR: Time to detection of the growth of *Mycobacterium tuberculosis* in MGIT 960 for determining the early bactericidal activity of antituberculosis agents. Eur J Clin Microbiol Infect Dis 2010;29:1561–1565.

35 Li L, Mahan CS, Palaci M, Horter L, Loeffelholz L, Johnson JL, Dietze R, Debanne SM, Joloba ML, Okwera A, Boom WH, Eisenach KD: Sputum *Mycobacterium tuberculosis* mRNA as a marker of bacteriologic clearance in response to anti-tuberculosis therapy. J Clin Microbiol 2010;48:46–51.

36 Mukamolova GV, Turapov O, Malkin J, Woltmann G, Barer MR: Resuscitation-promoting factors reveal an occult population of tubercle bacilli in sputum. Am J Respir Crit Care Med 2010;181:174–180.



Dr. Geraint Davies
Department of Pharmacology and Therapeutics
University of Liverpool
70 Pembroke Place, Liverpool L69 3GF (UK)
Tel. +44 0151 706 3036, E-Mail gerrydavies@doctors.org.uk

Donald PR, van Helden PD (eds): Antituberculosis Chemotherapy.
Prog Respir Res. Basel, Karger, 2011, vol 40, pp 235–242

# The Evaluation of New Antituberculosis Drugs in Children

David F. McNeeley[a] · Araz Raoof[b] · Jenny Lin[c] · Ben J. Marais[d]

[a]Medical Service Corporation International, Arlington, Va., USA; [b]Tibotec BVBA, Beerse, Belgium; [c]Tibotec Inc., Titusville, N.J., USA; [d]Department of Paediatrics and Child Health, Faculty of Health Sciences, Stellenbosch University and Tygerberg Children's Hospital, Tygerberg, South Africa

**Abstract**

For the first time in nearly a half century, several new tuberculosis (TB) drug candidates are in advanced clinical development. It is essential to ensure that new advances in TB chemotherapy are promptly made available to children. Current regulatory legislation encourages paediatric drug development by sponsors. A balanced benefit and risk assessment should be made with regard to both the imperative to provide children with the latest medications and the need to have a fundamental safety package that will protect the most vulnerable age groups. TB drug development in children is particularly challenging due to difficulties in disease diagnosis (obtaining adequate microbiological specimens), characterizing the extent of disease and monitoring treatment response. Fortunately, decades of experience in treating children supports extrapolation of efficacy data from adults to most children above 5 years of age. This in addition to the higher occurrence of extrapulmonary disease in younger children (below 5 years of age) suggests that paediatric studies should be primarily designed to collect pharmacokinetic and safety data to determine age-appropriate dosing regimens. This article reviews drug development issues and existing regulatory guidance pertinent to the development of new TB drugs for use in children.

Copyright © 2011 S. Karger AG, Basel

## Burden of Childhood Tuberculosis

Of all new tuberculosis (TB) cases diagnosed in 2000, 884,019 (11%) were estimated to be children aged less than 15 years [1]. More recent paediatric data are unavailable, and in all likelihood these outdated figures underestimate the current situation, since the number of diseased adults has increased greatly since 2000, particularly in areas with poor epidemic control [2]. Poor case ascertainment, absence of active case finding and limited surveillance data hamper efforts to accurately quantify the global burden of childhood TB [3]. In a comprehensive community-based survey performed in South Africa, children <13 years of age contributed 13.7% of the total disease burden with a calculated TB incidence of 408/100,000/year [4]. This equates to roughly 50% of the total adult TB incidence (840/100,000/year) in the same community, which seems a fair estimate of the paediatric disease burden to be expected in settings with poor epidemic control [5]. In non-endemic settings, the burden of childhood TB is greatly reduced due to minimal transmission of *Mycobacterium tuberculosis,* differences in population age structure with relatively fewer children compared to adults and adequate provision of preventive therapy following documented TB exposure.

There remains a misperception that children rarely develop life-threatening disease, which is the experience in areas where diligent contact tracing and active case finding ensures that they either receive adequate preventive therapy or are diagnosed early in their disease course. However, this is not the case in TB endemic areas where children frequently present with advanced disease and TB is a major contributor to under-5-year mortality. An autopsy study conducted in Zambia demonstrated that TB rivals bacterial pneumonia as a major cause of death in human immunodeficiency virus (HIV)-infected and -uninfected children [6]. A South African study documenting identifiable causes of respiratory disease in children with community-acquired pneumonia not responding to first-line antibiotics showed that *M. tuberculosis* is a common pathogen [7], while most children diagnosed in an endemic area had advanced and complicated disease [8].

The HIV epidemic has had a major negative impact on TB control efforts. In addition to increased absolute numbers of TB patients, HIV induced a marked age and gender shift among adult TB cases with more young people and women of childbearing age developing TB [9]. The implication for children is that more parents with young families at home are developing active TB, drastically increasing the TB exposure of young and vulnerable children in these communities [10, 11]. Since sputum smear-negative TB is more common among HIV-infected adults, efforts to improve access to chest radiograph and culture-based diagnosis have been greatly expanded, which should also assist to improve service delivery to children [12]. The Stop TB Strategy formulated a very inclusive goal: to treat 'all TB patients, infectious or non-infectious, adults and children, with/without HIV infection, with/without drug-resistant disease', which motivated the WHO to compile a guidance for the management of childhood TB in 2006 with a request for countries to include paediatric TB data in all future reports [13].

Due to the paucibacillary nature of paediatric TB (in those without cavitary disease or extensive lung infiltration), children are far less likely to acquire drug resistance and/or transmit TB than adults. However, since children are greatly affected by ongoing transmission of TB, drug resistance patterns observed among child TB cases reflect primary (transmitted) drug resistance within the community [14]. Globally the emergence of the drug-resistant TB epidemic has been identified as a major threat to TB control. The unavailability of effective second-line drugs and long delays before drug-resistant TB is identified, implies that many patients, including children, are initially treated with ineffective regimens, leading to acquisition of additional drug resistance (amplification) and continued transmission of drug-resistant organisms [15].

The impression that drug-resistant organisms are likely to be less fit and therefore less transmissible than drug-susceptible strains has been contradicted by recent observations. The fitness cost associated with the acquisition of drug resistance seems variable and strain dependent, while compensatory evolution may account for significantly higher fitness in clinical strains compared to their progenitors or laboratory strains [16]. Successful transmission is suggested by geographic clustering of drug-resistant cases, evidence of clonal expansion and drug-resistant disease in children [14–17]. A prospective surveillance study from South Africa documented a marked increase in drug-resistant, especially multidrug-resistant TB among children from 1994 to 2007, most likely reflecting increased multidrug-resistant TB among adults in the area [18]. Unless effective measures are urgently implemented to limit transmission, even greater numbers of children will be affected in future [15].

## Treating Children with Tuberculosis

Drug-susceptible TB responds remarkably well to standard first-line treatment, but until recently few resource-limited settings had access to child-friendly drug formulations; however, with funding support from UNITAID, the Global Drug Facility has approved grant applications from 55 countries for provision of child-friendly TB formulations and distributed approximately 115,000 treatments free of charge to children in poor countries during 2008 [19]. Indications are that the Global Drug Facility initiative will be sustained and expanded in future. Although these efforts improved the availability of child-friendly drug formulations, reliable access to quality-assured drugs remains a concern in many countries, and significant programmatic barriers still limit the availability of these drugs. In addition existing treatment guidelines and fixed-dose combination preparations for children may be suboptimal when age-dependent pharmacokinetic profiles are taken into account [20–22]. Guidance on optimal drug doses for first-line drugs was recently finalized [23], but it remains an indictment of drug development practices that optimal dosage recommendations for children and age-appropriate formulations were delayed for more than 50 years after first-line treatment regimens had beene optimized for adult patients.

## The Need for Access to New Drugs

It is clear that the large and previously unrecognized paediatric TB burden, the emergence of drug-resistant TB, the toxicity of second-line TB drugs and their lack of study in children (as well as adults) necessitate the involvement of children in the development of new TB drugs and drug regimens. Recognition of the need to involve children early in the development of new drugs is a recent phenomenon (discussed further below) that has grown along the trajectory of increased understanding of the ethical imperatives that has evolved since the publication of the Nuremberg Code in 1947 [24] and includes seminal documents and agreements such as the World Medical Association International Code of Medical Ethics [25], the Belmont Report [26] and specific guidelines adopted by the International Conference on Harmonization.

Fortunately most children respond well to current treatment regimens, but with the rising prevalence of drug-resistant TB and the need for shorter treatment durations it is essential that new drugs be made available to children as soon as possible. At the same time, due to the unique growth, development and metabolic nature of childhood, protection from unsafe and potentially toxic side effects of new drugs in children (and pregnant mothers) is an important obligation of both regulatory agencies and companies developing new drugs. The historical approach by which children were dosed off label by extrapolation from adult dosing information is clearly suboptimal and wrong. Current paediatric drug development seeks a balance both protecting vulnerable children and at the same time offering access to new therapies where the appropriate use within particular age groups has been clarified.

## The Regulatory Environment of Paediatric Drug Development

Regulatory agencies in both the USA and the European Community, namely the Food and Drug Administration (FDA) and the European Medicines Agency, have enacted legislation to redress the neglect of children in modern drug development. In the USA, two primary legislations govern the inclusion of children in modern drug development, the Pediatric Research Equity Act of 2003 and the Best Pharmaceuticals for Children Act of 2002. More recently, with the enactment of the FDA Amendments Act of 2007 [27], both Pediatric Research Equity Act and Best Pharmaceuticals for Children Act were reauthorized. The Pediatric Research Equity Act requires all applications (or supplements to an application) for a new active ingredient, new indication, new dosage form, new dosing regimen or new route of administration to contain a paediatric assessment unless the applicant has obtained a waiver or deferral. This assessment should include all relevant subpopulations of children, and the sponsor of a new drug is encouraged to submit a paediatric plan to the FDA as soon as possible during the drug development programme. According to the Best Pharmaceuticals for Children Act legislation, sponsors may obtain 6 months of additional paediatric exclusivity if studies were conducted in accordance with a written request issued by the FDA and submitted within the time frame specified in the written request. In Europe, paediatric drug development is currently governed by the Paediatric Regulation that came into force in the European Union on January 26, 2007 [28]. Similar to its US counterpart, this regulation requires paediatric studies conducted according to a paediatric investigation plan in order to have a valid application for marketing authorization, unless waived or deferred. The reward for conducting the paediatric development in compliance with a paediatric investigation plan is a 6-month extension of the supplementary protection certificate, provided that the results are included in product information and that authorization is obtained in all European Union member states.

## When to Initiate Paediatric Development

The existing paediatric regulations encourage sponsors to initiate the development of a paediatric investigation plan and discuss it with the respective regulatory agency 'as soon as possible' during drug development. Additionally, the timing of initiating paediatric trials with respect to the overall drug development programme should be evaluated. In general, paediatric patients can be considered for enrolment in clinical trials if age-appropriate dosing of the investigational drug has been confirmed and sufficient safety data (non-clinical and clinical) are available to support the initiation of a paediatric trial. This must also be approached with a balanced assessment between the benefit received by the child and the risks in what is considered a vulnerable population with unique growth, development (physical, neurological and psychological) and metabolic (drug distribution, metabolism and excretion) characteristics.

Several International Conference on Harmonization and region-specific regulatory guidelines provide recommendations on the required non-clinical studies to support clinical development and subsequent marketing approval of pharmaceuticals intended for human adult or paediatric use [29–33]. In general, a preclinical safety programme for marketing approval of a drug includes: pharmacology studies, general toxicity studies, toxicokinetic and non-clinical pharmacokinetic studies, reproductive toxicity studies, genotoxicity studies and carcinogenicity studies. On a case-by-case basis, other toxicity studies, including phototoxicity, immunotoxicity and juvenile animal toxicity studies, may also be required. The goal of these studies, collectively, is to comprehensively assess the product's safety profile and its potential toxic effects.

Non-clinical safety studies precede clinical trials in healthy volunteers or patients. The International Conference on Harmonization M3 guideline [34] recommends a typical

Table 1. Recommended duration of repeated-dose toxicity studies to support the conduct of clinical trials [34]

| Maximum duration of clinical trial | Recommended minimum duration of repeated-dose toxicity studies to support clinical trials | |
|---|---|---|
| | rodents | non-rodents |
| Up to 2 weeks | 2 weeks | 2 weeks |
| 2 weeks to 6 months | same as clinical trial | same as clinical trial |
| >6 months | 6 months | 9 months |

programme for non-biological small molecules as well as the timing of non-clinical studies relative to clinical development. Pharmacology studies are performed in the discovery phase of a drug and involve investigation of the mechanism of action, efficacy related to the target condition and safety profile to assess the potential effect on the cardiovascular, central nervous and respiratory systems. Various in vitro cell type screening assays and excised organs are used in addition to single-dose in vivo studies involving whole animals. Genotoxicity studies, i.e. assays of mutations and chromosomal aberration, must also be performed at an early stage of drug development; a complete battery of studies ought also to be available before the initiation of phase II studies. Subchronic repeated-dose toxicity studies, typically performed in 2 animal species (1 rodent and 1 non-rodent) are also performed at an early stage as the 'no observed adverse effect doses' established in these determine the starting dose for the first study in humans which is generally performed in healthy volunteers.

The duration of subsequent (chronic) repeated-dose toxicity studies is equal to or exceeds the duration of human clinical trials, up to a maximum of 6 months in rodent and 9 months in non-rodent species for human trials that may exceed 6 months of exposure to the new drug, For these studies, mice or rats are commonly used as rodent species and dogs or monkeys as non-rodents. Similarities to humans in relation to pharmacology targets and pharmacokinetic properties, most notably absorption and metabolism, are important considerations when selecting the appropriate animal species for safety assessment. Other studies, such as reproductive and developmental studies, are initiated before or during large-scale or long-duration clinical trials (e.g. phase III), subject also to the patient population involved (e.g. pregnant women). Carcinogenicity studies are conducted to support marketing authorization rather than clinical trials, unless there is significant cause for concern regarding carcinogenic risk.

## Children Are Not Small Adults

Children are often considered as small adults and are commonly given drugs evaluated for adult use only. There are, however, major biological (e.g. body composition, metabolic rate, organ functional capacity) and occasionally disease-related differences (e.g. receptor expression and function, immune maturity) between children and adults which could result in changes in drug activity and/or pharmacokinetic properties potentially causing exacerbated toxicity in children. In the past, drug development programmes have used safety data obtained from adult clinical trials and adult non-clinical studies (as outlined above) to support the use of drugs in a paediatric population. However, current regulations require that children be properly studied to directly collect safety, efficacy and pharmacokinetic information. Results from repeated-dose toxicity studies of appropriate duration in adult animals (table 1) and a complete package of safety pharmacology and genotoxicity studies are required prior to the initiation of clinical trials in paediatric populations. Reproduction toxicity studies, especially fertility and pre- and postnatal developmental studies are also important and yield valuable information on the age and gender of the paediatric population under study. Carcinogenicity data may also be required if there are strong reasons for concern, although generally such data are not required to support paediatric clinical trials.

Overall, human adult data are more relevant for children than non-clinical data, but several guidelines recommend that studies in juvenile animals be performed on a case-by-case basis, mainly when existing adult human and animal safety data are considered insufficient to support paediatric trials. Rats are commonly used in juvenile toxicity studies but other species can be used when there is sufficient scientific justification. The study design in juvenile animals should meet the age requirement and development stage to be investigated in the clinic. The timeline and the order in which various organs mature vary between animal species. Information on comparative developmental timing

**Table 2.** Paediatric age categories in humans and suggested corresponding ages in animal models for non-clinical studies to support paediatric drug development

| Species | Preterm | Newborn | Infant | Child | Adolescent |
|---|---|---|---|---|---|
| Human | | 0–28 days | 1–23 months | 2–12 years | 12–16 years |
| Monkey | – | 0–15 days | 0.5–6 months | 0.5–3 years | 3–4 years |
| Dog | – | 0–21 days | 3–6 weeks | 6–20 weeks | 5–7 months |
| Pig | – | 0–15 days | 2–4 weeks | 4–14 weeks | 4–6 months |
| Rabbit | 0–4 days | 0–10 days | 1.5–5 weeks | 5–12 weeks | 3–6 months |
| Rat | 0–4 days | 0–10 days | 1.5–3 weeks | 3–6 weeks | 7–11 weeks |
| Mouse | 0–4 days | 0–10 days | 1.5–3 weeks | 3–5 weeks | 5–7 weeks |

for certain functions and systems can be obtained in several guidelines and in the literature (table 2). For drugs that are excreted in milk, the lactation phase of the pre- and postnatal development study could meet the need for a formal juvenile toxicity study in weaning animals. In this phase, animals are exposed to the drug, sometimes in significant quantities, via milk, and assessment of several developmental/growth and toxicokinetic parameters can be performed, obviating the necessity for a separate study.

There are no specific guidelines that define the non-clinical and clinical requirements to support the development of paediatric TB drugs. The requirements seem similar to those outlined for other paediatric indications, but this is a discussion that must be held with regulatory agencies during consideration of the paediatric investigational plan. It is important, nevertheless, for those interested in paediatric TB drug development to understand that these non-clinical safety and toxicology studies are needed to ensure protection of the youngest and most vulnerable children, and these safety measures will of necessity delay the study of new drugs in the youngest age groups. On the other hand, it may be reasonable to consider the involvement of adolescents in phase II and phase III clinical trials since they are mature enough metabolically and developmentally to take adult doses of TB drugs and should be mature enough to provide informed consent to clinical trial participation. Table 3 summarizes some of the important considerations that should be taken into account in the clinical development programme of a new TB drug.

## Development of Child-Friendly Drug Formulations

Current paediatric drug development regulations require that paediatric investigational plans develop age-appropriate formulations for relevant paediatric age groups. Drug formulation and manufacturing is regulated by a series of legislative acts and guidances that are beyond the scope of this paper. It is important, however, to outline some principles since the development of an appropriate formulation for younger age groups may be a significant cause of delay in providing new therapies to young children.

Childhood is characterized by growth and development and many elements in the maturation of the growing child must be taken into consideration in the development of age-appropriate paediatric formulations, such as metabolic enzyme maturation, changes in renal function during kidney maturation, changes in total body water and volume of distribution, and maturation of the gastrointestinal tract. During the first 2 years of life, syrups and suspensions are frequently the mode of delivery, but liquids may not be the most desirable formulation in resource-limited settings due to their bulk (transportation and storage requirements), ease of contamination, limited shelf life and frequent need for refrigeration after opening. Other formulations such as sprinkles or granules that can be added to food or dispersible tablets are other possibilities; in slightly older children, minitabs, chewables and melt-aways are also an option. Adolescents usually do quite well with adult solid tablets or capsules.

## Tuberculosis Drug Development Guidance

Finally, it should be noted that the European Medicines Agency has recently adopted a new guidance to specifically address the development of new TB drugs [36]. The guidance takes into consideration some of the unique problems associated with TB drug development in young children, who have a higher incidence of extrapulmonary

**Table 3.** Clinical development considerations for new TB drugs, including initiation of a paediatric development programme

| |
|---|
| **Preclinical**<br>Development phase and animal studies<br>**Clinical**<br>Preclinical studies with animal models assist design of clinical trials in all phases of development |
| *Phase I*<br>First human trials (usually healthy adult volunteers)<br>Determine pharmacokinetic profile of drug and basic safety/tolerability<br>Drug interaction studies with companion background TB drugs |
| *Phase II*<br>First trials using adult TB patients<br>(a) Establish efficacy (small proof-of-concept trials)<br>Early bactericidal activity trials<br>(b) Establish optimal dose<br>Can be combined with expanded early bactericidal activity trials<br>Long follow-up period required to demonstrate durable cure (no reliable surrogate markers)<br>Exceptionally, conditional marketing approval can be granted on the basis of robust phase II data and phase III commitments negotiated with regulatory agencies; given the limited efficacy and significant toxicity associated with current second-line TB drugs, a new drug seeking an indication for treatment of multidrug-resistant TB would seem to be a reasonable candidate for this approach |
| *Phase III*<br>Definitive large-scale trials to 'prove efficacy and confirm safety' (traditional approval)<br>Well-controlled trials (usually randomized, placebo controlled, double blinded)<br>Long-term follow-up required to demonstrate durable cure; traditionally this has been 2 years after treatment completion, but may possibly be reduced to only 6–12 months [35]<br>**Initiation of paediatric development programme**<br>Paediatric studies usually not initiated until sufficient adult safety and efficacy data available; only after completion of phase IIb or in parallel with phase III trials<br>– Initiation of paediatric programme should be negotiated with regulatory authorities<br>– European Medicines Agency guidance recommends inclusion of adolescent children (≥10 years) in adult phase III trials (safety and efficacy; early completion of non-clinical safety/toxicity package for these age groups studied; see table 2)<br>*For younger age groups* (<10 years)<br>– Complete additional non-clinical safety/toxicity package for age groups to be<br>– Develop age-appropriate formulations<br>– Confirm stability and shelf life<br>– Trial design includes recruitment of successive age cohorts by descending age group<br>– Enrolment of the next younger age cohort proceeds when safety and pharmacokinetic data from preceding older age cohort is characterized to establish optimal dosing that will ensure drug exposure comparable to that achieved in adults (efficacy and safety)<br>– The primary objective for younger age groups is to define pharmacokinetics and safety; secondary objectives include demonstration of antimycobacterial activity and clinical benefit (e.g. resolution of infection, weight gain) |
| *Phase IV*<br>Undertaken after primary registration of a new drug to further explore alternative uses (e.g. latent TB infection or treatment of complicated extrapulmonary TB, such as tuberculous meningitis) |

disease and for whom pulmonary disease is difficult to confirm microbiologically due to difficulties in specimen collection and low bacteriological yields (Table 4). As suggested in the guidance, it seems reasonable to expect comparable antimycobacterial responses in adults and children, which allow for extrapolation of efficacy data from adults for most children. However, such extrapolation may be more difficult in younger children where the spectrum of disease is broader [37] but should still hold true since intrathoracic disease in children tends to be paucibacillary. As such, the focus of paediatric TB drug development becomes the development of age-appropriate formulations for use in young children, defining the optimal dosage recommendations to ensure adequate drug exposure, and demonstrating safety of the new drug in children [38].

**Table 4.** Studying new TB drugs in paediatric populations (from the European Medicines Evaluation Agency guidance on the clinical development of new agents to treat disease due to *M. tuberculosis* [36])

Some considerations for the development of paediatric investigation plans, taking into account existing Committee for Medicinal Products for Human Use guidance, may include the following:

- Whenever considered possible, taking into account what is known about the properties of the test agent, children and adolescents aged from approximately 10 years upwards should be included in studies that enrol adults; data on pharmacokinetics may be obtained from these subjects during treatment
- If adequately powered, randomized and controlled studies of efficacy are not considered to be feasible in children in specific age groups, there must be a justification for extrapolation of safety and efficacy data obtained from adults to children; the presentation of clinical disease may be different compared to adults but the response to treatment may be comparable at least from the age of 5 years upwards; below this age, an extrapolation of results from studies in adults may be more problematic due to higher rates of extrapulmonary TB
- If it is considered acceptable that safety and efficacy data obtained from adults can be extrapolated to children of specific age groups, it is required that age-specific dose regimens are identified based on pharmacokinetic studies conducted in children during therapy for TB; children should also be followed to obtain data on safety and efficacy
- The diagnosis of TB and the assessment of responses to treatment in children enrolled into these types of studies should be based on age-specific criteria recommended by internationally recognized expert bodies

## Conclusion

The current global TB epidemic poses an immense and imminent threat to the entire global community. Unfortunately, it is largely unrecognized in high-resource countries with effective TB control programmes. The TB burden suffered by children is even less appreciated, although childhood TB is fully treatable if diagnosed in time and if effective treatment is readily available. The development of novel TB drugs, for the first time in nearly half a century, is an exciting development that promises to shorten treatment duration and treat those with drug-resistant TB more effectively. Commitment from regulating authorities and drug developers should ensure that children will, at last, not be left behind during these developments. It is important for the paediatric community to realize that development of child-friendly drugs involves a series of steps and procedures, including lengthy non-clinical safety and toxicology studies to prevent harm to vulnerable children. However, we trust that the paediatric development plan of novel TB drugs will break new ground to achieve equity for children in the shortest time frame possible.

## Disclosure Statement

Jenny Lin and Araz Raoof work for subsidiaries of Johnson & Johnson that are developing a new drug for the treatment of TB.

## References


1 Nelson LJ, Wells CD: Global epidemiology of childhood tuberculosis. Int J Tuberc Lung Dis 2004;8:636–647.

2 World Health Organization: Global Tuberculosis Control: Epidemiology, Strategy, Financing. Geneva, World Health Organization, 2009.

3 Newton SM, Brent AJ, Anderson S, Whittaker E, Kampmann B: Paediatric tuberculosis. Lancet Infect Dis 2008;8:499–510.

4 Marais BJ, Hesseling AC, Gie RP, Schaaf HS, Beyers N: The burden of childhood tuberculosis and the accuracy of routine surveillance data in a high-burden setting. Int J Tuberc Lung Dis 2006;10:259–263.

5 Marais BJ, Schaaf HS: Childhood tuberculosis: an emerging and previously neglected problem. Infect Dis Clin North Am 2010;24:727–749.

6 Chintu C, Mudenda V, Lucas S, Nunn A, Lishimpi K, Maswahu D, Kasolo F, Mwaba P, Bhat G, Terunuma H, Zumla A: Lung diseases at necropsy in African children dying from respiratory illnesses: a descriptive necropsy study. Lancet 2002;360:985–990.

7 McNally LM, Jeena PM, Gajee K, Thula SA, Sturm AW, Cassol S, Tomkins AM, Coovadia HM, Goldblatt D: Effect of age, polymicrobial disease, and maternal HIV status on treatment response and cause of severe pneumonia in South African children: a prospective descriptive study. Lancet 2007;369:1440–1451.

8 Marais BJ, Gie RP, Schaaf HS, Hesseling AC, Enarson DA, Beyers N: The spectrum of childhood tuberculosis in a highly endemic area. Int J Tuberc Lung Dis 2006;10:732–738.

9 Lawn SD, Bekker LG, Middelkoop K, Myer L, Wood R: Impact of HIV infection on the epidemiology of tuberculosis in a peri-urban community in South Africa: the need for age-specific interventions. Clin Infect Dis 2006;42:1040–1047.

10 Marais BJ, Gupta A, Starke JR, El-Sony A: Tuberculosis in women and children. Lancet 2010;375:2057–2059.

11 Marais BJ, Rabie H, Cotton MF: TB and HIV in children – advances in prevention and management. Paediatr Respir Rev 2011;12:39–45.

12 Marais BJ, Raviglione M, Donald PR, Harries AD, Kritski AL, Graham SM, El-Sadr WM, Harrington M, Churchyard G, Mwaba P, Sanne I, Kaufmann SH, Whitty CJ, Atun R, Zumla A: Scale-up of services and research priorities for diagnosis, management and control of tuberculosis – Call to action. Lancet 2010;375:2179–2191.

13 World Health Organization: Guidance for National Tuberculosis Programmes on the Management of Tuberculosis in Children. WHO/HTM/TB/2006.371. Geneva, WHO, 2006.

14 Schaaf HS, Marais BJ, Hesseling AC, Gie RP, Beyers N, Donald PR: Childhood drug-resistant tuberculosis in the Western Cape Province of South Africa. Acta Paediatr 2006;95:523–528.

15 Gandhi N, Nunn P, Dheda K, Schaaf HS, Zignol M, van Soolingen D, Jensen P, Bayona J: Multidrug-resistant and extensively drug-resistant tuberculosis: a threat to global control of tuberculosis. Lancet 2010;375:1830–1843.

16 Gagneux G, Long CD, Small PM, Van T, Schoolnik GK, Bohannan BJM: The competitive cost of antibiotic resistance in *Mycobacterium tuberculosis*. Science 2006;312:1944–1946.

17 Marais BJ, Victor TC, Hesseling AC, Barnard M, Jordaan A, Brittle A, Reuter H, Beyers N, van Helden PD, Warren RM, Schaaf HS: Beijing and Haarlem genotypes are over-represented among children with drug resistant tuberculosis in the Western Cape Province of South Africa. J Clin Microbiol 2006;44:3539–3543.

18 Schaaf HS, Marais BJ, Hesseling AC, Brittle W, Donald PR: Surveillance of antituberculosis drug resistance among children from the Western Cape Province of South Africa – an upward trend. Am J Public Health 2009;99:1486–1490.

19 Gie RP, Matiru RH: Supplying quality-assured child-friendly anti-tuberculosis drugs to children. Int J Tuberc Lung Dis 2009;13:277–278.

20 McIlleron H, Willemse M, Werely CJ, Hussey GD, Schaaf HS, Smith PJ, Donald PR: Isoniazid plasma concentrations in a cohort of South African children with tuberculosis: implications for international pediatric dosing guidelines. Clin Infect Dis 2009;48:1547–1553.

21 Schaaf HS, Willemse M, Cilliers K, Labadarios D, Maritz JS, Hussey GD, McIlleron H, Smith P, Donald PR: Rifampin pharmacokinetics in children, with and without human immunodeficiency virus infection, hospitalized for the management of severe forms of tuberculosis. BMC Med 2009;7:19.

22 Graham SM, Bell DJ, Nyirongo S, Hartkorn R, Ward SA, Molyneux EM: Low levels of pyrazinamide and ethambutol in children with tuberculosis and impact of age, nutritional status and human immunodeficiency virus infection. Antimicrob Agents Chemother 2006;50:407–413.

23 Marais BJ, Schaaf HS, Donald PR: Pediatric tuberculosis: Issues related to current and future treatment options. Future Microbiol 2009;4:661–675.

24 http://ohsr.od.nih.gov/guidelines/nuremburg.html.

25 http://www.donoharm.org.uk/gendecl.htm.

26 http://ohsr.od.nih.gov/guidelines/belmont.html.

27 http://www.fda.gov/RegulatoryInformation/Legislation/FederalFoodDrugandCosmeticActFDCAct/SignificantAmendmentstotheFDCAct/FoodandDrugAdministrationAmendmentsActof2007/FullTextofFDAAALaw/default.htm.

28 http://ec.europa.eu/health/files/eudralex/vol-1/reg_2006_1901/reg_2006_1901_en.pdf.

29 Reich M, Stefano V, Compagni A: Orphan drug legislation: lessons for neglected tropical diseases. Int J Health Planning Manag, Wiley Interscience (April 24, 2008). http://www.wcfia.harvard.edu/sites/default/files/Reich_Orphan.pdf.

30 http://www.ema.europa.eu/docs/en_GB/document_library/Scientific_guideline/2009/09/WC500002926.pdf.

31 US FDA, Center for Drug Evaluation and Research: Guidance for industry, nonclinical safety evaluation of pediatric drug products. Rockville, US Department of Health and Human Services, February 2006.

32 European Medicines Evaluation Agency (EMEA), Committee for Human Medicinal Products (CHMP): Guideline on the need for non-clinical testing in juvenile animals on human pharmaceuticals for pediatric indications. January 2008.

33 USFDA: Guidance for industry: general considerations for pediatric pharmacokinetic studies for drugs and biological products. US Department of Health and Human Services, Food and Drug Administration Center for Drug Evaluation and Research, Center for Biologics Evaluation and Research, 1998.

34 International Conference on Harmonization of Technical Requirements for Registration of Pharmaceuticals for Human Use: Guidance on non-clinical safety studies for the conduct of human clinical trials marketing authorization for pharmaceuticals M3 (R2). 2008.

35 Marais BJ, van Helden PD, Donald PR: Adequacy of 6 month follow-up in chemotherapy therapy trials. Int J Tuberc Lung Dis 2010;14:927–930.

36 http://www.ema.europa.eu/docs/en_GB/document_library/Scientific_guideline/2010/01/WC500070049.pdf.

37 Donald PR: The assessment of new anti-tuberculosis drugs in children. Int J Tuberc Lung Dis 2007;11:1162–1165.

38 Burman WJ, Cotton MF, Gibb DA, Walker AS, Vernon AA, Donald PR: Ensuring the involvement of children in the evaluation of new tuberculosis treatment regimens. PLoS Med 2008;5:e176.



David F. McNeeley, MD
Medical Service Corporation International
2000 Clarendon Blvd., Suite 300
Arlington, VA 22201 (USA)
Tel. +1 730 276 3000, E-Mail dmcneeley@mscionline.com

Chapter 25

Donald PR, van Helden PD (eds): Antituberculosis Chemotherapy.
Prog Respir Res. Basel, Karger, 2011, vol 40, pp 243–246

# A New Era in Tuberculosis Treatment: What Does the Future Hold?

Ken Duncan

Global Health Discovery, Bill & Melinda Gates Foundation, Seattle, Wash., USA

**Abstract**

Antituberculosis drug discovery and development have increased dramatically over the last 2 decades following the declaration by the World Health Organization that tuberculosis (TB) was a 'global health emergency'. It is now clear that the current short-course 6-month regimen is not short enough or robust enough to contain the dual threat of HIV-influenced TB and multidrug-resistant TB. In the efforts to develop new drugs and regimens, the interplay between host and pathogen must be recognized and the role of the body's immune system explored in containing TB, but, possibly, at the same time encouraging features of persistence and thus complicating chemotherapy. Despite the potential pitfalls that lie ahead, the publication of the genome sequence of *Mycobacterium tuberculosis* and partnerships between pharmaceutical companies, biotechnology industries and academia are paving the way towards the development of new anti-TB drugs and regimens and give reason for cautious optimism.

Copyright © 2011 S. Karger AG, Basel

The papers in this volume of *Progress in Respiratory Research* provide a comprehensive retrospective analysis of the medicines available today for treating tuberculosis (TB), as well as a glimpse of what the future may hold. The landscape has evolved dramatically since the dark days of the early 1990s when the global TB epidemic was increasing in intensity and the emergence of multidrug-resistant (MDR) strains of *Mycobacterium tuberculosis* raised the spectre of a world in which TB would once again be an untreatable disease, leading the World Health Organization to declare TB 'a global health emergency' and to start developing programmes for the control of TB [1].

At that time there was very little activity in TB drug discovery and development. The world had been satisfied in the early 1970s when rifampicin was added to the TB drug armamentarium and the 'short-course' regimen we are familiar with today was introduced. It was assumed that the tools that had been created would be sufficient to control TB. This coincided with a period in which it was believed that infectious diseases had been conquered, following on from US Surgeon General William H. Stewart's reported statement in 1967 that we could 'close the book on infectious disease' [2]. It did not help that TB is a disease of poverty and had largely been controlled in countries that constitute the major markets for pharmaceuticals, and the drug industry concentrated its resources on more financially lucrative conditions. A further consequence of these factors was that many young researchers were actively discouraged from following a career in TB research of any kind. The only significant innovations to follow were development and widespread implementation of directly observed therapy, short course, which brought some order to the delivery of medicines and improved compliance and treatment completion rates, and the introduction of fixed-dose combinations, which ensured drug quality and guarded against monotherapy that can lead to drug resistance.

How wrong could we be to suppose that these tools would be sufficient to treat TB in all its forms? Coupled with the lack of an effective vaccine that protects adults from developing active pulmonary disease and the lack of selective and specific point-of-care diagnostic tests, the number of incident TB cases continues to rise, although in recent years mortality has begun to fall [3]. Co-infection with HIV has also had a devastating effect on the epidemic, particularly in sub-Saharan Africa [4]. MDR-TB continues to be a problem in many parts of the world [5], and although it can be treated with second-line agents, these are not always available, are expensive and cause significant side effects. The existence of even more broadly resistant ('extremely drug-resistant', XDR) TB strains highlights the need for new treatment options [6].

The greatest impediment to improving TB treatment outcome is surely the time it takes to cure a patient with active disease. The current complex multidrug regimen is highly effective with high cure rates, under well-defined conditions such as those encountered in well-managed programmes or under clinical trial conditions. But it takes a minimum of 6 months (the 'short' course) to achieve cure, and in general use, compliance cannot be assured and therefore treatment failure is common. The future of TB therapy must be one in which treatment time is reduced to only a few months or, better still, a few weeks. Why is this so difficult to achieve when we can cure other bacterial infections in a matter of days or weeks? The reasons are numerous and relate to the biology of the organism, the host response to infection and the properties of the available drugs [7].

## Barriers to Treatment Shortening

*M. tuberculosis* is slow-growing with a doubling time of around 20 h, in contrast to most bacterial pathogens, which divide much more rapidly. It would not be unreasonable to assume that, since antibiotics primarily work on cells that are actively dividing, the overall duration of therapy might somehow correlate with the length of the growth cycle. This raises doubt that a significantly faster cure might ever be achieved. During treatment we observe rapid initial reduction of bacterial numbers in sputum during the first few weeks of chemotherapy until bacteria can no longer be cultured, yet treatment must be continued because of 'persistence', an ill-defined phenomenon that describes the remaining bacilli that cause recurrence of disease.

The interplay between host and pathogen is a critical factor that cannot be ignored. *M. tuberculosis* is adept at escaping host defence mechanisms in macrophages, and the immune response to infection results in the formation of granulomatous lesions that become caseous and hypoxic, conditions in which the drugs are unable to penetrate or be effective. It is unclear whether chemotherapy helps the host clear the infection by killing the few damaged bacteria that remain after drug treatment, or hinders it by forcing the bacterium into a state in which it is not susceptible to drugs.

The 6-month treatment period represents a significant improvement over the 18–24 months it took to cure a patient when TB drugs were first introduced. In some respects it is not surprising that it still takes this long when the regimen comprises 4 'first-generation' agents. Although some efforts were made to improve current agents, no second-generation drugs were ever introduced. Contrast this with HIV therapy: the first agents introduced had poor pharmacokinetics, had to be dosed several times daily and had significant side effects limiting their acceptability. Today, many new medicines derived from those first agents, as well as drugs in new chemical classes, are available targeting multiple mechanisms and in fixed-dose combinations such that once-daily therapy can be tailored taking into account the drug resistance pattern in the infecting viral strain.

## The Present

Through the efforts of the pharmaceutical and biotechnology industries and academia, and supported by product development partnerships such as the Global Alliance for TB Drug Development (www.tballiance.org), there is a substantial pipeline of new drug candidates [8]. In preclinical studies, the potential to reduce the duration of chemotherapy has been demonstrated, and several drug candidates have been assessed in murine models of infection [9–11]. Recognizing that there needs to be a new regimen and that achieving this goal will take decades if it follows the established path of replacing and testing one drug sequentially in the current regimen, groups have come together to launch a broad effort, the Critical Path to TB Drug Regimens (www.c-path.org/cptr.cfm) to test new drug combinations at an earlier stage in clinical development than would normally be considered. Partnership with the US Food and Drug Administration is helping to develop regulatory science and define new guidelines for evaluating the safety and effectiveness of new combination products.

If we take an optimistic view of the current pipeline, there are sufficient candidates to ensure that a new combination regimen will be developed, and that this regimen will be able to shorten chemotherapy by 2, or perhaps 3, months. It should be noted, however, that the current drug candidates fall into relatively few drug classes and we should anticipate that due to attrition several drug candidates will fail to reach registration. Thus, the more pessimistic view is that the current pipeline is insufficient to meet our goal and we must continue efforts to replenish it. Fortunately, the drugs in development all show activity against MDR- and XDR-TB strains and should provide new options for treatment of patients infected with such strains, even if they fail to shorten the duration as would be required to change first-line therapy.

Our understanding of *M. tuberculosis* improved greatly with the publication of the genome sequence in 1998 [12] but this of itself is only one tool with which to advance drug discovery; although we know the primary sequence of every gene, we do not know which of the approximately 4,000 genes are the most vulnerable to inhibition, other than those that are the targets of today's drugs. Through genetic approaches, those genes that are essential for the viability of *M. tuberculosis* have been identified [13] but this only provides a starting point and further work is needed to validate potential drug targets. The promise of target-directed rational drug design was not fulfilled in other areas of antibacterial drug discovery [14], an important lesson for the TB community. New approaches that start with compounds having whole-cell activity against the pathogen have greatest promise but conversely provide the most difficult path to optimization. Fortunately we are now well positioned to take whole-cell hits, identify their targets rapidly and then deploy the full suite of structure-based design tools at our disposal to ensure success.

A feature of recent drug discovery efforts, particularly those aimed at solving the more intractable problems of persistence and latent TB, has been the formation of international, multidisciplinary partnerships between researchers in academia and industry, leveraging funds provided by governments and philanthropic donors. These consortia have succeeded in bringing together the diverse skills of researchers in academia with expertise found only in industry. An example of this aimed at identifying a new first-line drug is the 'New Medicines for Tuberculosis' programme (www.nm4tb.org), a consortium of European researchers funded by the European Commission 6th Framework Programme, in partnership with AstraZeneca scientists based in Bangalore, India. This team has identified and validated a number of drug targets, but its biggest success to date was the discovery of a new class of anti-TB agents, the benzothiazinones, and identification of the major target, decaprenylphosphoryl-β-D-ribose 2′-epimerase [15]. Another example is a consortium established to solve one of the 'Grand Challenges in Global Health' (www.gcgh.org), namely finding a more potent and rapidly acting treatment for latent TB. This consortium, funded jointly by the Bill & Melinda Gates Foundation and the Wellcome Trust, comprised academic groups from around the globe led by a team based at Imperial College, London, working in partnership with the Novartis Institute for Tropical Diseases, Singapore. Exploring the hypothesis that latent *M. tuberculosis* resides in hypoxic lesions, and that *M. tuberculosis* adapts its metabolism to cope with this environment, the team hopes to find agents that are effective under these conditions and thus can be used to eliminate latent infection, and it also aims to develop new tools and approaches needed for rapid evaluation of drugs in latently infected humans [16].

In spite of successes over the past decade, the paradox remains that if we continue to conduct TB drug discovery the way we always have, we risk only finding more of the same and not the breakthrough that we really need. In other words, current efforts may yield incremental improvement on therapy duration – which will nonetheless be welcomed with drugs that are easier to take and that combat MDR-TB – but will not provide a truly transformational medicine. With this in mind, the Bill & Melinda Gates Foundation embarked on a programme to address mycobacterial persistence. Various hypotheses were put forward to explain persistence, such as that the bacterium resides in a compartment where it responds to its micro-environment by altering its metabolism, thus remaining unaffected by current drugs, or that persistence is a stochastic phenomenon, that is at any one time a small fraction of bacteria are quiescent or dormant and not dividing and thus refractory to treatment. In a programme known as the 'TB Drug Accelerator', grants were made to investigate the underlying causes of persistence and to characterize the persistent organism in vivo, to generate robust and scalable whole-cell assays that mimic the conditions encountered by the persistent bacterium in the host, to generate new tools that would permit deconvolution of whole-cell active compounds to reveal their targets and thus engage the full suite of drug discovery tools, to determine which of the current animal models best predicts the ability of a drug to shorten therapy, and finally to apply state-of-the-art tools and technologies widely used elsewhere to facilitate preclinical discovery and clinical development, such as advances in imaging to monitor bacterial load in situ and in real time. At the time of writing, the programme is now generating data and tools that are opening new avenues of drug discovery in collaboration with a number of pharmaceutical companies.

## The Future

We can be optimistic that during the next decade new drugs will be registered and introduced that will augment or replace those that are currently in use. However, we must not be complacent and should strive to discover and develop a transformational therapy that will improve the outlook for newly diagnosed patients such that they are facing a course of treatment that lasts only a few weeks. We must increase the number and quality of drug candidates to ensure success and we must challenge the current paradigm of drug discovery to find agents working through new mechanisms. Finally, greater investment is required to understand the role played by the human immune system in order to identify ways in which this powerful weapon can be deployed with greater effect. To do all of this will require sustained financial and scientific commitment as there will surely be failures along the way, but we are well placed to achieve the breakthrough in therapy that will at last provide tools to control this disease more effectively.

## References


1 World Health Organization: Framework for Effective Tuberculosis Control. WHP/TB/94.179. Geneva, WHO, 1994.
2 Stewart WH: A mandate for state action. Washington, Association of State and Territorial Health Officers, December 4, 1967.
3 World Health Organization: Report 2009: Global Tuberculosis Control – Epidemiology, Strategy, Financing. WHO/HTM/TB/2009.411. Geneva, WHO, 2009.
4 World Health Organization: Global Tuberculosis Control: Surveillance, Planning, Financing. WHO/HTM/TB/2008.393. Geneva, WHO, 2008.
5 World Health Organization/International Union against Tuberculosis and Lung Disease: Global Project on Anti-Tuberculosis Drug Surveillance in the World. Report No 3: Anti-Tuberculosis Drug Resistance in the World. WHO/HTM/2004.343. Geneva, WHO, 2004.
6 Raviglione MC, Smith IM: XDR tuberculosis – implications for global public health. N Engl J Med 2007;356:656–659.
7 Connolly LE, Edelstein PH, Ramakrishnan L: Why is long-term therapy required to cure tuberculosis? PLoS Med 2007;4:e120.
8 Ginsberg AM: Drugs in development for tuberculosis. Drugs 2010;70:2201–2214.
9 Andries K, Verkasselt P, Guillemont J, Göhlmann HWH, Neefs JM, Winkler H, van Gestel J, Timmerman P, Zhu M, Lee E, Williams P, de Chaffoy D, Huitric E, Hoffner S, Cambau E, Truffot-Pernot C, Lounis N, Jarlier V. A diarylquinoline drug active on the ATP synthase of *Mycobacterium tuberculosis*. Science 2005;307:223–227.
10 Tyagi S, Nuermberger E, Yoshimatsu T, et al: Bactericidal activity of the nitroimidazopyran PA824 in a murine model of tuberculosis. Antimicrob Agents Chemother 2005;49:2289–2293.
11 Matsumoto M, Hashizume H, Tomishige T, Kawasaki M, Tsubouchi H, Sasaki H, Shimokawa Y, Komatsu M: OPC-67683, a nitro-dihydro-imidazooxazole derivative with promising action against tuberculosis in vitro in mice. PloS Med 2006;3:2131–2144.
**12** Cole ST, Brosch R, Parkhill J, Garnier T, Churcher C, Harris D, Gordon SV, Eiglmeier K, Gas S, Barry CE 3rd, Tekaia F, Badcock K, Basham D, Brown D, Chillingworth T, Connor R, Davies R, Devlin K, Feltwell T, Gentles S, Hamlin N, Holroyd S, Hornsby T, Jagels K, Krogh A, McLean J, Moule S, Murphy L, Oliver K, Osborne J, Quail MA, Rajandream MA, Rogers J, Rutter S, Seeger K, Skelton J, Squares R, Squares S, Sulston JE, Taylor K, Whitehead S, Barrell BG: Deciphering the biology of *Mycobacterium tuberculosis* from the complete genome sequence. Nature 1998;393:537–544.
13 Sassetti CM, Boyd DH, Rubin EJ: Genes required for mycobacterial growth defined by high density mutagenesis. Mol Microbiol 2003;48:77–84.
14 Payne DJ, Gwynn MN, Holmes DJ, Pompliano DL: Drugs for bad bugs: confronting the challenges of antibacterial drug discovery. Nat Rev Drug Discov 2007;6:29–40.
15 Makarov V, Manina G, Mikusova K, Möllmann U, Ryabova O, Saint-Joanis B, Dhar N, Pasca MR, Buroni S, Lucarelli AP, Milano A, De Rossi E, Belanova M, Bobovska A, Dianiskova P, Kordulakova J, Sala C, Fullam E, Schneider P, McKinney JD, Brodin P, Christophe T, Waddell S, Butcher P, Albrethsen J, Rosenkrands I, Brosch R, Nandi V, Bharath S, Gaonkar S, Shandil RK, Balasubramanian V, Balganesh T, Tyagi S, Grosset J, Riccardi G, Cole ST: Benzothiazinones kill *Mycobacterium tuberculosis* by blocking arabinan synthesis. Science 2009;324:801–804.
16 Barry CE, Boshoff HI, Dartois V, Dick T, Ehrt S, Flynn J, Schnappinger D, Wilkinson RJ, Young D: The spectrum of latent tuberculosis: rethinking the biology and intervention strategies. Nat Rev Microbiol 2009;7:845–855.



Ken Duncan
Deputy Director, Global Health Discovery
Bill & Melinda Gates Foundation
PO Box 23350, Seattle, WA 98102 (USA)
Tel. +1 206 709 3705, E-Mail ken.duncan@gatesfoundation.org

# Author Index

# Subject Index